Visit *www.wildernesspress.com*
for the latest updates for this book
(enter "PCT" in the "book search" box)

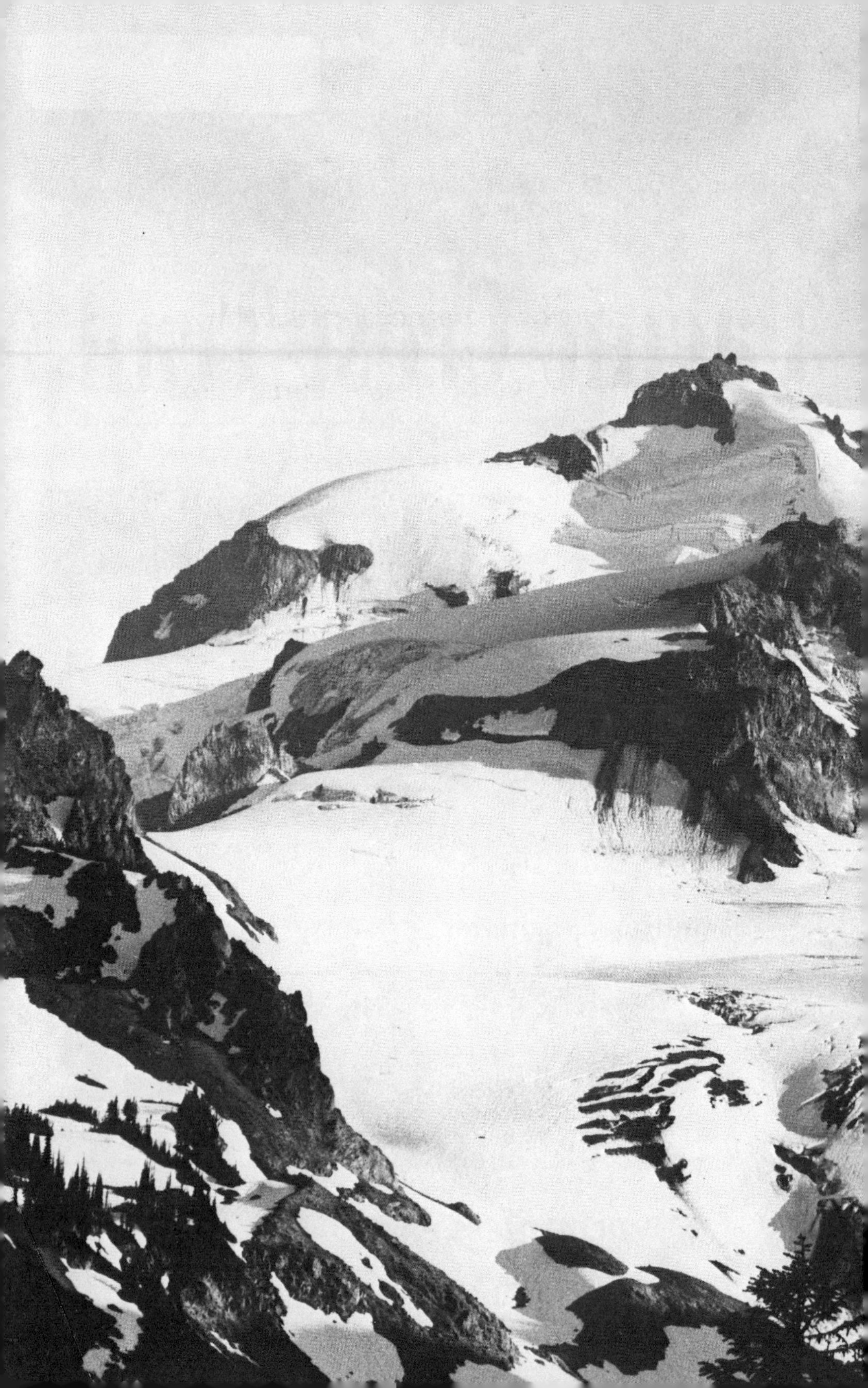

OREGON & WASHINGTON

Pacific Crest Trail

From the California Border to the Canadian Border

Jeffrey P. Schaffer Andy Selters

 WILDERNESS PRESS · BERKELEY, CA

Pacific Crest Trail: Oregon & Washington (From the California Border to the Canadian Border)

1st EDITION 1974
2nd EDITION 1976
3rd EDITION 1979
4th EDITION 1986
5th EDITION 1990
6th EDITION August 2000
7th EDITION October 2004
2nd printing February 2007

The Pacific Crest Trail is covered in three volumes: *Pacific Crest Trail: Southern California* (From the Mexican Border to Tuolumne Meadows); *Pacific Crest Trail: Northern California* (From Tuolumne Meadows to the Oregon Border); *Pacific Crest Trail: Oregon & Washington* (the Northwest part of the PCT to the Canadian Border).

Front cover photo copyright © 2004 by Jeffrey P. Schaffer
Interior photos, except where noted, by Jeffrey P. Schaffer
Maps: Jeffrey P. Schaffer and Kenneth R. Ng

ISBN-13: 978-0-89997-375-3
ISBN-10: 0-89997-375-2
UPC: 7-19609-97375-1

Manufactured in the United States of America

Published by: **Wilderness Press**
1200 5th Street
Berkeley, CA 94710
(800) 443-7227; FAX (510) 558-1696
info@wildernesspress.com
www.wildernesspress.com

Visit our website for a complete listing of our books and for ordering information.

Cover photo: Above Jefferson Park, Mount Jefferson
Frontispiece: Glacier Peak from the north

SAFETY NOTICE: Although Wilderness Press and the author have made every attempt to ensure that the information in this book is accurate at press time, they are not responsible for any loss, damage, injury, or inconvenience that may occur to anyone while using this book. You are responsible for your own safety and health while in the wilderness. The fact that a trail is described in this book does not mean that it will be safe for you. Be aware that trail conditions can change from day to day. Always check local conditions and know your own limitations.

Contents

Introductory Chapters

Trail Chapters

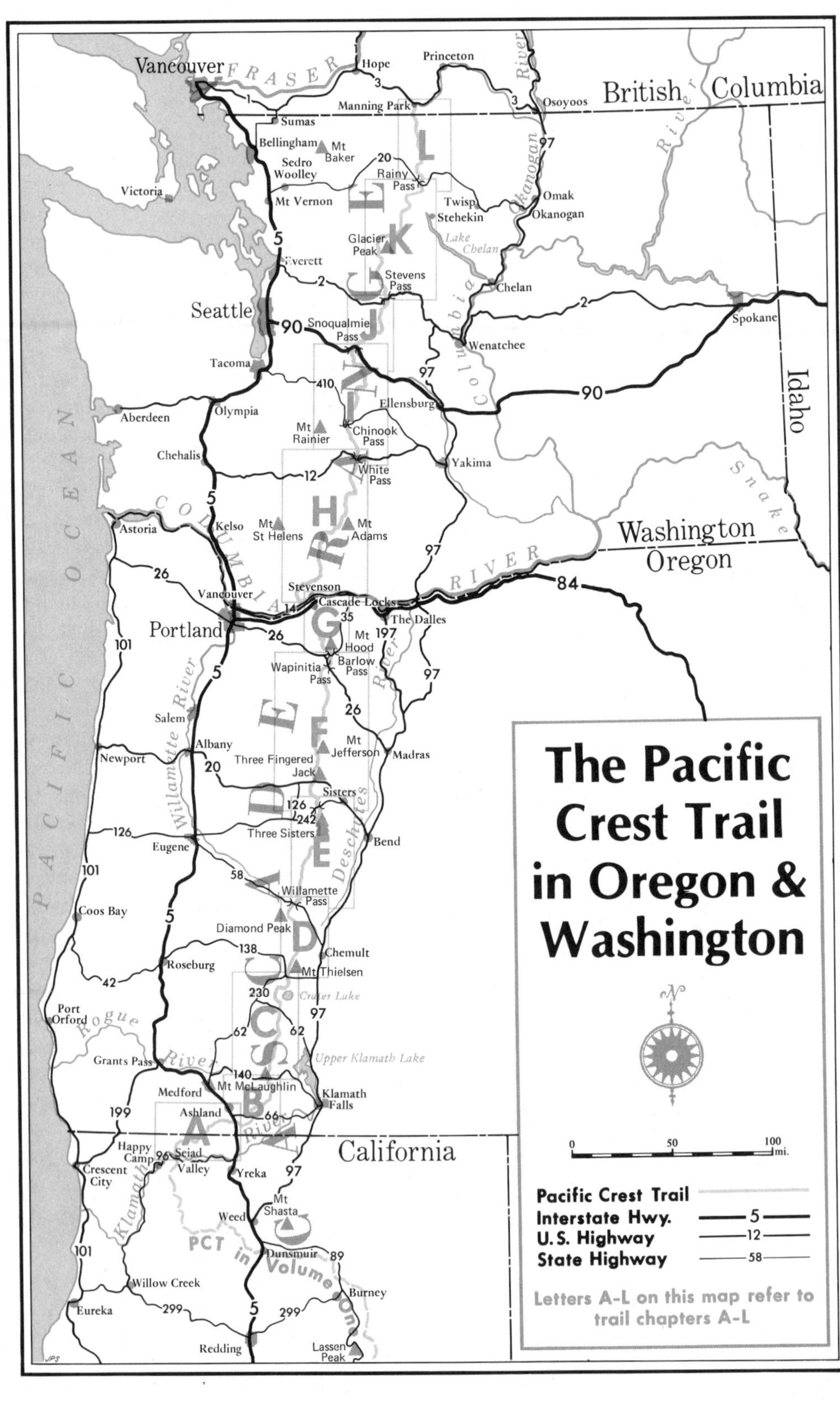

The Pacific Crest Trail in Oregon & Washington
Pacific Crest Trail
Interstate Hwy. 5
U.S. Highway 12
State Highway 58
Letters A-L on this map refer to trail chapters A-L
British Columbia
Washington
Oregon
California
Idaho
PACIFIC OCEAN
COLUMBIA RIVER
PCT in Volume 1
Vancouver
Victoria
Seattle
Tacoma
Olympia
Portland
Salem
Eugene
Bend
Medford
Ashland
Klamath Falls
Spokane
Yakima
Wenatchee
Ellensburg
Redding
Eureka

Chapter 1: History of the PCT

The first proposal for the creation of a Pacific Crest Trail (PCT) that we have been able to discover is contained in the book *Pacific Crest Trails* by Joseph T. Hazard (Superior Publishing Co.). He says that in 1926, he was just ending a business interview with a Miss Catherine Montgomery at the Western Washington College of Education in Bellingham when she said,

"Do you know what I've been thinking about, Mr. Hazard, for the last twenty minutes?"

"Just what have you in mind, Miss Montgomery?"

"A high trail winding down the heights of our western mountains with mile markers and shelter huts—like those pictures I'll show you of the 'Long Trail of the Appalachians'—from the Canadian Border to the Mexican Boundary Line!"

To go back six years in time, the Forest Service had by 1920 routed and posted a trail from Mt. Hood to Crater Lake in Oregon, named the Oregon Skyline Trail, and with hindsight we can say that it was the very first link in the PCT.

Hazard says that on that very night, he conveyed Miss Montgomery's suggestion to the Mt. Baker Club of Bellingham, which was enthusiastic about it. He says that soon a number of other mountain clubs and outdoor organizations in the Pacific Northwest adopted the idea and set about promoting it. Then, in 1928, Fred W. Cleator became Supervisor of Recreation for Region 6 (Oregon and Washington) of the U.S. Forest Service. Cleator proclaimed and began to develop the Cascade Crest Trail, a route down the spine of Washington from Canada to the Columbia River. Later, he extended the Oregon Skyline Trail at both ends so that it, too, traversed a whole state. In 1937, Region 6 of the Forest Service developed a design for PCT trail markers and posted them from the Canadian border to the California border.

But the Forest Service's Region 5 (California) did not follow his lead, and it remained for a private person to provide the real spark not only for a California segment of the PCT but indeed for the PCT itself. In the early 1930s, the idea of a Pacific Crest Trail entered the mind of Clinton C. Clarke of Pasadena, California, who was then chairman of the Executive Committee of the Mountain League of Los Angeles County. "In March 1932," wrote Clarke in *The Pacific Crest Trailway*, he "proposed to the United States

Forest and National Park Services the project of a continuous wilderness trail across the United States from Canada to Mexico. . . .The plan was to build a trail along the summit divides of the mountain ranges of these states, traversing the best scenic areas and maintaining an absolute wilderness character."

The proposal included formation of additional Mountain Leagues in Seattle, Portland, and San Francisco by representatives of youth organizations and hiking and mountaineering clubs similar to the one in Los Angeles. These Mountain Leagues would then take the lead in promoting the extension of the John Muir Trail northward and southward to complete a pathway from border to border. When it became evident that more than the Mountain Leagues were needed for such a major undertaking, Clarke took the lead in forming the Pacific Crest Trail System Conference, with representatives from the three Pacific Coast states. He served as its President for 25 years.

As early as January 1935, Clarke published a handbook-guide to the PCT, giving the route in rather sketchy terms ("the Trail goes east of Heart Lake, then south across granite fields to the junction of Piute and Evolution creeks"—this covers about 9 miles).

In the summer of 1935—and again the next three summers—groups of boys under the sponsorship of the YMCA explored the PCT route in relays, proceeding from Mexico on June 15, 1935, to Canada on August 12, 1938. This exploration was under the guidance of a YMCA secretary, Warren L. Rogers, who served as Executive Secretary of the Pacific Crest Trail System Conference (1932–1957) and who continued his interest in the PCT until his death in 1992.

During World War II, the PCT was generally ignored and its completion remained in a state of limbo until the 1960s, when backpacking began to appeal to large numbers of people. In 1965, the Bureau of Outdoor Recreation, a Federal agency, appointed a commission to make a nationwide trails study. The commission , noting that walking for pleasure was second only to driving for pleasure as the most popular recreation in America, recommended establishing a national system of trails of two kinds: long National Scenic Trails in the hinterlands and shorter National Recreation Trails in and near metropolitan areas. The commission recommended that Congress establish four Scenic Trails: the already existing Appalachian Trail, the partly existing PCT, a Potomac Heritage Trail, and a Continental Divide Trail. Congress responded by passing, in 1968, the National Trails System Act, which set the framework for a system of trails and specifically made the Appalachian Trail and the PCT the first two National Scenic Trails.

Meanwhile, in California, the Forest Service in 1965 had held a series of meetings about a route for the PCT in the state. These meetings involved people from the Forest Service, the Park Service, the State Division of Parks and Beaches, and other government bodies charged with responsibility over areas where the trail might go. These people decided that so much time had elapsed since Clarke had drawn his route that they should essentially start all over. Of course, it was pretty obvious that segments like the John Muir Trail would not be overlooked in choosing a new route through California. By the end of 1965, a proposed route had been drawn onto maps. (We don't say "mapped," for that would imply that someone actually had covered the route in the field.)

When Congress, in the 1968 law, created a citizens Advisory Council for the PCT, it was the route devised in 1965 that the Forest Service presented to the council as a "first draft" of a final PCT route. This body of citizens was to decide all the details of the final route; the Forest Service said it would adopt whatever the citizens wanted. The Advisory Council was also to concern itself with standards for the physical nature of the trail, markers to be erected along the trail, and the administration of the trail and its use.

In 1972, the Advisory Council agreed upon a route, and the Forest Service put it onto maps for internal use. Since much of the agreed-upon route in California, southern Oregon, and southern Washington was cross-country, these maps were sent to the various national forests along the route, for them to mark a temporary route in the places where no trail existed along the final PCT route. This they did—but not always after field work. The result was that the maps made available to the public in June 1972 showing the final proposed route and the temporary detours did not correspond to what was on the ground in many places. A common flaw was that the Forest Service showed a temporary or permanent PCT segment following a trail taken off a pre-existing Forest Service map, when in fact there *was no trail* where it was shown on that map in the first place.

Perfect or not, the final proposed route was sent to Washington for publication in the Federal Register, the next step toward its becoming official. A verbal description of the route was also published in the Federal Register on January 30, 1973. But the material in the register did not give a center line which could be precisely and unambiguously followed; it was only a *route*, and the details in many places remained to be settled. Furthermore, much private land along the route remained to be acquired, or at least an easement secured for using it.

At the time of the Register's publication, the PCT was more or less continuous from Canada's Manning Park to Highway 140 near Lake of the Woods in southern Oregon.

A portion of the Federal Register describing the PCT is reproduced below together with one of the register's PCT maps.

OREGON

At the south end of the Bridge of the Gods is the community of Cascade Locks, elevation 100 feet. This is the lowest elevation on the Pacific Crest Trail between the Canadian border and the Mexican border. A quarter of a mile south of the Bridge of the Gods, the Trail enters the Mt. Hood National Forest and ascends the rugged south side of the Columbia Gorge and quickly attains an elevation of 4,000 feet on Benson Plateau. It continues south, past Chinidere Mountain and Wahtum Lake, traversing the slopes high above Eagle Creek, the West Fork of Hood River and Lost Lake. The Trail then descends gently into Lolo Pass, crosses Forest Road N12 and ascends Bald Mountain where it is joined by Timberline Trail on Mt. Hood. Traversing Mt. Hood, the Trail then descends into the Muddy Fork, passes beneath Ramona Falls, and crosses the main fork of the Sandy River. Two miles south of the Sandy River, the Trail enters Mt. Hood Wilderness near Paradise Park at an elevation of 6,000 feet. It descends and crosses Zigzag Canyon, leaves the Mt. Hood Wilderness, and turns easterly to regain 1,000 feet in elevation and crosses just north of Timberline Lodge and the Mt. Hood Ski Area.

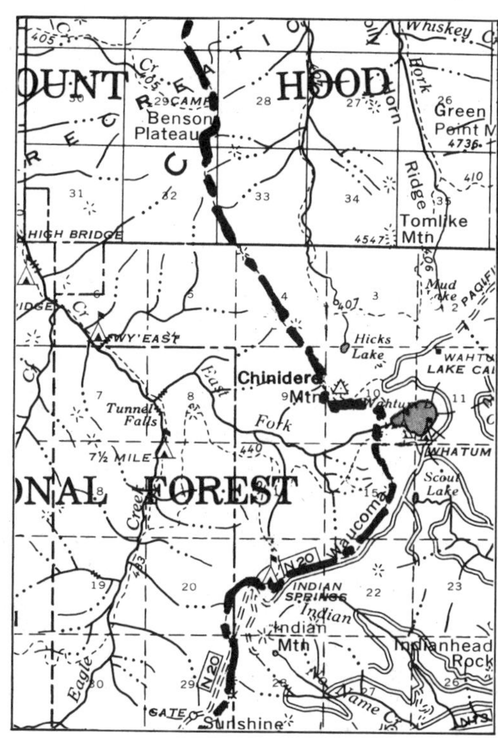

However, southwest from that highway, the 73-mile PCT route to the California border was *entirely* along roads. (Before the Register's publication of a route, the PCT route coincided with the old Oregon Skyline route, which headed south 40 miles from Highway 140 near Lake of the Woods over to the California border. Only 5 miles of trail existed along this older route.)

Of great importance, then, was the construction of the PCT to replace the 73-mile temporary route. In 1973, the PCT in the southern Sky Lakes Area was relocated so that it ended on Highway 140 near Fish Lake. Then, from 1974 until 1978, the trail was built southwest toward Interstate 5. During this time, another stretch of trail was built northeast from Seiad Valley toward Interstate 5. However, as late as 1985, private property stood in the way, and 3½ miles of route were still along roads.

Likewise, private property prevented the PCT in Washington from extending its last few miles south to the Columbia River. Its predecessor, the Cascade Crest Trail, had in fact been completed to the river in 1935, seven years after work on it had begun. However, that old trail ended 12½ miles east of a suitable river crossing, namely, the Bridge of the Gods. Likewise, the Oregon Skyline Trail ended not at a river crossing but rather at a trailhead 3 miles east of the bridge. An Oregon route to that bridge was built in 1974, but its Washington counterpart, across lands outside the National Forest, was not completed until 1984. This Washington stretch, making a roundabout route, takes 44 miles to reach Big Huckleberry Mountain; the old Cascade Crest Trail reached it in 20½ miles.

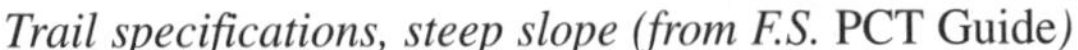
Trail specifications, steep slope (from F.S. PCT Guide*)*

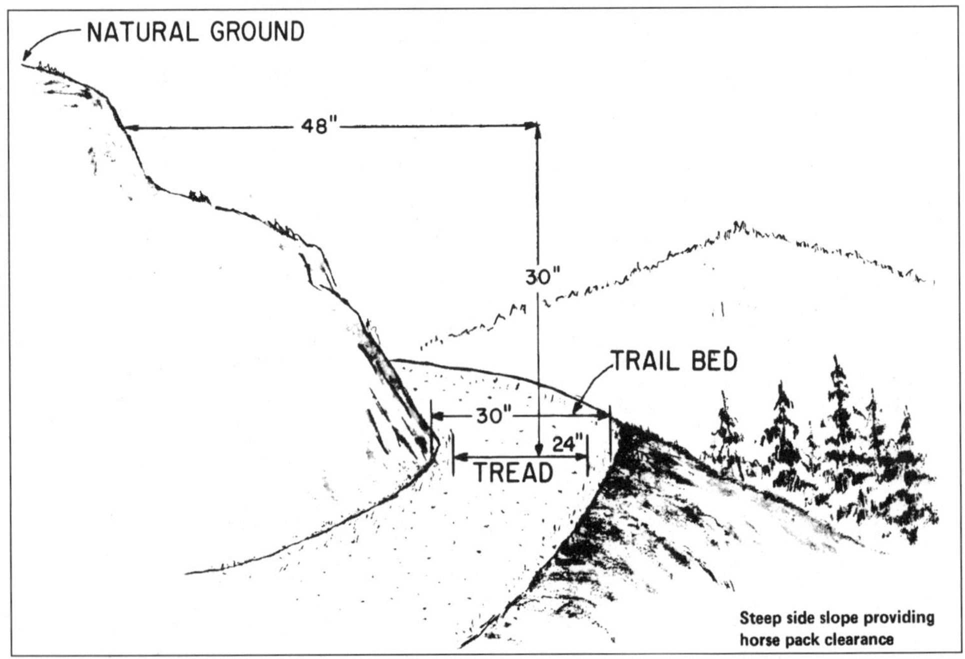

During the 1970s, the existing PCT also underwent changes. In May 1971, the Forest Service produced a *Pacific Crest Trail Guide for Location, Design, and Management*, which stipulated specific characteristics of the final trail. Perhaps the two most significant ones were that the trail should stay close to the crest and that its grade should not exceed 15 percent (a 15-foot rise for 100 horizontal feet). The old Cascade Crest and Oregon Skyline trails veered away from the crest in places, and in many places they were too steep.

In order to reduce the steepness, the trail had to either go around ridges rather than over them, or else it had to have switchbacks added to reduce the grade. Both changes led to increases in the PCT's overall length. The best example of such lengthening is along a stretch from Highway 138 north past Mt. Thielsen to Windigo Pass. Originally 24½ miles long, it was stretched to 30¼ miles by 1977, an increase of 23 percent. North of Windigo Pass, a new section of PCT was built because the old Oregon Skyline Trail veered too far east from the crest. This change also increased the overall PCT route length, replacing a 21-mile stretch with a winding, 30½-mile one, an increase of 45 percent! However, not all realignments are longer. For example, in Goat Rocks Wilderness, minor trail relocations in 1974 and 1978 both led to a small reduction in the PCT's length, as did a relocation in northern Sky Lakes Wilderness.

The PCT has also been relocated to avoid wet areas. One such area that gave hikers mosquito bites and muddy boots was a short stretch south from southern Washington's Sawtooth Huckleberry Field. The trail was rerouted along slopes above the area's boggy flats.

Publicity about the PCT, especially through Eric Ryback's popular, if inaccurate, account, inspired new waves of backpackers to trek along the route. Some parts of the route, however, were overused and therefore had to be relocated. One such area was the Twin Lakes area, just north of Wapinitia Pass. In Crater Lake National Park, a trail stretch was relocated for a similar reason. The Park's most scenic stretch crossed the Pumice Desert and gave the hiker views of both the Crater Lake rim and Mt. Thielsen. Decisionmakers, however, felt that hordes of hikers would trample the "desert's" fragile wildflowers into ruin—not very likely. Right or wrong, they relocated the trail to conform with the rest of the park's PCT—an essentially viewless, mosquito-infested traverse through a lodgepole forest.

To the consternation of PCT hikers, the decisionmakers did *not* relocate the stretch of the Crater Lake PCT that circumvents Crater Lake. This route, along abandoned roads, stays several miles away from the lake's view-packed rim, and therefore backpackers rarely take it. Surely, if any stretch of PCT deserves to be relocated, it is this stretch, which should be rebuilt so that it *at least* touches or approaches the rim in several places.

After new sections of the PCT were built and many others rebuilt or relocated, the Forest Service turned its attention to trailhead parking lots. Most PCT hikers, after all, do short stretches such as the 12 sections (A–L) found in this book, and virtually all of them park their cars near the PCT. In 1977 and 1978, the Forest Service constructed several large lots, just off the PCT and major roads, to fill the need. In the 1980s, most work was in the form of new trail construction in southern California. We hope the PCT will be completed, so that it exists as one continuous filament threading its way along the tops of mountain ranges from Mexico to Canada.

The trail's place in history is certainly minor when compared with today's world events, but generations from now, future historians may ponder its significance. During the middle of the 19th Century, pioneer trails were blazed across the continent to open up new lands and resources for a growing, young America. About a century later, trails of another kind appeared, which we now call National Scenic Trails. These are about as long as the pioneer trails, but, unlike them, they serve no economic purpose. At trails end, no fertile valleys, no gold mines, no thriving ports are reached. The PCT, like the other National Scenic Trails, is not a corridor to an economic end but rather is a process for individual change and growth. Although the trail's end is a desirable goal, it is not a necessary one, for travelers are enriched in a nonmaterial sense with every step they take along the way. Clinton Clarke saw the trail as a way to "lead people back to a simpler and more natural life and arouse a love for nature and the outdoors." The trail, then, is a prescription to improve the traveler's understanding of his or her place in the world. In a way, the trail is like a Norman Rockwell painting. This illustrator painted the American land and life not as it was but rather as it *should* have been. So, too, the PCT paints impressions on the hiker's mind, not of a world ravaged by man, but, rather, of a timeless, largely forgotten world where nature still exists as it was meant to be.

A trail-location drawing (from F.S. PCT Guide*)*

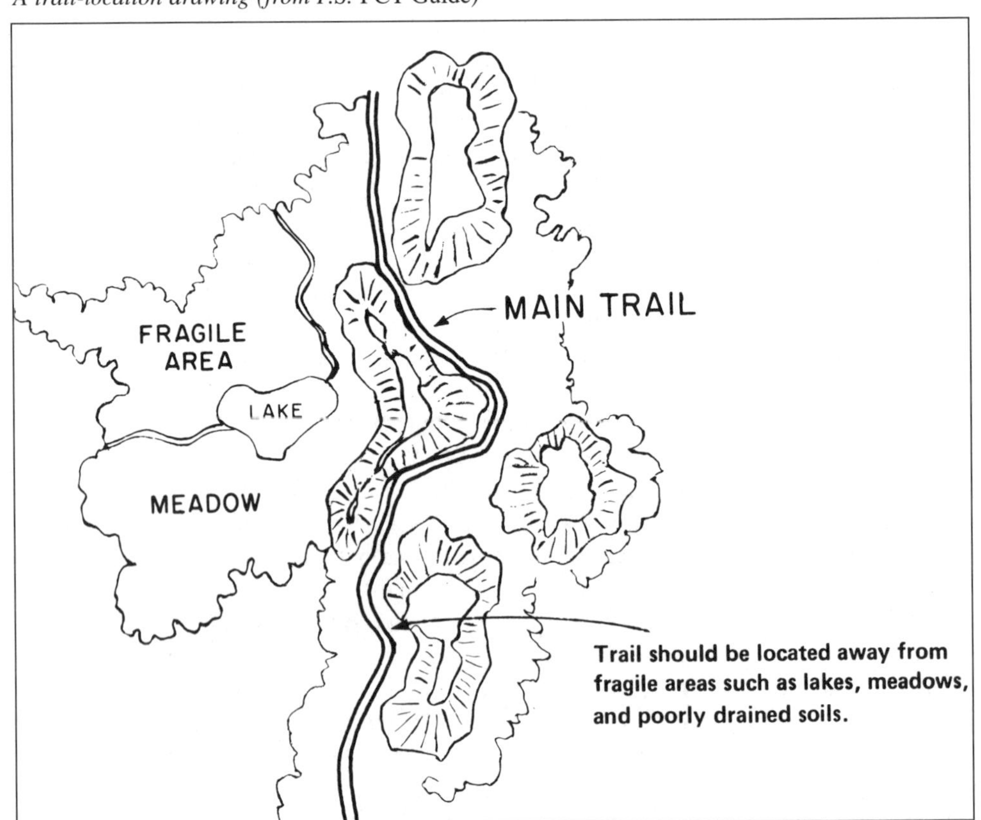
MAIN TRAIL
FRAGILE AREA
LAKE
MEADOW
Trail should be located away from fragile areas such as lakes, meadows, and poorly drained soils.

Chapter 2: Planning Your PCT Hike

WHAT TO EXPECT

Of the thousands of backpackers who will taste wilderness along the Pacific Crest Trail each year, probably a hundred or less will complete the Oregon-Washington section, and a few dozen will complete the entire tri-state route. Several hundred may hike either all of Oregon, which takes about 3½ weeks to hike, or all of Washington, which, being more rugged, takes a few days more. Probably the vast majority of the trail's travelers will confine their wilderness visit to two weeks or less and therefore will be able to carry all their needs on their backs without having to use resupply points. This guidebook divides the Oregon-Washington PCT into 12 convenient backpack trips (Sections A through L), each starting and ending at a highway. The shortest trip, Section B, is usually done in 2½ to 4 days, while the longest ones, Sections H and K, are usually done in 6 to 12 days.

Some readers will walk the whole trail, Mexico to Canada. This takes 5–6 months to complete if you do 14–17 miles of the PCT every day. Since most long-distance PCT hikers take layover days and also short side trips to supply points, they usually have to average about 20 miles per day when hiking along the trail. In past editions, we said that we hoped some readers would walk the whole trail in one long season. Some did, and some more certainly will. However, for several reasons, we no longer recommend it. Hiking 20 miles a day, you'll be too exhausted to appreciate the scenery. Also, during the first two months and the last month, you are likely to encounter plenty of bad weather, lots of snow-covered ground, or both. These detract from your enjoyment of the scenery as well as impede your progress. Finally, the human body was not meant to carry heavy packs continuously over a rugged, 2600-mile distance, and some hikers attempting this feat developed serious bone and ligament problems in their feet and legs.

Those still determined to hike the entire PCT continuously should start in early May (or sooner, if the Sierra Nevada snowpack has been light). The California section takes expert hikers about three months. You should try to complete the hottest part, south of the *southern* Sierra Nevada, by early June. However, you won't want to get into the High Sierra too early, for bad storms occurring as late as mid-June can bring your progress to a halt—or worse. If you're on schedule, you should cross into Oregon in early August and pass through Sky Lakes Wilderness and southern Three Sisters Wilderness in mid-to-late August. If you pass through these areas before late July, their seasonally superabundant mosquitoes will drive you almost insane. Perhaps by Labor Day, your labor of wilderness love will be celebrated with your entry into Washington. One month later, you should hope to consummate your hike, probably under the threat of rapidly deteriorating weather, in British Columbia's Ernest C. Manning Provincial Park.

If you are planning a short stretch and expect to encounter snow, hike from south to north. This way, you'll encounter more downhill snow slopes than uphill ones, since snow lingers longer on north slopes—the ones you'll be descending. It's more fun to slide down a snowbank than to climb up one.

If the Cascade Range in Oregon and Washington were a uniform, continuous range, you could expect the snowpack to retreat uniformly northward as the summer wore on, and you could plan a month-long trek north so that you would always have a dry trail, yet always have an adequate water source. However, this plan could have an undesired effect if you began at the height of the mosquito season: you'd have a continuous cloud of mosquitoes accompanying you north. The Cascade Range, however, is far from uniform, and often you will find yourself descending a snowbound pass into a warm, soothing, lake-dotted basin. If you are hiking the entire PCT, you are bound to encounter both pleasant and adverse trail conditions. If you want to avoid snow-clad trails, incessant mosquitoes, and severe water shortages, then hike the following segments at these recommended times (remembering, of course, that weather patterns vary considerably from year to year).

- Seiad Valley, Siskiyou Mountains, southern Oregon: *June through mid-September*
- Mt. McLoughlin, Sky Lakes basin, Seven Lakes basin: *mid-July through late August*
- Crater Lake: *July*
- Mt. Thielsen, Windigo Pass, Diamond Peak: *mid-July through late August*
- Three Sisters: *late July through early August*
- Mt. Washington, Three Fingered Jack: *late June through mid-July*
- Mt. Hood: *late July through mid-August*
- Columbia River gorge, southern Washington: *mid-June through early September*
- Mt. Adams, Goat Rocks, White Pass, Mt. Rainier, Stampede Pass, Snoqualmie Pass, Stevens Pass: *mid-July through mid-August*
- Glacier Peak, North Cascades, Manning Provincial Park: *late July through early August*

There are, of course, advantages and disadvantages to hiking in any season. In the North Cascades, for example,

- early June will present you with spectacular snow-clad alpine scenery—but also soft-snow walking and a slight avalanche hazard;
- early July will present you with a riotous display of wildflowers—plus sucking mosquitoes and biting flies;
- early August will present you with the best trail conditions—and lots of backpackers;
- early September will present you with fall colors and ripe huckleberries—but also nippy nights and sudden snowstorms.

WEATHER

With the foregoing information plus a scan through the introduction of each of this guide's 12 hiking chapters, you should be forming in your mind a vague idea of where and how long you expect to hike. Let's sharpen that idea by looking at the weather. The warmest temperatures are in mid-July through early August; they can vary from the 90s in southern Oregon to the 70s in the North Cascades. During this period, night temperatures for the entire two-state route are usually in the 40s but at times can be in the 50s or the 30s, and occasionally in the 20s.

In late June, with its long daylight hours, the maximum and minimum temperatures are almost as high as those in midsummer. In addition, you can expect to be plagued with mosquitoes through early August. *A tent is a necessity*—preferably one large enough for you and your friends to prepare meals in. During these warm summer nights, you'll want to sleep *atop* your sleeping bag, and, although the mosquitoes abate somewhat after dark, without a tent you won't get a mosquito-free sleep until later on in the season when the nights are cooler. Only when the wind picks up (late morning through late afternoon) or when a storm sets in are you afforded partial relief from these cursed insects. In Washington, you will also be exposed to at least three species of biting flies—*ouch!* But they are slower and easier to swat.

By late August, the days have got considerably shorter and the temperatures lower. The evenings and nights in southern Oregon are comfortable, but those in northern Washington are nippy, if not freezing. Expect to see morning frost on your tent, and prepare for brisk, "autumn" days. Too, there's likely to be a water shortage, particularly in most of Oregon. The national forests may be closed to backpacking, or they may require the backpacker to refrain from building campfires and use only a stove. A stove is also useful for boiling stagnant water and for melting snow. An advantage of a hike at this time, however, is that both Oregon and Washington will have a variety of berries ready for picking.

Another consideration is storms. Storm frequency increases northward. Northern California is virtually storm-free from mid-June through early September. In central Oregon, the period of good weather is only July through August, and even then occasional storms may be expected. If you visit southern Washington, be prepared for bad weather, even though you might get to hike a week or two at a time in beautiful midsummer weather. Expect bad or threatening weather in northern Washington. It is possible to hike two solid weeks in the North Cascades without receiving a drop of precipitation, but don't count on it—you might just receive a month of rain, as hikers did in the summer of 1978. Here, a tent is necessary to keep out the rain as well as to keep out the seasonal mosquitoes and flies.

Like storm frequency, lake temperature is influenced by the sun's apparent seasonal migratory pattern. Lakes are generally at their warmest in late July through early August. Also affecting a lake's temperature are its latitude, elevation, size, depth, inflow source, and the side of the mountain, if any, that it is on. Below are some representative *maximum* temperatures you can expect to find at certain lakes and rivers, south to north:

Klamath River, northern California	80°F
Emigrant Lake, near Ashland	78
Margurette Lake, Sky Lakes Wilderness	75
Dumbbell Lake, Three Sisters Wilderness	73

Scout Lake, Mt. Jefferson Wilderness	67
Wahtum Lake, northern Oregon	65
Eagle Creek, Columbia River gorge	57
Columbia River	65
Shoe Lake, Goat Rocks Wilderness	65
Pear Lake, Henry M. Jackson Wilderness	63
Lake Janus, Henry M. Jackson Wilderness	72
Mica Lake, Glacier Peak Wilderness	33
Stehekin River, North Cascades National Park	50

After you decide which segment of the PCT you want to do, next comes the question of transportation. Unlike round trips and loop trips, a hike along part of the PCT does not take you back to where you started. So if you take a car and leave it at the trailhead, you have a transportation problem. The solution may be any of several:

- walk back to where you started.
- take a bus back to where you started.
- hitchhike back to where you started.
- arrange for someone to drop you off and pick you up.
- arrange with another group to meet halfway along the trail and exchange car keys, or have duplicate sets made in advance.
- take at least 2 people and 2 cars, and leave one car at each end of your trek.
- take a bicycle or motorcycle in your vehicle, ride it to your starting trailhead, and, after walking your section, pick it up with your vehicle, which you left at the destination trailhead.

After you have decided on a solution to the car problem, write it down and put it in your pack. You might forget it if your trek is a long one.

LOGISTICS FOR THE LONG DISTANCE BACKPACKER

> *How can a book describe the psychological factors a person must prepare for. . . the despair, the alienation, the anxiety and especially the pain, both physical and mental, which slices to the very heart of the hiker's volition, which are the real things that must be planned for? No words can transmit those factors, which are more a part of planning than the elementary rituals of food, money and equipment, and how to get them.*
>
> —Jim Podlesney, in *Pacific Crest Hike Planning Guide*, edited by Chuck Long (Signpost Publications)

Chuck Long's book is long out of print, but *The PCT Hiker's Handbook* (3rd edition in 2000) does a commendable job in preparing you, mentally and physically (Adventure-Lore Press, Box 804, LaPine, OR 97739).

For up-to-the-minute trail conditions as well as accounts by hikers who've done all or major stretches of the trail, join the Pacific Crest Trail Association (PCTA, 5325 Elkhorn Blvd., PMB 256, Sacramento, CA 95842-2526; phone is (916) 349-2109 and (888) PCTRAIL = 728-7245; fax is (916) 349-1268; e-mail is info@pcta.org; web is www.pcta.org.). The Association publishes a journal, *Pacific Crest Trail Communicator*, six times per year, its office staff answers your questions, and they provide members with a wilderness permit for travel in excess of 500 miles on the PCT. Additionally, the PCTA organizes volunteer trail crews. The generally good condition of the Pacific Crest Trail is due in no small measure to the cadre of PCTA volunteers. If you enjoy your trek on the trail, consider joining the organization and doing some volunteer trail work.

The PCTA publishes two small books, each written by through-hikers (i.e., experts), that are very useful for the long-distance trekker. One is the *Pacific Crest Trail Data Book* by Benedict "Gentle Ben" Go, which presents the data from our two guidebooks (Volumes 1 and 2) in tabular form. His book is broken into five sections: Southern, Central, and Northern California, Oregon, and Washington, each with a general trail profile. In each section, Ben lists point-to-point distances, elevations, our guidebook maps, and water and facilities. The second book is the *Pacific Crest Trail Town Guide* by Leslie C. Croot, which covers resorts and lodges as well as towns. For each one, she presents a detailed map and a list of the following information: location, maildrop information, fuel availability, groceries, PCT Register, laundromat, lodging, restaurants, ATMs, outfitters, medical facilities, and special notes. Finally, she gives mileages between the sites, a table of the sites and services, maildrop addresses, and phone and fax numbers. In addition to these two books, the PCTA sells quite a complete assortment of books, videos, maps, etc., on the PCT.

Information not only on the PCT but on outdoor recreation in Oregon and Washington can be obtained at the Outdoor Recreation Information Center, which is located at the R.E.I. (Recreational Equipment, Inc.) site at 322 Yale Avenue North, Seattle, WA 98109-5429. Phone the center at: (206) 470-4060.

If you are going to be on the trail for more than a couple of weeks, you will want to have supplies waiting for you at one or more places along the route. For this, you can mail packages to yourself. Alternatively, you can drive to a place and leave a package with someone, if you are sure that person will be responsible for it. You can also hide caches in the wilderness, if you are willing to carry the heavy load in from the nearest road and carry all the packaging out—and if you trust the wildlife. There are a few towns near the PCT which will perhaps have adequate supplies and equipment—Ashland, Sisters, Cascade Locks, Stevenson, and Chelan. However, even those towns may not have an adequate selection of lightweight backpacking food. It is best to depend on post offices; see Leslie Croot's book.

Supplies

This discussion of supplies attempts to tell you what you will need and how best to get it. The discussion relies heavily on the experiences of Ben Schifrin (co-author of Volume 1) during his hike of the entire PCT.

The first thing to know about supplies along the PCT is that they are scarce. Too many young people try to do the PCT without pre-planning their food and other supplies. So they get to a resort and find that there is no white gas and its store is so limited that they will have to eat the same macaroni and cheese for the next five days. If you want to go light, the *only* choice is to pre-plan your menus and the rest of your needs and to mail things ahead to yourself.

Food

The main thing to have awaiting your arrival at a post office is food. When hiking long-distance on the PCT, food is the main concern. It causes more daydreaming and more bickering than anything else, even sex. As for the bickering, most people hike in groups, and much of the friction in a group is due to different eating habits. Some hikers don't eat breakfast; others won't hike an inch until they've had their steak and eggs. Some people eat every hour; others take the traditional three meal breaks. Many of these problems can be cured if each hiker carries his/her own food and suits his/her own prejudices. This arrangement also allows flexibility in pace and in hiking partners.

As for the daydreaming, it comes to focus on delicious food, and lots of it. Schifrin's first rule is that it won't hurt to take too much, because it will turn out to be too little, anyway. He and his two companions ate over 6000 calories a day out of their packs and still lost weight. The mental stresses, as well as the obvious physical ones, use up energy. So food serves two purposes: to provide fuel and to bolster morale. Take the things you crave. Most goodies—Hershey bars, beer, double fudgies, fresh cheese, mint cakes—are great energy sources and also provide variety and what Schifrin calls a "body con." At the bottom of some horrible ascent, you say to yourself, "You get a double helping of Hershey bar when you get to the top." It's something to sweat for.

Then there's the usual egregious gluttony upon reaching a town (which are so scarce along the Oregon-Washington PCT)—steaks, quarts of ice cream, gallons of chocolate milk, giant shrimp salads. Besides being good for morale and filling you up, these binges can give you a good idea of what's been missing from your diet, namely, whatever you craved and stuffed yourself on. For the next trail segment, correct the deficiency insofar as you can. And for the whole trek, take a supply of multivitamin pills, just in case your diet is deficient in important vitamins.

Other hikers seem to think that wild foods are theirs for the taking. Berries—huckleberries in particular—certainly are, but they won't sustain you. Remember that Indians spent most of their waking hours in search of foodstuffs, not just an hour a day. Besides, if hikers gorged themselves at every berry patch, there would be that much less for other hikers and the wild animals. Sample the berries, don't feast on them. Similarly with trout: don't plan to live off trout—they may not be biting during the time you have free to devote to fishing. View a fresh catch as a bonus, not an essential.

You won't have to rely on "Mother Nature" in Oregon or Washington since, if you're an "average" long-distance PCT hiker, you'll never have to carry more than an 8-day food supply, even on the longest stretches between supply points. Therefore, with careful shopping, you can buy all the food you'll need at your local supermarket, rather than buy expensive, freeze-dried food. (In California's John Muir Trail section of the PCT, lightweight, freeze-dried food is a *must*.) Freeze-dried food, despite its high cost, is preferred by some hikers since, in the Oregon-Washington PCT, using it can cut your pack's weight by 5–15 pounds, depending on how much food you typically eat and how far you are going to hike.

Regardless of whether you carry regular or lightweight food, you will most likely want a balance between cold and hot foods. Cold foods are of course more appropriate for lunch, though we meet hikers who go 100 miles without cooking. Some people refuse to face the dawn without hot drinks. Those who dispense with hot foods to save weight and time may suffer mentally on a freezing evening in the North Cascades. Variety is the key. No matter how much time you spend planning your food, however, you are sure to be dissatisfied, somewhere down the trail, with what you brought or with how much of it you brought. You may find that eventually, all freeze-dried dinners taste the same to you. You may find that you can never get a full feeling. You may lose 30 pounds. Or you may find that you brought too much. Just be prepared for such things to happen. Fortunately, you are not totally locked into your planned menus. You can mail back—or properly dispose of—what you can't stand, and buy something else at towns and resorts along the way, although it will not be cheap in such places. You can even ask your contact at home to buy some new food items and mail them to you.

In planning menus, remember that at 5000 feet of elevation, cooking time is double what it is at sea level and triple at 7500 feet. So don't bring foods that take long to cook at sea level.

Wood won't always be available, and if you are hiking 15+ miles a day, you'll find neither the time nor the energy to gather wood and start a fire. Anyway, wood is getting too scarce to use, due to the large number of backpackers, so we strongly recommend you bring a stove instead. You should know the rate at which your stove consumes fuel, for you will need lots of it if you do the whole PCT. Cartridge stoves, such as the Bluet, do not burn as hot as white-gas stoves, particularly when the cartridge is low on fuel, but they do have several advantages: they are very easy to start and virtually foolproof, and you can mail propane cartridges, whereas you can't mail white gas. (Unleaded gasoline, purchased at gas stations, works adequately in white-gas stoves, but be ready for more clogging and shorter stove life.)

Water

Usually, you can hike most stretches of the PCT carrying no more than a quart of water. But is it safe to drink? You can't tell. Clear lakes and streams in the continental U.S. may contain *Giardia lamblia* or *Cryptosporidium* or both, microscopic organisms that cause intestinal diseases. While these diseases are usually not life-threatening, they can make you feel absolutely rotten with diarrhea, cramps, gas, and the like. To be safe, always treat water from any open source. There are only two means effective against both *Giardia* and *Cryptosporidium*: boiling and filtering. Most authorities now agree that bringing water to a rolling boil suffices to kill both microorganisms, though boiling a minute is even surer. Boiling, however, is time-consuming, can use a lot of fuel, and can leave you with unpleasantly warm drinking water. Most people use water filters. Water filters need to strain out particles as small as 0.4 micron in order to catch both *Giardia* and the much smaller *Cryptosporidium*. If you depend on a filter, make sure it can be cleaned to maintain its flow with repeated use in turbid water. No known chemical treatment is effective against *Cryptosporidium*. However, *Giardia* can be killed by iodine tablets and crystals *if the chemical is used correctly*, which includes letting the mixture take effect for 30 minutes. Some hikers carry iodine to treat water in emergencies, such as when their primary water-treatment choice is unavailable.

Clothing

In planning what clothes to take, realize that rain, and sometimes snow, is possible at any time at any point along the Oregon-Washington PCT. Therefore, have good protection against wet and cold, whatever it costs. Remember that cotton clothing is useless when wet. Play it safe and assume there will be a storm. Bring along appropriate clothing and *know* how to keep it—and your sleeping bag—dry.

Boots are the most important piece of clothing. They must be broken in before the trip. Otherwise, they may turn out not to fit, and they will surely give you a crop of blisters. For the entire PCT, it's best to have two pairs of boots in the same size and same style. Mail one pair ahead. Schifrin broke his foot because his two pairs were of two different styles, and one pair didn't give his feet the support the other pair had accustomed them to. You might go all the way on just one pair, after one or two resolings, but if you try to make the entire PCT through the North Cascades with the boots you started with, you will be sticking your neck out—and maybe your toes. Treat the boots with Snoseal or another effective compound often, to keep them waterproof and to prevent cracking from heat.

It may not occur to you in advance how tough walking will be on your socks, too. One PCT trekker said he wore out one pair every 125 miles on the average, though we think that's a little extreme. Still, you will need replacements. You might start out with a three-day supply of socks—three pairs of heavy wool socks and three (or six, if you wear double inners) pairs of inner socks (polypropylene is preferable). Schaffer has gone 1000+ miles with this combination. If you hope to equal that, you must change socks daily and wash them daily. Note also that clean socks are less likely to give you blisters.

Besides boot soles and socks, you are going to wear out some underwear, shirts, and, probably, pants. The less often you wash them, the faster they will wear out, due to rotting. In choosing your clothes to start with, remember that as you hike, your waist will get smaller and legs bigger.

Light footwear is very nice to have for fording streams and for comfort in camp. It's damn near heaven to take off those heavy boots after a 20-mile day. Tennis shoes are traditional, but gymnastic slippers work almost as well around camp (not in streams), and they weigh only a few ounces. SCUBA diving booties may be the best of the three: they wear well, can be worn in bed, don't absorb water, have great traction, are warmer than down booties, can be worn inside your boots, and can even keep your socks dry in stream fords. But they don't breathe, so wear them with clean feet and socks. Finally, sport sandals have become popular for camp wear, and buckled models are good for stream crossings, especially if worn with diving booties.

With all this said about footgear, you might consider going much lighter, as mentioned earlier. Schaffer usually backpacks in jogging shoes, carrying as much as 40 pounds (25% of his weight). Only if his pack is going to be considerably heavier, or if the route is going to be quite snowbound, does he consider wearing boots. Obviously, if you expect to use ice ax and crampons, you'll want to wear boots.

Equipment

Spare no expense. Mistakes and shortcuts in equipment mean lost time, lost money, lost sleep, and lost health.

Besides your usual summer backpacking equipment, you may need a tent, skis or snowshoes, an ice ax, and a rope. You'll need a guidebook with maps—this one. And even if you don't normally carry a camera, PCT trekkers say you'll be sorry if you don't take one on the BIG hike.

Almost all PCT hikers carry a *tent* and are glad they did. A tent is important for warmth in the snowy parts and for dryness in all the parts. In Oregon, a tent allows you to sleep by keeping the mosquitoes off you. We recommend a quality 2-person mountain tent—on the large side, or you and your companion may become less than friends.

The question of *skis* versus *snowshoes* for early season in the high mountains remains under debate, and some PCT hikers say they'd rather take their chances without either, considering the cost and the weight. The main advantage of skis, of course, is that you can cover a lot of ground downhill in a hurry—if you know how to ski with a pack. We suspect many of the trekkers who chose snowshoes would have used skis if they had been better cross-country-with-pack skiers. The main disadvantage of skis is that you can't mail them; you have to ship them by Greyhound or some other way.

Many PCT through-hikers say an *ice ax* is definitely a necessity, and others say it is at least worth its weight for the many different things it will do. We recommend one for any segment where you expect to be in snow. You should take a *rope* for belaying on steep snow or on ice and for difficult fords at the height of the snowmelt.

You'll probably want to record your trip with photos. If that's all you want to do, then the inexpensive, recyclable cameras, about 5 ounces light, may do. You get better results with zoom cameras, which are almost as small but twice the weight for, say, a 28-70 mm zoom. You may want a longer zoom in a few cases, but that can double the cost and can double the weight—not worth it, in Schaffer's opinion. Finally, if you want quality photos, you'll have to purchase a single-lens reflex camera and one or more lenses. If just one, choose about a 35–100 mm zoom with "macro," which is not a true macro but nevertheless is good enough for shooting wildflowers. In a few years, digital cameras may replace all of these. At the start of the millennium, they are too heavy, and, except for a few very pricey ones, they lack sufficient resolution.

The cost

You can expect to spend several thousand *dollars* for the whole PCT unless you already have almost all the equipment you will need. Take plenty of money in traveler's checks. You won't be able to resist the food when you are in civilization, and you will find yourself with unforeseen needs for equipment. In addition, you will want to be able to correct some original decisions that you have later found unwise or unworkable, and to do so usually takes money.

In addition, things change—for example, Forest Service campgrounds. In the past, they were free, but increasingly, trekkers are required to pay a few dollars for each night's stay at them. Perhaps in the near future they may all charge a fee. (If so, you may plan to stop at them for water and rest but then move onward and make camp farther along the trail.) Also, the late 1990s saw some National Forests charge to drive on their roads and/or park at their trailheads, and the trend was increasing. Finally, the Eldorado National Forest started charging fees to camp in Desolation Wilderness (California). There, at the start of the millennium, you'll pay a reservation fee of $5 per party, then $5 per night per person, for the first two nights (free beyond that). If all these policies take effect in Oregon and Washington, then $5 here, $10 there, and before you're through you could spend well over $100.

Mailing tips

You can mail yourself almost any food, clothing, or equipment. Before you leave home, you won't know whether you are going to run out of, say, molefoam, but you will have a good idea of your rate of consumption of food, clothing, and fuel for your stove. You can arrange for mailings of quantities of these things, purchased at home, where they are probably cheaper than in the towns along the way.

Address your package to:

Yourself
General Delivery
P.O., state ZIP
HOLD UNTIL (date)

Also, **boldly** write somewhere on the package "Pacific Crest Trail Hiker." Don't mail perishables. Make your packages strong, sturdy, and tight. You are *really* depending on their contents. Have your home contact mail packages at least 24 days before you expect to get them, and, even then, pay for the postal service called "Special Handling." By sending "Priority Mail," in addition, you can have the parcel forwarded or returned without an additional charge. Do not seal the packages when you pack them, because you are likely to have second thoughts. You can then phone your mail contact and ask him or her to add certain things to (or take certain things out of) the box that goes to X place, or wherever. Before you leave home, phone the resupply sites you will be sending packages to in order to make sure they will hold them until your arrival. Leslie Croot's book, mentioned above, gives their phone numbers. Be aware that some sites accept US mail, while others require UPS, and her book tells you which one to use as well as when each site will be open for package pick-up. (You don't want to waste a day or two simply because you arrived at a resupply site and it was closed.) Finally, in previous editions, we listed post offices along the route, but this list was made obsolete by Leslie's book; she does a much more thorough job.

HYPOTHERMIA

Every year you can read accounts of hikers freezing to death in the mountains. They die of hypothermia, the #1 killer of outdoor recreationists. You, too, may be exposed to it, particularly if you start hiking the PCT in April in order to do all three states. Because it is so easy to die from hypothermia, we are including the following information, which is endorsed by the Forest Service and by mountain-rescue groups. Read it. It may save your life.

Hypothermia is subnormal body temperature, which is caused outdoors by exposure to cold, usually aggravated by wetness, wind, and exhaustion. The moment your body begins to lose heat faster than it produces it, your body makes involuntary adjustments to preserve the normal temperature in its vital organs. Uncontrolled shivering is one way your body attempts to maintain its vital temperature. *If you've begun uncontrolled shivering, you must consider yourself a prime candidate for hypothermia and act accordingly.* When this happens, cold reaches your brain, depriving you of judgment and reasoning power. You will not realize this is happening. You will lose control of your hands. Your internal body temperature is sliding downward. Without treatment, this slide leads to stupor, collapse, and death. Learn the four lines of defense against hypothermia.

Your first line of defense: avoid exposure.

1. Stay dry. When clothes get wet, they lose about 90% of their insulating value. Wool loses less; cotton and down lose more. Synthetics are best.

2. Beware of wind. A slight breeze carries heat away from bare skin much faster than still air does. Wind drives cold air under and through clothing. Wind refrigerates wet clothes by evaporating moisture from the surface.

3. Understand cold. Most hypothermia cases develop in air temperatures between 30° and 50°. Most outdoors persons simply can't believe such temperatures can be dangerous. They fatally underestimate the danger of being wet at such temperatures. But just jump in a cold lakelet, and you'll agree that 50° water is unbearably cold. The cold that kills is cold water running down neck and legs, cold water held against the body by sopping clothes, cold water flushing body heat from the surface of the clothes.

4. Continue to eat and drink. It is very hard for fit outdoors persons to develop hypothermia, unless they become dehydrated and run out of energy.

Your second line of defense: terminate exposure.

If you cannot stay dry and warm under existing weather conditions, using the clothes you have with you, *terminate exposure.*

1. Be brave enough to give up reaching your destination or whatever you had in mind. That one extra mile might be your last.

2. Get out of the wind and rain. Build a fire. Concentrate on making your camp or bivouac as secure and comfortable as possible.

3. Never ignore shivering. Initial shivering is a clue that you're getting cold, and this is when it is important to take action to get warmer. Persistent or violent shivering is clear warning that you are on the verge of hypothermia. *Make camp.*

4. Forestall exhaustion. Make camp while you still have a reserve of energy. Allow for the fact that exposure greatly reduces your normal endurance. You may think you are doing fine when the fact that you are exercising is the only thing preventing your going into hypothermia. If exhaustion forces you to stop, however briefly, your rate of body heat production instantly drops by 50% or more; violent, incapacitating shivering may begin immediately; you may slip into hypothermia *in a matter of minutes.*

5. Appoint a foul-weather leader. Make the best-protected member of your party responsible for calling a halt before the least-protected member becomes exhausted or goes into violent shivering.

Your third line of defense: detect hypothermia.

If your party is exposed to wind, cold and wetness, *think hypothermia.* Watch yourself and others for hypothermia's symptoms:

1. Uncontrollable fits of shivering.
2. Vague, slow, slurred speech.
3. Memory lapses; incoherence.
4. Immobile or fumbling hands.
5. Frequent stumbling; lurching gait.
6. Drowsiness—to sleep is to die.
7. Apparent exhaustion, such as inability to get up after a rest.

Your fourth and last line of defense: treatment.

Victims may deny being in trouble. Believe the symptoms, *not* the victim. Even mild symptoms demand immediate, drastic treatment.

1. Get victims out of the wind and rain.
2. Strip off *all* wet clothes.
3. If victims are only mildly impaired:
   a. Give them warm drinks.
   b. Get them into dry clothes and a warm sleeping bag. Well-wrapped, warm (not hot) rocks or canteens will hasten recovery.
4. If victims are semiconscious or worse:
   a. Don't give hot drinks unless they are capable of holding a cup and drinking from it. Forcing drinks on semiconscious persons could cause them to gag and *drown* (unfortunately, this is quite common with inexperienced would-be rescuers)!
   b. Leave them stripped. Put them in a sleeping bag with another person (also stripped). If you have double bag or can zip two together, put the victim between two warmth donors. *Skin-to-skin contact* is the most effective treatment. Never leave victims as long as they are alive. To do so is to kill them—it's just that simple!
5. Build a fire to warm the camp.

Other notes on avoiding hypothermia.

1. Choose rainclothes that are effective against *wind-driven* rain and that cover head, neck, body and legs. Gore-Tex, Sympatex, and other laminates work the best, more so when new. Sympatex seems to work better for longer. Many serious rain-walkers prefer completely sealed and waterproof shell gear, figuring that with synthetic insulation, some condensation is better than a leaky jacket.

2. Take clothing that retains its insulation even when wet, such as polypropylene, capilene, or dacron fabrics. These hold even less water than the traditional wet-weather favorite, wool, and so make it easier for your body to keep warm. Always carry a two-piece underwear set, and a heavier pair of pants, plus a sweater or pullover (synthetic "fleece" and "pile" designs are rugged and perform well). Never forget a knit wool or fleece headpiece that can protect the head, neck, and chin. *Cotton underwear and down-filled parkas are worse than useless when wet, as are cotton shirts and pants.* As early Americans long ago discovered, one stays warmer in a cold rain when stark naked than when bundled up in wet clothes. Some folks in the drippy North Cascade forests carry umbrellas.

3. Carry a stormproof tent with a good rain fly and set it up *before* you need it.

4. Carry trail food rich in calories, such as nuts, jerky, and candy, and keep nibbling during hypothermia weather.

5. Take a gas stove or a plumber's candle, flammable paste, or other reliable fire starter.

6. Never abandon survival gear under any circumstances. If you didn't bring along the above items, stay put and make the best of it. An all-too-common fatal mistake is for victims to abandon everything so that, unburdened, they can run for help.

7. "It never happens to me. I'm Joe Athlete." Don't you believe it. It can be you, even if you are in fantastic shape and are carrying the proper equipment. Be alert for hypothermia conditions and hypothermia symptoms.

OUTDOOR COURTESY

Traveling a wild trail, away from centers of civilization, is a unique experience. It brings intimate association with nature—communion with the earth, the forest, the chaparral, the wildlife, the clear sky. A great responsibility accompanies this experience—the obligation to keep the wilderness as you found it. Being considerate of the wilderness rights of others will make the mountain adventures of those who follow equally rewarding. As a wilderness visitor, you should become familiar with the rules of wilderness courtesy outlined below.

Trails. Never cut switchbacks. This practice breaks down trails and hastens erosion. Take care not to dislodge rocks that might fall on hikers below you. Improve and preserve trails, as by clearing away loose rocks (carefully) and removing branches. Report any trail damage and broken or misplaced signs to a ranger or mention them in a PCTA register.

Off trail. Restrain the impulse to blaze trees or to build ducks where not essential. Let the next person find the way as you did.

Campsites. This guidebook mentions campsites you will find along the trail, but you perhaps will not use them. Indeed, in his handbook, the author argues against their use and instead promotes "stealth camping," which is camping away from both trail and water and leaving minimal evidence that you were there. Most hikers probably prefer a scenic lakeside campsite, and if it is beside the PCT, so much the better. Jardine, however, does make a legitimate point: many existing campsites have degraded the local environment.

Minimize your impact at any campsite by not building a fire, even if it is legal. Defecate and urinate well away from water, not in a convenient, close-by spot perhaps used by many who have camped before you. The widespread giardiasis problem and the spreading *Cryptosporidium* problem seem to stem more from poor bathroom habits than from anything else. (We cannot blame the horses and cattle for this problem.) The campsite should be left in as good condition as you found it, or even better.

Environmentally-conscious equestrians need to choose carefully the location of each campsite, since evidence of their visit will be hard to miss, given all the urine, manure, and feed that will accumulate during the stay. Ideally, equestrians should make every effort to camp outside the wilderness, but that is not always possible and generally not desirable. Equestrians need to make an extra effort to clean up their campsites, partly to avert the wrath of irate backpackers, who have become increasingly anti-horse (due in no small measure to real or perceived localized heavy environmental impact in the mountains by professional packers).

Litter. Along the trail, place candy wrappers, raisin boxes, orange peels, etc., in your pocket or pack for later disposal; throw nothing on the trail. Pick up litter you find along the trail or in camp. More than almost anything else (with the possible exception of abundant, fresh manure), litter detracts from the wilderness scene. Remember, you *can* take it with you.

Noise. Boisterous conduct is out of harmony in a wilderness experience. Be a considerate hiker and camper. Don't ruin another's enjoyment of the wilderness.

Good Samaritanship. Human life and well-being take precedence over everything else—in the wilderness as elsewhere. If a hiker or camper is in trouble, help in any way you can. Indifference is a moral crime. Give comfort or first aid; then seek help.

LAND-USE REGULATIONS

The Oregon-Washington PCT passes through national parks, national forests, Indian land, land administered by the Bureau of Land Management, state land, and private land. All these areas have their own regulations, which you ignore only at your risk—risk of physical difficulty as well as of the possibility of being cited for violations.

On private land, of course, the regulations are what the owner says they are. The same is true on Indian land. In particular, don't build a fire on private land without the owner's written permission. Regulations on U.S. Bureau of Land Management land are not of major consequence for users of this book, since the route passes through only a few miles of it, in Section B. The same is true of state land, in southernmost Washington.

The Forest Service and the Park Service have more regulations. These are not uniform throughout the states or between the two services. We list below the Forest Service and Park Service regulations that *are* uniform along the trail, plus some that are peculiar to the Park Service. Special regulations in particular places are mentioned in the trail description when it "arrives" at those places.

1. *Wilderness permits.* Unlike in California, where wilderness permits are required for most of the wildernesses the PCT trekker camps in, they are not required in the national forests of Oregon and Washington. (In the Siskiyou Mountains of northern California, in which this guidebook begins, the trail doesn't enter any wilderness.) However, wilderness permits are required for a backcountry stay overnight in national parks, and in Oregon and Washington there are three: Crater Lake, Mt. Rainier, and North Cascades. Your traverse through Crater Lake National Park is sufficiently long that you'll probably camp one or two nights in it. See the start of Chapter C for permit information. The PCT briefly enters and exits Mt. Rainier National Park several times, and the only place you may want to camp within the park would be at Anderson Lake (Map I4). There, you won't need a permit, but should you stray from the trail and camp in the park's backcountry, you will. As in Crater Lake National Park, in North Cascades National Park you'll likely camp one or more nights See the start of Chapter K for permit information.

As with wilderness permits, campfire permits are no longer required in the two states in both national forests and national parks. However, while allowing campfires, both services discourage them and prefer that you carry a stove instead. In Mt. Rainier National Park, campfires are prohibited at all but the park's lowest backcountry sites, so bring a stove or eat cold food. Except for emergencies, you shouldn't make a campfire anywhere along the PCT, since downed wood hosts organisms on which larger animals feed, and, as the wood decays, it adds nutrients to the soil.

2. *Parking at trailheads* used to be free, but in the late 1990s, an increasing number of trailheads required parking fees. If you are going to park a vehicle at (or near) any PCT trailhead, there's a good chance there will be a fee of several dollars per day, so be prepared. Oregon and Washington residents generally are aware of this, and those that ride and hike often save considerable money by purchasing an annual Trail Park Pass.

These are quite readily available at ranger stations, at any R.E.I. store, and at numerous retail outlets.

3. *A fishing license* is required in Oregon for those 14 or older and in Washington for those 15 or older. Both states have a variety of fishing licenses (and fees), based on your age, state of residency, and length of fishing excursion. For further information, contact:

Oregon Department of Fish and Wildlife
2501 S.W. 1st Street—P.O. Box 59
Portland, OR 97207
(503) 872-5268

or

Washington Department of Fish and Wildlife
600 Capitol Way North
Olympia, WA 98501
(360) 902-2200

4. *Destruction*, injury, defacement, removal, or disturbance in any manner of any natural feature of public property is prohibited. This includes:

a. Molesting any animal;
b. Picking flowers or other plants;
c. Cutting, blazing, marking, driving nails in, or otherwise damaging growing trees or standing snags;
d. Writing, carving, or painting of name or other inscription anywhere;
e. Destruction, defacement, or moving of signs.

5. *Collecting specimens* of minerals, plants, animals, or historical objects is prohibited without written authorization, obtained in advance, from the Park Service or Forest Service. Permits are not issued for personal collections.

6. *Smoking* is not permitted while traveling through vegetated areas. You may stop and smoke in a safe place.

7. *Pack and saddle animals* have the right-of-way on trails. Hikers should get completely off the trail, on the downhill side if possible, and remain quiet until the stock has passed.

8. It is illegal to cut *switchbacks.*

9. *Use existing campsites* if there are any. If not, camp away from the trail and at least 100 feet from lakes and streams, on mineral soil or unvegetated forest floor—never in meadows or other soft, vegetated spots. Unfortunately, in many popular areas—Jefferso Park, in particular—almost all the good campsites are within 100 feet of water. Until t Forest Service builds or recommends alternate campsites, the hiker will have little ch but to use one of the existing illegal sites.

10. *Construction of improvements* such as rock walls, large fireplaces, boug tables, and rock-and-log stream crossings is prohibited.

11. *Soap and other pollutants* should be kept out of lakes and streams. Us gents is not recommended, since they affect the water detrimentally.

12. *Toilets* should be in soft soil away from camps and water. Dig a sha bury it.

13. You are required to *clean up your camp* before you leave. Tin worn-out or useless gear, and other unburnables must be carried out.

14. *National Parks but not Forests* prohibit dogs and cats on the trail and prohibit carrying or using firearms.

15. *Horses* and other pack or saddle animals should be kept at least 200 feet from any lake, stream, or spring, except when watering, loading, unloading, or traveling on established trail routes. Forage may be limited, so you should carry feed. Avoid tying horses to trees at campsites for prolonged periods. Hobble, stake, or use a picket line with your stock.

BORDER CROSSING

Most PCT hikers do not cross the United States/Canada border. Those that do may find it easier going north into Canada than heading south into the United States.

PCT north from United States into Canada

If you're doing this, request an "Application for entry to Canada via the Pacific Crest Trail." You can get an application by writing the Canada Immigration Centre, 2 Sumas Way, Abbotsford, B.C. V2S 7L9 (phone: 604/504-4688; fax: 504-4693). However, it may be simpler to just copy the application from the PCTA website (www.pcta.org), which is more likely to have the latest information on this matter. Follow the simple instructions and mail it in. If your trip is merely one into Canada to Manning Park and then a prompt return to the United States by vehicle or other transportation (e.g., bus), then you won't have to report to Canada Customs.

Hopefully, when you get the application form, you'll also get an information sheet. Basically, what you need to know is the following. Foremost, you need identification with a photo, such as a driver's license (non-US citizens, a passport). Guns and most other weapons are banned, but either a hunting knife or pocket knife (no switchblades) is okay. Don't take your pet dog or fresh fruit and vegetables across the border.

If you're an equestrian, you'll need a USDA Export Health Certificate for your stock. Get this from a USDA accredited veterinarian, who will send it to the USDA veterinary service in Olympia, Washington, reached at (360) 753-9430. They will return it to your veterinarian. You should do this within 30 days of your border crossing, which is very inconvenient for those planning to spend several months on the trail. Once in Canada, you must take your stock directly to Canada Customs at Huntingdon, B.C. or Osoyoos, B.C.

…th from Canada into United States

… in this direction and attempting to deal with Customs is an exercise in frus- …ffer was told to contact the headquarters of North Cascades National Park. …ere said that those crossing the border need to report to the District Office …but once there, no employee would know what to do. This seems true. …ffer to US Customs Service in Seattle, and the employee he talked …e trail's existence (!) and said that it was illegal to enter the United …was no US Customs port of entry. (Never mind that folks have …r decades!) He did, however, refer Schaffer to a western port … originally begun his quest for legal entry into the United …contact the headquarters of North Cascades National …ths to hike the trail from end to end and longer to get an …s.

Since the greatest country in the world seems either totally incompetent and/or impotent with regard to answering a simple question, Schaffer suggests you simply check in with US Customs at Sumas or Oroville. Then head over to Manning Provincial Park and start your trek south. Make sure you have proper identification and follow the brief guidelines above for entry into Canada.

GOVERNMENT ADMINISTRATIVE HEADQUARTERS

If you couldn't get the necessary information from the Pacific Crest Trail Association or the Outdoor Recreation Information Center (both mentioned earlier, at the start of "Logistics for the Long Distance Backpacker"), then as a last resort you can turn to government administrative headquarters, which are listed here. Generally, each agency won't be able to answer specific questions, but you'll likely be referred to one of their subunits, such as a ranger station, where someone may know the answer. Also visit their websites on the Internet.

General

Regional Forester
Pacific Southwest Region
1323 Club Drive
Vallejo, CA 94592
(707) 562-8737

Regional Forester
Pacific Northwest Region
P.O. Box 3623
Portland, OR 97208
(503) 808-2201

Bureau of Land Mgmt.
P.O. Box 2965
Portland, OR 97208
(503) 952-6287

Specific, South to North

Klamath National Forest
1312 Fairlane Road
Yreka, CA 96097
(916) 842-6131

Rogue River Natl. Forest
P.O. Box 520
Medford, OR 97501
(541) 858-2200

Winema National Forest
2819 Dahlia Street
Klamath Falls, OR 97601
(541) 883-6714

Crater Lake National Park
P.O. Box 7
Crater Lake, OR 97604
(541) 594-2211

Umpqua National Forest
P.O. Box 1008
Roseburg, OR 97470
(541) 672-6601

Deschutes National Forest
1645 Highway 20 East
Bend, OR 97701
(541) 383-5300

Willamette National Forest
P.O. Box 10607
Eugene, OR 97440
(541) 465-6521

Mt. Hood National Forest
16400 Champion Way
Sandy, OR 97055
(503) 668-1700

Gifford Pinchot Natl. Forest
10600 N.E. 51st Circle
Vancouver, WA 98682
(360) 891-5000

Mt. Baker-Snoqualmie National Forest
64th Avenue West
Mountlake Terrace, WA 98043
(425) 775-9702

Specific, South to North ***(cont.)***

Mt. Rainier National Park
Tahoma Woods, Star Rte.
Ashford, WA 98304
(360) 569-2211

North Cascades Natl. Park
2105 State Route 20
Sedro Woolley, WA 98284
(360) 856-5700

Okanogan & Wenatchee
Natl. Forest
215 Melody Lane
Wenatchee, WA 98801
(509) 662-4335

Manning Provincial Park
Box 3
Manning Park, B.C.
V0X 1R0, Canada
(250) 840-8836

FORGOTTEN ANYTHING?

Here is a checklist of items we feel you should *consider* bringing along. You might prefer to bring other things, too.

wallet
keys
watch
travelers checks
wilderness permit
this guidebook
nature guides
pencil and notepad
camera
camera accessories
film
fishing gear
fishing license
mountaineering gear
other special gear (e.g., ice ax)
walking stick(s)
pack
sleeping bag
foam pad or air mattress
ground cloth
tent or tube tent
rain gear
down vest or down parka
windbreaker and/or sweatshirt
shirts (wool or synthetic)
pants (wool or synthetic)
shorts
swimsuit
towel and/or washcloth
underwear (polypropylene)
socks
gaiters
boots and boot laces
camp shoes
wool cap and/or brimmed hat
dark glasses
gloves
sewing kit
toilet paper
personal hygiene items
aspirin
prescription medicine
molefoam
first-aid kit
snakebite kit
insect repellent (lots of it)
sunscreen
lip balm
toothbrush, toothpaste
compass
altimeter
flashlight
extra batteries
pocket knife
can opener
food and drink
bearproof food container
salt and pepper
stove and fuel
matches in waterproof container
pots, bowls, and utensils
drinking mug
soap: leave it home!
water bottles (½ gallon is sufficient)
several trash bags
stuffsacks for sleeping bag and/or bearbagging
50 feet of parachute cord for bearbagging
50 feet of parachute cord for emergencies (tent lines, pack repairs, shoelaces)
100 feet of lightweight nylon rope for stream fords and risky snow-slope traverses

Chapter 3: PCT Natural History

INTRODUCTION

The California section of the Pacific Crest Trail (PCT) is noted for its great diversity of plants and animals, minerals and rocks, climates and landscapes. The Oregon section of the PCT provides quite a contrast, having the most homogenous vegetation and landscape of this tri-state route. The Washington section falls between these two extremes. Along the route covered by this volume, certain rocks, plants, and animals appear time and time again. The most common entities appear to be—

Rock: andesite, basalt
Flower: lupine
Shrub: huckleberry
Tree: mountain hemlock, subalpine fir, western white pine
Invertebrate: mosquito
Fish: trout
Amphibian: western toad, tree frog (but all amphibians are faring poorly)
Reptile: garter snake
Bird: Dark-eyed junco
Mammal:
Small: chipmunk, golden-mantled ground squirrel
Large: human, deer

The average elevation of Oregon's section of PCT is about 5120 feet, whereas Washington's section is about 4550 feet—lower in part because the weathering and erosional processes farther north are more intense (contrast Washington's 4550 to California's 6120). Not only is the average trail elevation different between these two northwest states, so too is the typical terrain that the trail traverses. The Oregon section is flatter, drier, more volcanic, and less glaciated than Washington's section. In Oregon, a typical hike is through a mountain-hemlock forest while traversing rolling ridges and crossing lake-bound basins. In Washington, a typical hike is through alternating forests of mountain hemlock and subalpine species while climbing over passes and dropping somewhat into glaciated canyons. Both states, of course, have many distinctive features worth investigating.

GEOLOGY

We can thank the existence of western America's mountains for the existence of the PCT. Without these mountains, we'd have instead the Pacific *Coast* Trail. But why should we have mountains in the first place? The answer lies with plate tectonics—the ceaseless movements of the earth's crust and its associated upper mantle. This composite outer layer is made up of a few giant plates plus more abundant, smaller plates, all interacting with one another. Some movements lead to the formation of mountain ranges, others to ocean basins.

Although plate tectonics has been occurring for several billion years, we need concern ourselves only with the last 50 million or so years. Back then, oceanic plates were diving under continental plates, much as they do today. One oceanic plate, the Farallon plate, was diving east under the continental North American plate, and it was being consumed in the process, particularly in its midsection. About 29 million years ago, the midsection had been totally consumed, leaving a southern part and a northern part. It is the northern part we are interested in, now known as the Juan de Fuca plate. Like the larger Farallon plate, the Juan de Fuca plate continued diving under the North American plate. Also like that plate, it continued drifting north with respect to North America (see illustration).

When one plate dives beneath another, it eventually melts, due to increasing temperature. This typically happens at depths of about 60 to 90 miles. The melt doesn't have the same chemical composition as the plate, for overlying oceanic sediments, laden with water, have been dragged down with the descending plate, and these sediments are incorporated into the melt. The resulting melt, or magma, is relatively light in density, and it works its way up toward the earth's surface. If it reaches the surface, a volcanic eruption occurs, such as the devastating eruption of Mt. St. Helens on May 18, 1980. If it doesn't reach the surface, it solidifies at depth as granitic rock. Erosion over millions of years strips off overlying rocks to expose the granitic rock, which is what we see in the North Cascades.

The continual diving of the Juan de Fuca plate insures continual production of magma, thus guaranteeing a future for the Cascade Range. Note, however, that because the plate is drifting north, so too will the zone of active Cascade volcanoes. In the future, new volcanoes will erupt in British Columbia, while the old ones in southern Oregon and northern California will cease to erupt.

While the foregoing discourse describes the dynamics of the Cascade Range, it does not describe its history. That history is fairly well known from the mid-Tertiary period onward (see Geologic Time Table on page 28). In the late Eocene and early Miocene epochs, deposits from the ancient Cascade Range reached a thickness of six miles in some places. For such an accumulation to occur, the regional crust must have been relatively stable for some time. By the mid-Miocene, the range experienced folding, faulting, and, in the north, intrusion by granitic batholiths, plutons, stocks, and dikes. (These intrusive masses are distinguished by their relative size; a batholith may be tens of miles across, whereas a dike may be only a few feet or a few inches across.) During the mid-Miocene, linear vents east of the Cascades opened and poured forth the very fluid

Columbia River basalts, which flooded much of the terrain of southern Washington and northern Oregon. The many flows from the fiery episodes are best seen by hikers as they descend north toward the Columbia River along the lower half of the Eagle Creek Trail.

Plant fossils collected east of the Cascades indicate the environment was considerably more humid than it is today. From this knowledge, the paleobotanist infers that the Cascades were lower in elevation, or, more likely, the pre-faulted eastern lands were higher, since there was no evidence of a rain shadow. One need only drive to Sisters or Wenatchee to notice how much drier the east slopes of today's Cascades are compared to their west slopes.

After the partial flooding of the range by the Columbia River basalts, the earth's internal forces, quite likely due to the interaction between the North American and Juan de Fuca plates, uplifted the range and initiated a series of active volcanoes. Uplift and eruptions continued during the Quaternary, but in this epoch, the higher peaks were subjected to repeated glaciations brought on by changes in the world-wide climatic pattern. Some paleoclimatologists have speculated that the moving plates have rearranged the

Western North America, about 15 million years ago (left) and today (right). The Juan de Fuca plate (gray) is producing new oceanic crust along its western edge, causing sea-floor spreading (large, dark arrows). This plate is bordered by the Pacific plate on its west and south edges, and by the North American plate on its east edge. Note that in the 15-million-year time lapse, the Juan de Fuca plate has changed its orientation with respect to North America, and that it has migrated considerably eastward and northward while diving under the continent (open arrows). Note that the directions of sea-floor spreading and plate diving are very different. In another 15 million years, the Juan de Fuca plate will all but disappear beneath the North American plate. In the map on the right the stars are major Cascade Range volcanoes and the small rectangle is this chapter's geologic map.

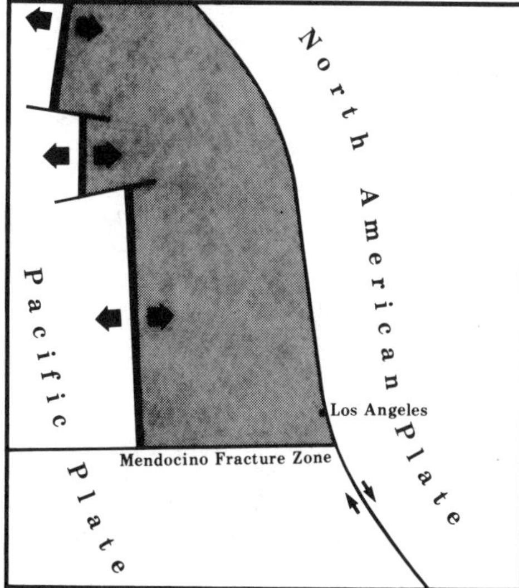

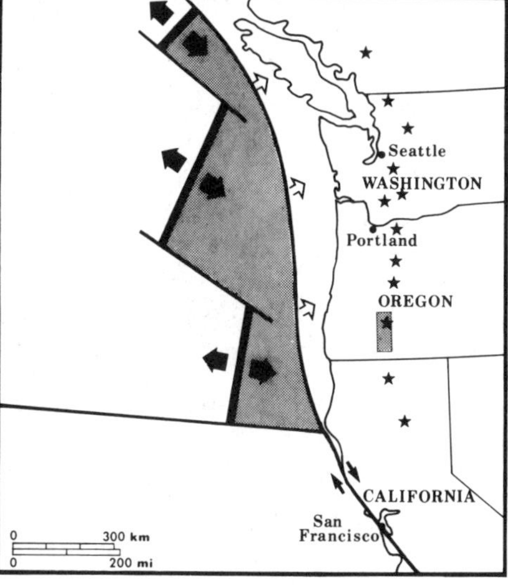

ocean basins, thereby affecting ocean currents and also major weather patterns, but the influences that initiated the Ice Age (the Pleistocene epoch) are still debated.

The same processes at work in the past are at work today. Volcanoes attempt to grow ever upward, but they are checked by the forces of gravity, weathering, and erosion. The higher a peak grows, the more it is attacked by the icy fingers of glaciers. Gravity pulls loose particles downward; the right snow conditions initiate avalanches; and minor eruptions and near-surface intrusions melt snowpacks, thereby creating enormous mudflows. Particularly good examples of the destructive power of such mudflows may be seen in the Mt. St. Helens environs.

The major volcanoes we see today are quite young—definitely late Quaternary. Many of them have erupted in geologically recent times, and there is every reason to believe they will erupt again. The PCT traverses most of these "dormant" volcanoes, including,

GEOLOGIC TIME SCALE

Era	Period	Epoch	Began (years ago)	Duration (years)
	Quaternary	Holocene	10,000	10,000
		Pleistocene	2,480,000	2,470,000
Cenozoic	Tertiary	Pliocene	5,200,000	2,720,000
		Miocene	23,300,000	18,100,000
		Oligocene	34,000,000	10,700,000
		Eocene	56,500,000	22,500,000
		Paleocene	65,000,000	8,500,000
Mesozoic	Cretaceous	*Numerous epochs recognized*	145,000,000	80,000,000
	Jurassic		208,000,000	63,000,000
	Triassic		245,000,000	37,000,000
Paleozoic	Permian	*Numerous epochs recognized*	286,000,000	41,000,000
	Carboniferous		360,000,000	74,000,000
	Devonian		408,000,000	48,000,000
	Silurian		438,000,000	30,000,000
	Ordovician		505,000,000	67,000,000
	Cambrian		540,000,000	35,000,000
Precambrian	No defined periods or epochs; oldest known rocks are about 4.2 billion years old; Earth's crust solidified about 4.6 million years ago.			

Derived from sources available in the 1990s. Most earth scientists still recognize the Tertiary-Quaternary boundary at 1,600,000 years, which is a poor choice except in Italy (where the boundary was so defined). The 2,480,000-year date is that of the Gauss-Matuyama reversal of the earth's magnetic poles, and this date is virtually synonymous with the commencement of the dozens of cycles of major glaciations in the northern hemisphere; it also marks the approximate date of earliest man (origin of genus *Homo*). Thus it accommodates the two classic concepts of the Quaternary, this period originally being the Ice Age and the Age of Man.

south to north, Mt. McLoughlin (9495), Crater Lake (11,500-foot-high Mt. Mazama until 6900 years ago), the Three Sisters (10,358, 10,047, 10,085), Mt. Jefferson (10,497), Mt. Hood (11,235), Mt. Adams (12,276), Mt. Rainier (14,410), and Glacier Peak (10,541). Geologic vignettes of these and other summits are included in our trail descriptions.

During the Ice Age, which has *temporarily* abated, an almost continuous mantle of ice covered the Cascades from Mt. McLoughlin north into Canada. From this mantle, huge fingers of glacier ice extended downcanyon, sometimes for tens of miles, and some gave rise to enormous lakes, such as Lake Chelan in the North Cascades. Evidence of large southern glaciers can be found near Crater Lake, even though Mt. Mazama, their source, was later blown out of existence. When hikers climb east from Diamond Lake on the Howlock Mountain Trail, about 16 miles north of Crater Lake, they climb up a large lateral moraine left by a Mt. Mazama glacier when it retreated about 10,000 years ago, at the time when most of the Cascades' glaciers melted back.

Today we are living in an interglacial period that could come to an end relatively soon. The hiker trekking along the PCT today thus sees the Cascade Range in its "atypical" form, for in the last million years, most of the range lay under an ice sheet about 95% of the time. So, if you experience chilly, wet weather along your PCT hike, be grateful it isn't worse: 20,000 years ago, your hike would have resembled a trek across today's icy Greenland.

BIOLOGY

Your first guess about the PCT—a high adventure rich in magnificent alpine scenery and sweeping panoramas—turns out to be incorrect along some parts of the trail. The real-life trail hike will sometimes seem to consist of enduring many repetitious miles through viewless forests, battling hordes of mosquitoes, or even hiking up to a whole day at a time without reaching fresh water. If you get bogged down in such unpleasant impressions, it may be because you haven't developed an appreciation of the natural history of this remarkable route. There is a great variety of plants and animals, rocks and minerals, landscapes and climates along the PCT, and the more you know about each, the more you will enjoy your trek.

Flora

A backpacker who has just completed the California section of the PCT might conclude that southern Oregon's forests form a more integrated "neighborhood" of species than California's forests did. Passing through different environments of the Sierra Nevada, you may have noticed the segregation of tree species and concluded that as you ascend toward the range's crest, you pass through a sequence of forests: Douglas-fir, white fir, red fir, mountain hemlock. Near the Oregon border, however, you discover that these four species and others reside together. Certainly, this aggregation would never be seen in the Sierra. The great diversity of environments found within that range has allowed each species to adapt to the environment most suitable for it.

In contrast, the southern Oregon environments, and therefore the plant communities, are not as sharply defined. Still, each plant species is found within a certain elevation range and over a certain geographic area. The general elevation and north-south range of 21 Cascade Range conifers are shown on profiles on the following pages. These species

South north profiles of the Cascade Range approximately along the Pacific Crest Trail. Each profile shows the altitudinal and latitudinal range of one or two conifers.

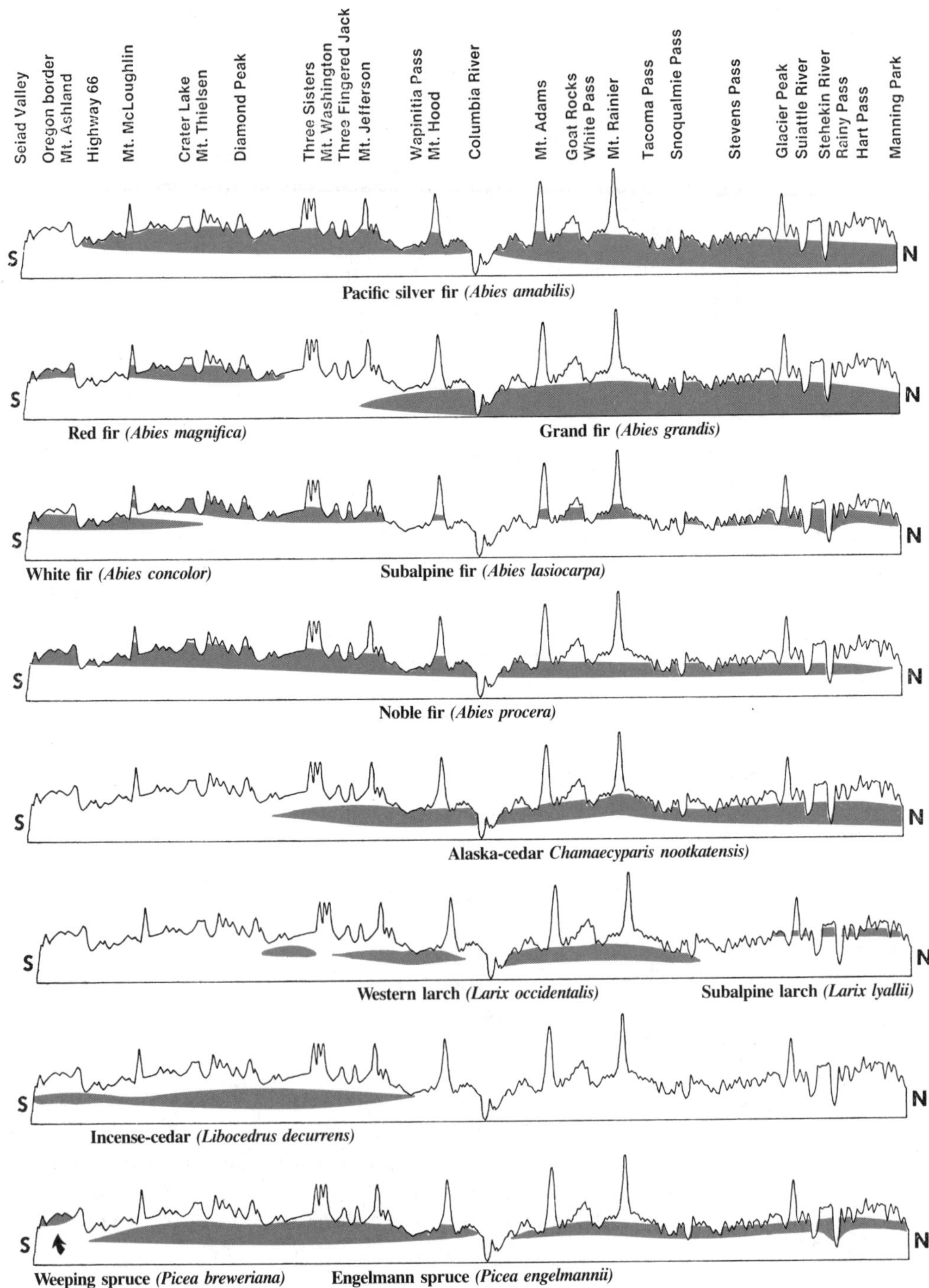

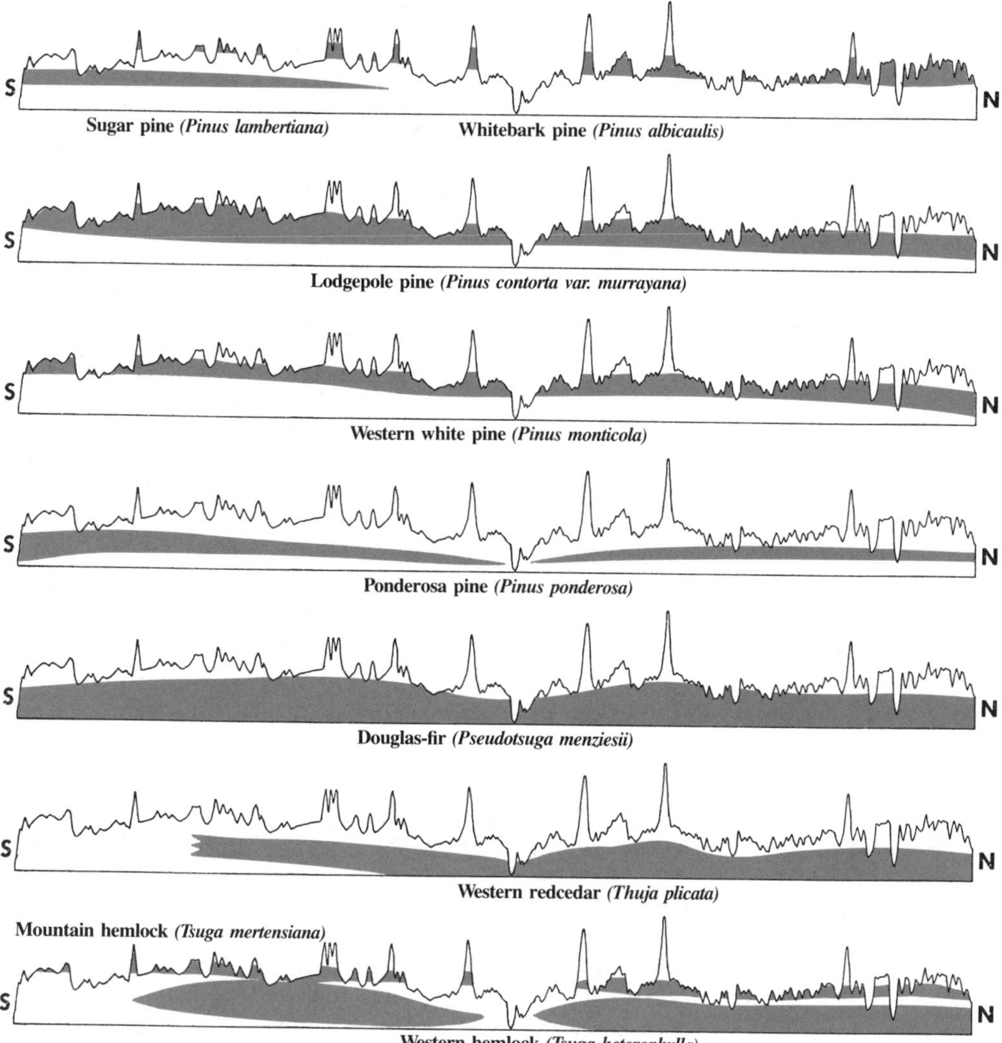

make up virtually all the forest cover you'll pass through on your Oregon-Washington trek. Note how the species vary in distribution, both horizontally and vertically.

If you've hiked through California's rugged Sierra Nevada, you'll find southern Oregon a much gentler, more uniform landscape. But despite its relatively subdued topography, it still supports a diverse assemblage of plants, and the discerning hiker soon learns what species to expect around the next bend. Ponderosa pines thrive in the drier southern Oregon forests, yet they are nonexistent in the dry pumice soils of the Crater Lake vicinity. Here, you'll find lodgepole pines which, ironically, are water-loving trees. These are usually seen growing in boggy soils near lakes, creeks, and wet meadows, where they often edge out the mountain hemlocks, which are by far the most common tree you'll see along the PCT in Oregon and Washington. The most suitable habitat for hemlocks appears to be shady north slopes, on which pure stands of tall, straight specimens grow. At lower elevations, mountain hemlocks give way to western hemlocks and Douglas-firs, and, as the environment becomes drier southward and eastward, these two species yield to ponderosa pines. The harder you look at a forest, even a small piece of it, the more you realize that this seemingly uniform stand of trees is in fact a complex assemblage of particular plants, animals, soils, rocks, and microclimates all influencing each other.

The trail description in this book commences at Seiad Valley, a manmade ranchland carved from a Douglas-fir forest. Near the end of the odyssey, along Agnes Creek and the Stehekin River, you also encounter a Douglas-fir forest. The two are hardly alike. The Douglas-fir forest of northern California and southern Oregon contains, among other trees, incense-cedar, ponderosa pine, white fir, Oregon oak, and madrone. Its counterpart in northern Washington contains, among others, western redcedar, western white pine, grand fir, vine maple, and Engelmann spruce.

The two forests vary considerably in the density of their vegetation. Not only does the rain-laden northern forest have a denser stand of taller conifers, but it also has a denser understory. Its huckleberries, thimbleberries, Devil's club, and other moisture-loving shrubs are quite a contrast to the stiff, dry manzanita, ceanothus, and scrub oaks seen in the southern forest. Wildflowers in the northern forest are more abundant than their counterparts to the south. During rainstorms, they are too abundant, for their thick growth along the trail ensures that you'll be soaked by them from as high as your waist on down. Both forests have quite a number of species in common, but from central Oregon northward, the moisture-oriented species become prominent. Now you find bunchberry, dogwood, Oregon grape, Lewis monkeyflower, and other species growing on the dark, damp forest floor.

In contrast to trees, which are quite specific in their habitat selection, flowers can tolerate a broad range of environments. You'll find, for example, yarrow, a sunflower, at timberline on the slopes of Mt. Hood and also on the Douglas-fir forest floor that borders the southern shore of the Columbia River. Both environments are moist, but the Mt. Hood alpine meadows, at 6000 feet above the bottom of the Columbia River gorge, are a considerably harsher environment.

Some flowers prefer open meadows to shady forests; others prefer dry environments. Thistle, lupine, and phlox are found along the sunnier portions of the trail. Growing from crevices among rocks are the aptly named stonecrops, and on the pumice flats too dry for even the lodgepole pines to pioneer, the Newberry knotweed thrives.

In addition to adapting to specific climatic conditions, a plant may also adapt to a specific soil condition. Thus, you see on the otherwise-barren mica schist slopes of Condrey Mountain, near the southern Oregon border, acre after acre of pink, prostrate pussypaws.

Lastly, a species may have a distribution governed by the presence of other species. Corn lilies thrive in wet meadows, but lodgepoles invade these lands and shade them out. Mountain hemlocks may soon follow and eventually achieve dominance over the lodgepoles. Then the careless camper comes along, lets the campfire escape, and the forest burns. Among the charred stumps of the desolate ruins rises the tall, blazing, magenta

From top, left to right: fireweed, paintbrush, tiger lily; Newberry knotweed, corn lily (false hellebore, skunk cabbage), pasqueflower; pearly everlasting, phlox, Sitka valerian

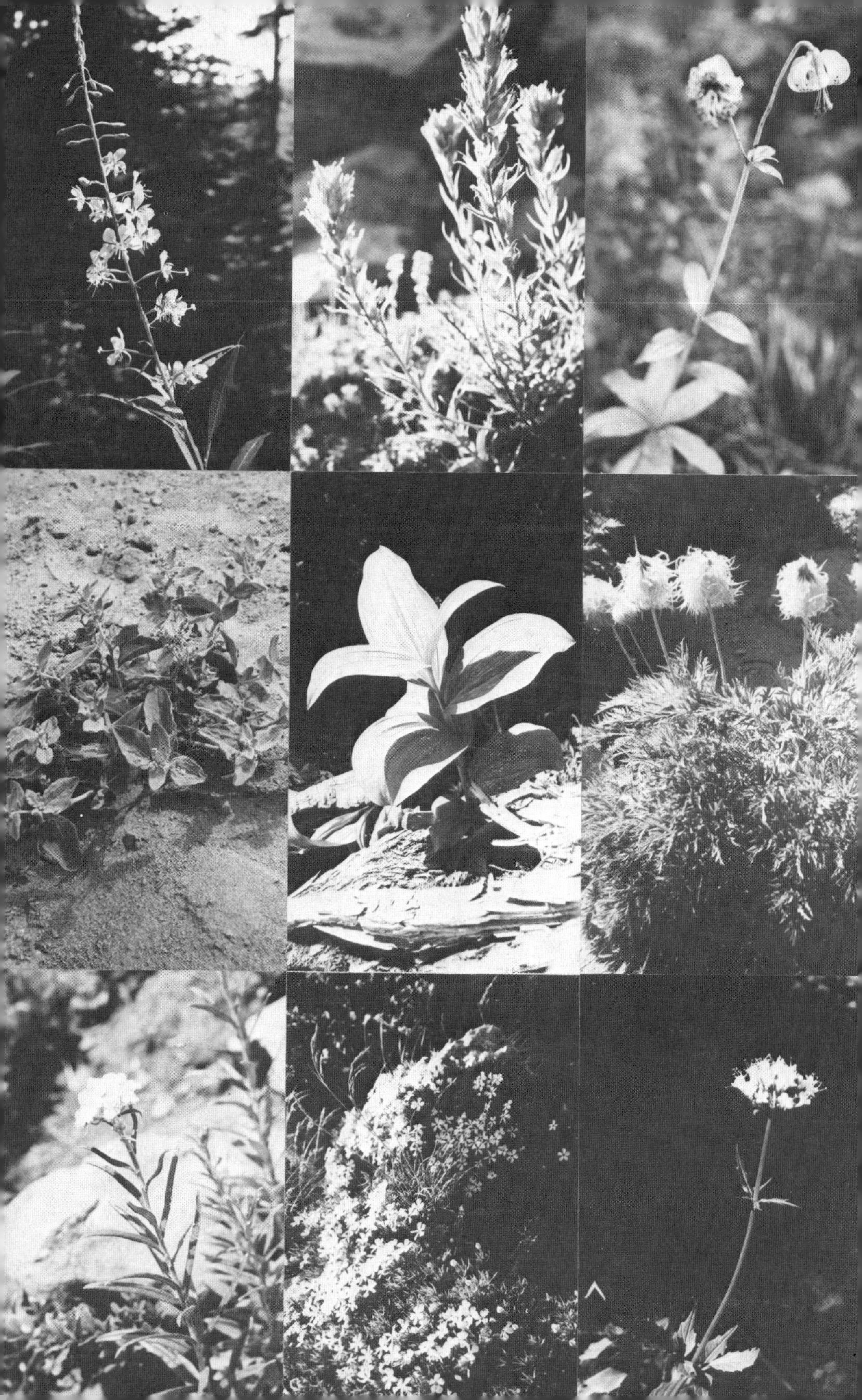

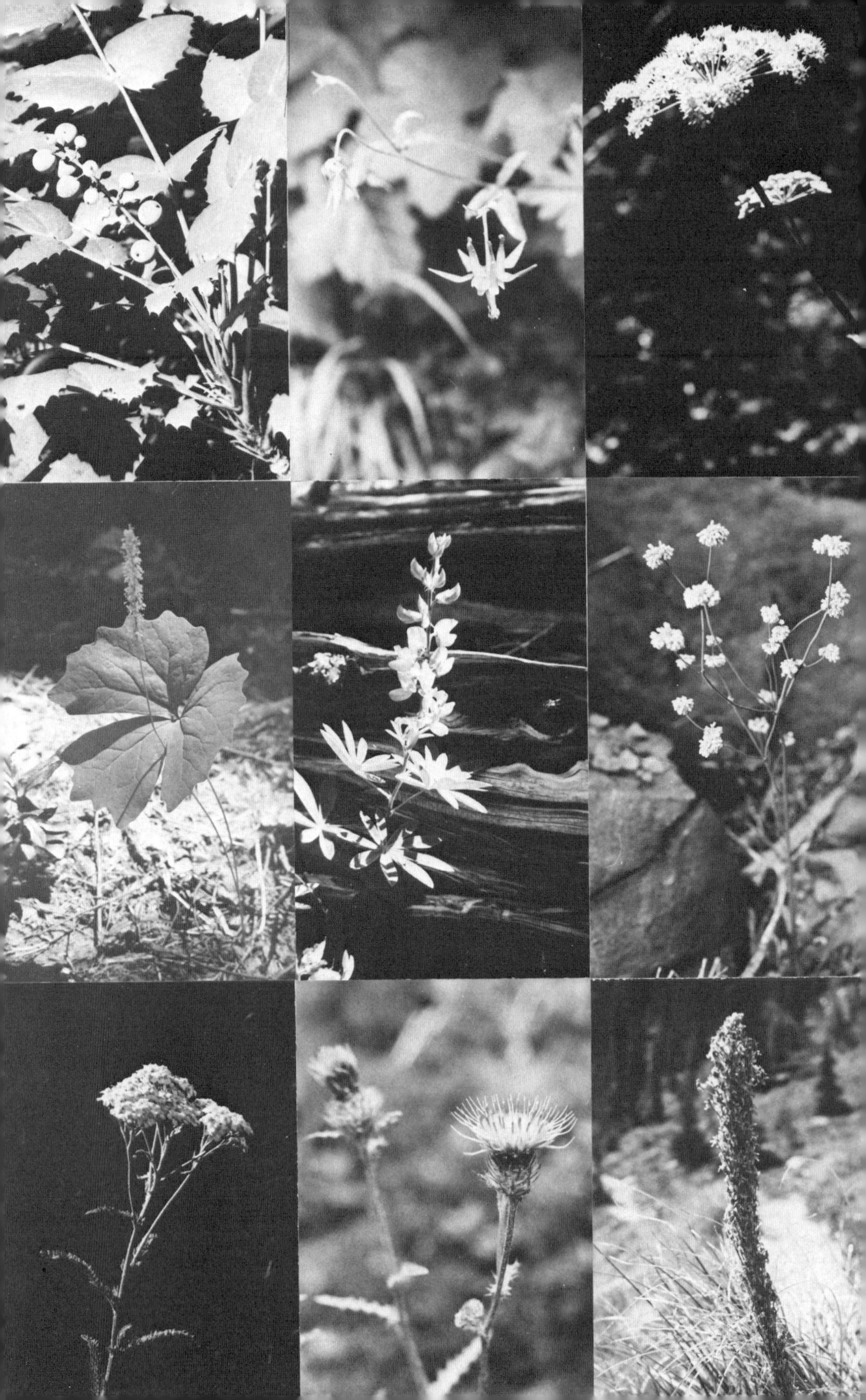

fireweed, and Nature once again strives to transform this landscape back into a mature forest.

Fauna

We have seen that plants adapt to a variety of conditions imposed by the environment and by other species. Animals, like plants, are also subject to a variety of conditions, but they have the added advantage of mobility. On a hot summer day, a beetle under a scant forest cover can escape the merciless sun by seeking protection under a loose stone or under a mat of dry needles.

Larger animals, of course, have greater mobility and therefore can better overcome the difficulties of the environment. Amphibians, reptiles, birds, and mammals may frequent the trail, but they scamper away when you, the intruder, approach. At popular campsites, however, the animals come out to meet you, or, more exactly, to obtain your food. Of course, almost anywhere along the trail you may encounter the ubiquitous mosquito, always looking for a free meal. But in popular campsites, you'll meet the robin, the gray jay, the Clark's nutcracker, the Townsend and yellow-pine chipmunks, the golden-mantled ground squirrel, and, at night, mice and black bears. You may be tempted to feed them, or they may try to help themselves, but please protect them from your food; they will survive better on the "real, organic" food Mother Nature produces. Furthermore, an artificially large population supported by generous summer backpackers may in winter overgraze the vegetation. In the following paragraphs, we'll take a closer look at three species.

Mule deer. Two subspecies of this large mammal can be found along much of the Oregon-Washington PCT. Mule deer, like other herbivores, do not eat every type of plant they encounter but tend to be quite specific in their search for food. Their primary browse is new growth on huckleberry, salal, blackberry, bitterbrush, and snowbrush, although they also eat certain grasses and forbs. Together with other herbivores, parasites, and saprophytes (organisms feeding on decaying organic matter), they consume a small portion of the 100 billion tons of organic matter produced annually on the earth by plants.

Mule deer face a considerable population problem because some of their predators have disappeared. After the arrival of "civilized" people, the wolves and grizzly bears were exterminated except in some remote areas of northern Washington. In their places, coyotes and black bears have increased in numbers. Coyotes, however, feed principally on rabbits and rodents and only occasionally attack a fawn or a sick deer. Black bears occasionally kill fawns. The mountain lion, a true specialist in feeding habits, preys mainly on deer and may kill 50 of them in a year. This magnificent mammal, unfortunately, has been unjustly persecuted by people, and many deer that are saved from the big cat are lost to starvation and disease. Increasing human population compounds the problem. The expansion of settlements causes the big cats to retreat farther, which leaves them farther from the suburban deer. Forests must be logged to feed this expansion of settlements, and then the logged-over areas sprout an assemblage of shrubs that are a feast for deer. The deer population responds to this new food supply by increasing in number. Then the shrubs mature or the forest grows back, and there is less food for the

From top, left to right: Oregon grape, columbine, ligusticum; vanilla-leaf, lupine, eriogonum; yarrow, thistle, beargrass

larger deer population, which is now faced with starvation. Forest fires produce the same feast-followed-by-famine effect.

Golden-mantled ground squirrel. There are two species of these ground squirrels, the Sierra Nevada golden-mantled ground squirrel, which ranges from the southern Sierra north to the Columbia River, and the Cascades golden-mantled ground squirrel, which ranges from the Columbia River north into British Columbia. On the eastern Cascade slopes of Washington, the Cascades golden-mantled ground squirrel lives in the same habitat as the yellow-pine chipmunk, but they have slightly different niches, or roles, to carry out in their pine-and-fir-forest environment. Both have the same food and the same burrowing habits, but the ground squirrel obtains nuts and seeds that have fallen to the forest floor, whereas the chipmunk obtains these morsels by extracting them from their source. The ground squirrel, like its distant cousin the marmot, puts on a thick layer of fat to provide it with enough energy to last through winter hibernation. The chipmunk, like the black bear, only partly hibernates. During the winter, it awakens periodically to feed on the nuts and seeds it has stored in its ground burrow.

Western toad. Every Westerner is familiar with this drab, chunky amphibian. Along the Oregon-Washington PCT, you encounter its subspecies know as the boreal toad. This cold-blooded animal is amazingly adaptable, being found among rock crevices in dry, desolate lava flows as well as in subalpine wildflower gardens in the North Cascades. Its main environmental requirement appears to be the presence of at least one early-summer seasonal pond in which it can breed and lay eggs.

Although you may encounter dozens of boreal toads along a stretch of trail in one day (they occur in clusters), they prefer to actively hop or crawl about at night. Should you bed down near one of their breeding ponds, you may hear the weak chirps (they have no "croaking" vocal sacs) from dozens of males. Rolling over on one won't give you warts, but later you might feel the puncture, bite, or sting of a mosquito, ant, or yellowjacket that otherwise would have made a tasty meal for the toad.

mule deer

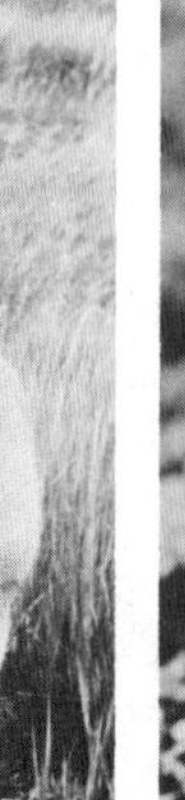

ground squirrel

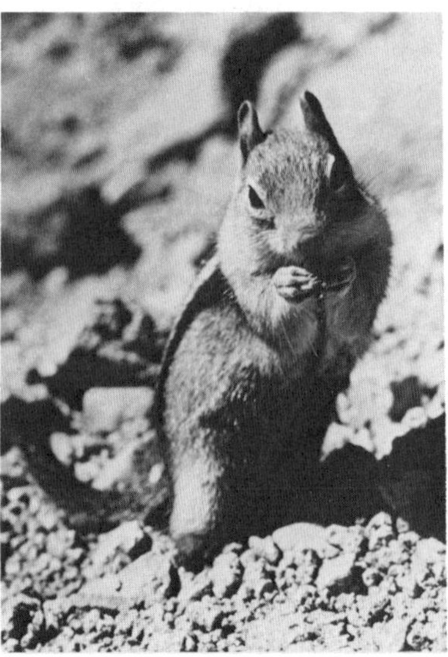

western toad

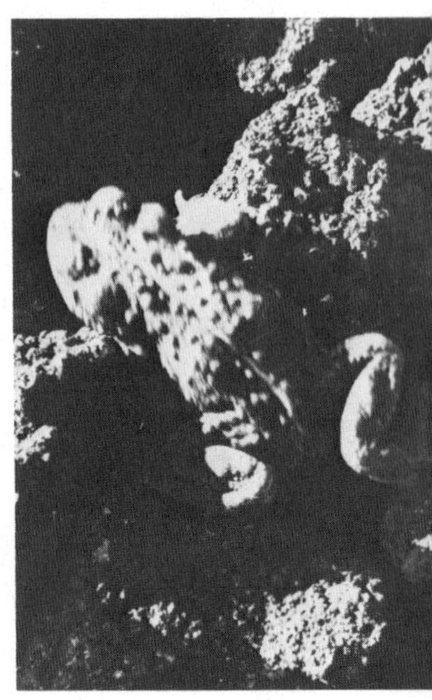

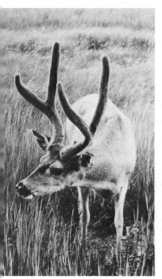

Chapter 4: Using This Guide

TWELVE HIKING CHAPTERS

The bulk of this guide is composed of trail descriptions and accompanying topographic maps of the PCT. In 12 chapters, Sections A through L, this guide covers the PCT from Highway 96 in northern California to Highway 3 in British Columbia. Readers familiar with this guide's companion volume will note that its Section R is essentially the same as this one's Section A (for an explanation of this duplication, see Section A's *Introduction*. We have divided the Oregon-Washington PCT into 12 sections because the vast majority of hikers will be walking only a part of the trail, not all of it. Each section starts and ends at a highway, and often at or near a supply center such as a town, resort, or park. All the sections are short enough to make comfortable backpacking trips ranging from about 4 to 12 days for the average backpacker. Each of these sections could be conveniently broken into two or more shorter sections to provide even shorter hikes. However, we've refrained from making a new chapter beginning at every road crossing since this could unnecessarily increase the size and weight—and price—of the book.

PRE-HIKE INFORMATION

At the beginning of each section, you'll find pre-hike information that mentions: 1) the attractions and natural features of that section, 2) the declination setting for your compass, 3) a mileage table between points within that section, 4) supply points on or near the route, 5) wilderness-permit information, if applicable, and 6) special problems. This pre-hike information also includes a map of the entire section.

Features. At the start of each section, an introduction briefly mentions the features—both good and bad—that you'll encounter while hiking through that section. These introductions will help you decide which section or sections are right for you.

Declination. The declination setting for your compass is important if you have to get an accurate reading. Actually, the declination changes very little throughout this whole two-state section, being, at the start of the millennium, about 16¾°E in northernmost California and increasing to about 19¾°E in southernmost British Columbia. Trekkers can set their compasses at about 18°E and manage fine for this book's two-state stretch. By 2020, however, declination will have declined a bit, and then 17½°E may be a better average.

If your compass does not correct for declination, you'll have to add the appropriate declination to get the true bearing. For example, if your compass indicates that a prominent hill lies along a bearing of 70°, and if the section you're hiking has a declination of 20°E, then you should add 20°, getting 90° (due east) as the true bearing of that hill. If you can identify that hill on a map, you can find where *you* are on the PCT by adding 180°, getting 270° (due west) in this example. By drawing a line due west from the hill to an intersection of the PCT, you'll determine your position.

This example is correct only for true-bearing compasses, which list degrees from 0 to 360 in a counterclockwise direction. However, almost everyone uses reverse-bearing compasses (e.g., Silva and Suunto), which list degrees in a clockwise direction. With these backsighting compasses, you subtract. If you get a bearing of 110°, you subtract 20° to get a true bearing of 90°.

Most hikers will agree it's easier to carry a compass with a declination setting than to try and remember if you should add or subtract declination. Regardless of which type of compass you use, you *should not* attempt a major section of the PCT without a thorough understanding of your compass *and* of map interpretation. On a long hike, you could be caught in a whiteout and your trail could be buried under snow. Then, your navigation skills, or lack thereof, might determine whether you lived or died. Until you master both map and compass, take only short hikes in good weather.

Mileage Table. Each mileage table lists distances between major points found within its PCT section. Both distances between points and cumulative mileages are given. We list cumulative mileages south to north *and* north to south so that no matter which direction you are hiking the PCT, you can easily determine the mileages you plan to hike. Many of the points listed in the tables are at or near good campsites. If you typically average 17 miles a day—the on-route rate you'll need to complete the tri-state PCT in under 6 months—then you can determine where you should camp to maintain this rate, and you can estimate when you should arrive at a certain supply point. Of course, in reality your time schedule may turn out to be quite different from your planned schedule, due to unforeseen circumstances.

At the end of this short chapter we've included a mileage table for the entire Oregon-Washington PCT. By scanning this table's *distances between points*, you can tell at a glance just how long each section is. You can then select one or more of appropriate length, turn to that section's **Introduction**, and see if it sounds appealing. Then read its **Problems** (if any) and see if it still sounds appealing. Of course, you need not start at the beginning of any section, since *every* PCT section is cut by one or more access roads.

Supplies. If you're going to be on the trail for more than two weeks, you'll probably want to stop somewhere to resupply. This pre-trail section mentions the resorts, stores, post offices, and towns that are readily accessible to the hiker. In most cases, the supply point is just a resort or small store with minimal food supplies and perhaps with a post office. By "minimal" we mean a few odds and ends that typically cater to passing motorists, e.g., beer and potato chips. Therefore, it is best to make your own "CARE" packages and send them to appropriate locations. For some, you use the US Postal Service; for others, UPS, and we specify which.

Wilderness Permits. In sections C, I, and K, you'll pass through a national park. In these, you'll need a permit if you camp in their backcountry, and their pre-trail paragraphs tell you where you can write for one or pick up one. This wilderness-permit information is mentioned only in sections C, I and K, since only in them might you need to get a permit.

Problems. In every section but B, you can expect early-season snow patches to hinder your progress, while later you can expect pursuing mosquitoes to speed it up. This pre-trail paragraph, not found in every section, mentions these two problems when they are found in superabundance. It also mentions extensive waterless stretches, which are amazingly frequent for such a wet mountain range. After reading about a section's special problems, you may decide to reschedule the time you plan to hike through it, or perhaps you may choose a more appealing section.

Section Map. Early editions of the two-volume *Pacific Crest Trail* guides contained only a long sequence of narrow topographic maps. Hikers using them reasonably complained of these maps' "tunnel vision": without a Forest Service map, you couldn't tell what lay more than a few miles east or west of the PCT; you could only look ahead or behind. In response to this problem, we've widened the maps so they are up to 46% wider than in the early editions, thus permitting you to take compass readings on more-distant topographic features. With its expanded lateral coverage, you can locate yourself faster and better.

Still, there are instances when you'd like to see miles of lateral coverage, particularly when your trek has gone afoul due to bad weather, injury, or other disaster. Then you'll want to know the quickest way out to civilization. Hence, we've included section maps to show you the trails, roads, towns, and other features you should know about if you must abort your hike. Because we've included these large-area section maps, you should be able to get along entirely without Forest Service maps or any other aids.

Topographic Maps. Finally, we list the US Geological Survey's 7.5′ topographic maps (scale 1:24,000) that cover the PCT in each section. Being large-scale maps, they are quite bulky and would add about a pound or so for each section. This amounts to about 10 pounds for the two states, and they'd set you back hundreds of dollars. Obviously, the book in your hand is much lighter and cheaper than about 100 topo maps.

ROUTE DESCRIPTION

When you start reading the text of a PCT section, you will notice that a pair of numbers follows each of the more important trail points. For example, at Russell Creek in Mt. Jefferson Wilderness, this pair is (5520–2.8), which means that you cross this creek at an elevation of 5520 *feet* and at a distance of 2.8 *miles* from your last given point, which in this example is at a junction with the Woodpecker Trail. By studying these figures along the section you are hiking, you can easily determine the distance you'll have to hike from point A to point B, and by noting the elevation changes, you'll get a good idea of how much climbing and descending you'll have to do. Along this guide's *alternate* routes, there are occasional second mileage figures, each of which represents the cumulative mileage along the alternate route to that point.

In addition to giving accurate directions, the route description tells you where you can camp, where you can get water, what hazards you should be aware of, how streams and trail conditions may change with the season, and other useful hiking information.

Where alternate routes, side routes, resupply-access routes and off-trail water access occur, we set it off with an icon (following), boldface its title, and set it in a different typeface:

Side route:...

Alternate route:...

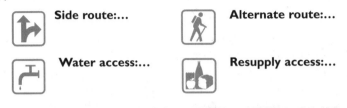

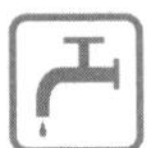

Water access:...

Resupply access:...

In addition, the description also tells you something about the country you are walking through—the scenery, the geology, the biology, and sometimes a bit of history. We hope this added information will increase your outdoor perception and add to your enjoyment of your trek. If the passage is about a sentence or longer, we set it off with a gray rectangle ▮ *before and after it* ▮ and *italicize* it. By identifying these various routes and passages, we hope to help you follow the PCT trail description more smoothly, jumping over other information you do not need.

THE TOPOGRAPHIC MAPS

East hiking section contains all the topographic maps you'll need to hike that part of the PCT. All these maps are at a scale of 1:50,000, or about 0.8 mile per inch (1 mile per 1¼ inches). Most hikers are acquainted with 7.5′ maps (1:24,000) and 15′ maps (1:62,500). Since our topos are based on these two map sizes, we chose an intermediate scale of 1:50,000 because if 7.5′ maps are reduced any farther, say to 1:62,000, the names and numbers on them become too difficult to read. Yet, if we were to enlarge the 15′ maps to 1:24,000, the size, weight, and price of the book would increase by about 25% and the lateral coverage of each map would be cut in half. We think the 1:50,000 scale has the best cost:benefit ratio.

Many of this guide's topos show township-and-range sections, which are *usually* square and *usually* measure one mile on a side. Topos with these sections thus have a one-mile grid pattern, which aids in judging distances.

On the topos, the PCT route appears as a solid black line. Any alternate route that is set apart in the text by the icon and typeface, as described above, is also shown on the maps, and it is indicated by an alternating dot-dash black line. A map legend at the end of this chapter lists most of the symbols you'll find on this guide's topographic maps.

TEXT AND MAP CROSS-REFERENCES

To make this guide as functional as possible, we've tried to place the maps as close as possible to the appropriate columns of trail description, and we've included four reference systems. Perhaps the most obvious system is the one composed of a set of large, bold-italic letters and numbers—***See maps A1, A2***—centered at the bottom of the text on each route-description page. These identify the appropriate map (map Al, map A2, etc.) that shows the section of PCT being described in the page of route description. In most cases, that map is no more than a page or two away.

But what if you see a feature on a map and you want to find where it is mentioned in the text? In that case, turn to the Index, which lists entries for both text and maps.

The last two reference systems deal with maps only. Since the PCT is not an arrow-straight north-south path, neither is the sequence of topo maps that show it. Therefore, along the border of each map, we list the maps that touch it. For example, turn to map C3. Note that three maps border this map: C1, C2, and C4. The blue tick mark between "see MAP C1" and "see MAP C2" tells you where map C1 ends and map C2 begins. The blue tick mark to the right of "see MAP C4" tells you where the right border of map C4 is. (Its left border is off the page, hence the tick mark lies flat, indicating that the map continues in that direction.) By learning the significance of the topos' tick marks, you should be able to go from map to map with a minimum of orientation problems.

But if you still have problems in determining the location of one map with respect to another, then use our fourth reference system, the large-area section map at the beginning of each hiking chapter. On it, all the topo map borders for that chapter are printed in light blue. In like manner, the Oregon-Washington map, opposite the start of Chapter 1, shows all the large-area maps for this book's hiking sections, A through L. Thus, if you want to hike, say, Sections E through G, you can easily visualize how much of the entire Oregon-Washington stretch you're going to be doing.

FOLLOWING THE TRAIL

The PCT is usually a trail, though in a few places—notably Goat Rocks' Packwood Glacier and Glacier Peak's Red and Fire Creek passes—it is usually a snowfield. On a clear midsummer's day, the PCT is easy to follow, even if it is a snowfield. However, in early season or in a storm, the trail could be buried under snow. If the snow is a foot or more deep, then the trail's course may be obscure. When this happens, you may have to watch for other visual clues: PCT emblems, posts, blazes, and ducks. (A blaze is a place on a tree trunk where someone has carved away a patch or two of bark to leave a conspicuous, manmade scar; a duck is an obviously manmade pile of rocks.) Since all these markers can be ephemeral, our route descriptions do not emphasize them.

In fact, we're even reluctant to state that a trail junction is "signed," since the sign may disappear in a year or two. Where we mention trail junctions (or road junctions, for that matter), we give the trail's official name and number, if it has both (for example, Jefferson Park Trail 3429). Some trails have only official names or official numbers. Others have neither, and for these we say "trail" instead of "Trail." If a trail once had a trail number but no longer does, we still prefer to state it, since we can fit numbers onto the book's topo maps far more easily than lengthy trail names. When the PCT came into prominence in the early 1970s, it received a lot more hiker use, and consequently, it has been kept up very well. With all the signs and markers along it, the PCT can almost be followed without map or guide through Oregon and Washington—if you have good weather and no emergencies.

LEGEND

Heavy-duty road
Medium-duty road
Improved light-duty road
Unimproved dirt road
Jeep road or trail
Railroad: single track
Railroad: multiple track

PCT route along trails
PCT route along roads
Authors' alternate route

Year-round streams
Seasonal streams

Scale of maps, 1:50,000

1 0 1 MILE

Oregon-Washington PCT Mileage Table

Start/*Section*/End	**S→N**	**Section Length**	**N→S**
Highway 96 in Seiad Valley	0.0		1005.5
Section A		64.5	
Interstate 5 near Siskiyou Pass	64.5		941.0
Section B		54.0	
Highway 140 near Fish Lake	118.5		887.0
Section C		76.0	
Highway 138 near the Cascade Crest	194.5		811.0
Section D		61.3	
Highway 58 near Willamette Pass	255.8		749.7
Section E		76.0	
Highway 242 at McKenzie Pass	331.8		673.7
Section F		112.5	
Highway 35 near Barlow Pass	444.3		561.2
Section G		51.7	
Interstate 84 at Bridge of the Gods	496.0		509.5
Walk across Bridge of the Gods		0.5	
Highway 14 at Bridge of the Gods	496.5		509.0
Section H		147.5	
Highway 12 near White Pass	644.0		361.5
Section I		99.0	
Interstate 90 at Snoqualmie Pass	743.0		262.5
Section J		74.7	
Highway 2 at Stevens Pass	817.7		187.8
Section K		117.5	
Highway 20 at Rainy Pass	935.2		70.3
Section L		70.3	
Highway 3 in Manning Provincial Park	1005.5		0.0

Old and new PCT diamonds plus a duck with post and plastic streamer

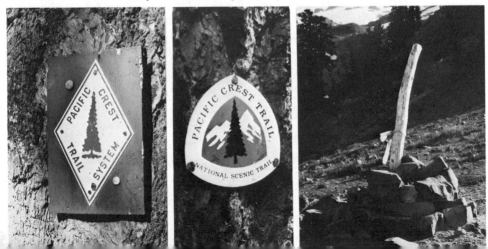

12 Trail Chapters

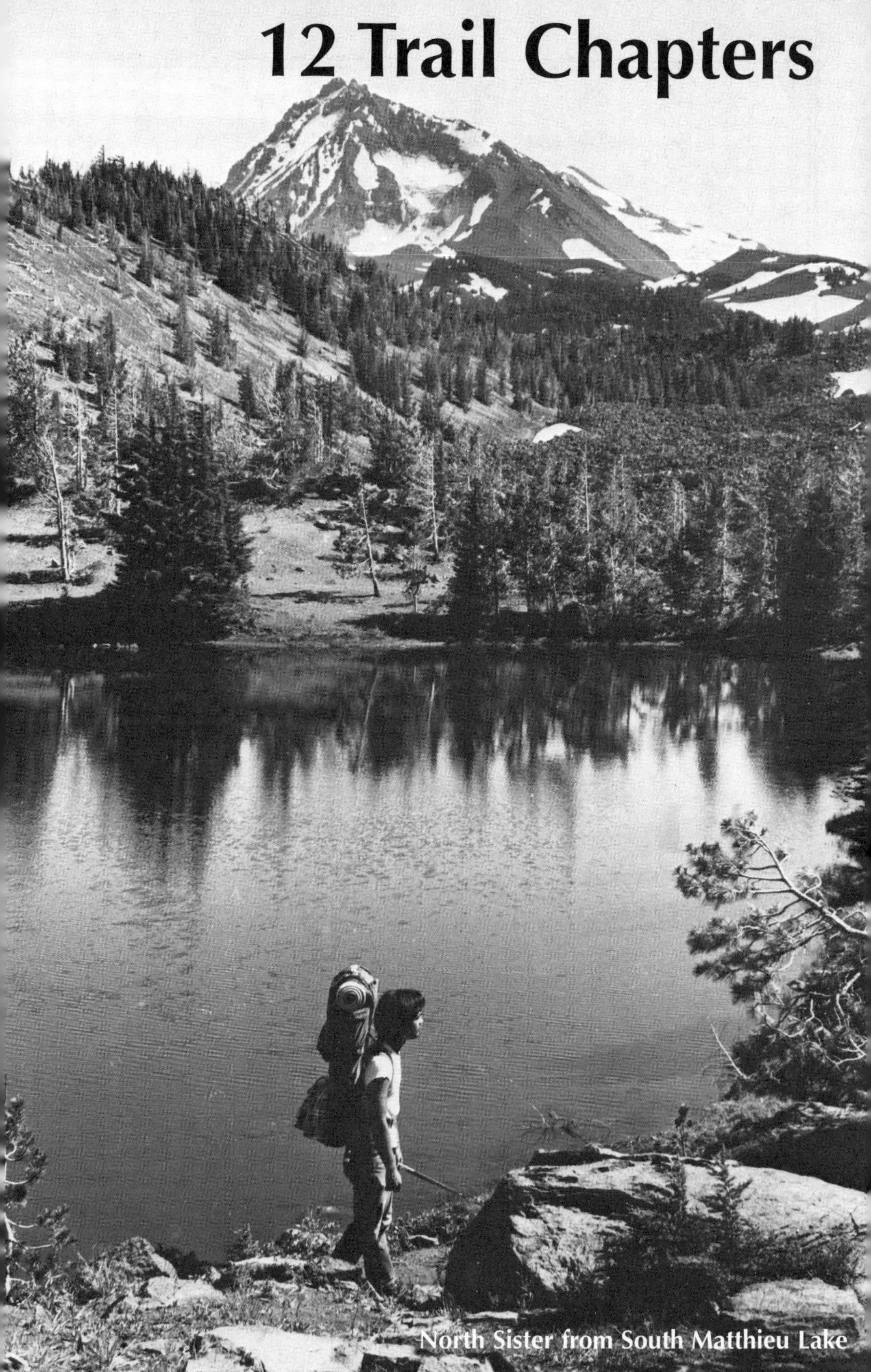

North Sister from South Matthieu Lake

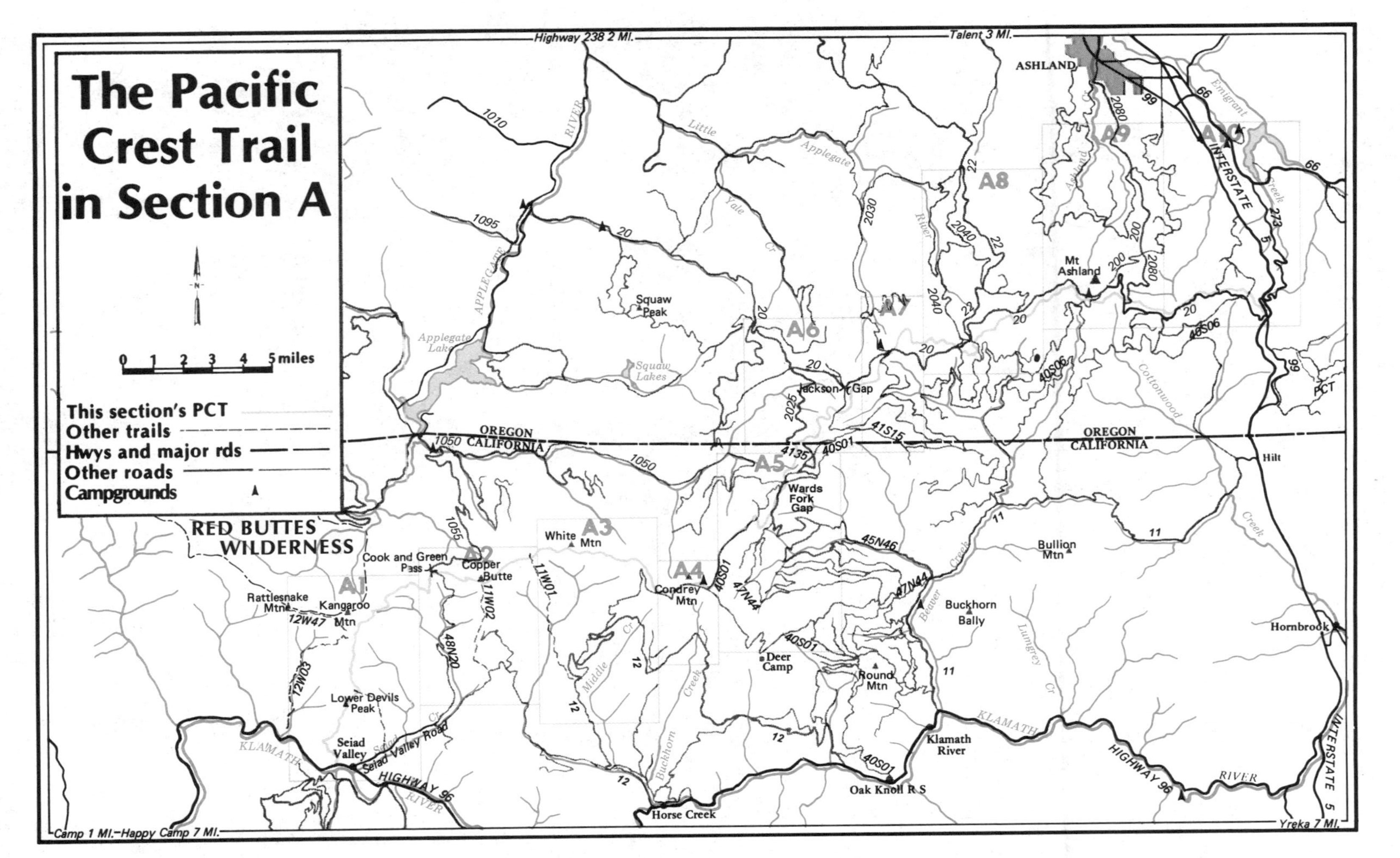

The Pacific Crest Trail in Section A
0 1 2 3 4 5 miles
This section's PCT
Other trails
Hwys and major rds
Other roads
Campgrounds
Highway 238 2 MI.
Talent 3 MI.
ASHLAND
Mt Ashland
Squaw Peak
Squaw Lakes
Applegate Lake
Jackson Gap
Wards Fork Gap
OREGON
CALIFORNIA
Hilt
Hornbrook
RED BUTTES WILDERNESS
Cook and Green Pass
Copper Butte
White Mtn
Condrey Mtn
Rattlesnake Mtn
Kangaroo Mtn
Lower Devils Peak
Seiad Valley
Seiad Valley Road
Deer Camp
Round Mtn
Bullion Mtn
Buckhorn Bally
Klamath River
Oak Knoll R S
Horse Creek
HIGHWAY 96
INTERSTATE 5
PCT
Camp 1 MI.–Happy Camp 7 MI.
Yreka 7 MI.

Section A: Highway 96 in Seiad Valley to Interstate 5 near Siskiyou Pass

Introduction: PCT hikers who have used the *Volume 1: California* guide will note that its Section R is essentially the same as this volume's Section A. The reason for this duplication is that the Pacific Crest Trail crosses the California-Oregon border in the middle of nowhere, roughly midway between Seiad Valley, on Highway 96, and Ashland, on Interstate 5. Hence, hikers wanting to do every foot of California will logically continue northeast toward Ashland (or at least to Interstate 5), while those wanting to hike north along every foot of Oregon will logically start near Seiad Valley.

Actually, you can drive to within a short walk of the point where the Pacific Crest Trail enters Oregon. To do this, drive west from Medford, Oregon, on Highway 238, passing through Jacksonville in about 5 miles. The route then goes 7 miles southwest to the tiny community of Ruch, where you leave 238 and head south on a road up the Applegate River. In 6½ miles you'll pass the Star Work Center, then in an additional 2½ miles you'll cross to the east bank of the Applegate River and immediately branch left on Road 20. This road climbs 14½ miles to Silver Fork Gap, located at the east end of Yellowjacket Ridge. From here, Road 20 climbs east to Jackson Gap, but you descend southeast on Road 2025, which winds 4¼ miles to a gap just east of Donomore Peak. Just 40 yards south of this gap, the PCT crosses your road, and if you follow the trail about 200 yards southwest, to where it turns abruptly northeast, you'll be a few feet inside California. By starting north here, you'll save 2–3 days of hiking.

In this guide's Section A, the hiker makes a long traverse east to get over to the Cascade Range. The long traverse west in California, from Burney Falls to Marble Mountain, was quite necessary, though inconveniently long, since a route going north from Burney Falls past Mt. Shasta would be a dry, hot one indeed. Before the Pacific Crest Trail route became final, this sun-drenched corridor was the one most hikers followed to the Oregon Skyline Trail—Oregon's section of the Pacific Crest Trail. Section A's route stays remarkably high for most of its length, dropping significantly only at each end. Although high, it has been only mildly glaciated, and because glaciers haven't scoured away the soil, thick forests abound. These, unfortunately, are rampant with logging roads. From Reeves Ranch eastward you are always paralleling one road or another, so you certainly lose the wilderness feeling this high-crest hike is supposed to offer, Views, however, are pleasing enough, and surprisingly few logging operations are seen from the trail. Before early July these roads are an advantage, for significant stretches of trail are still snowbound. The roads, being more open, are quite easy to follow, though they still have enough snow patches on them to stop motor vehicles. As you progress east on trail or road, you walk across increasingly younger rocks, first late-Paleozoic/early-Mesozoic metamorphic rocks, then mid-Mesozoic granite rocks of the Mt. Ashland area and finally mid-to-late Cenozoic volcanic rocks of the Interstate 5 area.

Declination: 17¼°E

Points on Route:	S→N	Mi. Btwn. Pts.	N→S
Highway 96 at Seiad Valley	0.0		64.5
		6.5	
Lower Devils Peak saddle	6.5		58.0
		8.6	
Cook and Green Pass	15.1		49.4
		5.3	
Lowdens Cabin site spur trail	20.4		44.1
		7.5	
Alex Hole Camp entrance	27.9		36.6
		2.3	
Mud Springs spur road	30.2		34.3
		2.4	
Bearground Spring	32.6		31.9
		1.3	
Wards Fork Gap	33.9		30.6
		2.8	
California-Oregon border	36.7		27.8
		4.4	
Sheep Camp Spring	41.1		23.4
		2.3	
Wrangle Gap	43.4		21.1
		5.4	
Long John Saddle	48.8		15.7
		5.0	
Grouse Gap	53.8		10.7
		3.8	
Road 2080	57.6		6.9
		6.9	
Interstate 5 near Mt. Ashland Road 20	64.5		0.0

Supplies: No supplies are available once you leave Seiad Valley. Along this crest route virtually all roads south will get you down to Highway 96, which has a smattering of hamlets, and virtually all roads north will ultimately channel you down to the Ashland-Medford area. However, we don't think you should descend either direction since you would then be way off route. Even in an emergency situation, you're likely to get help from people driving along the near-crest roads long before you could reach any settlement. If you're continuing through Oregon, you'll want to end Section A in Ashland, and three routes to it are described in this chapter. You won't find any more sizable towns within an easy day's walk of the PCT until you reach the Oregon-Washington border area, more than 400 miles beyond this section's end. If you think you'll need a new pack, a camera, or a pair of boots, certainly stop in Ashland.

Maps:

Seiad Valley, CA
Kangaroo Mountain, CA
Dutch Creek, CA
Condrey Mountain, CA
Dutchman Peak, OR
Siskiyou Peak, OR
Mt. Ashland, OR
Siskiyou Pass, OR

THE ROUTE

You begin this section at the Seiad Store and post office (1371′ elevation, 46 miles west of Interstate 5 via Highway 96). Walking west along the highway, you immediately cross Seiad Valley Road, which heads northeast up to Horse Tail Falls and beyond to Cook and Green Pass. Not much farther on, you reach School House Gulch (1380–0.5), from which the PCT route once started. Following the road as it curves west, you quickly reach a newer trailhead for Lower Devils Peak Lookout Trail 12W04 (1380–0.3). Since it is an exhausting 4400-foot ascent to potential campsites by the Kangaroo Mountain meadows, one is prudent to start this strenuous trek in the cool shade of the morning.

Under a cover of madrone, Douglas-fir, incense-cedar, and Oregon oak, your trail

See map A1

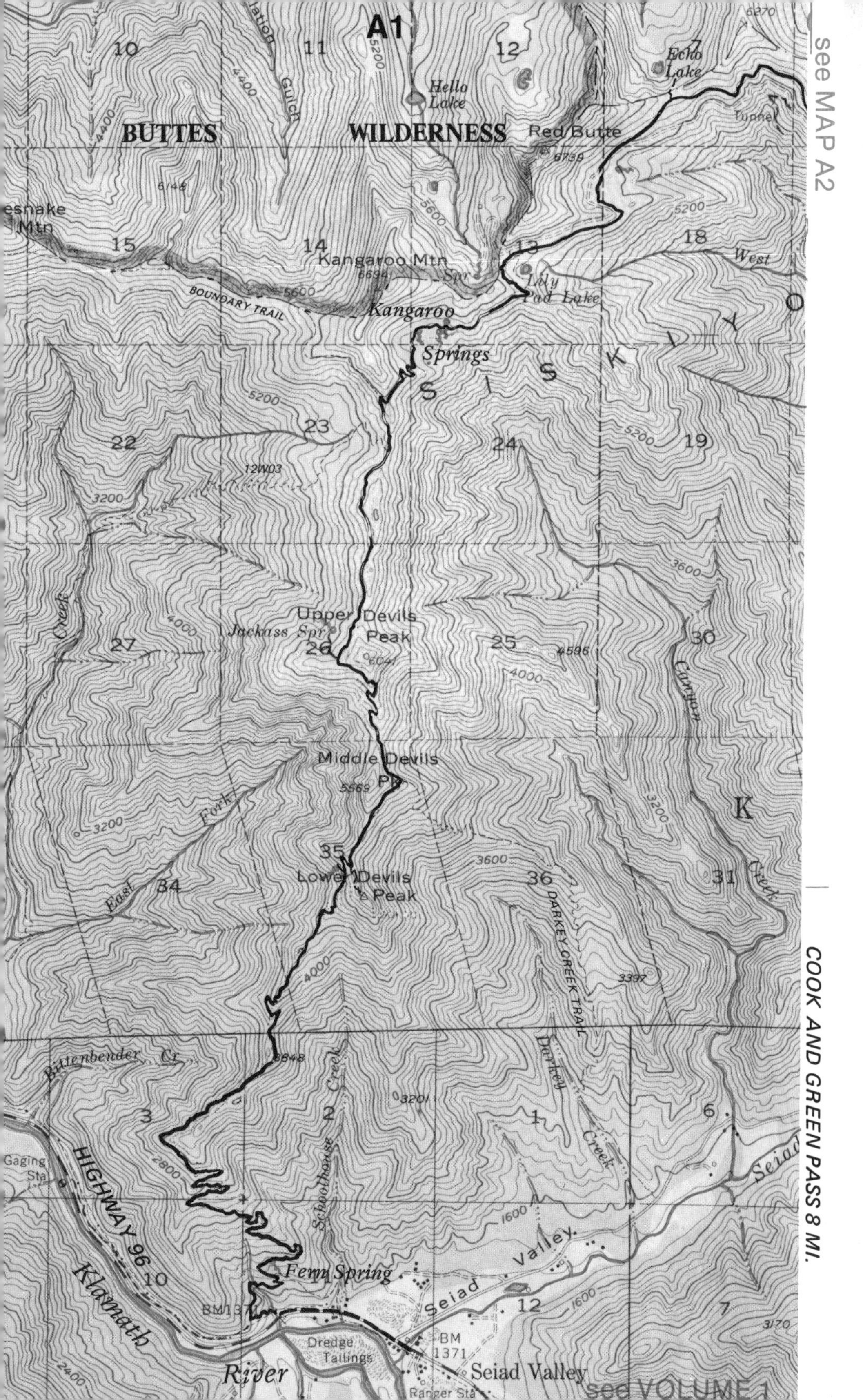
A1
BUTTES
WILDERNESS
Hello Lake
Echo Lake
Red Butte
Tunnel
Gulch
Kangaroo Mtn
Spr
Lily Pad Lake
BOUNDARY TRAIL
Kangaroo Springs
S I S K I Y O
West
12W03
Upper Devils Peak
Jackass Spr
Middle Devils Pk
Lower Devils Peak
Creek
East Fork
Canyon Creek
K
DARKEY CREEK TRAIL
Darkey Creek
Bittenbender Cr
Schoolhouse Creek
Gaging Sta
HIGHWAY 96
Klamath River
Fern Spring
Seiad Valley
Seiad
Dredge Tailings
BM 1371
Ranger Sta
see VOLUME 1
see MAP A2
COOK AND GREEN PASS 8 MI.

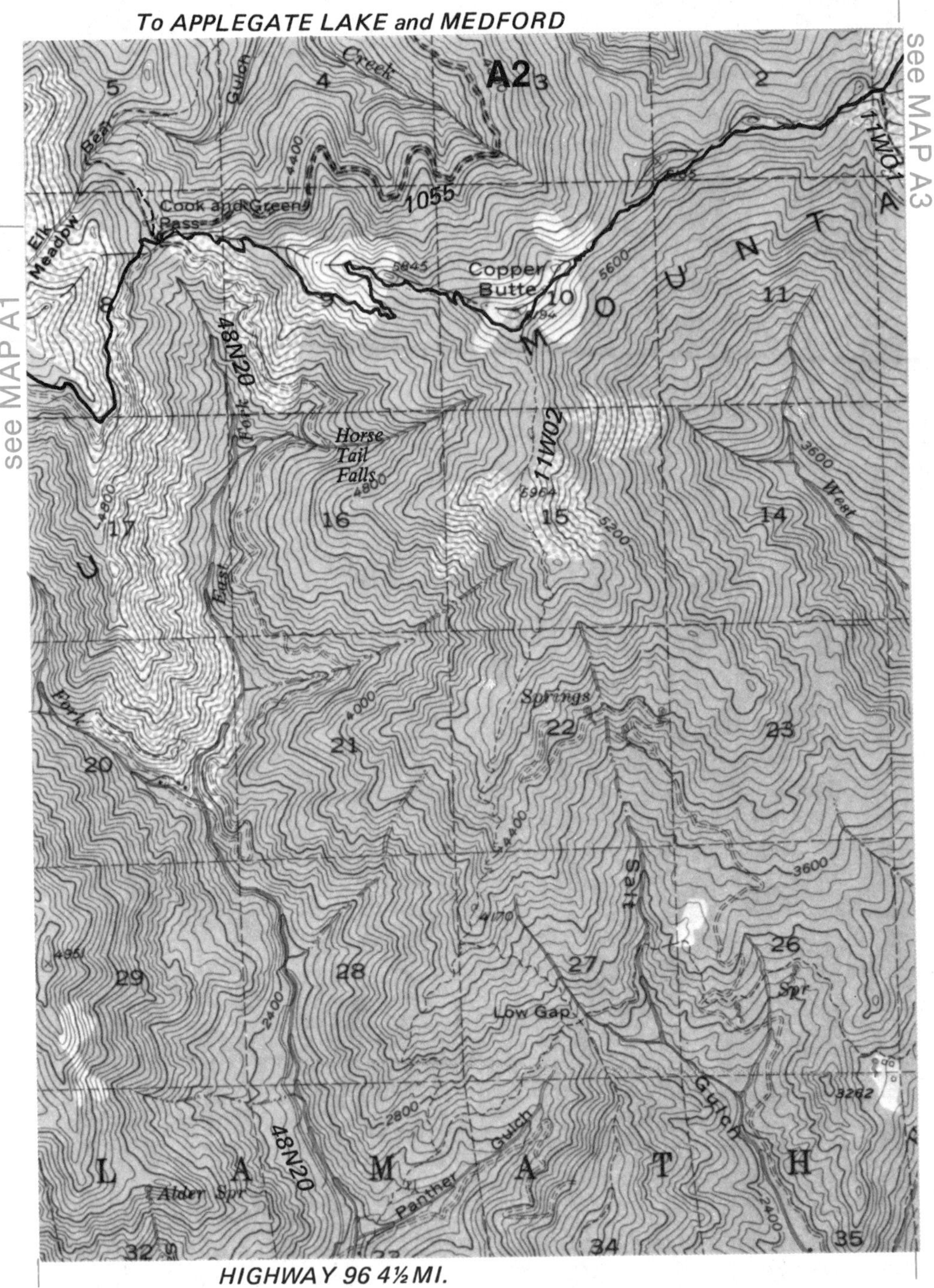

curves west and climbs moderately to reach a junction (1600–0.2) with a trail that parallels Highway 96 west for 1.4 miles before ending close to a stream-gaging cable that spans the mighty Klamath River. ▮ *The PCT was supposed to cross there, rather than on the Highway 96 bridge east of Seiad Valley, but this plan was abandoned.* ▮

From the junction with the trail paralleling Highway 96, where you cross under some

See map A1

minor powerlines, your trail heads north into a shaded gully with its poison oak, and you soon reach a junction with the original Devils Peak Lookout Trail, now abandoned. About ¼ mile beyond this junction you reach Fern Spring (1900–0.7), a small seep trickling from a pipe into a concrete cistern. You may find a trail register here.

The well-engineered trail switchbacks up shady, though fly-infested, south-facing slopes, then follows a ridge system northeast up toward Lower Devils Peak. ▮ *Along this stretch you'll see some trees scorched in a widespread fire started by lightning in the summer of 1987. The damage here is minor compared to that north of Lower Devils Peak.* ▮ Where the ridge fuses with the peak's flank, you climb up some short switchbacks and then traverse north across west-facing slopes to a junction.

Water access. From here, a 40-yard-long trail goes over to Lookout Spring. This trickling spring is *usually* reliable, though one has to marvel at how any water flows at all, since the spring is so close to the Devils Peaks crest.

From the junction you climb about 300 yards in a final push up to Lower Devils Peak saddle (5020–4.8), on the Devils Peaks crest.

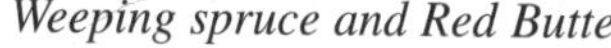

Weeping spruce and Red Butte

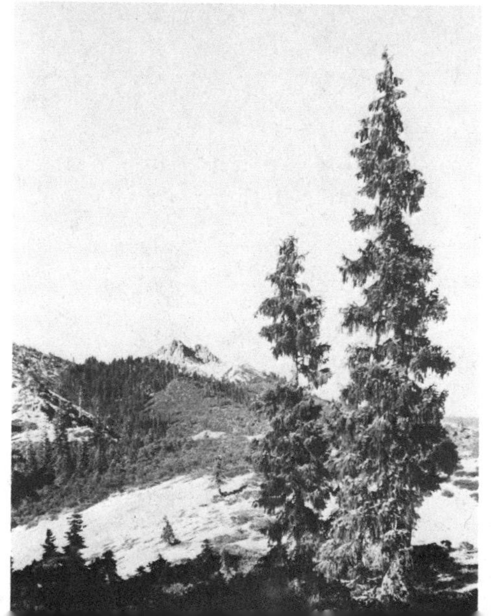

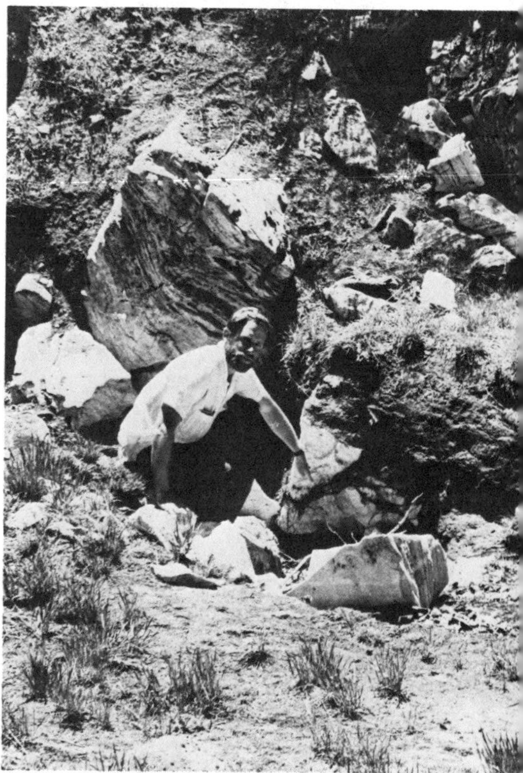

Schaffer at sinkhole

Side route. From the saddle you can follow a faint, rocky trail ¼ mile over to the remains of Lower Devils Peak Lookout, which was dismantled in 1976. The views you may obtain from it are fine, but the many views ahead equal those from the lookout site. The lower room of the lookout still remains, albeit roofless, and it does offer a flat, fairly wind-free campsite.

From the crest saddle, you start across the first of several major burns you'll traverse before Lily Pad Lake. ▮ *Note the knobcone pines here. These pines need a major fire, whose heat opens their cones, to release the seeds. These short-lived pines die in the process, but new pines soon sprout. Without periodic fires, the population would die out.* ▮ On the east ridge of Middle Devils Peak, you meet the Darkey Creek Trail (5170–0.6), starting down the burned-over ridge. ▮ *As you traverse the northeast-facing slopes of Middle Devils Peak, you pass the first of several small*

See map A1

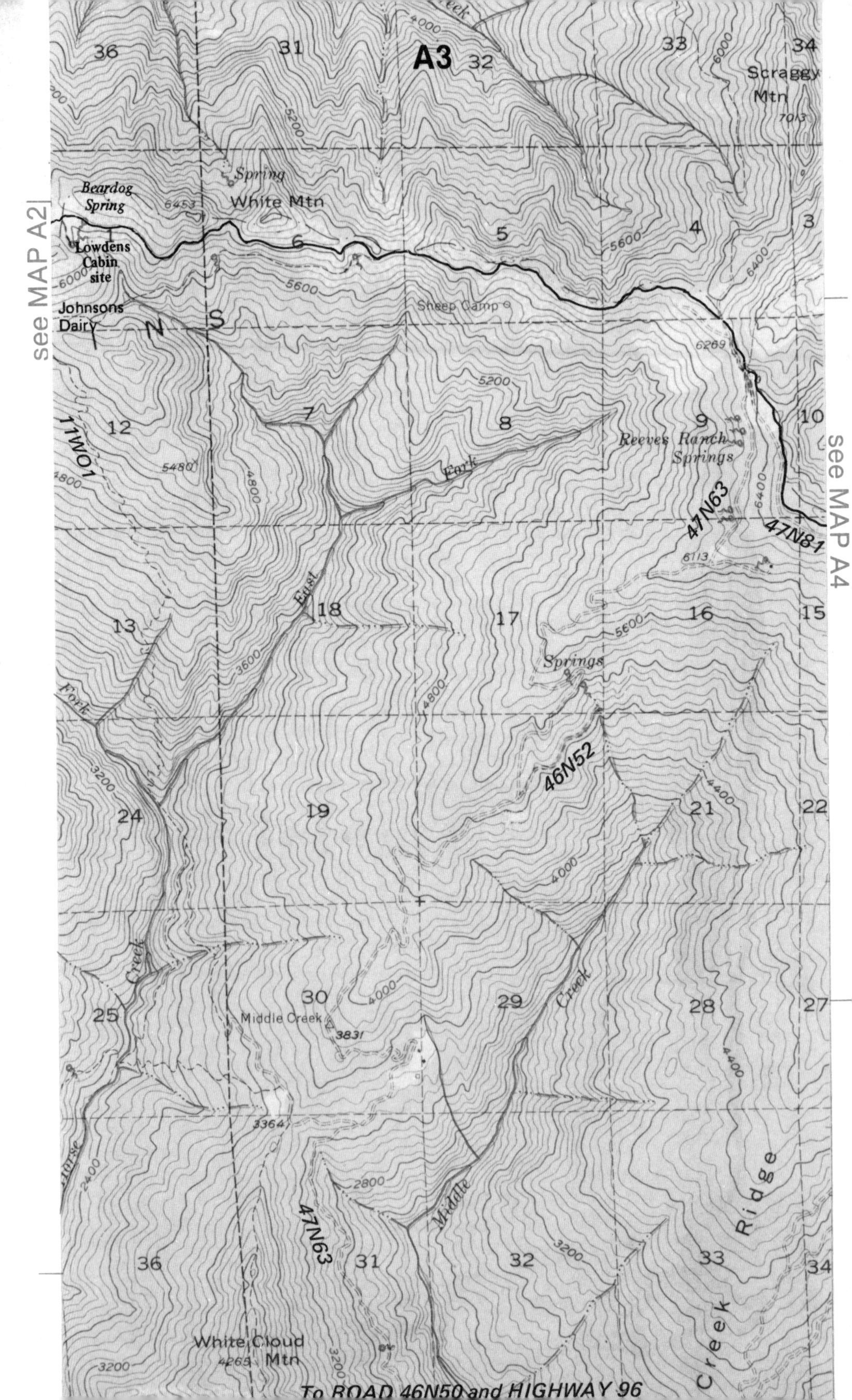

A3
Scraggy Mtn
7013
Beardog Spring
Spring
White Mtn
6453
Lowdens Cabin site
Johnsons Dairy
Sheep Camp
see MAP A2
see MAP A4
11W01
Fork
Reeves Ranch Springs
47N63
47N81
6269
6113
East
Springs
46N52
5480
Middle Creek
3831
3364
Creek
Middle
Creek Ridge
White Cloud Mtn
4265
47N63
To ROAD 46N50 and HIGHWAY 96

groves of weeping spruce, spared from the conflagration. Note the trees' drooping "Douglas-fir" branches, their oversize "hemlock" cones, and their scaly "lodgepole" bark. ▮

North of the peak you reach a saddle, and from here, as well as from short switchbacks above it, you can pause for views of snow-capped Mt. Shasta (14,162′) to the east and Marble Mountain Wilderness to the south. Beyond the switchbacks you reach Upper Devils Peak's western arm (5820–1.0).

Water access. From here, a spur trail once descended 330 steep yards past western white pines to seeping Jackass Spring amid a cluster of alders. The pines and the trail are largely gone, but if you bear about 330° downslope, you should have very little trouble finding the spring.

Your trail now makes a traverse north, and along it you pass the charred remains of a forest before coming to a small grove of weeping spruce. Just past it, you descend briefly to a saddle, which has a junction with faint Portuguese Creek Trail 12W03 (5760–1.2).

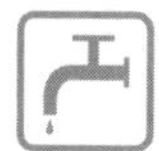

Water access. If you need water, you can drop west about 300 vertical feet along it to the seasonal headwaters of Portuguese Creek and then follow the creek down another 300–600 feet in elevation to find flowing water.

The PCT next climbs north up to a quickly reached junction with Boundary Trail 12W47 (5940–0.3). ▮ *Before the creation of Red Buttes Wilderness in 1984, this was known as the Rattlesnake Mountain Trail. As you can see on this section's first map, the trail stays quite close to the south boundary of Red Buttes Wilderness. You'll likely have noted by now a high, often snowy peak along the western skyline, 7309-foot Preston Peak.* ▮

Now you head 100 yards southeast to a minor saddle on nearby Devils Peaks crest, which also happens to be the south ridge of rusty Kangaroo Mountain. The mountain's glaciated, broad-floored basin greets you as you start a short, switchbacking descent, and along it you may see two tiny ponds, each having a nearby campsite. Head north from the switchbacks. ▮ *You'll discover a creek that disappears into a sinkhole dissolved from a layer of light-gray marble that contrasts strongly with the ancient, orange, ultramafic intrusives of this area. These rocks are likely the northern extension of the rock types one sees along the PCT in Marble Mountain Wilderness, on the distant southern skyline.* ▮

Likely because of the often damp nature of the basin's floor, the basin was largely spared from the 1987 fire. The basin's western lands are drier, and if you need to camp, look for a site there. Heading east, you reach a spring (5760–0.8) in spongy ground. From this spring—the easternmost of the Kangaroo Springs—the trail soon reaches a southeast slope. This the trail traverses, and soon you reach Kangaroo Mountain's east ridge (5900–0.5) and leave burned, *trailside* vegetation behind, although you'll see burned slopes on lands south of you all the way to Cook and Green Pass.

From the east ridge you can gaze down at Lily Pad Lake, with its small, poor, adjacent campsites and its multitude of frogs. Your trail stays high above this lake and arcs northwest over to a narrow ridge, which is a small part of the Red Buttes Wilderness boundary. Along this ridge you may find a trail register, and just past it is a junction with a spur trail (5900–0.2). This goes 115 yards north along the boundary ridge to a jeep road, on which you could pitch a tent. Westward, within the wilderness, the jeep road is closed, but eastward it is still open and is definitely used. The PCT will parallel it at a distance down to Cook and Green Pass.

With that goal in mind, you go but 200 yards northeast on the PCT before intersecting an old trail that starts from the jeep road just above you and drops to Lily Pad Lake. Now you descend gently east to a ridge that provides views down into the lake's glaciated canyon. From the ridge you circle a shallower, mildly glaciated canyon and cross the jeep road (5710–1.0), which has been staying just above you.

Side route. Just several yards before this crossing, a spur trail leads about 20 yards downslope to an excellent campsite. Hopefully, the nearby spring will be flowing when you arrive here, but don't count on it.

See map A1

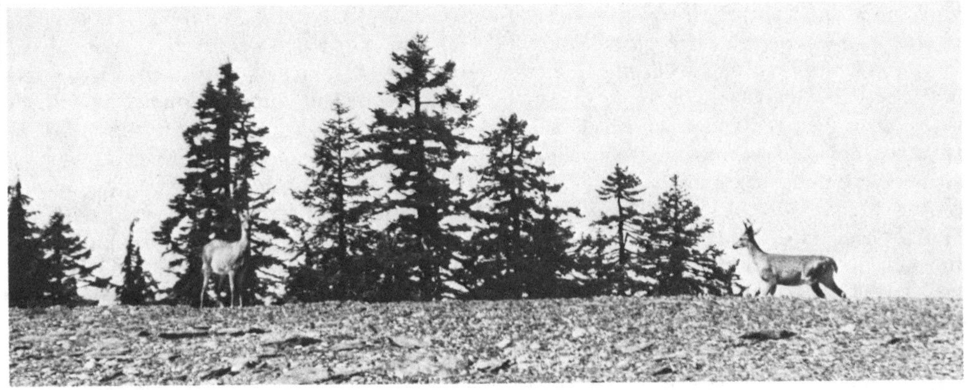

Deer on crest near Mud Springs

The PCT has kept below the road to avoid the Chrome King Mine, which lies just southwest of the road crossing. Next you traverse through a stand of timber and then climb past more brush to a junction on a crest saddle (5900–0.5).

Side route. From it Horse Camp Trail 958 descends northeast toward nearby Echo Lake, whose environs provide camping superior to that at Lily Pad Lake.

Leaving the saddle and the last outcrop of marble you'll encounter on this northbound trek, you make a long, mostly brushy descent, first east and then north, down to Cook and Green Pass (4770–2.5). There is room for at least several hiking parties on the forested, nearly flat crest immediately west of the road that crosses the pass.

Water access. Get water by going along a trail that leads northwest from the pass. You'll reach a spring in 150 yards; if it's dry, continue another 225 yards to a creeklet. Here, along the crest border between Klamath National Forest to the south and Rogue River National Forest to the north, a major USFS road crosses the pass and then descends about 12½ miles to the start of this section's route, Seiad Store. The PCT route is about 2½ miles longer. Northbound from Cook and Green Pass, the USFS road snakes its way about 10 miles down to Hutton Campground, which is situated about a mile from a large reservoir, Applegate Lake. After severe storms, parts of this road can be closed for a year or more to vehicles.

See maps A1, A2

See map A2

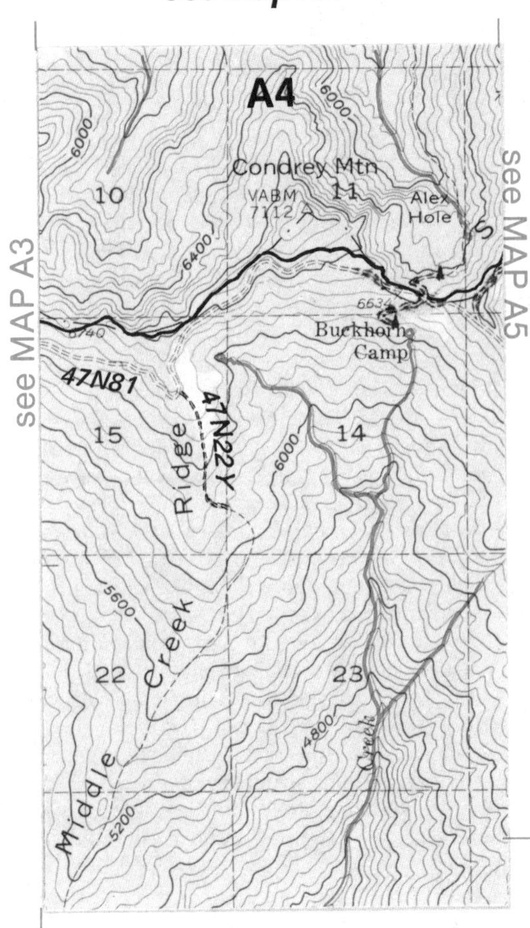

see MAP A6

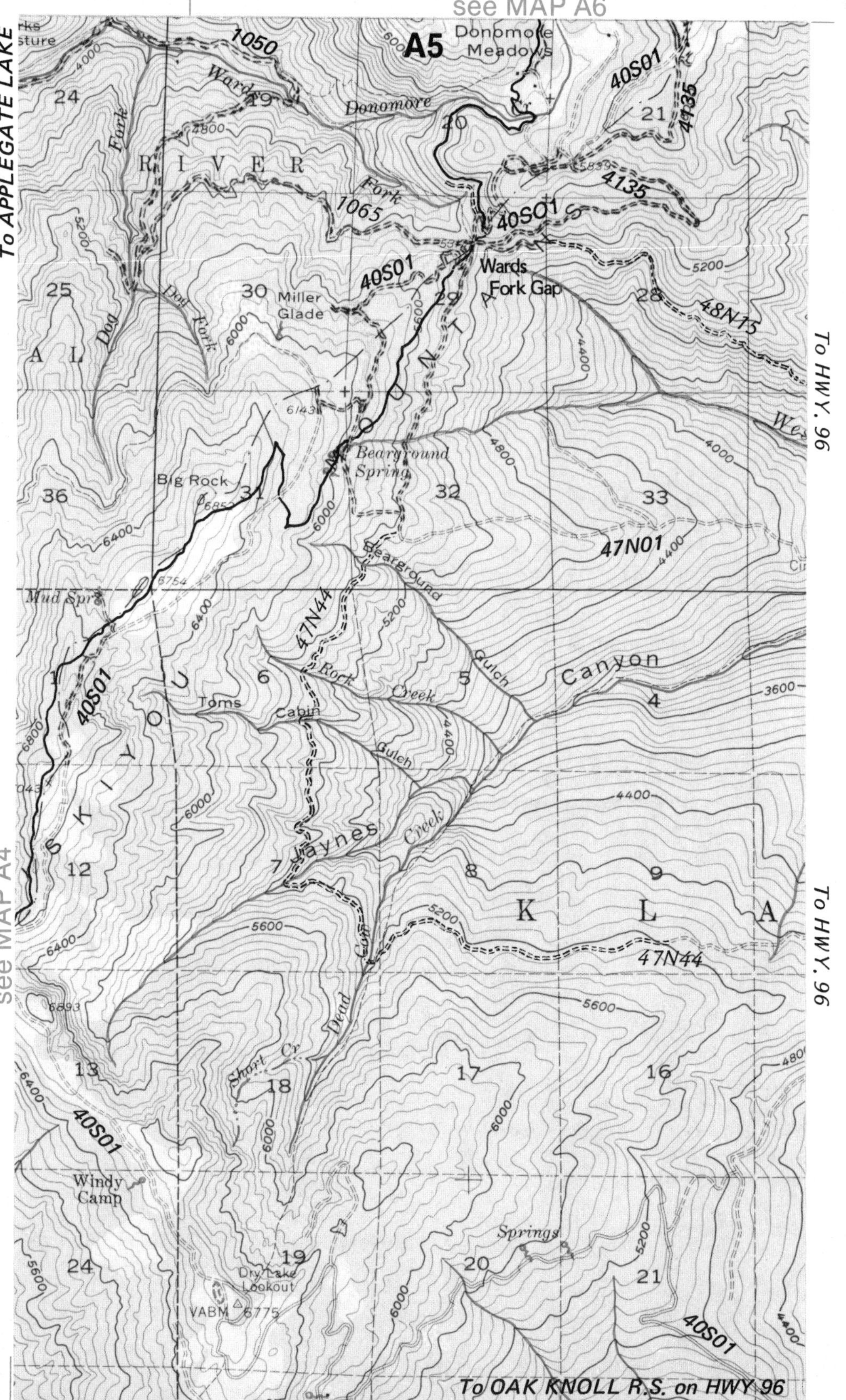

see MAP A4

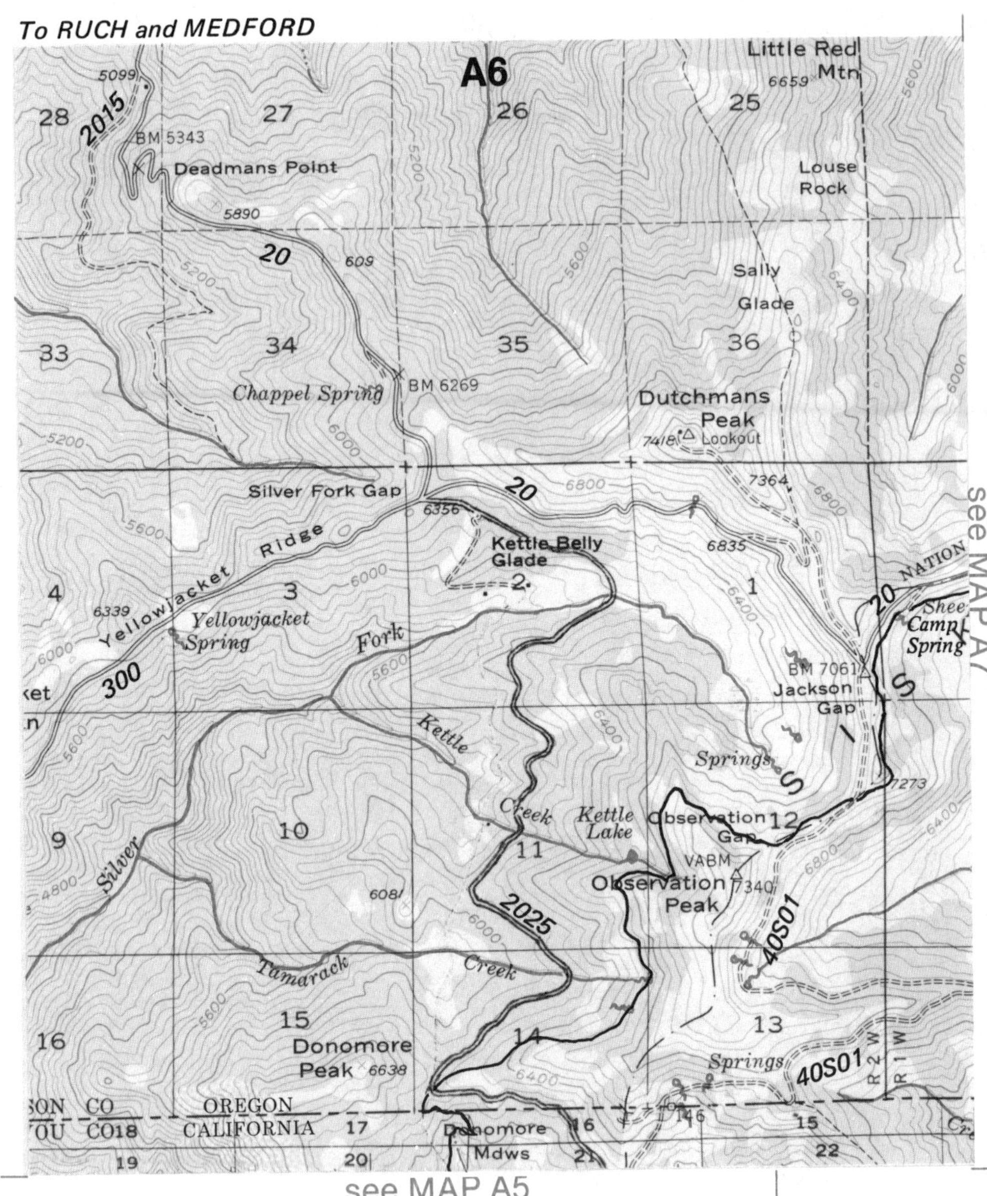

From this pass, you follow an obvious trail east up the ridge toward Copper Butte. ▮ *On it you pass scattered knobcone pines in a vegetative cover that includes manzanita, western serviceberry, tobacco brush, and Sadler's oak. Like tombstones, slabs of greenish-gray, foliated mica schist stand erect along the trail and, in the proper light, reflect the sun's rays as glacially polished rocks do.* ▮ The trail makes a long switchback up to the crest, passing a clearcut in the process. ▮ *There are other clearcuts to the south, on slopes east of Seiad Creek, and this patchwork landscape of forest and clearing contrasts with the burned slopes, which are mostly west of the creek. Remember that this section is logging country, and one may run into ongoing logging operations along the route east.* ▮

Once back on the crest, the PCT enters a stand of white fir, red fir, mountain hemlock, Douglas-fir, ponderosa pine, and knobcone pine. ▮ *This is a combination you'd never see in the Sierra Nevada, where these trees are altitudinally zoned to a much greater extent. On the north slopes just below the crest, you'll also find weeping spruce.* ▮ Rather than struggle to

See map A2

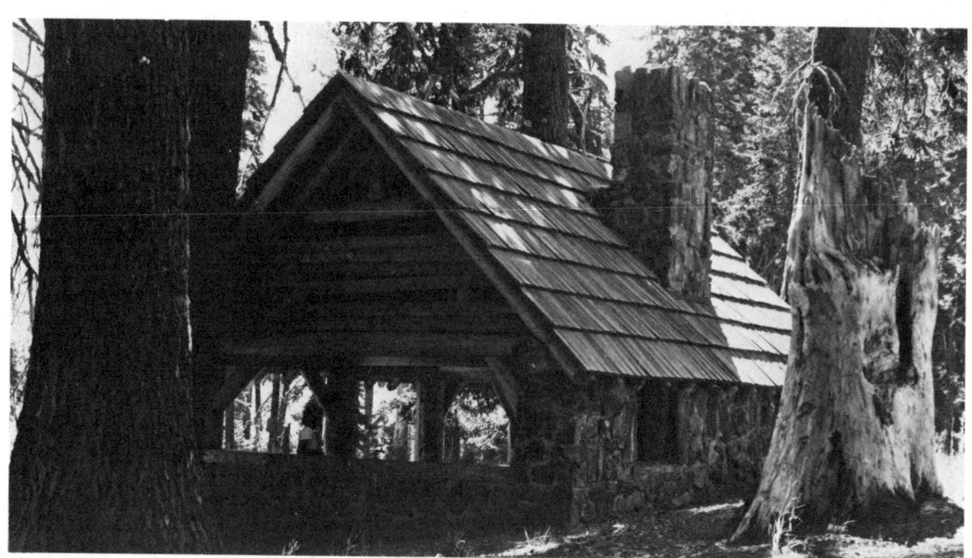

Wrangle Campground shelter

the top of Copper Butte, as early PCT hikers did on the old trail, you make a slight ascent to its south ridge, on which you meet Trail 11W02 (6080–2.8), which descends south to Low Gap, Salt Gulch, and Seiad Valley. The course now becomes a northeast one, and you keep close to the crest, crossing several forested crest saddles before arriving at an open one (6040–2.2), from which Horse Creek Trail 11W01 begins a brushy descent south to Middle Creek Road 46N50. This road descends southeast to the hamlet of Horse Creek on Highway 96. You continue northeast to another saddle (6040–0.3).

Side routes. Here you'll find a spur trail, hopefully marked, which heads 230 yards southeast to a small spring with an equally small campsite at the Lowdens Cabin site. It is better to camp at the saddle, where there is more room. Northward from it, Tin Cup Trail 961 descends 1.6 miles to Road 600.

Leaving the saddle, you start a contour east and from brushy slopes can identify the spring area, across the meadow south of you, by noting a large log near the forest's edge. By Beardog Spring, immediately below the trail, this brushy contour becomes a forested one of Douglas-fir, Jeffrey pine and incense-cedar. Beyond a deep crest saddle, you soon start along the south slope of White Mountain. You cross somewhat open slopes again, reach its spur ridge, and then arc east across the upper limits of a meadowy hollow. At its east end is a junction (5950–2.0) with the old PCT.

Water access. This trail will lead you to a seasonal seep near the hollow's west edge. Late-season hikers will have to descend the hollow a short distance to get their water.

Just beyond this junction, you reach another saddle and from it climb east up to a higher crest. Stay close to it on a path that glitters with mica flakes before you eventually curve southeast and descend an open slope. On it, you cross, then parallel, a crest road that takes you across a long saddle, then almost touches the hairpin turn of Road 47N81 (6310–2.4).

Water access. You can take the lower road branch south ½ mile to Reeves Ranch Springs, located below the road. The northernmost spring is seasonal, but the two others appear to be perennial. Dense groves of alders give away their location but also make reaching them an effort.

The PCT parallels the east side of the road's upper branch, climbing first south, then east, and eventually traversing the south slopes of

See maps A2, A3, A4

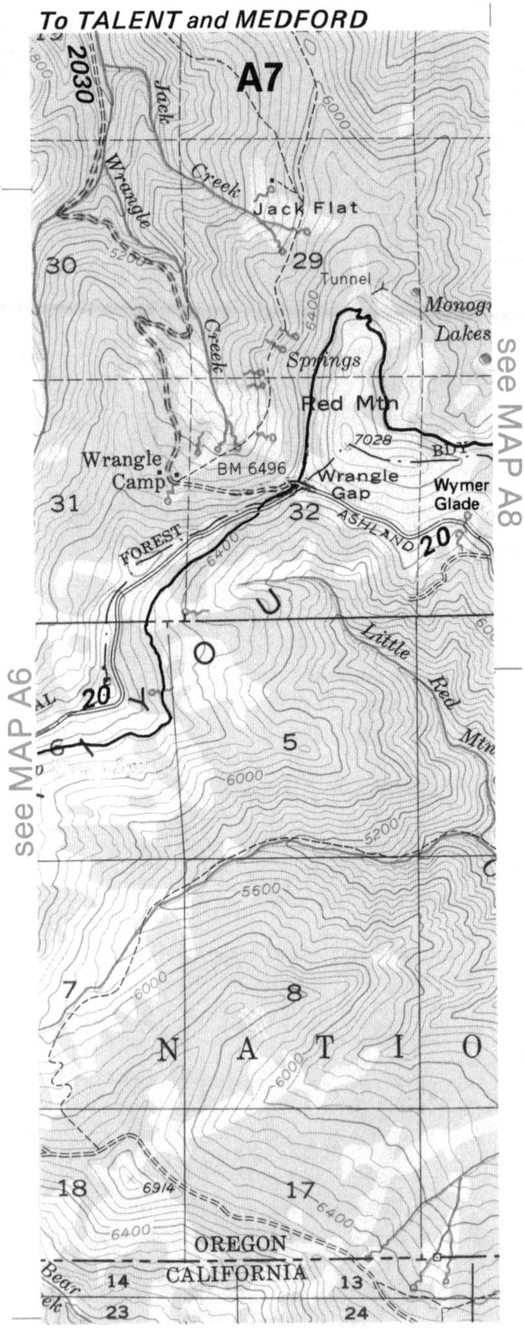

To TALENT and MEDFORD

see MAP A6

see MAP A8

Condrey Mountain before descending ¾ mile to a saddle (6630–3.1).

Side routes. From here, a spur road leaves Road 47N81 to descend west-southwest 0.3 mile to Buckhorn Camp, a poor campsite beside a trickling spring a few yards farther east. Another spur road leaves the saddle, this one descending north ¼ mile to delightful Alex Hole Camp, located near a willow-lined spring. Here, where your far-reaching view north is framed by cliffs of mica schist, your only neighbors may be deer, chipmunks, and mountain bluebirds.

Back on the PCT, you start to parallel ascending Road 47N81 and then veer north away from it to climb the main Siskiyou crest. You almost top Peak 7043 before descending into a mountain-hemlock forest. Long-lasting snow patches can make the next mile to the Mud Springs spur road difficult to follow, but, if so, you can take the crest road, just east of you, to the same destination. If you encounter snow along here, you are certain to encounter more snow to the east. Just yards away from Road 40S01, the PCT crosses the Mud Springs spur road (6730–2.3).

Water access. You can continue northwest 0.2 mile down this road to its end, where there are several very refreshing clear-water springs and a couple of small campsites on sloping ground. You may prefer to camp on level ground by the PCT.

Past the spur road you have a wonderful, open, near-crest traverse that passes a prominent rock midway in the approach to less imposing, misnamed Big Rock. Descend northeast across its open, gravelly east slope of glistening mica, briefly enter a patch of firs, leave it, and head south back into forest as you descend to a crossing of Road 40S01 (6250–1.6). The trail now enters an old logging area as it first continues southward, turns northeast, and descends to cross a road (5930–0.8), which lies immediately north of Bearground Spring. As you'll see, this is an area of several springs. In this vicinity, which in former days was heavily used by car campers, you should be able to find a decent campsite.

From the Bearground Spring road, you start among shady Shasta red firs and make a steady descent northeast, crossing an abandoned logging road midway to a saddle. Nearing this saddle, you cross narrow Road 40S01 at its hairpin turn, immediately recross the road, and

See maps A4, A5

in a couple of minutes reach a 6-way road junction on the saddle, Wards Fork Gap (5317–1.3). Southbound Road 47N01 traverses over to Road 47N44, and from that junction both descend to Beaver Creek. Along the creek, Road 48N01 descends to Highway 96, reaching it just 0.7 mile northeast of Klamath River, a small community with store and post office. Road 48N15, descending east from the saddle, also will get you to Beaver Creek. Road 1065 traverses west from the saddle but later drops to Road 1050, which makes a long, leisurely descent west to Hutton Campground and the nearby Applegate Lake area.

Between north-climbing Road 48N16 and east-climbing 40S01, the PCT starts to climb northeast from Wards Fork Gap. This short stretch can be overgrown and hard to follow. If you can't, then from the saddle head north briefly up Road 48N16 to a bend, from which a logging spur continues north. You'll see the PCT just above it, paralleling it first north, then west. Walk south up Road 48N16 midway to its second bend, and you should be able to find the northbound PCT without much trouble.

On it, you make a short climb north before embarking on a long traverse that circles clockwise around a knoll to Donomore Creek. This you parallel east to within 100 yards of the Donomore Meadows road, then bridge the creek (5600–1.5) and wind northward up an amorphous ridge that may be crisscrossed with misleading cow paths. In ½ mile you cross this road at a point about 80 yards east of a cabin, then parallel a jeep road, immediately below you, which follows the meadow's edge north. At the meadow's upper end, the trail curves east above it, then switchbacks west for a short, partly steep ascent northwest into Oregon, and soon veers north up to a logging-road saddle (6210–1.4).

Here you cross wide Road 2025, then climb east up a clearcut crest, and leave it to make a long, curving traverse northward to the west ridge (6750–1.6) of twin-topped Observation Peak. Kettle Lake, below you, immediately comes into view as you start an uphill traverse east. Unfortunately, it lacks level land suitable for camping. Climb east to Kettle Creek and then climb north from it, high above Kettle Lake, before rounding the large northwest ridge of Observation Peak. A southeast traverse through stands of mountain hemlocks—snowbound until mid-July—gets you to Observation Gap (7030–1.2), a shallow saddle just west of and above 40S01.1. From the gap, go ½ mile

See maps A5, A6

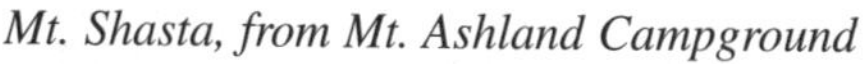

Mt. Shasta, from Mt. Ashland Campground

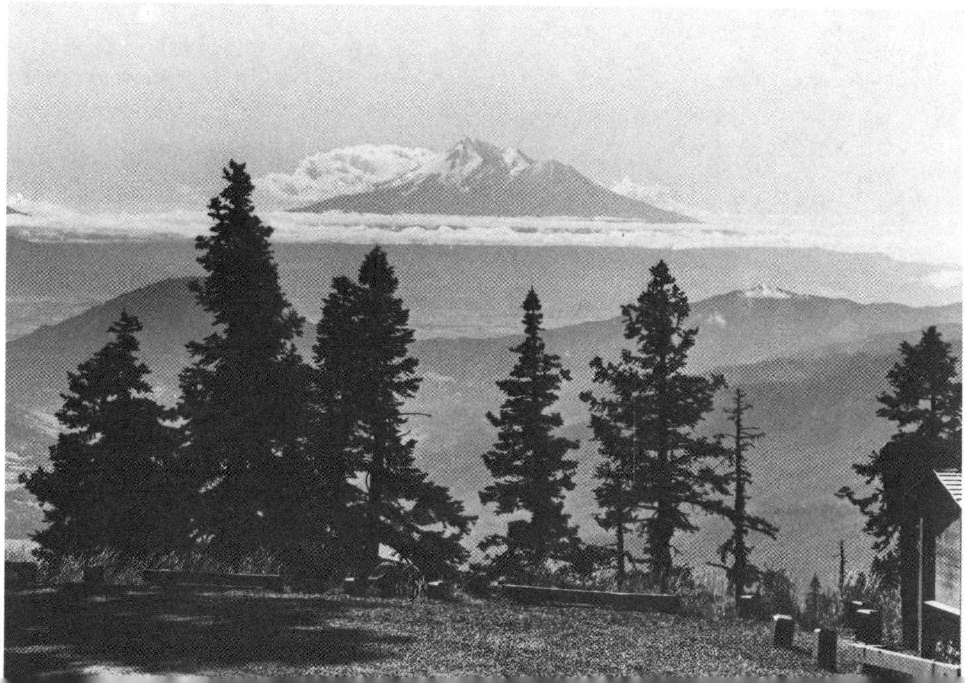

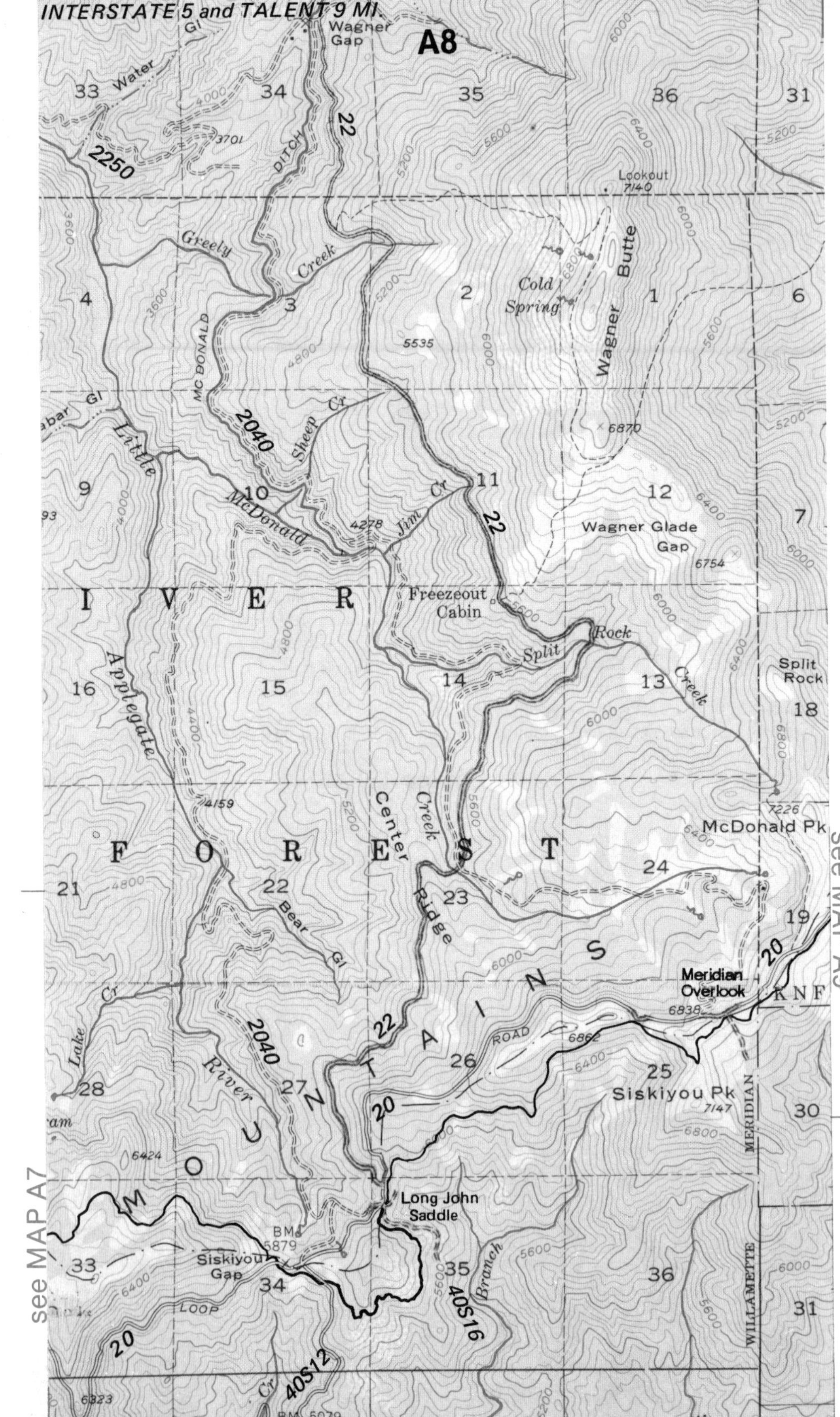

INTERSTATE 5 and TALENT 9 MI.
A8
Wagner Gap
Wagner Butte
Lookout 7140
Cold Spring
Greely Creek
Sheep Cr
Little McDonald
Jim Cr
Freezeout Cabin
Wagner Glade Gap
Split Rock Creek
Split Rock
McDonald Pk
Applegate
Center Creek
Center Ridge
Bear Gl
Lake Cr
River
Meridian Overlook
Siskiyou Pk
Long John Saddle
Siskiyou Gap
Branch
ROAD
LOOP
MERIDIAN
WILLAMETTE
KNF
ROGUE RIVER NATIONAL FOREST
SISKIYOU MOUNTAINS
see MAP A7
see MAP A9

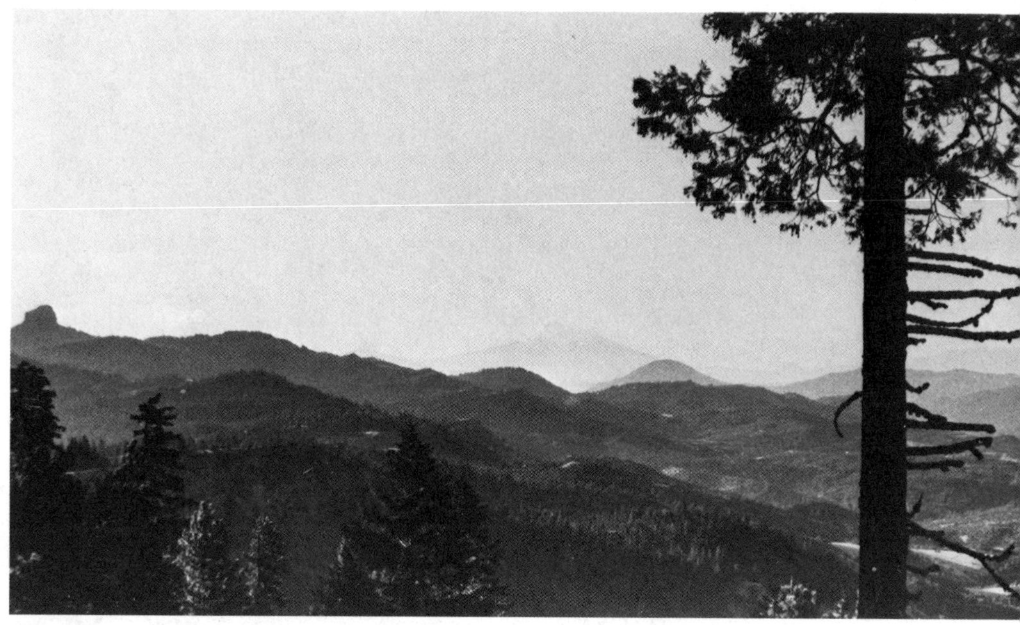

Pilot Rock and distant Mt. Shasta, from PCT above Mt. Ashland Road

on the crest trail, cross Road 40S01.1, traverse around the east slopes of Peak 7273, and then parallel the crest north toward Jackson Gap (7040–1.2). ▮ *Before reaching this gap you'll certainly notice landscape terracing in the Jackson Gap area, done to prevent erosion on the burned-over slopes.* ▮ Crossing this gap about 100 feet above you is broad Road 20, which you'll parallel all the way to the end of Section A. Before mid-July, snow drifts will probably force you to take this road rather than the PCT.

Leaving the cover of hemlocks and firs, arc clockwise across the upper slopes of a huge open bowl, soon reaching a spur road (6920–0.3) to Sheep Camp Spring, located 10 yards south on it. Camp space is very limited, and since it lacks tree cover, you would probably greet next morning's sunrise from a very wet sleeping bag. Departing east from the spur road, you gradually descend, with unobstructed views, to a spur ridge, then arc northeast to Wrangle Gap (6496–2.3), reaching it ¼ mile after crossing to the north side of Road 20.

Side route. From here, a spur road descends steeply west to Wrangle Campground. This little-used recreation site, nestled among Shasta red firs, has a large stone shelter complete with fireplace, two stoves, and tables. In the 1970s it also had tap water. Unless the USFS decides to reinstate piped-in water, you'll have to get some at the upper end of a small bowl, where you'll find a spring that is about 150 yards south-southwest from the shelter.

From Wrangle Gap, the PCT route could have gone east, but instead it makes a long climb north to the end of Red Mountain ridge and starts to wind southeast up it. The route does have the advantage of giving you sweeping panoramas of southern Oregon and its pointed landmark, Mt. McLoughlin—an Ice Age volcano. After crossing the ridge, contour south and then east, leaving Red Mountain's slopes for a winding, moderate descent to the west end of open Siskiyou Gap (5890–3.8), where you cross Road 20. ▮ *The northeast quarter of Section 34 lies in private land, and for many years the owner resisted attempts at building a direct trail, paralleling Road 20, over to nearby Long John Saddle. Finally, in desperation, the USFS built a trail twice as long to that goal.* ▮ It first parallels Road 20 briefly over to its junction with Road 40S12,

See maps A6, A7, A8

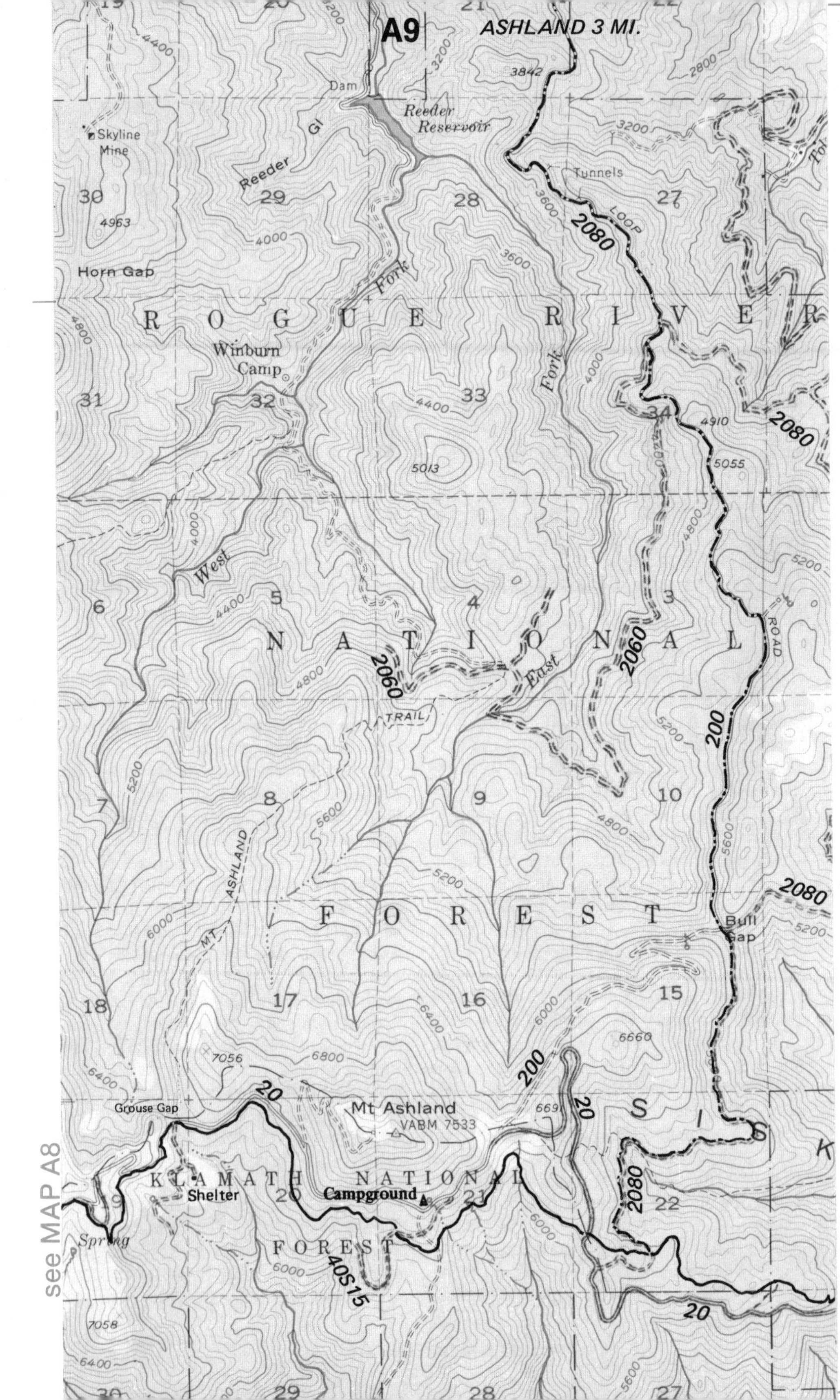

A9
ASHLAND 3 MI.
Dam
Reeder Reservoir
Reeder Gl
Skyline Mine
Horn Gap
Tunnels
LOOP
2080
ROGUE RIVER
Winburn Camp
West
Fork
East
NATIONAL
2060
TRAIL
ROAD
200
MT ASHLAND
FOREST
Bull Gap
Grouse Gap
Mt Ashland
VABM 7533
KLAMATH NATIONAL FOREST
Shelter
Campground
Spring
40S15
20
SISK
see MAP A8

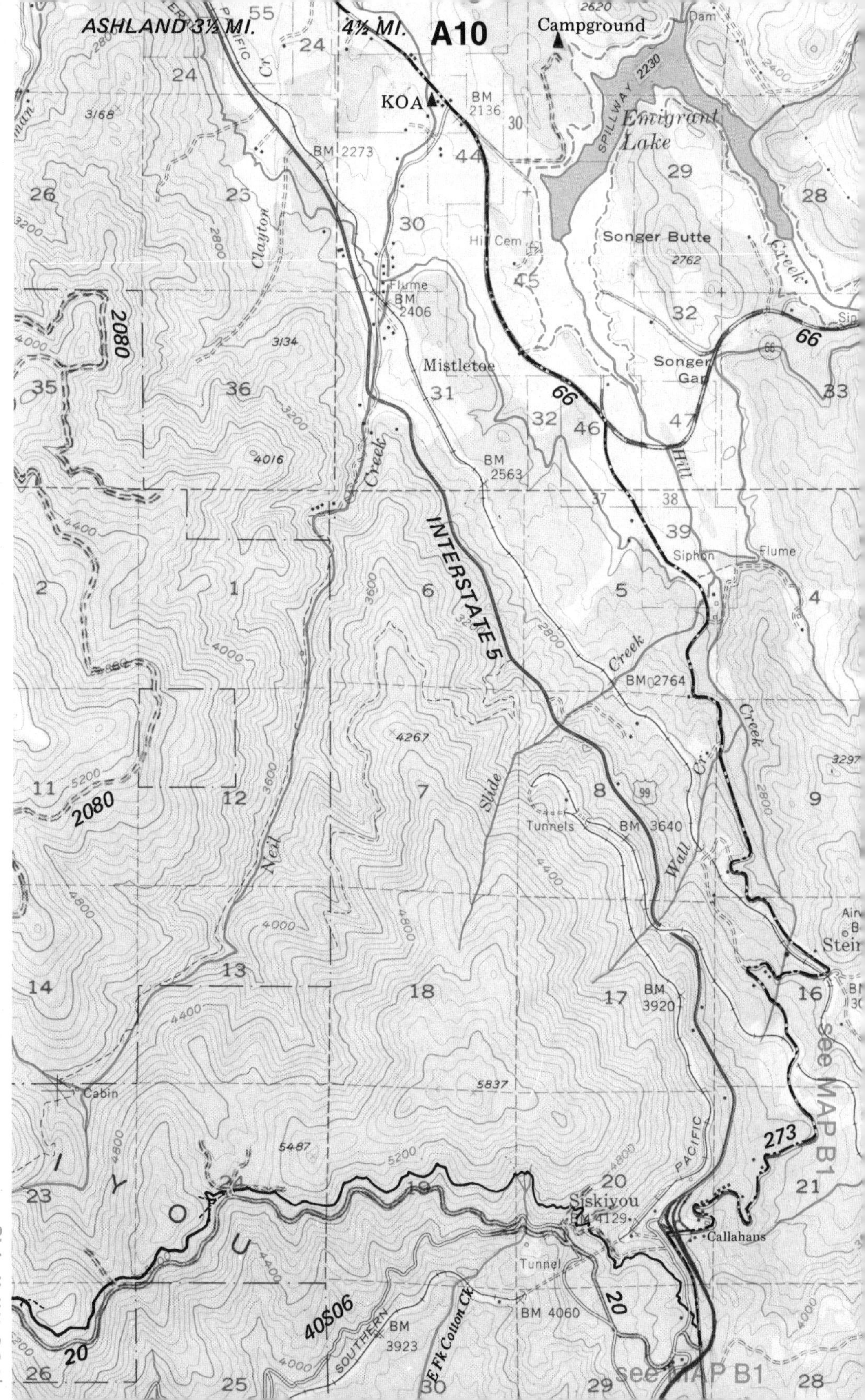

ASHLAND 3½ MI.
4½ MI.
A10
Campground
Dam
KOA
Emigrant Lake
SPILLWAY 2230
Songer Butte
Mistletoe
Hill Cem
Flume
Songer Gap
66
INTERSTATE 5
Clayton
Creek
Neil
Slide
Wall Cr.
Hill
Siphon
Tunnels
Cabin
Siskiyou
Callahans
Tunnel
E Fk Cotton Ck
SOUTHERN PACIFIC
2080
40S06
20
273
99
See MAP B1

then parallels that road briefly over to a crossing (5800–0.3). Then it makes a long swing around a hill, offering some Mt. Shasta views in partial compensation for the added hiking effort before finally reaching a 5-way road junction (5880–1.3) on forested Long John Saddle.

Road 20 traverses north across the level saddle, and a minor logging road descends northeast. Between the two, the PCT starts to parallel Road 20 north and then climbs northeast through an old logging area. After a mile of progress, you come to a spur ridge and exchange this scarred landscape for a shady forest climb north. From a gully, the gradient eases to give you a pleasant stroll northeast to an open crest saddle (6710–2.1). On it, the tread almost disappears as it parallels Road 20 for a few yards, and then it becomes prominent again and climbs a short ½ mile up to a saddle just north of Siskiyou Peak. From this saddle you'll see chunky Pilot Peak on the eastern skyline—a guiding beacon for early pioneers and for you. If you're continuing through Oregon, you should pass by the peak in a few days. The road now winds ⅓ mile northeast toward a saddle on the main crest, crossing a spur road (6900–0.8) that is just 25 yards below its departure from crest-hugging Road 20. ▮ *The saddle is signed as the Meridian Overlook, since it is a viewpoint close to the Willamette Meridian.* ▮

You parallel Road 20 northeast, sometimes below it and sometimes above it, to another saddle (7030–1.1) south of the main crest. Here the road bends north to descend, but the PCT first goes south briefly before switchbacking to descend northeast to reach Road

See maps A8, A9

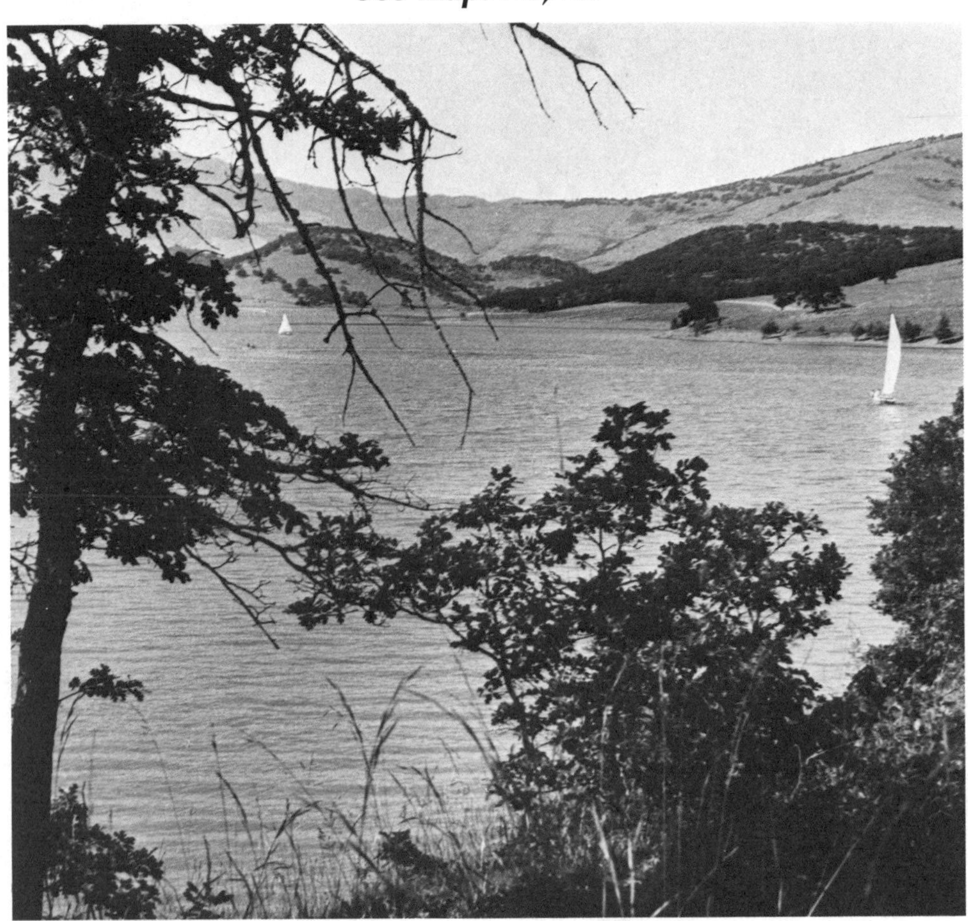

Ashland's Emigrant Lake, along alternate route

40S30 (6630–1.0) at its junction with Road 20 on expansive Grouse Gap.

Side route. This road takes you 0.2 mile south to a fork, from where you branch left on Road 40S30A for a minute's walk to Grouse Gap Shelter. Built in the mid-1970s, it was finally fenced in two decades later (1994) to keep the local residents (cattle) out. The shelter provides protection from the elements, and it offers dramatic sunrise views of Mt. Shasta. You can usually get water from the creeklet just northeast of and below the shelter, but late-season trekkers will likely have to backtrack on 40S30A to 40S30, and then take that road ⅓ mile southwest down to an obvious gully with a spring-fed creeklet.

From Grouse Gap, the PCT parallels Road 20 and passes several seeping springs before it gradually drops away from that road down to a crossing of Road 40S15 (6480–1.9), which climbs ½ mile northeast up to this crest road. From their junction, Road 20 contours ½ mile northeast to the Mt. Ashland Ski Area, and eastward the road is paved.

Side route. An alternative to camping at Grouse Gap Shelter is to camp at Mt. Ashland Campground, which straddles both sides of Road 20. To reach it, leave the PCT and follow Road 40S15 about 250 yards up to its bend left, from where you'll see an abandoned logging road that climbs directly upslope to the campground. The piped water isn't always flowing, and when it's not, get water in a little gully just above the campground's upper (north) sites.

From Road 40S15, the PCT contours southeast to the bend and then traverses northeast to an open bowl below the ski area. From this, the trail traverses southeast to a saddle, where you cross Road 20 (6160–1.5). Continuing southeast down-ridge, you follow the PCT down to Road 2080 (6060–0.4).

Resupply access. From this ridge, you can take a supply route by following Road 2080 north down to Bull Gap (5500–2.8), where you meet Road 200, which climbs southwest up to the Mt. Ashland Ski Area. Continuing north, take Road 200, which in 3 miles rejoins Road 2080, all the way down to Glenview Drive (2200–8.5) in Ashland. Descend this road north, then descend Fork Street. You quickly reach Pioneer Street and follow it two blocks to C Street. The Ashland Post Office is one block southeast on it, at the corner of First and C streets (1920–1.1). To get back to the PCT, head southwest one block to East Main and walk southeast. It quickly becomes two-way Siskiyou Boulevard (1950–0.3), and you continue southeast on it to Highway 66 (Ashland Street) (2010–2.2). Take this east past the Ashland Shopping Center to Washington Street, which has the Ashland Ranger Station at its end. Just east of this short street you reach Interstate 5 (1980–1.3–15.1). Since hitchhiking on freeways is legal in Oregon, you can hitchhike up it 9 miles to the Mt. Ashland exit. Alternately, you can continue on Highway 66, then go south up Highway 273 to that exit, about a 12-mile route. This route is described in the opposite direction at the end of this chapter.

Back at Siskiyou Boulevard you can also keep to East Main and follow it 1.0 mile east to the Pacific Northwest Museum of Natural History. It is a fitting introduction to your hike north through Oregon and Washington. From the museum, continue 0.9 mile east to Tolman Creek road, and on it curve south ½ mile back to Highway 66, meeting it at the Ashland Shopping Center (supermarket, superdrug, bank, etc., etc.).

If you decide against the supply route, then continue east down the forested trail. The PCT stays on or north of the crest, but after 0.7 mile it crosses to the south side and in ¼ mile crosses a jeep road that climbs northeast back to the nearby crest. ▮ *Not until 1987 was the next stretch—through sections 23, 24, and 26—completed. Rights-of-way across private property held up PCT construction for more than a decade.* ▮

The PCT continues its eastern descent, first past grass and bracken ferns, and then mostly past brush. Soon the trail switchbacks and then quickly reaches the shady grounds of Mt. Ashland Inn, a bed-and-breakfast establishment opened Christmas 1987. ▮ *The rates are very reasonable, as such establishments go, but they*

See maps A9, A10

are nevertheless far too high for the average long-distance hiker. However, the owners do freely offer water to passing hikers. ▮

A minute's walk below the inn, you cross a saddle (5490–1.5) and then parallel Road 20 for a generally brushy traverse over to another saddle (5110–0.8). Next you make a similar traverse, this one to a saddle with 4 roads radiating from it (4990–0.8). Eastbound, the PCT is confined between an old crest road and Road 20 for the first ⅓ mile, and then it parallels the latter as both descend east around ridges and across gullies. Three closely spaced gullies near the end of this descent provide spring-fed water before they coalesce to flow into East Fork Cotton Creek.

Because you are on private land, you're not allowed to deviate from the trail's tread and aren't allowed to camp. Thick brush prevents you from doing either, anyway. About 0.4 mile past the last spring-fed gully, you cross a road (4610–2.5) that descends steeply southeast to nearby Road 20, which here turns southeast to cross a broad saddle. Then, after a short, steep descent of your own, you cross a road (4470–0.1) that climbs gently west up to a union with the first road at paved Road 20. Both dirt roads are private—off limits—as is a third road that you parallel east before momentarily turning south to cross (4360–0.1). Now you parallel this road, staying just above it, dip in and out of a gully with a sometimes-flowing freshet, and soon curve away from the road as you glimpse busy, nearby Interstate 5. The path ends (4250–0.8) at an abandoned segment of old Highway 99, which you take for 140 yards around a hollow to a fork. Here you go left and descend an old, closed road 150 yards to trail's end on Highway 99. This trailhead is 250 yards north of where Mt. Ashland Road 20 ends at Highway 99 (4240–0.3), and that junction in turn is immediately north of where Interstate 5 crosses over the highway. Here, at the junction of Road 20 and Highway 99, this section ends. ▮ *The Mesozoic granitic rocks you've traversed along the eastern crest of the Siskiyou Mountains are here overlain by mid-Tertiary, thick, basaltic andesite flows, and the Shasta red firs and mountain hemlocks have yielded to Douglas-firs and orange-barked madrones.*

Resupply access. If you've hiked the PCT through much or all of California, you may want to celebrate your entry into Oregon by visiting Callahan's Restaurant. Go north on Highway 99 for ⅔ mile to Highway 273 and on it cross under Interstate 5 at its Mt. Ashland exit. The restaurant is just east of it. This ever-popular place, closed on Mondays, serves only dinners, and though Callahan's is expensive by backpackers' standards, it is one of the better dining places along or near the entire PCT. If you've been starving these last few miles, you'll be glad to know that each of their dinners includes all the salad, soup, and spaghetti you can eat. When the restaurant is closed, Callahan's Country Store, also on the grounds, usually is open. It has "emergency supplies": beer, chips, candy, more beer.

To resupply for another stretch of the PCT in southern Oregon, you can hitchhike 9 miles down Interstate 5 to the Highway 66 interchange and take the highway west into downtown Ashland.

Resupply access. An old, temporary PCT route offers you another way down to Ashland. From Callahan's (3950–0.9 mile from end of Road 20), you can go down tree-lined Highway 273 to a junction with Highway 66 (2290–6.7). Just east of it is the shallow upper end of Emigrant Lake, a popular fishing area: the deeper parts are relegated to water skiers, boaters, and swimmers. Northwest, Highway 66 leads you to the main entrance to the Emigrant Lake Recreation Area (2150–1.8). Here a paved road heads southeast 0.4 mile up to a lateral dam, then curves north 0.6 mile to a public campground. Past the recreation area's entrance you'll come to fairly expensive but well-equipped Glenyan KOA campground (2140–0.2) with showers and a store. It caters to backpackers as well as to car campers, and the larger your hiking group, the cheaper your per-person camp fee will be.

Continuing north on Highway 66, you meet Dead Indian Road (1920–2.6) before your highway turns west and climbs to cross Interstate 5 (1980–0.7–12.9) at the outskirts of

See map A10

Ashland. Some backpackers prefer to celebrate in Ashland rather than at Callahan's, for there is quite a selection of good-to-excellent cafés and restaurants. In addition, more cultured backpackers take in one or more performances of Ashland's Oregon Shakespearean Festival, which runs most of the year. If the weather has been dreary or snow patches abundant, then perhaps a Shakespearean comedy will lift your spirits. Just north of the festival's grounds is the Ashland Hostel (150 N. Main), which welcomes PCT hikers and even has a PCT register.

See map A10

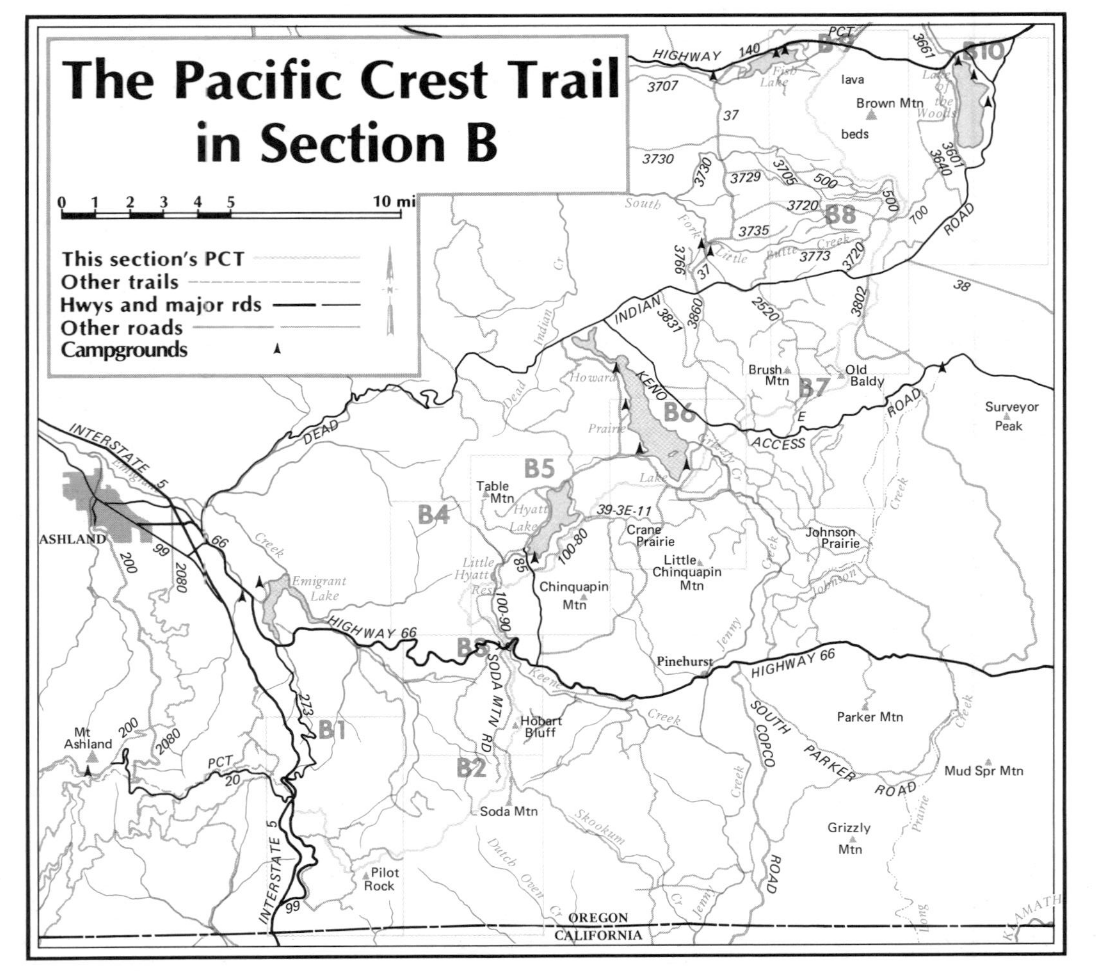
The Pacific Crest Trail in Section B
0 1 2 3 4 5 10 mi
This section's PCT
Other trails
Hwys and major rds
Other roads
Campgrounds
HIGHWAY 140
PCT
B9
B10
3661
Fish Lake
Lake of the Woods
lava
Brown Mtn
beds
3707
37
3730
3729
3705
500
3601
3640
3720
B8
700
ROAD
South Fork
Little Butte Creek
3735
3773
3766
38
INDIAN
3831
3860
2520
3802
Howard Prairie Lake
KENO
B6
Brush Mtn
B7
Old Baldy
E
ACCESS
ROAD
Surveyor Peak
INTERSTATE 5
DEAD
Dead Indian Cr
ASHLAND
99
200
2080
66
Emigrant Creek
Emigrant Lake
B5
Table Mtn
Hyatt Lake
B4
39-3E-11
Crane Prairie
Little Chinquapin Mtn
Johnson Prairie
Johnson
Grizzly Cr
Creek
Little Hyatt Res
85
100-80
100-90
Chinquapin Mtn
Jenny
HIGHWAY 66
B3
SODA MTN RD
Keene Creek
Pinehurst
Hobart Bluff
Parker Mtn
SOUTH COPCO ROAD
PARKER ROAD
Mud Spr Mtn
273
B1
Mt Ashland
PCT
20
B2
Soda Mtn
Skookum
Dutch Oven Cr
Grizzly Mtn
Prairie Creek
Long
Jenny Cr
Pilot Rock
OREGON
CALIFORNIA
KLAMATH

Section B: Interstate 5 near Siskiyou Pass to Highway 140 near Fish Lake

Introduction: Sections A and C are among the highest stretches of PCT to be found in either Oregon or Washington. In contrast, Section B, between them, is one of the lowest, and it is certainly the driest, least scenic section to be found in either state. This section abounds with logged lands that the PCT often passes through or skirts around. If these don't detract from this section's appeal, the lack of wilderness sensation will: often you are closely paralleling logging roads or jeep roads. Furthermore, although two sizable lakes are approached—Hyatt and Howard Prairie—both are dammed and both lack any alpine or subalpine character. And there is a *notable* lack of drinking water. With such a list of detractions, Section B will certainly be shunned by many and its trail will likely be taken mainly by long-distance hikers passing through to a more scenic section.

Declination: 17¼°E

Points on Route:	S→N	Mi. Btwn. Pts.	N→S
Interstate 5 near Mt. Ashland Road 20	0.0		54.0
		4.6	
Cross upper Pilot Rock Jeep Road	4.6		49.4
		5.0	
Fenced-in spring	9.6		44.4
		4.3	
Hobart Bluff spur trail	13.9		40.1
		3.4	
Highway 66 at Green Springs Summit	17.3		36.7
		4.8	
Little Hyatt Reservoir	22.1		31.9
		1.5	
Hyatt Lake Campground spur trail	23.6		30.4
		7.9	
Road to Klum Landing Campground	31.5		22.5
		1.9	
Keno Access Road	33.4		20.6
		9.1	
Dead Indian Road	42.5		11.5
		11.5	
Highway 140 near Fish Lake	54.0		0.0

Supplies: If you need major supplies, get them in Ashland before you start hiking this section. Directions to this city are given at the end of the previous section. Since this section is short, the need for supplies will be minimal, and minimal supplies is all you'll find at Hyatt Lake, Howard Prairie Lake, Lake of the Woods, and Fish Lake resorts. All but Hyatt Lake Resort are somewhat out of your way, especially Lake of the Woods Resort. Three resorts accept packages from UPS, not from the US Postal Service. Their UPS addresses are: Hyatt Lake Resort, 7979 Hyatt Prairie Road, Ashland, OR 97520; Fish Lake Resort, Highway 140, Mile Marker 30, Medford, OR 97501; and Lake of the Woods Resort, 950 Harriman Route, Klamath Falls, OR 97601.

Problems: In this section you'll have to hike up to 22 miles between on-route water sources. If you intend to do this hiking section, then try to do it in June, when snow problems are minimal, yet seasonal creeks are flowing.

Maps:

Siskiyou Pass, OR
Soda Mountain, OR
Hyatt Reservoir, OR
Emigrant Lake, OR (PCT barely enters map)
Little Chinquapin Mountain, OR
Brown Mountain, OR
Mount McLoughlin, OR
Lake of the Woods South, OR (alternate route)
Lake of the Woods North, OR (alternate route)

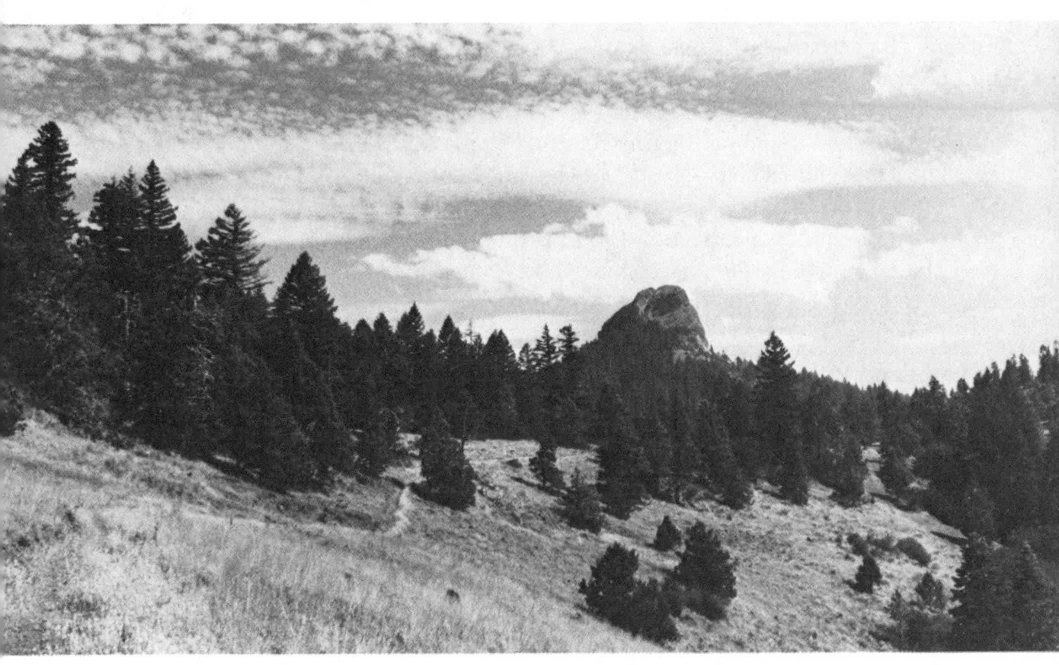

PCT striking east toward Pilot Rock

THE ROUTE

Section B's starting point is at the junction of Mt. Ashland Road 20 and Highway 99 (4240), this point being immediately north of Interstate 5. To reach it by car, start in Ashland at the Highway 66 exit and drive 9 miles south on I5 up to the Mt. Ashland exit. If you're driving north, note that this exit is 16½ miles past the Highway 96 exit in northern California. From the exit proceed ⅔ mile south on Highway 99 to the Road 20 junction.

From this junction, start hiking south up the highway, immediately crossing under noisy I5. You hike straight for ⅓ mile and then start to curve right. In about 250 more yards, you should see the resumption of PCT tread (4380–0.5), which crosses a gully that runs down the highway's east side. If you reach a road branching east, you've gone about 120 yards too far.

On the PCT, you cross the gully and then momentarily cross the road. On private land, you traverse eastward about ¾ mile across Section 28, and then your winding path angles north at a spring (4490–0.9) but quickly switchbacks. On a southward track, climb moderately up toward a ridge, passing close to another spring almost a half mile after the first, just before leaving Section 28. In Section 33, you wind gently ⅓ mile south up to a crest and, after a moment's walk down a spur ridge, reach a road junction. One of the roads descends to a broad saddle, and you do the same, keeping east of the road as the path, an abandoned jeep road, winds 0.2 mile down to a major intersec-

See map B1

see MAP A10

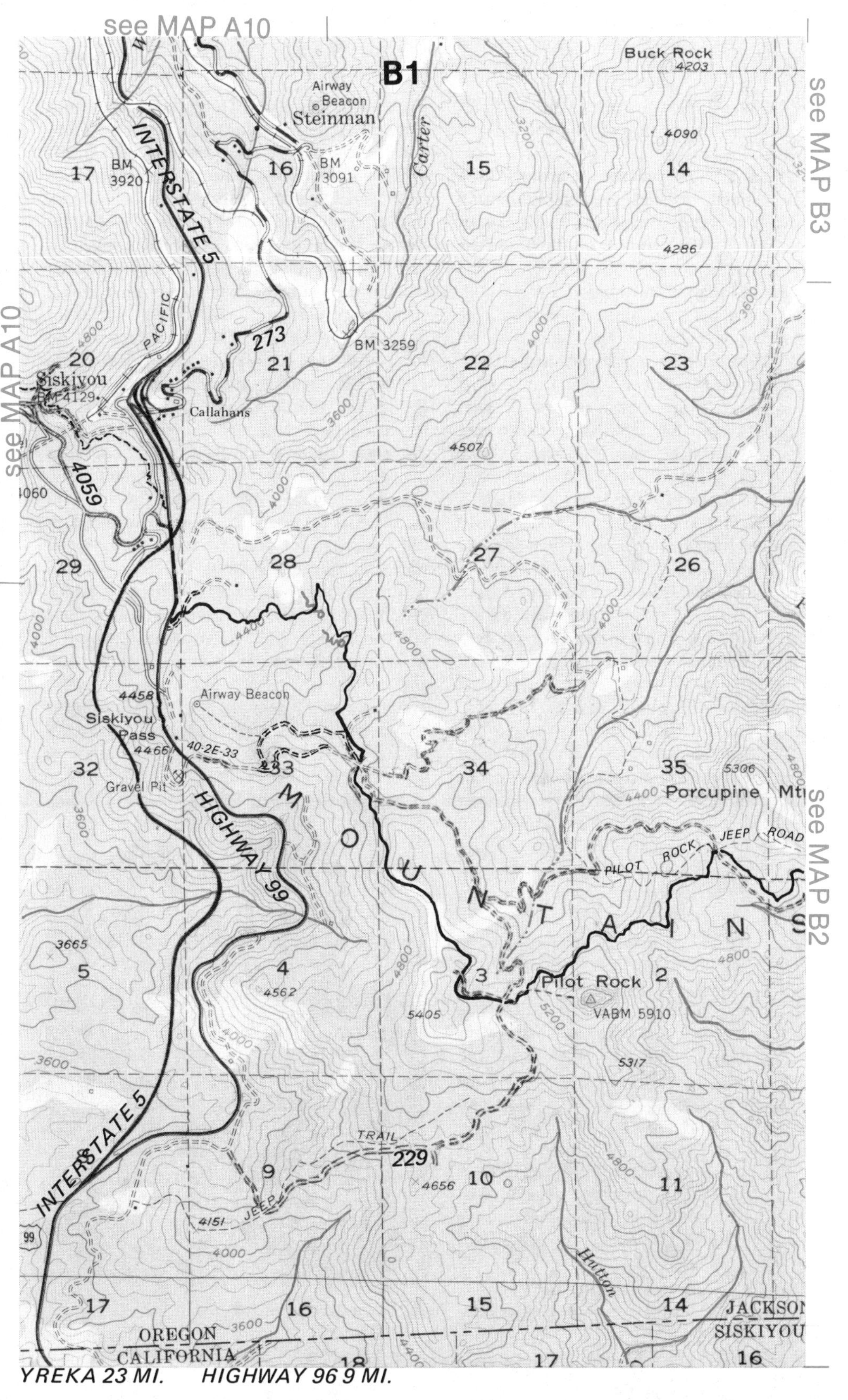

see MAP B3

see MAP A10

see MAP B2

YREKA 23 MI. HIGHWAY 96 9 MI.

tion (4420–1.3). Here, roads go in all directions, two of them leading south along the east side of a crest.

Starting on lumber-company land, the PCT begins beside the western southbound road. In 0.2 mile, however, it almost touches the wider, eastern one and then climbs ⅓ mile through a cool forest of Douglas-fir and white fir. As the trail emerges onto public land and southwest-facing slopes, the forest thins rapidly, junipers appear, and temperatures rise. Hike southeast across a long, open crest; past its low point, the trail, mixing with old jeep tracks, can become rather vague. However, head toward a cluster of trees, through which your faint trail passes, bearing toward steep-sided Pilot Rock. In a few minutes you cross a secondary crest, bend southwest, and traverse to a minor road, which you cross and then parallel as it curves east to a prominent intersection atop a broad saddle (5080–1.7).

The Pilot Rock Jeep Road starts east from this saddle, soon climbing steeply toward the base of Pilot Rock. The trail makes an obscure start along this road's south edge and after 270 yards (5120–0.2) crosses it for a northeast climb to a nearby volcanic point.

Side route. If you have the time, you might first make an excursion to the summit of Pilot Rock. The jeep road ends at the rock's base, from which you'll see an obvious chute up to the top. This route is relatively safe and no rope is required. However, acrophobics or careless climbers could get into trouble.

From the volcanic point beyond the Pilot Rock Jeep Road, the PCT goes briefly east along an abandoned road and then descends northeast 180 yards to a trailside outcrop with a summit that provides fair views across the northern landscape. Continuing your northeast descent, you round a ridge in ¼ mile and momentarily reach a crest. Parallel this northeast for a few minutes before turning east across it at a gate (5160–0.9)—the first of many. Immediately, a dramatic volcanic landscape unfolds before you, with a huge blocky pinnacle in the foreground and towering Pilot Rock to the south.

Beyond the pinnacle, the trail quickly angles north and then makes a pleasant, winding descent through a Douglas-fir forest to a large gate only a few yards south of a crest saddle (4990–0.7). A road from the southeast climbs up to this saddle, crosses it, and swings west, eventually joining the Pilot Rock Road, which climbs east from Highway 99. Also at this crest is a reappearance of the Pilot Rock Jeep Road, which seems to be quite abandoned west of the saddle. East of it, however, it is in good shape, as you'll see, for you'll cross it again and again. On the next stretch, as on most of Section B, the route alternates between private land—usually lumber companies—and Bureau of Land Management (BLM) land.

From the crest saddle, the trail first descends southeast and then curves northeast over to a gully. The PCT is now routed on an abandoned, overgrown roadbed, which you follow east for a few minutes and then climb north to a crest (5020–1.2). A short segment of trail leads east across north-facing slopes to a road, up which you walk 65 yards to a minor crest saddle and the trail's resumption, on your left (5040–0.2). This trail segment goes but 110 yards, and then you cross the jeep road and

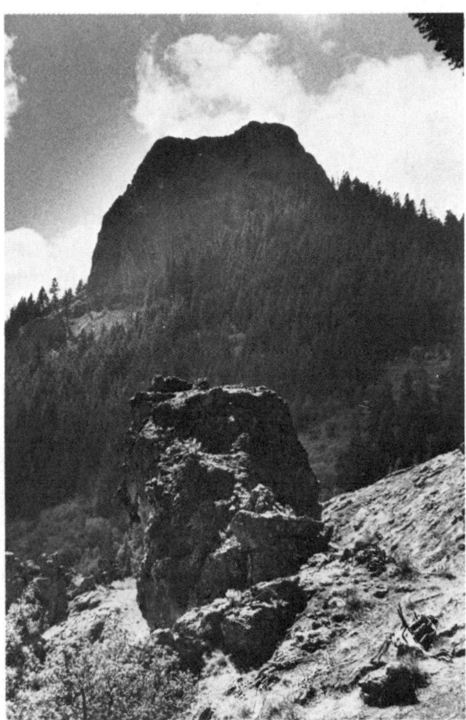

Pilot Rock and trailside pinnacle

See maps B1, B2

see MAP B3

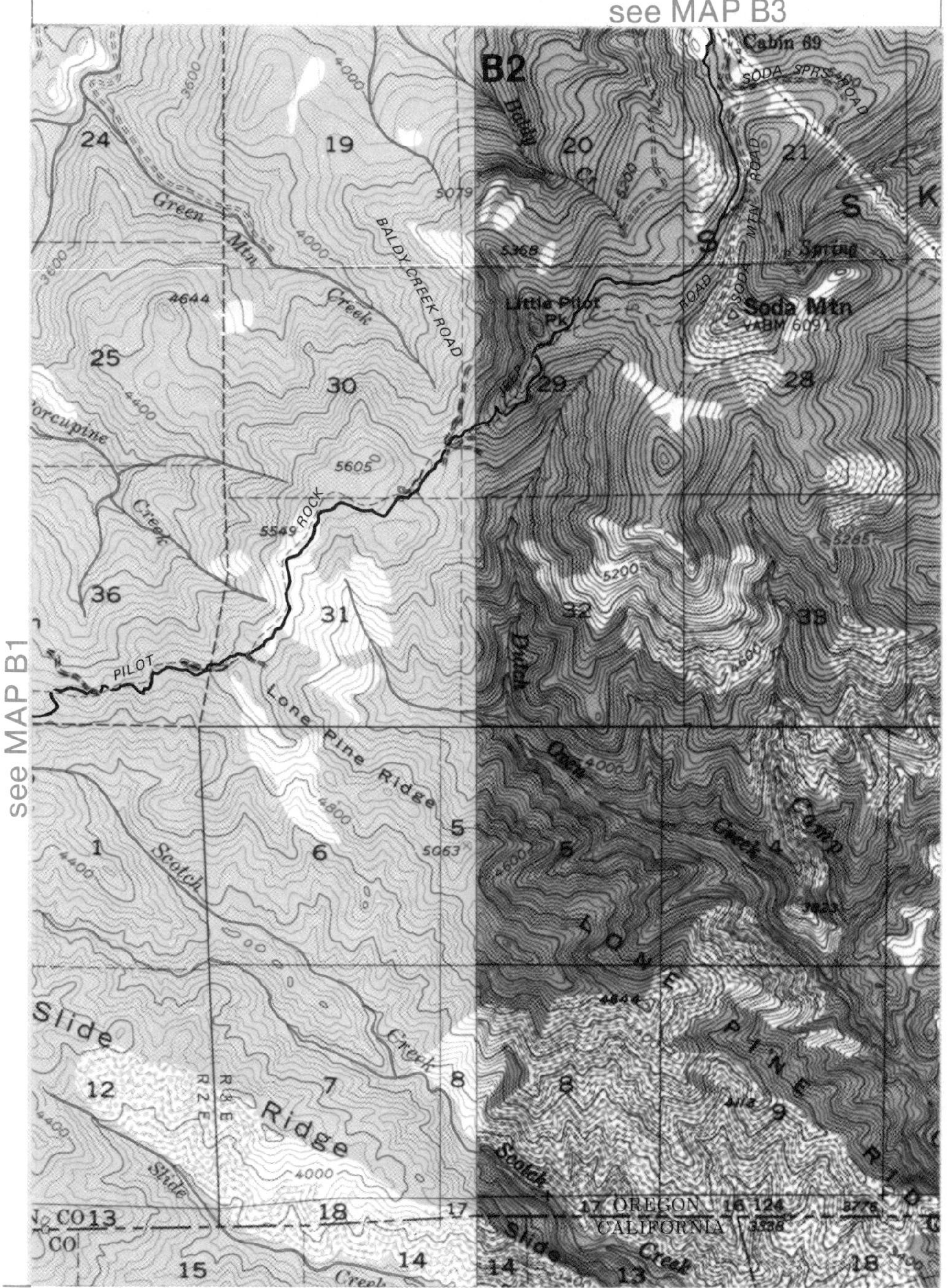

see MAP B1

parallel it east. Twice more you cross this road, the second time where a minor road (5270–0.8) starts a descent southeast.

The trail now parallels the jeep road northeast, and after ¼ mile it provides a half mile of almost continuous views of Mt. Shasta. Pilot Rock, your former guiding beacon, is now hidden. Beyond the views, the trail enters forest and descends gently east, crossing a broad saddle just before it turns northeast to enter a fenced-in compound with a refreshing spring (5290–1.2). This spring, complete with cistern and water faucet, is a full 7.7 miles from the upper spring near the southeast corner of

See map B2

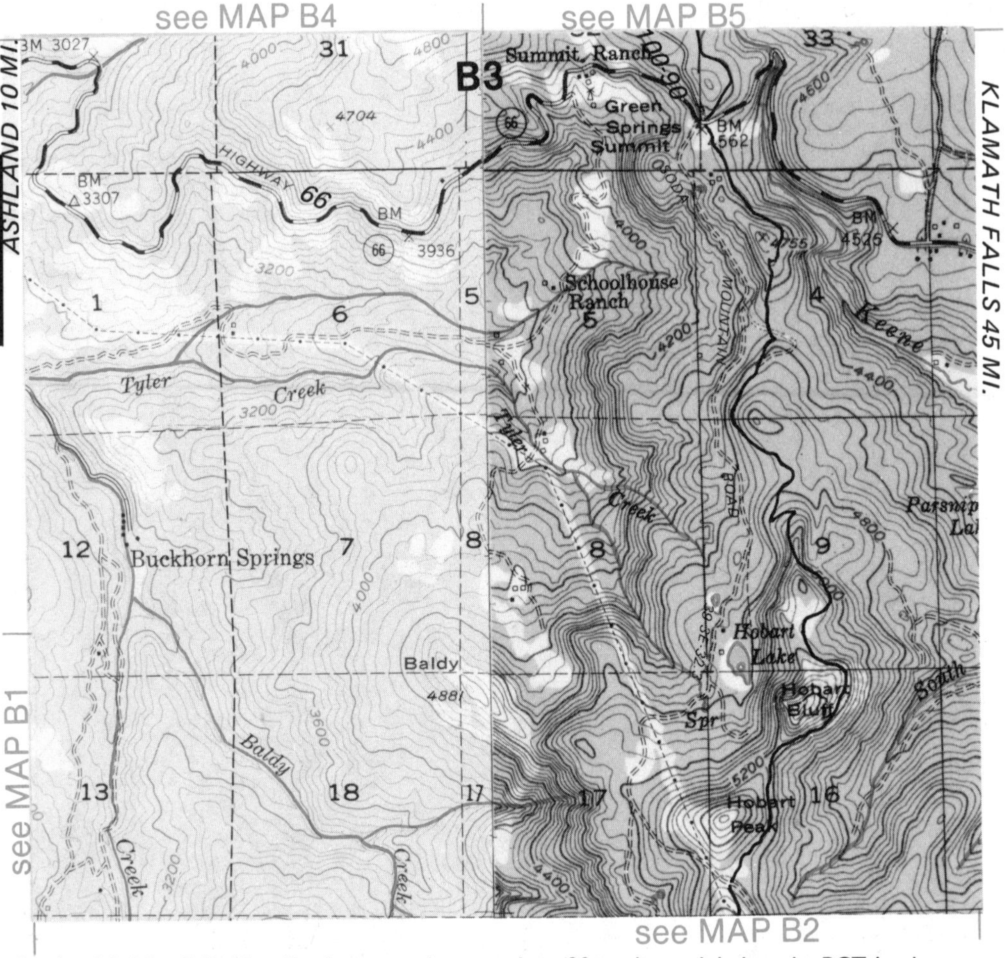

Section 28 (Map B1). Happily, the water situation ahead starts out much better. Since this fenced-in spring is your first reliable water in many miles, you might plan to camp here. The fence keeps out cows—a definite plus—but all the enclosed area is gently sloping—a definite minus.

Still following the jeep road, the PCT descends northeast to a saddle (5140–0.3). From it the Baldy Creek Road descends north, another descends east, a third contours northeast, and just above it your jeep road climbs northeast. The PCT parallels this road's northwest side, twice crosses it, skirts past the south slope (5550–0.9) of unassuming Little Pilot Peak, and then dips to the north side of a saddle (5550–0.1). On this saddle, you could make a small camp by or on the jeep road.

Water access. Here you'll see a tiny, man-made pond on an open slope 90 yards north below the PCT. As always, treat the water before drinking it.

Continue northeast for a ¼-mile traverse and then bend east for a continuing traverse, passing a seeping spring found between two open slopes. Past the second slope, the trail curves northeast, and you quickly see a pond and an adjacent spring-fed tub 80 yards northwest down from the trail (5550–0.8). Before leaving here, tank up, for your next reliable water will be at a spring north of Green Springs Mountain, a dry 8.8 miles away.

Continuing the traverse, you meet an old trail (5560–0.2) that climbs 300 yards to a saddle junction with the Soda Mountain Road. Your companion, the Pilot Rock Jeep Road, ends at this road about 0.3 mile south of the saddle. The PCT stays below the saddle, traversing open slopes that give you views west to Mt. Ashland and all the countryside below. Beyond the views, the trail drops to a shaded

See map B2

saddle (5420–0.6), traverses north along a crest, and then drops past powerlines to a crossing of Soda Springs Road (5300–0.5).

Just east of an open saddle, you start north-northeast through a meadow with vegetation that sometimes obscures the trail, but in 100 yards you re-enter forest cover for a shady traverse around Hobart Peak to a long saddle. One-third mile past it you'll meet the Hobart Bluff spur trail (5220–0.9).

Side route. This trail climbs ⅓ mile to the juniper-capped summit. From it you'll see distant Mt. Shasta to the south-southeast, Soda Mountain to the near south, Pilot Rock behind Hobart Peak to the southwest, Mt. Ashland to the west, the spacious Ashland-Medford Valley to the northwest, and pyramidal Mt. McLoughlin, which you'll see close-up at the start of Section C, to the north-northeast.

From the Hobart Bluff spur trail, the PCT traverses through a woodland of pygmy Oregon oaks before emerging on more-open slopes and then curving northwest down into forest cover. This temporarily gives way to a dry-grassland slope; then the PCT descends north-northeast, giving you a last view of the Ashland environs. You climb again and almost top Peak 4755 and then descend north-northwest, spying Keene Creek reservoir before crossing Highway 66 at Green Springs Summit (4551–3.4).

Water access. You can reach the tempting reservoir by hiking ¼ mile northeast along Highway 66 and then dropping to the nearby shore. Spots of ground are level enough for camping (no campfires, please).

Immediately east of north-climbing Hyatt Lake Recreation Road 100-90, the PCT climbs gently northeast from Green Springs Summit and then rolls northwest across private land, crossing a one-lane road about 90 yards past a small powerline.

Water access. If you need water, head 0.2 mile north down the road to private cattleland, leave the road, and, staying west of a fence, drop to nearby grass-bordered Keene Creek.

Just 0.2 mile past the road crossing on private land, you cross Road 100-90 (4700–1.4) and then climb south-southwest up to a crossing of the Greensprings Mountain Road (4840–0.5). The PCT then continues briefly to the meadow's head, curves north around it, and then closely follows the road almost to a saddle. By the saddle, you cross a spur road (4940–0.7) that climbs briefly west from the main road. Then you cross immediately north of the actual saddle and descend gently northwest to open slopes with views west. The trail quickly turns northeast, and through a shady forest it contours over to, hopefully, a water faucet (4800–0.6), fed by an uphill spring. (Southbound hikers take note: this spring is your last on-route, reliable water until a spring-fed tub of water 8.8 miles away.)

Beyond the faucet, the PCT drops 300 yards to the Greensprings Mountain Road, which you follow northeast for 150 yards and then leave immediately before this road curves northwest for a moderate descent. Back on trail, you descend briefly northeast to jeep tracks beside the Ashland lateral canal (4600–0.5), now a dry gully. ▮ *It once diverted water from Keene Creek west down to Ashland and thence to the Rogue River, but today Keene Creek flows as it used to, ultimately down to the Klamath River.* ▮

The PCT has made a westward diversion of its own—to avoid private property—and it now climbs east to a ridge, drops into a gully, crosses a second ridge, and in a second gully meets a trail (4670–0.9) that climbs northward ¼ mile to Little Hyatt Reservoir. Head east down to the nearby canal, cross it, and then follow it momentarily up to the reservoir's dam and adjacent Hyatt Lake Recreation Road 100-90 (4610–0.2). Under ponderosa pines along the reservoir's east shore, you can fish or just stretch out and relax. Swimming is best near the dam, from which you can dive into the tranquil water. It is a great place for a layover day, for it lacks the noise and congestion found at larger Hyatt and Howard Prairie lakes. At Little Hyatt Reservoir you can camp in the *de facto* campground (with toilet) above the east shore.

Moving along, you find the PCT's resumption 25 yards south of where it ended at Road 100-90. The trail first climbs southeast and barely pokes into Section 28's private land—a totally unnecessary intrusion—and then it

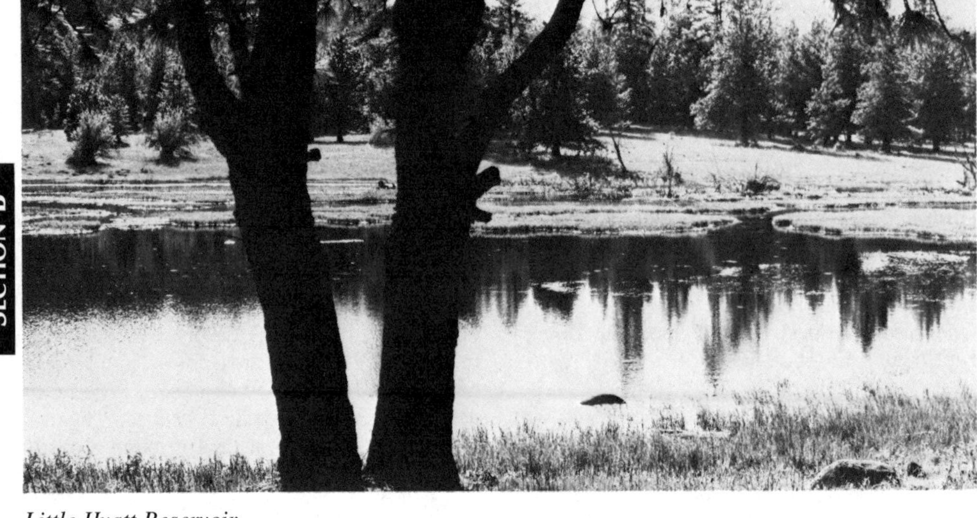

Little Hyatt Reservoir

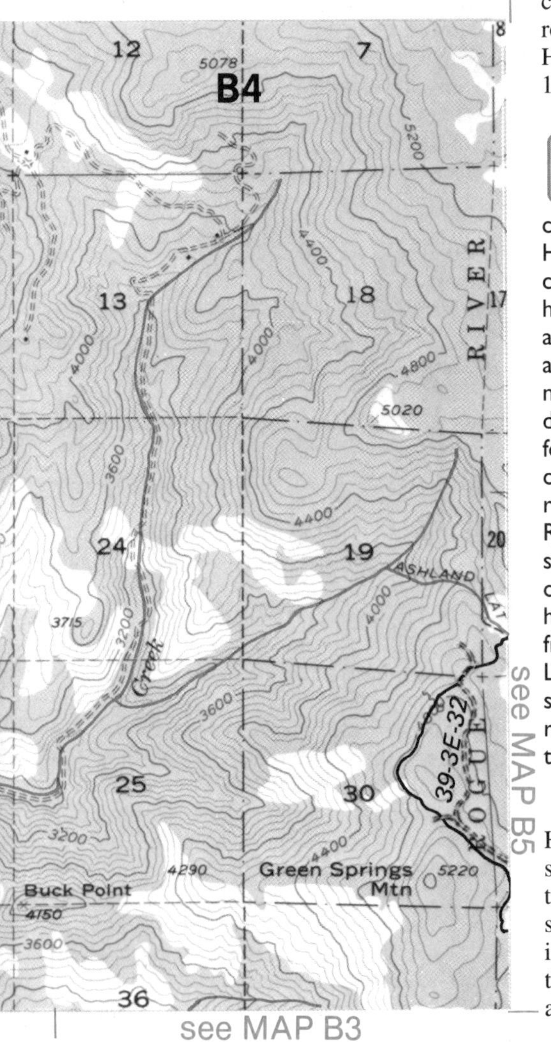

climbs generally northeast past old roads to a road fork (5090–1.5) at which the northbound Hyatt Lake Road branches northwest as Road 100-85 and northeast as Road 100-80.

Resupply access. From this fork, you can follow steps *over* a fence and then follow a trail north ¼ mile to a campsite that is 80 yards west-southwest of Hyatt Lake Campground's shower rooms. The campsite was specifically established for PCT hikers, but because the trail to it is vague, the authors prefer to take the automobile approach. From the road fork, walk 170 yards northeast down to the entrance road, descend another 170 yards to a sign-in, *pay* for a shower, and then take the camp's west-climbing road over to the nearby shower rooms. If you don't camp at Little Hyatt Reservoir, you'll almost certainly want to do so at Hyatt Lake Campground. From the campground's north end, a shoreline trail heads west over to the lake's nearby dam, and from its far side, you can walk over to Hyatt Lake Resort, which has a café and a limited supply of groceries plus showers and a laundry room. By this route, the resort is a ¾ mile side trip from the road fork.

Back at the road fork, the PCT crosses the Hyatt Lake Road and curves east around the south side of the recreation area's administration building. After 280 trail yards, you reach a spur trail that heads north 140 yards to a drinking fountain—installed for PCT hikers—and then continues 100 yards along the building's access road to Road 100-80. The campground

See map B5

entrance road is found 100 yards west on this road. The drinking fountain is your last reliable source of water until Grizzly Creek and its adjacent canal, about 8.5 miles farther.

Beyond the spur trail, the PCT climbs east to a usually dry gully and then traverses northeast, crossing gullies and rounding ridges. The tread stays above usually visible Road 100-80 and snag-tarnished Hyatt Lake. Cross southeast-climbing Road 39-3E-15 (5100–2.1), down which you could walk 160 yards to the main, paved road and then follow it 220 yards west to the entrance road of the Hyatt Lake Overflow Camping Area. Next you wind over to east-climbing Wildcat Glades Road 39-3E-11 (5090–0.9). You could briefly descend this road to the main, paved road and then follow it (or the shoreline) westward to Hyatt Lake North Overflow Camping Area on the lake's peninsula. Heading east on the PCT, you soon cross an older road (5100–0.2) to Wildcat Glades and immediately reach a seeping creek that drains the nearby glades.

Along the seeping creek's north bank, the trail starts upstream but quickly veers north and passes two sets of jeep tracks as it climbs up a ridge. After a switchback, the trail swings to the east side of a secondary summit and then in 200 yards approaches the main one (5540–1.0). The scramble up to it (5610) gives you a disappointing view. Now halfway through this book's Section B, you descend northeast along a crest, almost touch a saddle (5310–0.5), and then turn east for a long descent. Midway along it, a jeep road climbs south across your trail up to a nearby saddle. Just past this road is a fair view of Mt. McLoughlin and Howard Prairie Lake. The descent ends when you cross a road (4620–2.0) that climbs southwest to a nearby rock quarry.

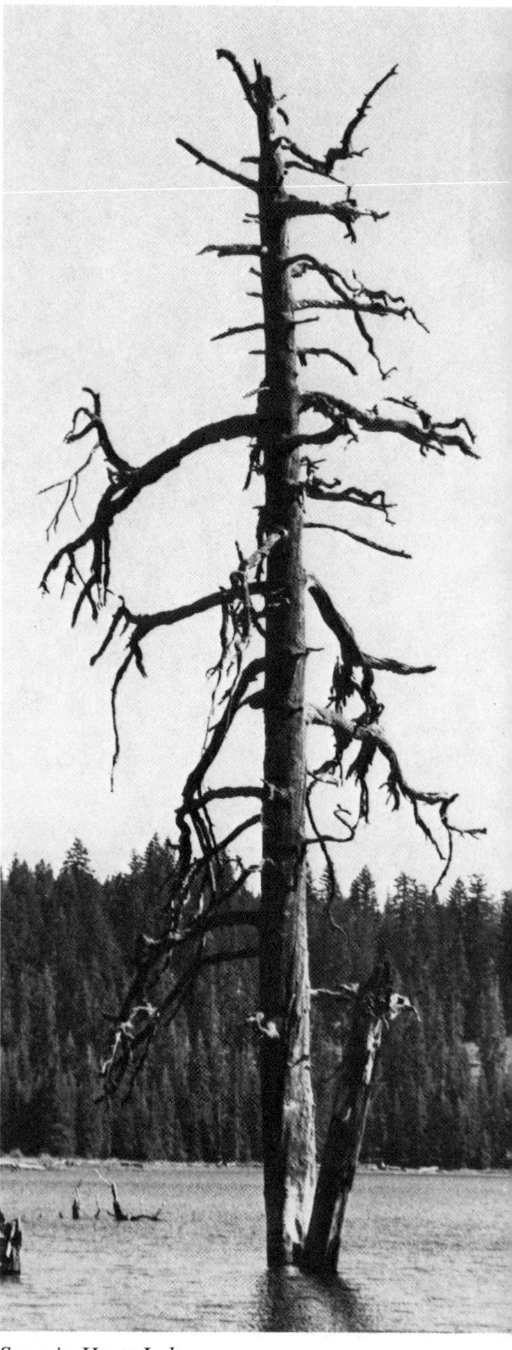

Snag in Hyatt Lake

Side route. At this crossing, you are only a few yards south of a major forest road. You can take it 1.6 miles northwest to a spur road that descends ¼ mile to Howard Prairie Lake and the Willow Point Campground. Just off this spur road, you'll also find a ranger station. From the spur-road junction, you can hike 0.7 mile west up to a paved road, follow it north 1.0 mile, and then branch right 0.4 mile down to bustling Howard Prairie Lake Resort, which logically caters more to boating enthusiasts than to backpackers. However, meals and limited supplies can be bought. Howard Prairie Lake, though shallower than Hyatt Lake, is considerably better

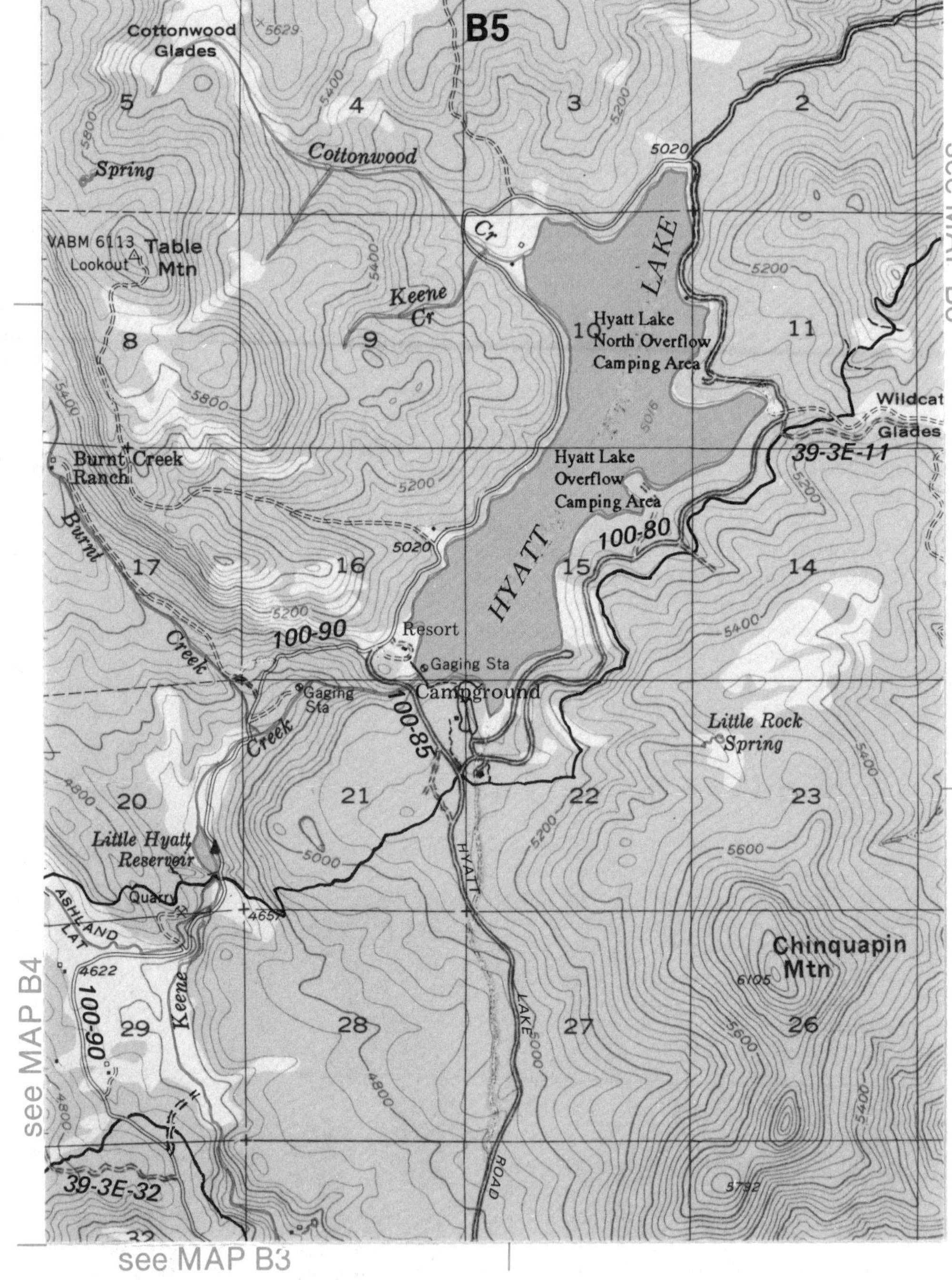

in appearance, since all the trees were removed before its basin was flooded.

From the quarry-road crossing, the PCT parallels the major forest road east to a quick junction (4620–0.1) with a road that descends an easy ½ mile to Soda Creek before climbing ¾ mile to the Wildcat Glades Road. Water obtained from Soda Creek is certainly better than that in Grizzly Creek, your next on-route source. Beyond the Soda Creek road, the PCT crosses a broad, open saddle. At its far end

See map B6

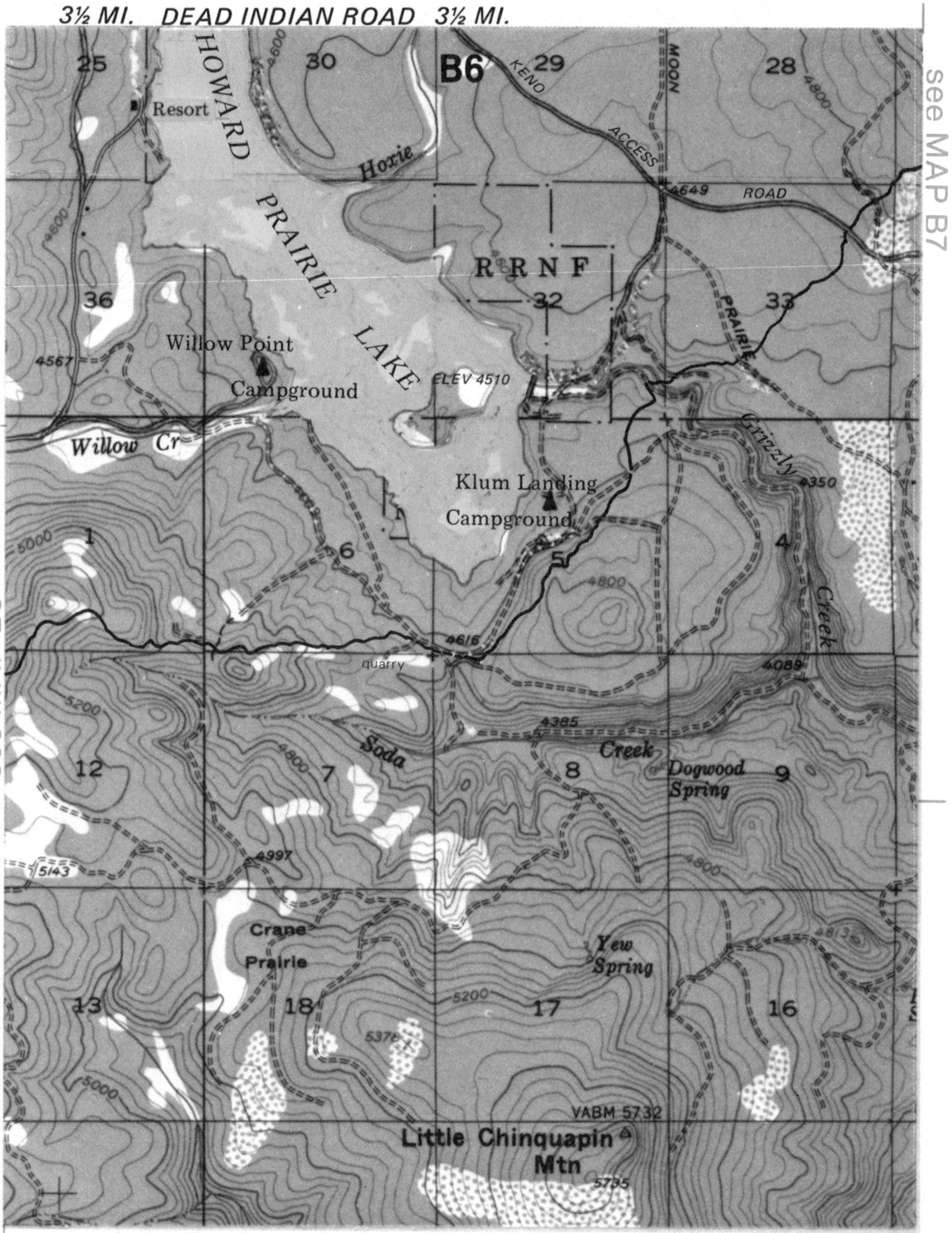

3½ MI. DEAD INDIAN ROAD 3½ MI.

see MAP B7

see MAP B5

(4620–0.2), where a secondary road starts a climb east, the PCT starts a climb northeast and quickly leaves the company of the major forest road.

On the ascent, you get a couple of views down the length of Howard Prairie Lake, but these disappear before the trail's high point, the views being blocked by Douglas-firs, grand firs, sugar pines, and incense-cedars. The easy ascent is mirrored by an equally easy drop to a crossing of a little-used road (4670–0.9).

Side route. You can follow this road 250 yards southwest down to the major forest road and then go an equal distance north on that road to the Klum

see MAP B8

see MAP B6

HIGHWAY 66 18 MI.

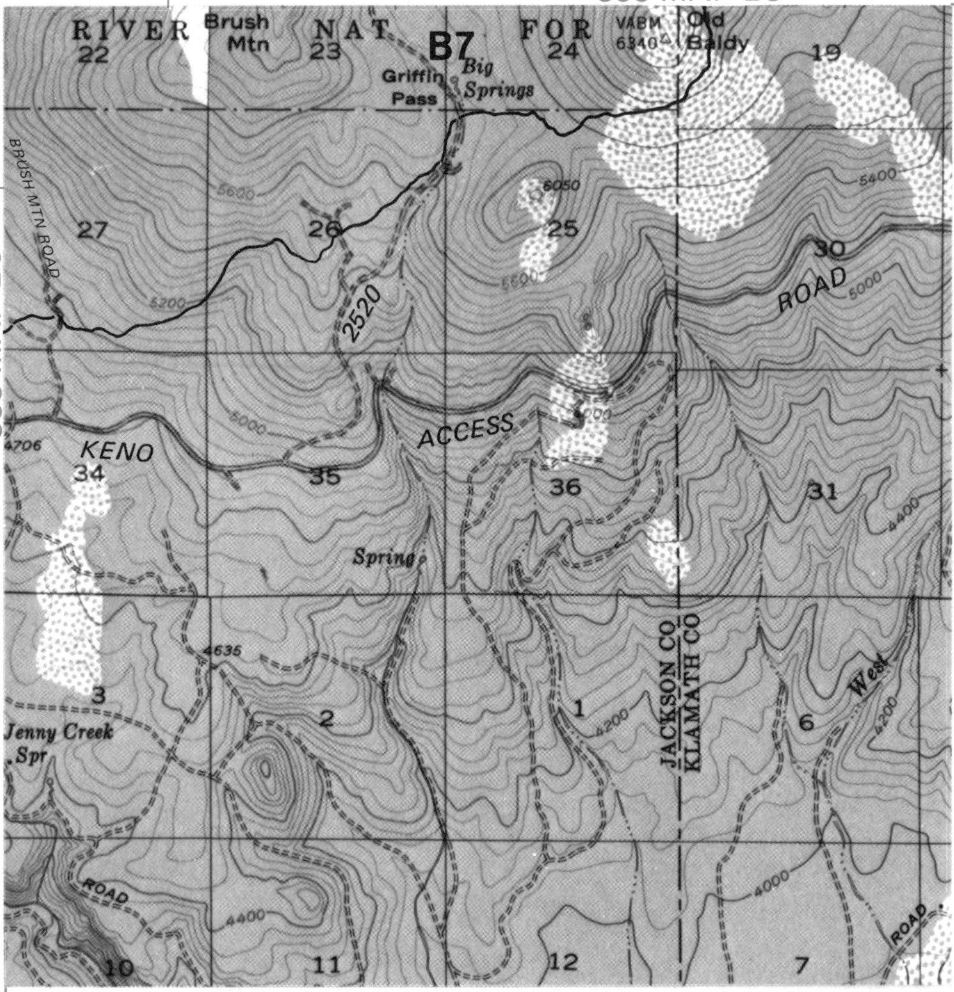

B7

RIVER NAT FOR
Brush Mtn
22 23 24
VABM 6340 Old Baldy
19
Griffin Pass
Big Springs
BRUSH MTN ROAD
5600
6050
27 26 25
5400
30
ROAD
5000
2520
5200
5500
5000
4706
KENO
ACCESS
34 35 36 31
4400
Spring
JACKSON CO
KLAMATH CO
4635
3 2 1 6
West
Jenny Creek Spr
4200
4000
ROAD
4400
10 11 12 7

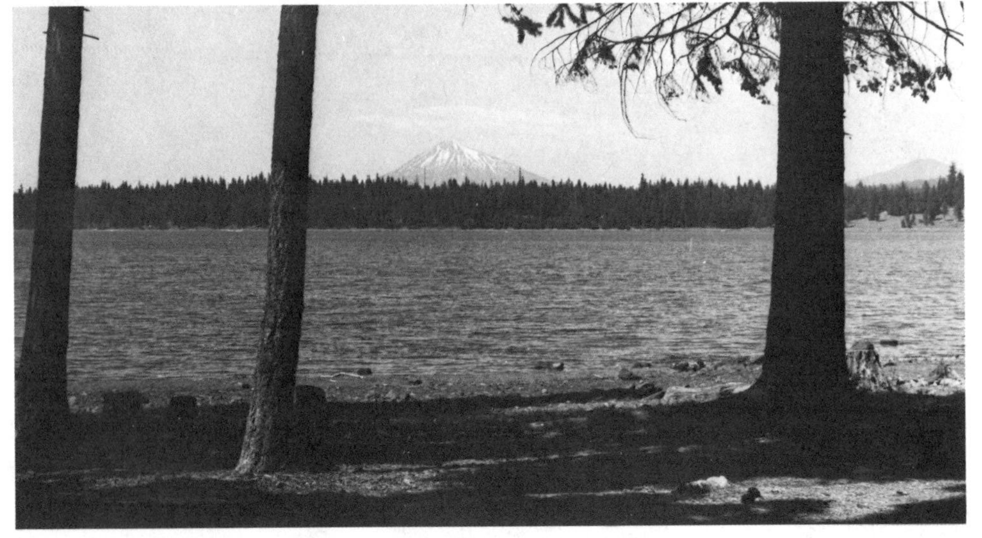

Mt. McLoughlin rising above Howard Prairie Lake

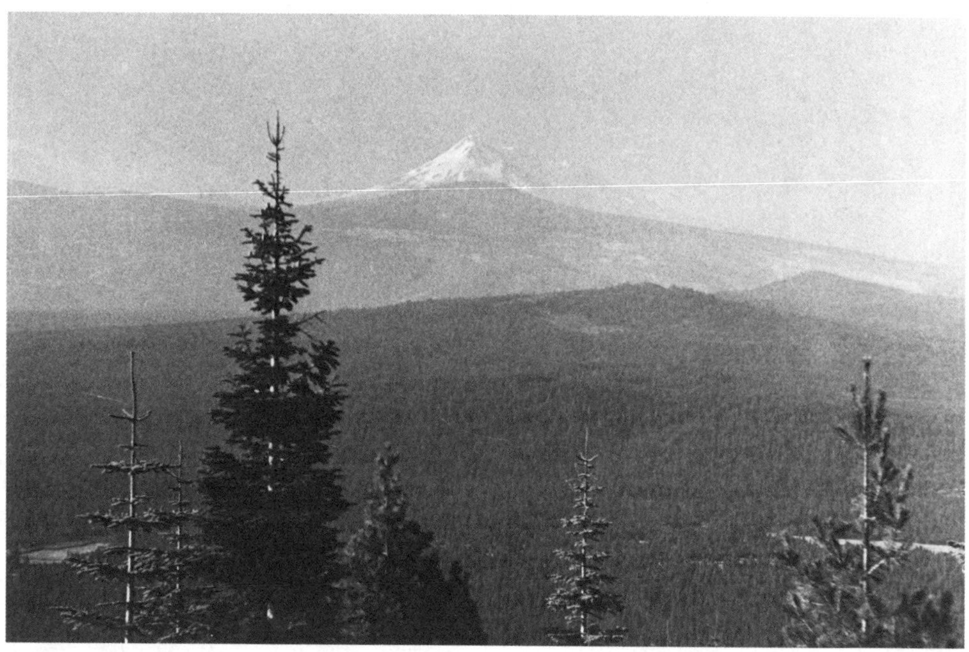

Distant Mt. Shasta, from slopes of Old Baldy

Landing Campground entrance. Like the Little Hyatt Reservoir *de facto* campground, this campground is a good place to spend a layover day. Relax, fish, or perhaps swim out to Howard Prairie Lake's interesting island.

Past the little-used road, the PCT drops northeast to a well-maintained road (4610–0.2) that traverses southwest to the start of the little-used road.

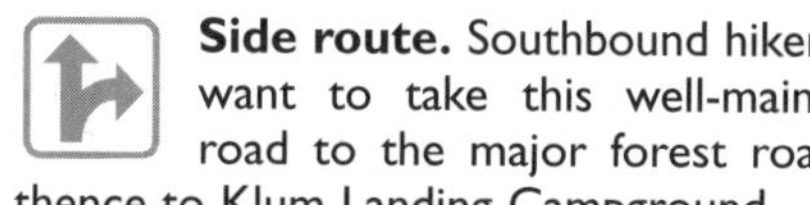

Side route. Southbound hikers may want to take this well-maintained road to the major forest road and thence to Klum Landing Campground.

The PCT now heads north through a meadow whose seasonally tall grasses and herbs can hide the tread. Quickly, however, the trail enters forest cover, the tread becomes obvious, and you wind down to a canal, cross it and its maintenance road, and then drop in 90 yards to a long bridge over Grizzly Creek (4440–0.5). You *could* camp in this area, which is within BLM boundaries, but all too often you would smell the water in both the canal and the creek. Klum Landing Campground is certainly more desirable, even if it is ⅓ mile off route. You are now 8.5 miles past your last on-route water, near Hyatt Lake, and your next reliable on-route water, northeast below Devils Peak, is a ludicrous 48½ miles away. Fortunately, a near-trail source, with plenty of room for camping, lies only 4.0 miles distant.

Working toward the next near-trail water source, you climb east, cross a forgotten road in 160 yards, and then continue up to a crossing of the Moon Prairie Road (4580–0.4). The trail now turns northeast and climbs gently to a crossing of paved Keno Access Road (4720–0.8), a major trans-Cascade route for logging trucks bound for Klamath Falls. The PCT continues northeast and climbs to an old road (4790–0.2) whose traffic was pre-empted by the newer logging road. From it, you round the northwest corner of a clearcut, pass a minor spur road, and then curve east to a bend in the Brush Mountain Road (4960–0.6). Westbound hikers: please note that the last few yards of trail can be hidden by mulleins, thistles, and other "weeds" that characteristically spring up in logging areas; therefore, just plow west from the bend.

You initially climb southeast from the bend but gradually curve northeast up through a shady forest of Douglas-fir and grand fir, cross

See maps B6, B7

see MAP B9

see MAP B10

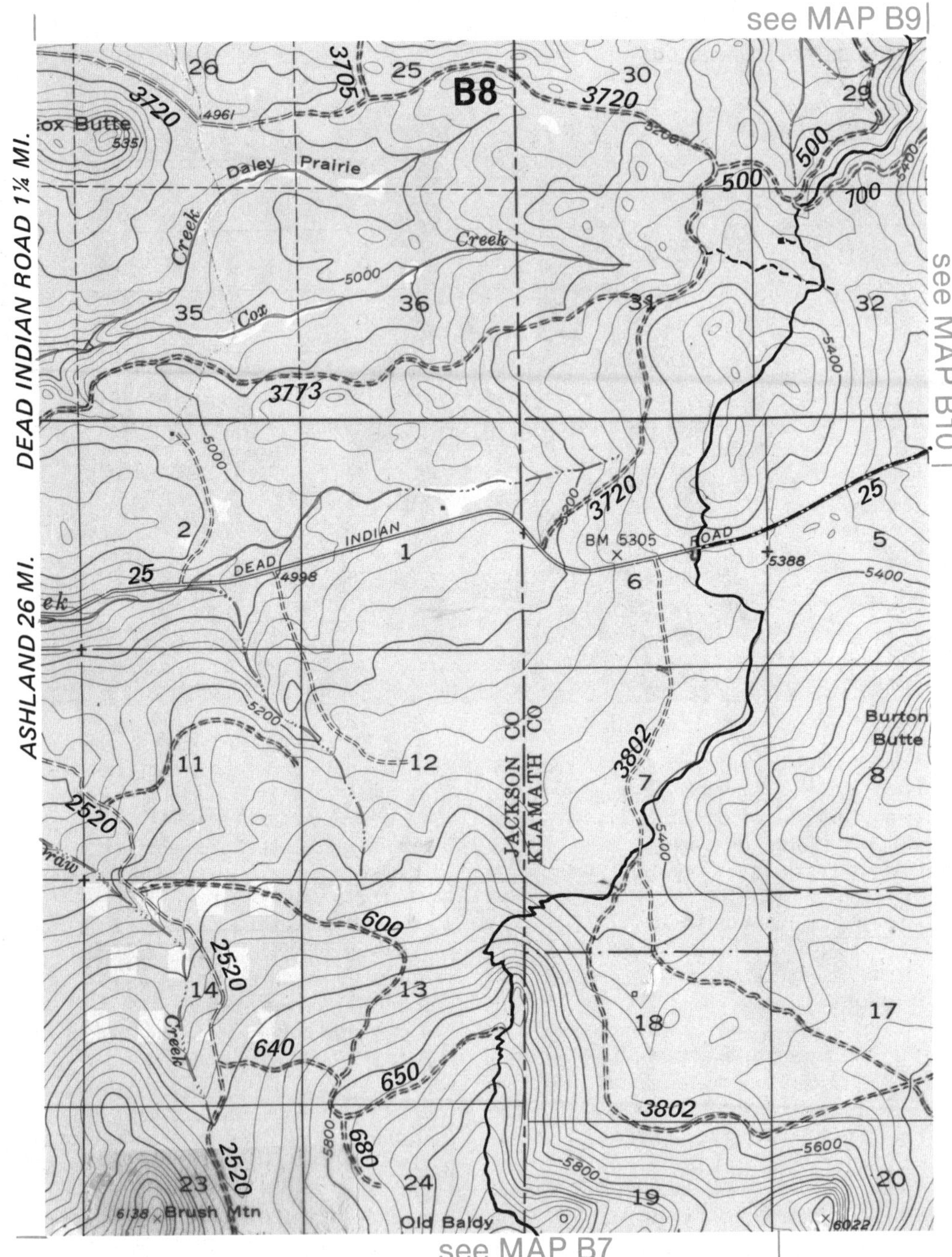

see MAP B7

a broad gully, climb to an adjacent ridge, and just beyond it reach an old logging road (5480–1.5). This descends 0.3 mile to Griffin Pass Road 2520, which is also your immediate objective. Resume a moderate climb northeast and soon approach that road (5640–0.5). The PCT bends north beside this road.

Water access. You should seriously consider walking 25 yards over to the road and down it 75 yards to an eastbound spur road. This spur road immediately crosses a creeklet that has been dammed, thus providing the hiker with a pond of fresh water, the last reliable source until the

See map B7

off-route Fish Lake Resort, a long 19.4 miles ahead. Since most long-distance backpackers average 15–20 miles a day, they should plan to camp here one night and then at Fish Lake the following night.

Where the PCT turns north, it parallels Road 2520 up to a crossing (5670–0.2) that is 250 yards short of ill-defined Griffin Pass. Still on BLM land, you parallel the Rogue River National Forest boundary east, immediately crossing the seasonal Big Springs creeklet. In ⅓ mile, the trail bends southeast for a brief climb to a broad, shady saddle; then it angles northeast for a brief, moderate climb to Old Baldy's clearcut slopes. The ascent east around this conical landmark is an easy one, and its brushy terrain allows plenty of views south across miles of forest to majestic Mt. Shasta.

Chinquapin, tobacco brush, and greenleaf manzanita yield to noble fir as the curving trail climbs to a northeast spur ridge, from which you traverse 140 yards northwest to the Rogue River National Forest boundary (6190–1.7). ▮ *Before 1972, the PCT route followed the old Oregon Skyline Trail route—mostly roads in southern Oregon—and it came up to a now-abandoned trail to the boundary. In pre-1972 days, the "PCT" headed north directly from Shasta rather than making the giant swing west to the Marble Mountains as it does today.* ▮

Side route. You can scramble south to Old Baldy's nearby summit (6340′) for 360° views. Abandoned by fire lookouts, it is now under the watchful eyes of turkey vultures. From it you can see Mt. Shasta (bearing 176°), Yreka (185°), Soda Mountain (217°), Pilot Rock (223°), Hyatt Reservoir and Mt. Ashland (242°), and Mt. McLoughlin (354°). With these landmarks identified, a careful observer should be able to trace the PCT route over miles of country.

Now within Forest Service land, as you'll be almost continually to the Washington border, you start northwest and quickly bend north to descend a pleasant, forested ridge. Approaching a ridge saddle, you come upon a faint spur trail (5880–1.0), which heads 140 yards west to Road 650. Beyond the spur trail, the PCT touches upon the saddle and then switchbacks down the northwest slopes of the ridge, swings east almost to Road 3802, turns north, and quickly crosses a closed road (5390–1.2). Parallel Road 3802, soon cross it (5390–0.3), and then wind north to a trailhead parking area by a crossing of Dead Indian Road (5360–1.9). The parking area is about 300 yards east of the road's junction with Road 3802. If you are covering hundreds of miles of PCT rather than just Section B, you may want to follow Dead Indian Road over to Lake of the Woods Resort. This alternate route is described at the end of this section.

Northbound, the PCT climbs away from Dead Indian Road, cuts northeast across a broad ridgecrest, and then descends through an old logging area to a broad saddle traversed by an abandoned road, a route now used in winter by snowmobilers. About 0.3 mile north of it, you reach an important junction (5330–1.7).

Water access. The spur trail west goes a mere 180 yards to the 12-foot-square Brown Shelter, with space for five. More important is an obvious well, situated about 10 yards from the shelter.

Onward, the PCT winds north briefly down to a crossing of Road 700 (5270–0.2). This crossing is about 100 yards south of the road's junction with Road 500, which makes a loop—as your trail does—round the headwaters of South Fork Little Butte Creek.

From Road 740, the PCT first contours northeast and then north, paralleling Road 500, which you sometimes see below as you cross an old logging area. Some gullies you cross may contain water, particularly if you are hiking through in the mosquito-plagued month of June. Finally, the trail drops to cross the Brown Mountain Trail branch of South Fork Little Butte Creek (5180–2.2).

The PCT follows the seasonal creek westward until the stream angles south; then the trail traverses west for ½ mile before turning northwest and dropping 20 feet to a hollow. A 60-foot gain northwest from it takes you to a minor ridge (5210–1.4).

Water access. Should you need water, you can either leave the trail in the hollow and head about 300 yards south-southwest to the nearby creek, or else

See maps B7, B8, B9

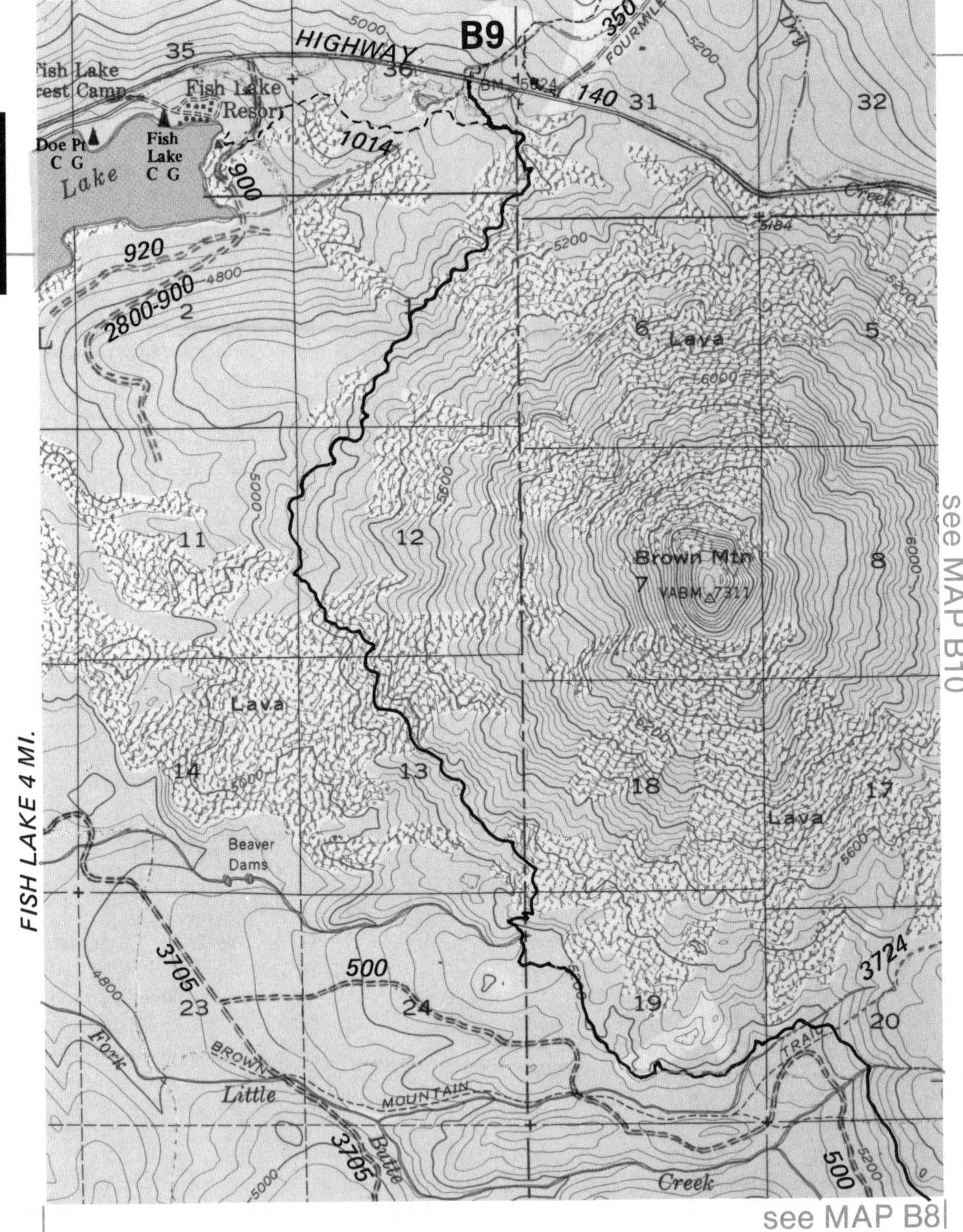

leave the trail from the minor ridge and descend about 200 yards southwest to Road 500, and then follow it ¼ mile south to the creek.

From the ridge, the trail continues its long, irregular arc around the lower slopes of Brown Mountain. Although the trail on the map superficially appears to be an easy traverse, careful study of it reveals that it has plenty of ups and downs—some of them steep—as you'll find out. Traversing the northwest slopes of Brown Mountain, views of Mt. McLoughlin—a dormant volcano—appear and disappear. Nearing Highway 140, you reach a junction with Fish Lake Trail 1014 (4940–5.8).

See map B9

Resupply access. Unless you are ending your hike at Highway 140, you'll want to visit the Fish Lake environs both for water and for supplies. A layover day wouldn't hurt. Trail 1014 winds ⅓ mile down to a seasonal pond, soon crosses the equally seasonal Cascade Canal, rambles across varied slopes, and then treads a stringer separating a youthful upper lava flow from an equally youthful lower one. Next, it descends more or less alongside the lower flow and intersections Road 900 just before that road starts a traverse across the flow. With 1.5 miles between you and the PCT, you wind 100 yards west to a junction just before Fish Lake. Here, a spur trail branches left, going 55 yards to a PCT campsite perched above the lake's shore. However, you might want to head 300 yards, first north and then west over to Fish Lake Resort's campground. Note the trail's end, for it may not be too obvious, and you'll want to find it later when you return to the PCT. But first, head over to the resort's office and café, located just above the boat dock. Food and supplies cater to the beer-drinking fishing crowd, though a beer (or two) will probably sound very tempting after your long, dry haul. Pick up your parcel if you've mailed one to the resort. You can get a hot meal and a shower (or take a swim) and then perhaps do some laundry before returning to the PCT campsite.

See map B9

Mt. McLoughlin and Lake of the Woods early in the morning

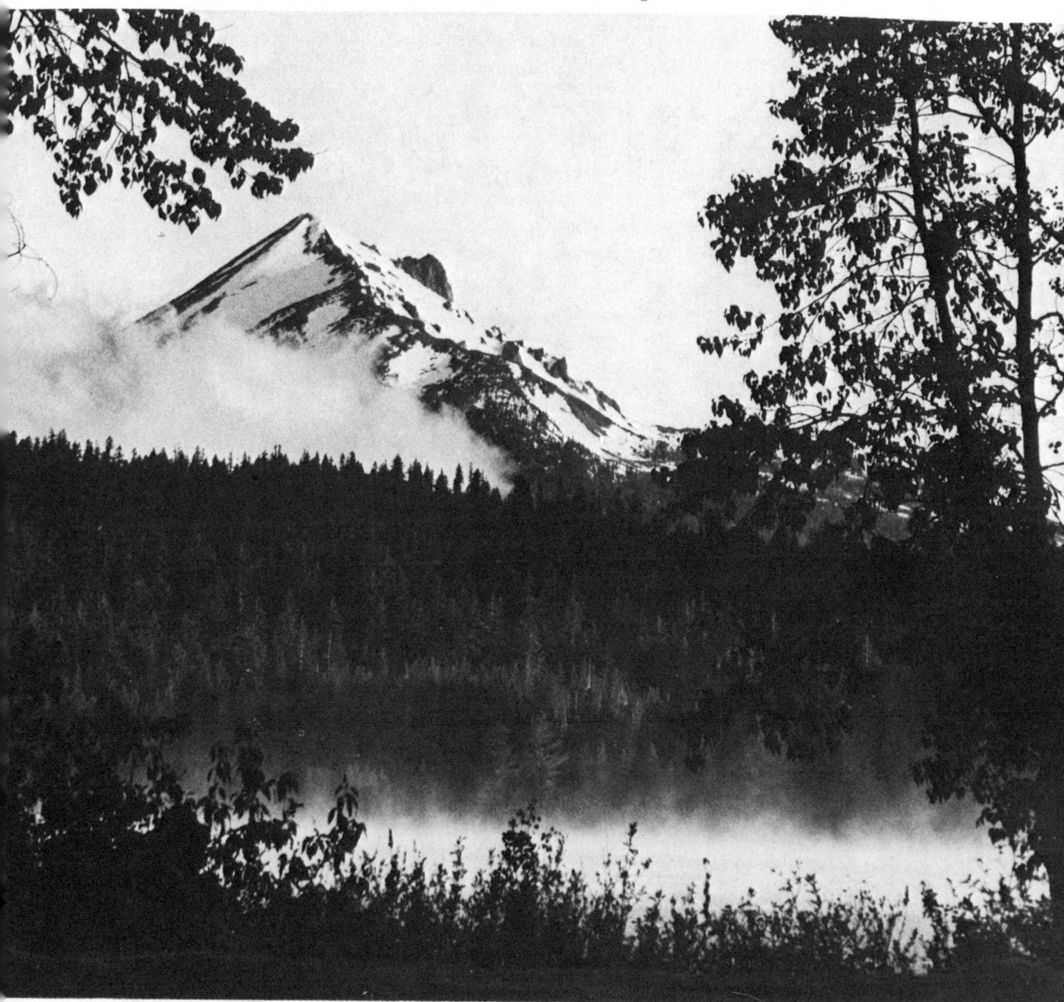

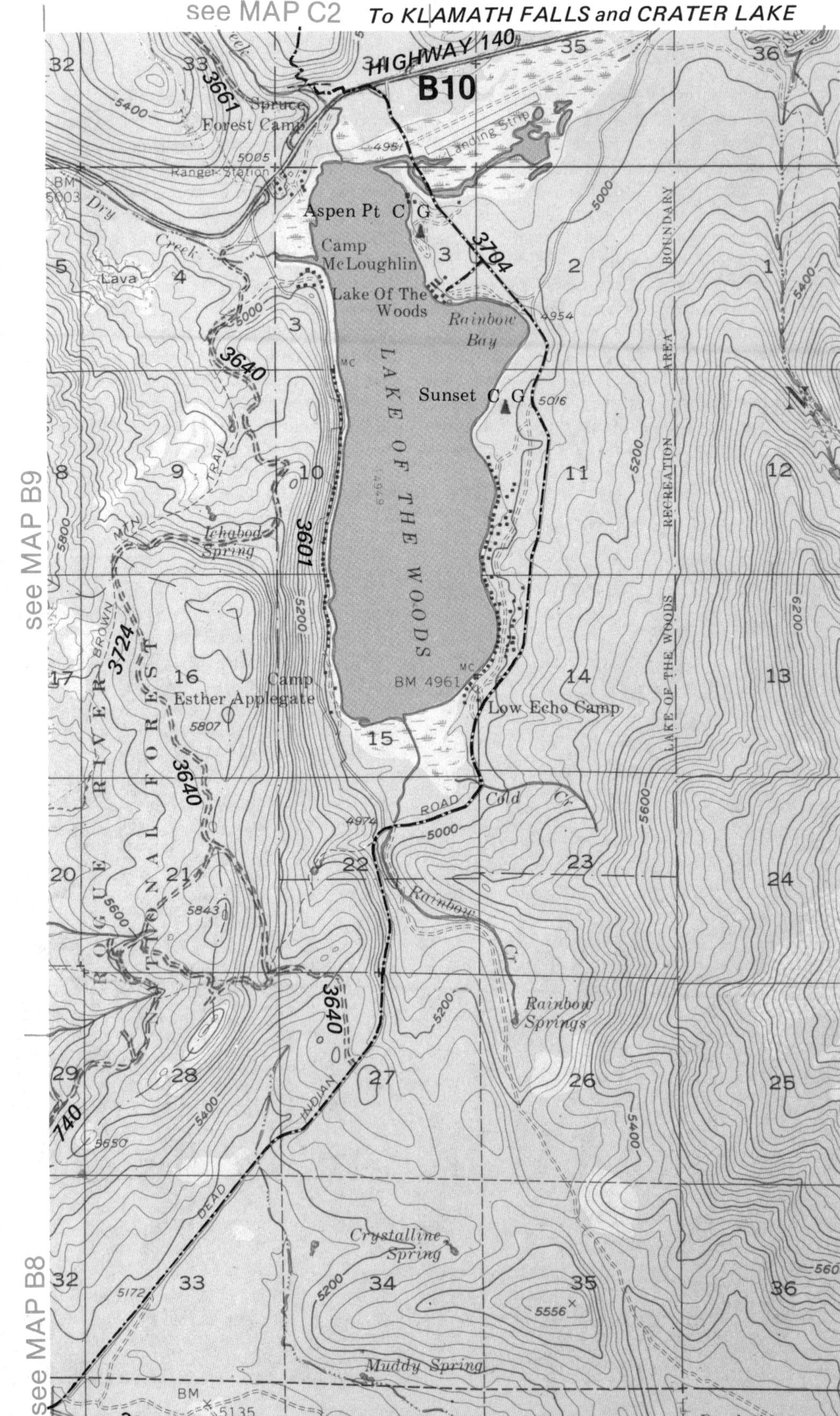

see MAP C2
To KLAMATH FALLS and CRATER LAKE
HIGHWAY 140
B10
Spruce Forest Camp
Ranger Station
Landing Strip
Dry Creek
Lava
Aspen Pt C G
Camp McLoughlin
Lake Of The Woods
Rainbow Bay
Sunset C G
LAKE OF THE WOODS
Ichabod Spring
Camp Esther Applegate
Low Echo Camp
Cold Cr.
Rainbow Cr.
Rainbow Springs
Crystalline Spring
Muddy Spring
ROGUE RIVER NATIONAL FOREST
LAKE OF THE WOODS RECREATION AREA BOUNDARY
DEAD INDIAN ROAD
see MAP B9
see MAP B8
3661
3704
3640
3601
3724
740

After your stay at Fish Lake, return via Trail 1014 to the PCT. In 85 yards along the PCT you cross an old, abandoned highway bed and then soon reach broad, straight Highway 140 (4980–0.2). Cascade Canal crosses under Highway 140 about 40 yards west of your crossing. You'll meet the canal just beyond the highway. Don't expect any water flowing in it after midsummer. The first near-trail water will be at Freye Lake, ¼ mile off the PCT and 4¾ miles from the highway.

Alternate route. Those who take the Lake of the Woods alternate route will reach Highway 140 about 4½ miles east of the PCT's highway crossing. However, rather than traverse west to it, they will climb north to meet it in popular Sky Lakes Wilderness. By climbing north you pass more than a dozen lakes worth camping at, plus about two dozen trailside ponds—quite a contrast with the virtually waterless PCT segment to which this is an alternate.

The alternate route begins where the PCT crosses Dead Indian Road. It climbs east ¼ mile from the PCT to the Cascade crest and then descends to a junction with Lake of the Woods' West Shore Road 3601 (4974–4.7).

The hungry PCT trekker bears east from the junction and then curves north to pass the Winema National Forest East Side Recreation Residences along the shore, before reaching the entrance to Sunset Campground (4990–2.2). In summer this is crowded with water-skiers, swimmers, campers, and anglers. You'll find the lake's waters are stocked with Kokanee salmon, rainbow and eastern brook trout, and brown bullhead.

Continuing north, you reach a junction with Road 3704 (4954–1.0), along which you trek northwest to a spur road (5000–0.3) that heads ¼ mile southwest down to the lakeshore and the Lake of the Woods Resort. Here you can restock with enough supplies to last you until Crater Lake Post Office, 52 miles away by this alternate route. The resort also serves good meals, and its store has a small post office at which you can pick up goodies you've mailed to yourself.

Back on Road 3704, continue northwest past the entrance to Aspen Point Campground (4970–0.4), which is also the entrance to a picnic area and a safe swimming area. If you haven't yet taken a dip, do so here. Onward, you reach Highway 140 (4980–0.7), which you then take 0.2 mile west to a pole-line road. Start north but in 5 yards branch right from it, making a hairpin turn onto a minor road. Follow it 100 yards to the start of Rye Spur Trail 3771 (4990–0.3). Measuring 9.6 miles from the PCT crossing at Dead Indian Road, this alternate route to a Highway 140 trailhead is about 2 miles shorter than the PCT route. A continuation of this alternate route, which is also shorter than the continued PCT route, is described in the early part of Section C.

See maps B8, B9, B10

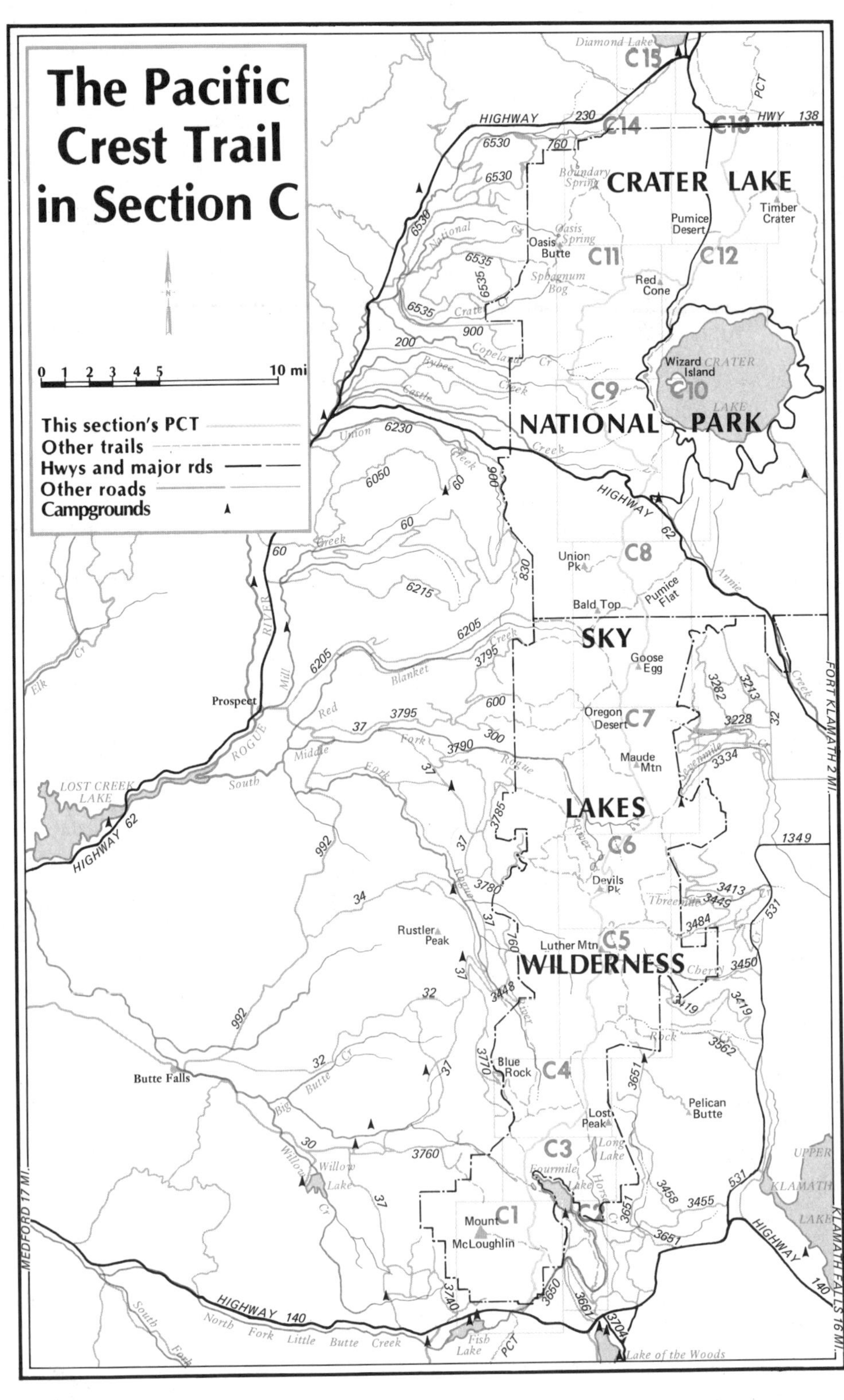
The Pacific Crest Trail in Section C
0 1 2 3 4 5 10 mi
This section's PCT
Other trails
Hwys and major rds
Other roads
Campgrounds
Diamond Lake
C15
PCT
HIGHWAY 230
HWY 138
C14
C13
760
6530
Boundary Spring
CRATER LAKE
Timber Crater
Pumice Desert
Oasis Butte
Oasis Spring
C11
C12
6535
National Cr
Sphagnum Bog
Red Cone
Crater
900
200
Copeland Cr
Bybee Creek
Castle
Wizard Island
CRATER LAKE
C9
C10
NATIONAL PARK
Union 6230
Creek
6050
60
HIGHWAY 62
C8
Union Pk
Pumice Flat
Bald Top
Annie
830
6215
6205
SKY
Goose Egg
Elk Cr
RIVER
Mill
Prospect
Blanket
Red
3795
600
300
Oregon Desert
C7
3282
3213
3228
32
FORT KLAMATH 2 MI.
37
3790
Fork
Middle Fork
Rogue
Sevenmile Cr
3334
Maude Mtn
ROGUE
South
LOST CREEK LAKE
LAKES
3785
C6
1349
HIGHWAY 62
992
Devils Pk
34
3780
3413
3445
Threemile
3484
531
Rustler Peak
Luther Mtn
C5
WILDERNESS
Cherry
3450
32
3448
River
3419
Rock Cr
3562
Butte Falls
3770
Blue Rock
C4
3651
Big Butte Cr
Lost Peak
Pelican Butte
30
3760
C3
Long Lake
Willow Cr
Willow Lake
Fourmile Lake
Horse Cr
3458
3455
UPPER KLAMATH LAKE
Mount McLoughlin
C1
C2
HIGHWAY 140
KLAMATH FALLS 16 MI.
MEDFORD 17 MI.
South Fork
3740
3650
3661
3704
North Fork Little Butte Creek
Fish Lake
Lake of the Woods

Section C: Highway 140 near Fish Lake Highway 138 near the Cascade Crest

Introduction: Both Sections A and B have a paucity of lakes and a surplus of roads, but in Section C the scenery changes, and at last you feel you are in a mountain wilderness. In fact, before the mid-1970s, the scenery south of Highway 140 was deemed too poor to have a crest trail, and in those days, anyone who hiked from northern California to southern Oregon had to follow a route that was almost entirely along roads.

The bulk of Section C is composed of two attractive areas: Sky Lakes Wilderness and inspiring Crater Lake National Park. The number of lakes in the wilderness rivals that in any other mountain area to be found anywhere along the PCT, while the beauty and depth of Crater Lake make it a worldwide attraction.

Unfortunately, the original PCT route avoided Crater Lake entirely, taking a low route, mostly along old closed roads, along the lower slopes of the former volcano, Mt. Mazama. So back in our first edition (1974), we recommended an alternate, soon to become popular, route, mostly along paved Rim Drive, that traversed Crater Lake's west rim. Some use trails existed along the rim, and in the 1990s the Park Service linked these with new tread to produce an alternate, hiker-only PCT rim route. Equestrians, unfortunately, still must take the low route. These alternate routes and others in Sky Lakes Wilderness are described along with the regular PCT route.

Declination: 17½°E

Points on Route	S➤N	Mi. Btwn. Pts.	N➤S
Highway 140 near Fish Lake	0.0		76.0
Mt. McLoughlin Trail, westbound	4.7	4.7	71.3
Red Lake Trail (cross the alternate route)	13.9	9.2	62.1
Snow Lakes Trail (end of alternate route)	23.5	9.6	52.5
Devils Peak/Lee Peak saddle	25.9	2.4	50.1
Middle Fork Basin Trail to Ranger Springs	31.8	5.9	44.2
Jack Spring spur trail	36.4	4.6	39.8
Stuart Falls Trail, northeast end	3.7	7.3	32.3
Highway 62	8.9	5.2	27.1
Lightning Springs Trail	55.4	6.5	20.6
Red Cone Spring	63.3	7.9	12.7
North-rim access road	67.2	3.9	8.8
Highway 138 near the Cascade crest	76.0	8.8	0.0

Supplies: There are no on-route supply points, but an alternate route is described that takes you past the Crater Lake Post Office (97604), which is found in the same building as the Park Headquarters. This building is about 55½ trail miles north of Fish Lake Resort, in northern Section B, and about 29 miles south of Diamond Lake Resort, in southern Section D. On your mailed parcels, mark your estimated time of arrival, because the post office does not like to hold them very long. Below the post office is Mazama Village, which has an inn, campground, store, and coin-operated laundry and showers. Above the post office is the Rim Village, with meals and limited supplies.

Wilderness Permits and Special Restrictions: To camp in the Crater Lake National Park backcountry, you'll need a wilderness permit. It doesn't matter whether you are on foot, horseback, or skis, or whether you are entering on a popular summer weekend or in the dead of winter—they are still required. In person, you can get a permit either at the Park Headquarters or at the Rim Village Visitor Center. You can also get a permit in advance by writing to Superintendent, P.O. Box 7, Crater Lake National Park, Crater Lake, OR 97604, or you can phone park personnel at (503) 594-2211. Note that if you're trekking north or south through the park, you should find self-registration stations.

There are specific camping restrictions at the park. No camping is allowed within one mile of any paved road, nature trail, or developed area, and none is allowed within 1½ miles of Sphagnum Bog or Boundary Springs. As in any wilderness area, no camping is allowed in meadows or within 100 feet of any water source. The size of each backcountry party is limited to a maximum of 12 persons and 8 head of stock.

Problems: Sky Lakes Wilderness is an area of abundant precipitation and abundant lakelets. Both combine to ensure a tremendous mosquito population that will ruin your hike if you're caught without a tent. However, by mid-July the mosquito population begins to drop, and by early August a tent may not be necessary.

Since Crater Lake National Park lacks ponds and lakelets and also has a paucity of flowing streams, you would expect it to also be mosquito-free, right? Sorry, it isn't. This is because the lake's rim receives a yearly average of 48 feet of snowfall, and the resulting snowpack provides moist, mosquito-bearing ground through most of July. This same snowpack also can make hiking difficult before mid-July, but in early August, after the snowpack has disappeared, drinking water may become scarce. From midsummer onward, the stretch from Red Cone Spring to Section D's Thielsen Creek, a 21-mile stretch, may be dry.

Maps:

Mount McLoughlin, OR
Lake of the Woods North, OR
Pelican Butte, OR
Devils Peak, OR
Union Peak, OR
Crater Lake West, OR
Pumice Desert West, OR
Pumice Desert East, OR

THE ROUTE

Official PCT route. A large trailhead parking lot is provided for those hikers who plan to leave their vehicles along Highway 140. There is a signed road to this lot that begins 0.4 mile east of the PCT's highway crossing. From the sign, you go 15 yards north on Fourmile Lake Road 3650, turn left, and parallel the highway west to the nearby lot. From the lot's northwest corner a trail goes 0.2 mile north to the PCT. Don't park at the small space where the PCT crosses the highway, since long-distance backpackers may want to camp there when water is available in the adjacent Cascade Canal.

This description begins where the PCT starts north from Highway 140 (4980). This point is just 0.2 mile west of the Jackson/Klamath county line and 40 yards east of the Cascade Canal. Just after you start up this trail, you bridge this seasonally flowing canal and then parallel it northeast to a junction (5100–0.3) with the short trail back to the large

See maps C1

trailhead parking lot. Just past this junction, the trail almost touches the canal before it angles away and ascends open slopes that provide a view south toward Brown Mountain and its basalt flows. As the PCT climbs, it enters Sky Lakes Wilderness, where it crosses lava flows, and then it enters a white-fir forest and continues up to a junction with Mt. McLoughlin Trail 3716 (6110–4.0) in a forest of red firs and mountain hemlocks.

Side route (from official PCT only). Southeast, this heavily used trail descends 1.0 mile to a trailhead at Road 3650. Years ago it was used to descend 3.0 additional miles to the Highway 140/Road 3601 intersection near the Lake of the Woods Work Center/Visitor Center. As in the past, those hiking the last part of Section B along the lake's west shore, would take this trail to regain the PCT.

On the PCT, which briefly doubles as the Mt. McLoughlin Trail, climb shortly west on an easier grade to the Freye Lake spur trail (6190–0.2), which is just 50 yards past a gully; this trail goes ¼ mile over to the shallow, semi-stagnant lake and its camps. Walk an equally short distance west on the PCT (6240–0.2).

Side route (from official PCT only). Here, the Mt. McLoughlin Trail takes its leave, climbing 3½ miles up to the summit of this dormant stratovolcano. The views you get from it are among the best obtained from any peak situated near the tri-state PCT. If you have good weather, don't pass up the opportunity to climb it. Drop your heavy backpack nearby and take 2 or 3 hours to reach the often-snowy summit. On your return, you can sometimes use tempting snowfields to speed your descent, but be forewarned that these can lead you astray, as they diverge south-southeast from the east-descending trail.

Leaving the west-climbing Mt. McLoughlin Trail, the PCT quickly tops a ridge, then winds slowly down through the forest, not once offering a view, and comes to a junction with the Twin Ponds Trail (5840–3.7). This junction lies between two shallow ponds that by late summer are no more than dry, grassy meadows.

Side route (from official PCT only). Small campsites can be found at Summit Lake, 0.4 mile northwest down this trail, but beyond the lake, the trail, which is numbered 993, becomes very brushy. To the southeast the trail is numbered 3715, and it winds 2.5 miles to a trailhead at the west end of Fourmile Lake Campground.

From the junction your trail starts northeast, quickly veers north past a stagnant pond, climbs steadily up a ridge, and then descends slightly to a junction with Cat Hill Way Trail 992 (6100–1.6).

Side route (from official PCT only). This path climbs 3.6 miles north to a popular trailhead, which also serves more-popular Blue Canyon Trail 982. Southward from your junction, note the abandoned tread of deteriorating Blue Rock Trail 3737, which can still be followed 2.0 miles, passing Fourmile Lake before ending at the Twin Ponds Trail, along the south shore of Squaw Lake.

Your trail heads north to a gully that is snowbound until late June and then veers east up to a gentle slope before curving northeast and climbing to a broad saddle (6300–1.6). The route now contours across a slope forested with mountain hemlock, red fir, and western white pine. You round a north ridge, descend southeast to another saddle (6240–1.2), and by going about 50 yards north can find a spring. Ahead on the PCT, you bear northeast down toward a saddle to reach the PCT's southern junction with Red Lake Trail 987 (6020–1.1), where the alternate route from Section B, below, rejoins the official PCT.

Alternate route (continued from Section B). Some hikers may have taken Section B's alternate route that guides them first to Lake of the Woods Resort for supplies and then north to Highway 140. The following description takes them on an 11.2-mile route north back to the Red Lake Trail junction with the PCT. This stretch, 2.7 miles shorter than the comparable stretch of PCT, provides you with a lower, lake-dotted alternate route from Highway 140.

See maps C1, C3, C4, B10

see MAP C3

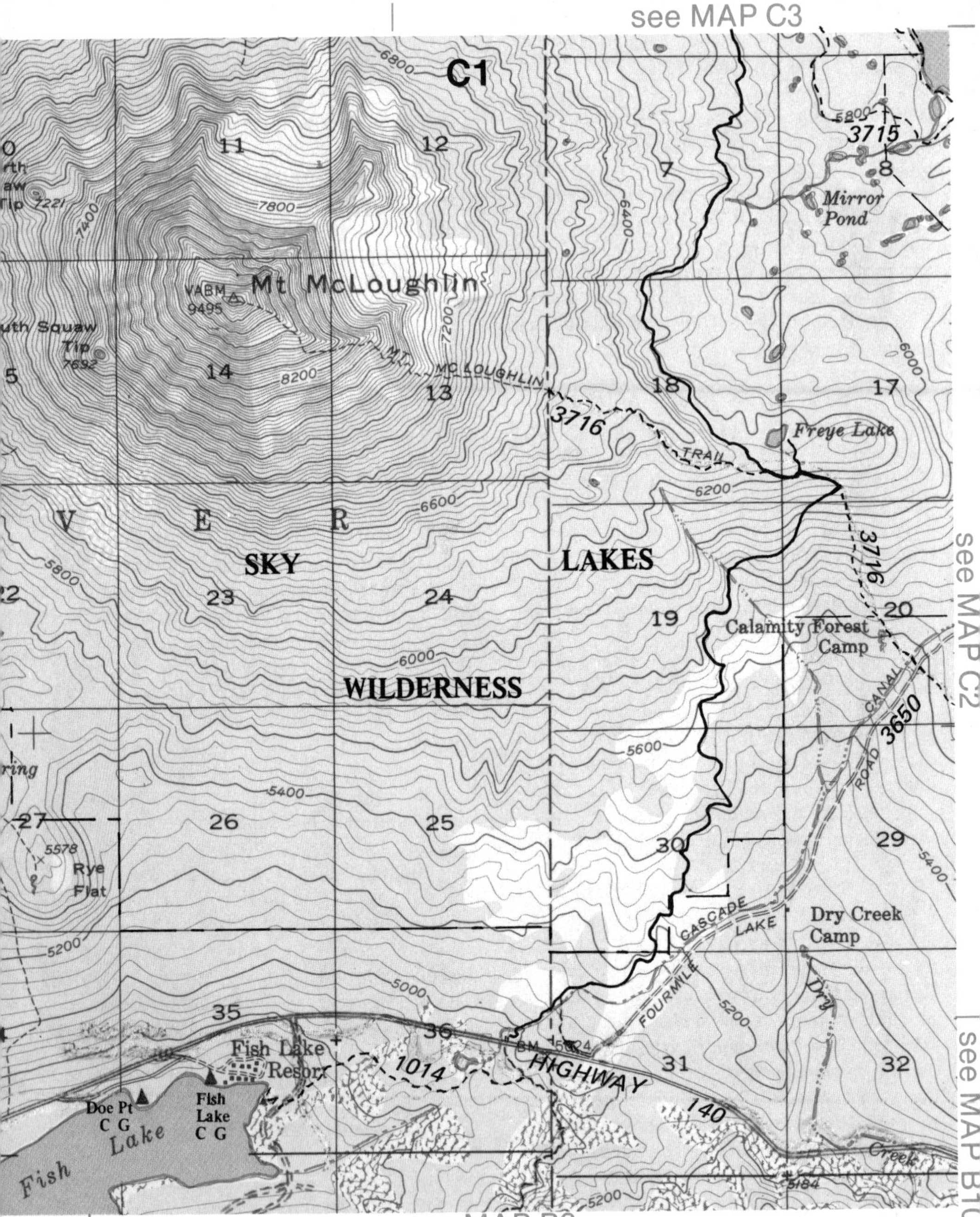

see MAP C2

see MAP B10

see MAP B9

To reach the trailhead, start from the north end of Lake of the Woods' east-shore Road 3704, which ends at Highway 140. Walk 0.2 mile west on the highway and then branch north onto a pole-line road. (If you're eastbound on the highway, you'll find this road about 250 yards east of Billie Creek.) You go but 5 yards north on the road and then branch right, making a hairpin turn onto a minor road. Follow it 100 yards to the trailhead, located just before the pole line. Your mileage begins from here (4990).

Rye Spur Trail 3771 starts west and quickly meets the Billie Creek Nature Trail (5000–0.2), which continues west for a loop around a part of Billie Creek. Your Rye Spur Trail switchbacks

See map B10

steeply northward and then climbs at an easier pace to Road 3633 (5290–0.5). Walk 160 yards northwest up it to the Cascade Canal (5701–0.8); in early summer the canal flows swiftly, but by August it can be bone-dry. The Rye Spur Trail continues climbing northward until it reaches the first of three clustered outcrops (6230–1.2). ▌ *Here you get some fine views of the scenery from Pelican Butte to the northeast, across to Mountain Lakes Wilderness to the southeast.* ▌ Beyond the outcrops, your views disappear, and you hike at a leisurely pace to a recrossing of the Cascade Canal (5730–3.3). This point is but 30 yards down the canal's road from a parking area by Fourmile Lake's dam. Had you hiked north along the canal road to this point, rather than taking the Rye Spur Trail, you'd have saved yourself 0.2 mile distance and about 500 feet of climbing effort. If evening is fast approaching, you can mosey west a short ½ mile to the lake's campground and then on the next day either continue along the alternate route or take Twin Ponds Trail 3715 a rolling 2.5 miles over to the PCT.

Keeping to the alternate route, you walk but 30 yards east down the canal's road to the start of Long Lake Trail 3759. Just 35 yards up this trail you meet Fourmile Creek Trail 3714, forking right. The Long Lake Trail visits two of Fourmile Lake's lodgepole-snag bays, presenting views of Mt. McLoughlin and its avalanche-prone lower slopes. Now entering Sky Lakes Wilderness, you climb ½ mile to Woodpecker Lake, which is mostly less than chest deep. In ¼ mile you reach more appealing Badger Lake (5910–1.6), with better fishing and swimming than its neighbor; look for a fairly nice campsite by the lake's northeast edge. Next the trail passes knee-deep Lilly Pond and then passes a marshy meadow, both of interest to wildflower enthusiasts. Northward, there's seasonally boggy terrain to traverse, and then you climb ½ mile northeast to a junction with Long Lake Trail 3713 (6050–1.7). This winds 0.3 mile east to a junction near the south shore of Long Lake. From it, abandoned Horse Creek Trail 3741 departs south down Long Creek, while a spur trail shoots east to a good south-shore campsite. The lake is quite shallow, though deep enough to support trout and to offer some fair swimming.

This alternate route, part of the defunct Oregon Skyline Trail, immediately begins a ½-mile easy descent northeast to the west shore of Long Lake and then continues north along it to a junction (6050–0.8) by the lake's north shore. Eastward, a spur trail goes over to Long Lake Camp, spacious enough for group camping. Be aware that mosquitoes can plague the site as late as early August. North of Long Lake, this fault-line trail crosses an unnoticeable gentle divide and then descends past a marshy meadow on its way down to a junction with Lost Creek Trail 3712 (6000–1.0). This

See maps B10, C2

see MAP C3

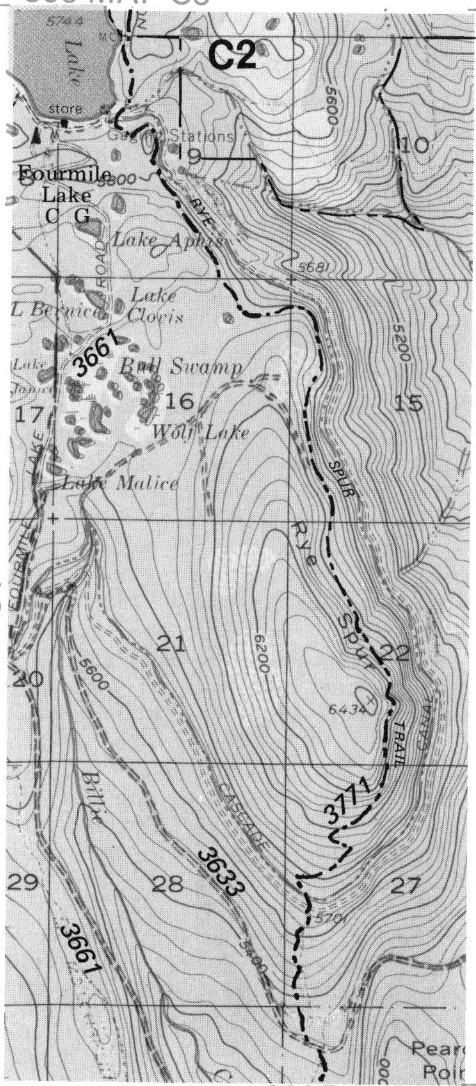

see MAP C1

see MAP B10

See maps C2, C3, C4

trail quickly rounds Center Lake, which is knee-deep in its prime but only a grassy meadow in late summer; then Trail 3712 descends 1⅓ easy miles to a switchback in Road 3659 (just off Map C4). Eastward, this road goes 1.3 miles to a main road, 3659, which northward ends in 1.7 miles at Cold Springs Campground.

At the Lost Creek Trail junction, Long Lake Trail 3759 ends and Red Lake Trail 987 begins. Climb over an adjacent ridge and immediately intersect the PCT (6020–0.1–11.2).

Official PCT and alternate route from Section B rejoined. You're immediately confronted with a choice between the official PCT route, following, and another alternate route, below, which the authors recommend.

Official PCT route. From its southern junction with the Red Lake Trail, the PCT makes a quite level, easy traverse north, staying close to a fault-line crest, until it reaches its northern junction with the Red Lake Trail (6070–2.7).

Alternate route. A more rewarding alternate to the PCT's essentially viewless traverse is to continue along the Red Lake Trail to this junction. Along this route, you first make a short, moderate descent to the east end of Blue Canyon Trail 982 (5900–0.2). Westward, you can follow it 0.4 mile to a good spur trail that goes 130 yards north to Island Lake's most abundant campsites. Secluded ones lie above the lake's west shore. Onward, the Red Lake Trail heads through huckleberry bogs to a junction by the northeast corner of Island Lake (5910–0.5). From an adjacent campsite, a *de facto* trail goes 0.4 mile west to very pleasing Dee Lake. You'll find an improved horse camp on the low ridge separating Dee and Island lakes. Dee is an excellent lake for swimming—shallow enough to have warm water, yet deep enough that it isn't an oversized swamp like the north half of Island Lake, which is mostly less than waist-deep.

Beyond Island Lake your boggy, huckleberry-laden route north passes several ponds that are more suited to mosquitoes than to humans and then arrives at large but grassy and extremely shallow Red Lake, with possible camping and fishing. After another ½ mile walk north past this lake, you reach a junction (5870–1.4). Ahead, the old Red Lake Trail is abandoned, so climb east moderately up the new Red Lake Trail to rejoin the PCT (6070–0.7–2.8).

With the official PCT and the alternate route rejoined at this junction, the PCT makes an easy, viewless, uneventful climb northeast to the start of another lake-studded route, the southwest end of Sky Lakes Trail 3762 (6140–1.0). At this junction, you have a choice of routes, the official PCT route, following, or several alternate routes that all begin on the Sky Lakes Trail, below. The authors highly recommend the alternate routes.

Official PCT route. Where the Sky Lakes Trail departs from the PCT toward the escarpment above Deer Lake, the PCT heads north-northwest in a forest of lodgepole pines and mountain hemlocks, ascends a gentle slope past several nearby ponds, and then reaches an open forest as it approaches a cliff above the Dwarf Lakes Area. ▮ *Glaciated Pelican Butte (8036) is the prominent summit in the southeast; the more subdued Cherry Peak (6623) is directly east. You can't see the lakes below because the area so forested.* ▮ The trail switchbacks slightly up to avoid the cliff, switchbacks slightly down the west side, and soon encounters a 100-yard spur trail (6600–2.5) to an overlook with a view that encompasses most of the rolling hills to the west. Now you switchback several times up to a small summit before descending the ridgeline to a saddle and an intersection of abandoned Wickiup Trail 986/3728 (6585–1.0).

The PCT now takes you northeast up to a ridge where the views east of the Sky Lakes Basin really begin to open up. ▮ *Along the trail segment that crosses a barren slope of volcanic blocks, you are likely to find, sprouting in the thin volcanic soil, numerous creamy-white western pasqueflowers (also called anemones), which are readily identified by their finely dissected leaves, hairy stems, and dozens of stamens. By August, their flowers are transformed into balls of silky plumes.* ▮ The trail contours north-northeast to the west edge of a saddle and reaches Divide Trail 3717 (6840–1.2). If you have the time, climb nearby Luther Mountain for stupendous views of the Sky Lakes Area; see the end of "Diverting to the Divide Trail to Luther Mountain and the PCT" in the Alternate routes, below.

see MAP C5

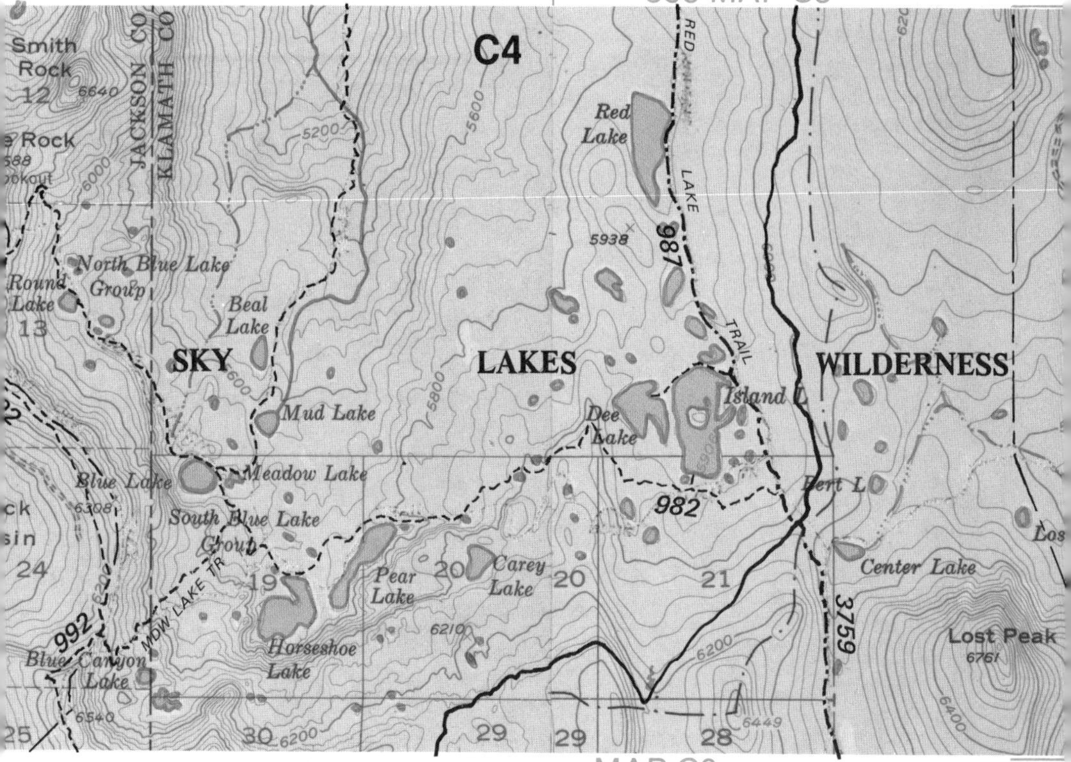
C4
Smith Rock
12
6640
JACKSON CO
KLAMATH CO
Rock
Lookout
5200
5600
Red Lake
RED LAKE TRAIL
987
5938
North Blue Lake Group
Round Lake
13
Beal Lake
SKY
LAKES
WILDERNESS
Mud Lake
5800
Dee Lake
Island L
Meadow Lake
Blue Lake
6308
Bert L
South Blue Lake Group
982
24
MDW LAKE TR
19
Pear Lake
20
Carey Lake
20
21
Center Lake
3759
992
6210
Horseshoe Lake
Lost Peak
6761
Blue Canyon Lake
6200
6540
6400
25
30
6200
29
29
28
6449

see MAP C3

see MAP C4

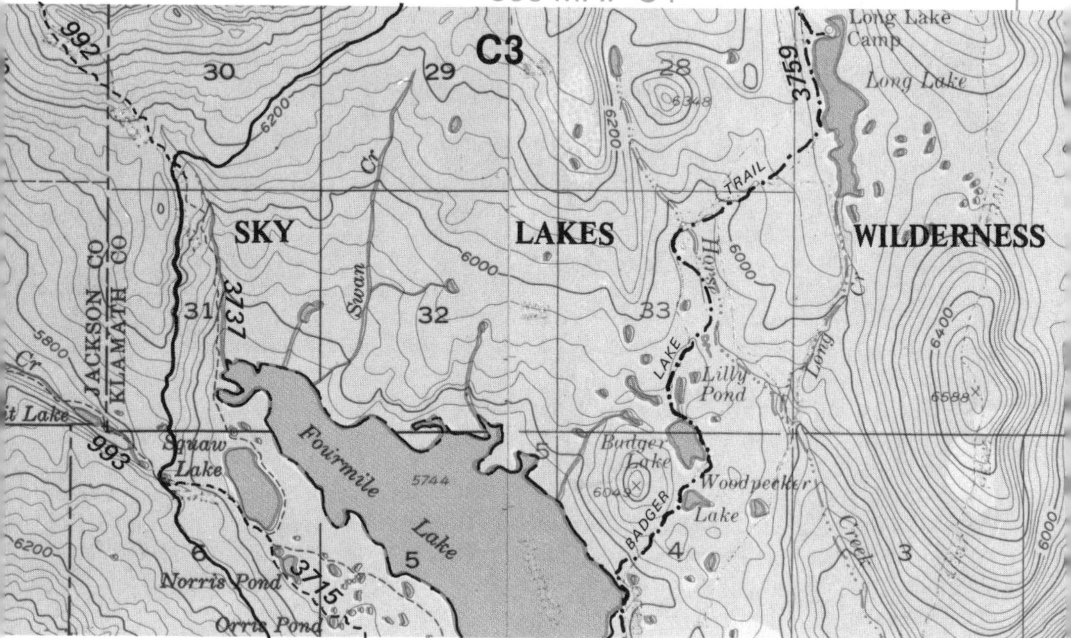
C3
992
30
29
28
6348
Long Lake Camp
Long Lake
3759
6200
TRAIL
SKY
LAKES
WILDERNESS
6000
Swan Cr
Horse
6000
JACKSON CO
KLAMATH CO
31
3737
32
33
6400
5800
LAKE
Lilly Pond
Long Cr
6588
993
Squaw Lake
Fourmile Lake
5744
Budger Lake
6049
Woodpecker Lake
BADGER
6200
6
5
4
3
Creek
6000
Norris Pond
3715
Orris Pond

see MAP C1
see MAP C2

see MAP C6

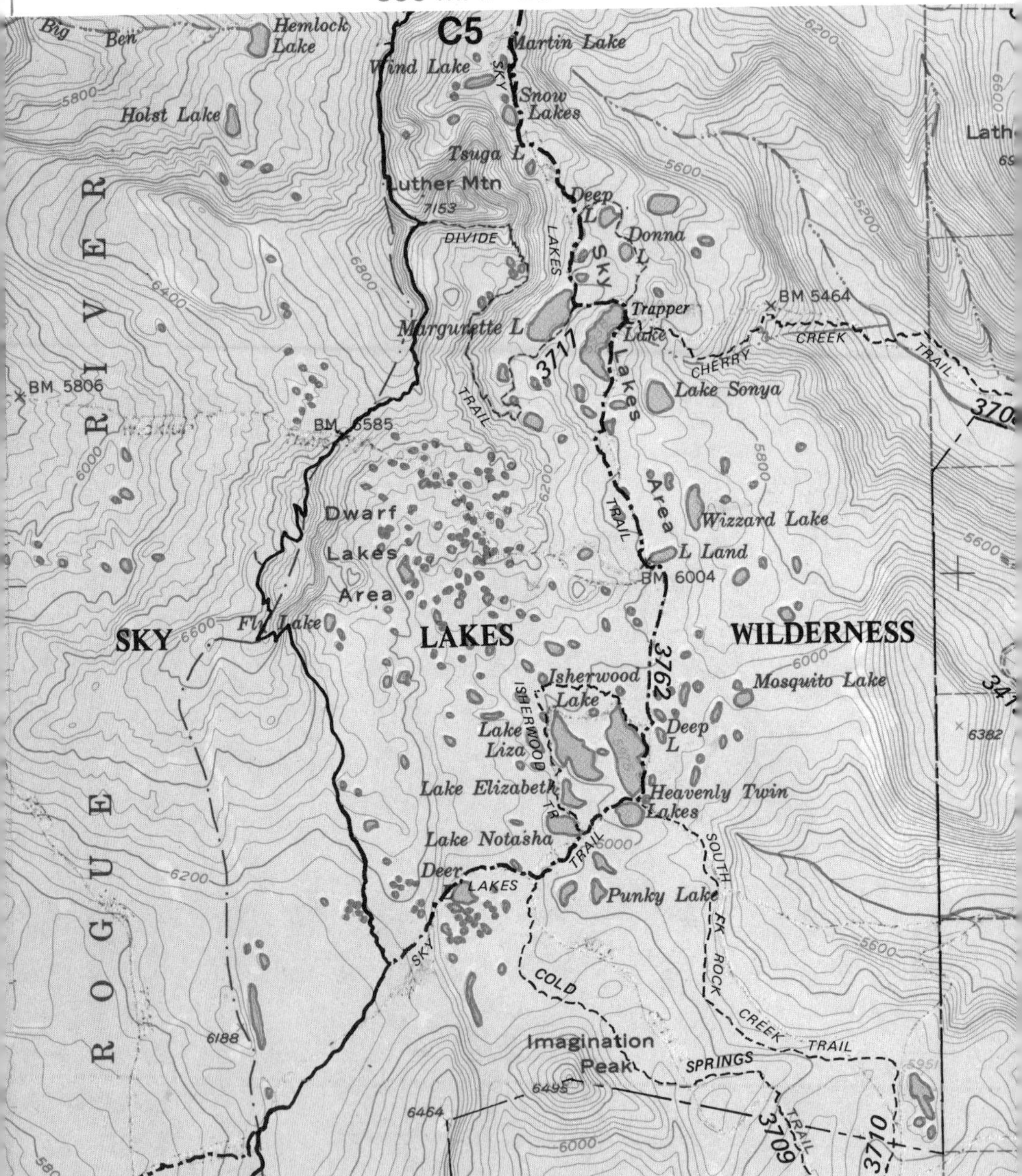

C5

see MAP C4

COLD SPR. C.G. and ROAD 3651 ¼ MI.

Side route (from official PCT only). The 2.6-mile Divide Trail strikes due east across the rocky slopes of this peak (7153), makes ten switchbacks down to three presentable ponds, and then winds gradually down to the Sky Lakes Trail junction at Margurette Lake (6010), but not before passing virtually every body of water in the vicinity. This is quite a lovely side trip to take if you are not in a hurry.

From the Divide Trail saddle, you descend moderately to a ridge and follow it north as it gradually levels off to a junction with abandoned Hemlock Lake Trail 985 (6600–1.0). After starting up the crest, you quickly meet

Snow Lakes Trail 3739 (6670–0.2). This junction is not only the end of the highly recommended alternate route, it offers those who've stayed on the official PCT a little side route that happens to be the last bit of the alternate route.

Side route (from official PCT only). A 0.2-mile traverse on Snow Lakes Trail 3739 takes you over to the first of a pair of Snow Lakes, the environs offering scenic, relatively mosquito-free camps.

Alternate routes. Several optional routes are possible, and they'll add 2–3 miles to your hiking distance as compared to the PCT.

Start northeast on the Sky Lakes Trail, which was once part of the now-defunct Oregon Skyline Trail. Soon you crest a broad divide and then make a moderate ¼-mile diagonal down a fault escarpment before leveling off near mostly shallow Deer Lake (6070–0.5). Some folks camp here, but far better camping, fishing, and swimming lie ahead. Eastward, you arc past a pond to a junction with Cold Springs Trail 3710 (6050– 0.4), which winds 2.6 miles over to Cold Springs Campground. Next, your trail winds northeast to a junction with Isherwood Trail 3729 (6030–0.3).

Diverting to the Isherwood Trail. The 1.5-mile Isherwood Trail is 0.8 mile longer than the Sky Lakes Trail counterpart, but it passes five lakes and a greater number of campsites. Just a stone's throw over a low ridge, the Isherwood Trail comes to Lake Notasha. This lake, with a camp above its east shore, is the deepest of the five lakes, and it is the only one stocked with both rainbow and brook trout. Another low ridge separates Notasha from Elizabeth, which is shallow enough for warm swimming, yet deep enough to sustain trout. Next, you drop to the brink of a fault escarpment along the west shore of Isherwood Lake, one of the few lakes in the wilderness you can dive directly into; for most lakes, you have to wade out into deep water. From a horse camp midway along the escarpment, you can walk due west to adjacent, chest-deep Lake Liza, with marginal appeal. Beyond Isherwood, the trail winds north to a meadow and then veers east to the north tip of north Heavenly Twin Lake. For isolated camps, look for sites above its west shore. After passing a northeast-shore camp, the Isherwood Trail ends at the Sky Lakes Trail just southwest of shallow Deep Lake.

Staying on the Sky Lakes Trail. If you shun the Isherwood Trail, your Sky Lakes Trail soon passes between the Heavenly Twin Lakes, the smaller, deeper southern one being far less attractive than the northern one. Look for secluded camps along the latter's west shore. By these two lakes, you reach a junction with misnamed South Rock Creek Trail 3709 (5980–0.3), which traverses 3.1 miles over to Cold Springs Campground. The Sky Lakes Trail turns north, skirts along the east shore of northern Heavenly Twin Lake, and then meets the northeast end of the Isherwood Trail (5980–0.4).

Sky Lakes and Isherwood trails rejoin. From this junction, you continue north past chest-deep "Deep" Lake and its seasonal satellites and reach abandoned Wickiup Trail 3728 (6004–0.9). Shallow, uninviting Lake Land lies just below the trail's east end. The lake at best provides some warm swimming; however, you'd be better off visiting Wizzard Lake, a fairly deep lake just 200 yards northeast below Lake Land's outlet. Next, you soon pass a knee-deep pond on the right and then, past a low ridge, two waist-deep lakelets. The south shore of Trapper Lake lies just ahead, and from the point where you see it, you could go 250 yards cross-country southeast to 38-foot-deep Lake Sonya, easily the basin's deepest lake. More likely, you'll want to camp at the east-shore sites of scenic Trapper Lake. By this lake's outlet, you meet Cherry Creek Trail 3708 (5940–1.2), which descends 5.2 miles to a trailhead at Road 3450. This road in turn descends 1.9 miles to heavily traveled County Route 531, should you need to vacate the wilderness. From the upper end of the Cherry Creek Trail, you walk but a minute north along Trapper Lake to its northeast corner, where you meet Donna Lake Trail 3734.

Diverting to the Donna Lake Trail. This 0.9-mile trail makes an initial ascent northeast before curving past Donna and Deep lakes and then climbing back to the Sky Lakes Trail as described in "Sky Lakes and Donna Lake trails rejoin," below.

Staying on the Sky Lakes Trail. The Sky Lakes Trail next climbs briefly west to a ridge junction with the Divide Trail 3717 (6010–0.3)

See maps C5, C6

see MAP C7

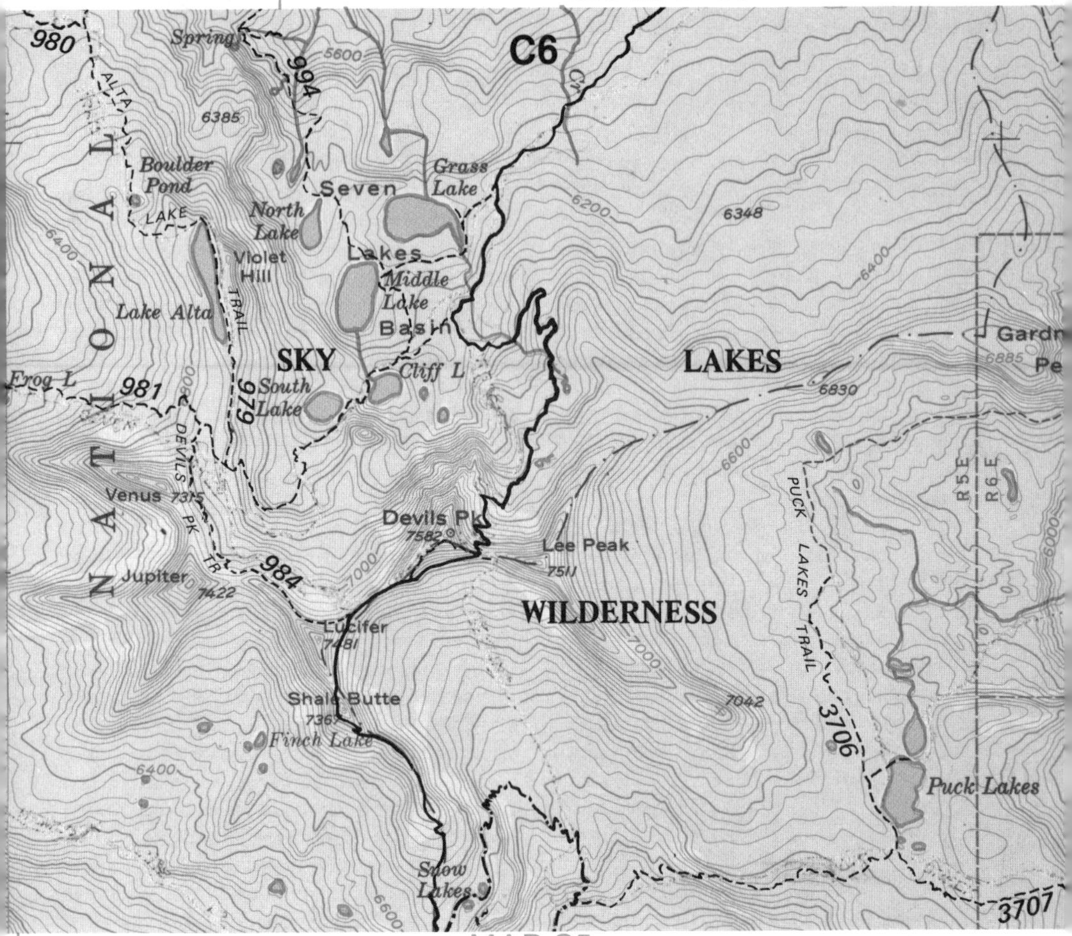

see MAP C5

just above Margurette Lake. You'll find a couple of camps both north and south of this junction.

Diverting to the Divide Trail to Luther Mountain and the PCT. Starting southwest, Divide Trail 3717 is your first route back to the PCT. It is well-graded, but at 2.6 miles unnecessarily long. It ends at a junction with the PCT on a saddle immediately west of Luther Mountain. ▮ *That peak, which is the throat of an old volcano, is well worth climbing. Scramble east up to the summit to get a commanding view of the entire Sky Lakes Area plus an aerial view down Cherry Creek canyon.* ▮

Staying on the Sky Lakes Trail. Beyond the Divide Trail, the Sky Lakes Trail skirts past attractive Margurette Lake. With a prominent

See map C5

Mt. McLoughlin, from PCT on Shale Butte

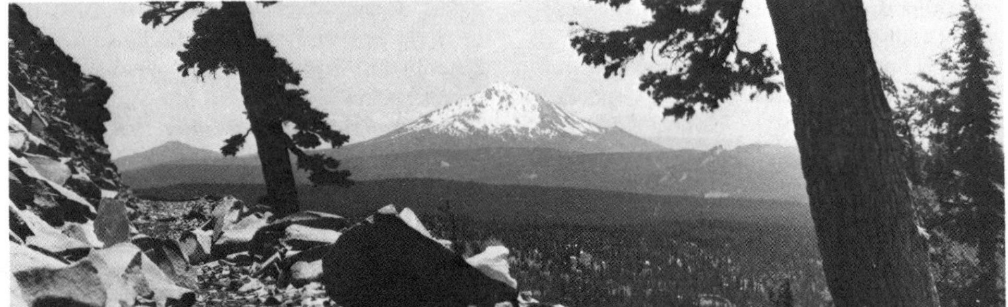

cliff for a tapestry and Luther Mountain for a crown, this deep lake reigns as queen of the Sky Lakes. In quick time, you pass two lakelets and then meet the northwest end of Donna Lake Trail 3734 (6010–0.4).

Sky Lakes and Donna Lake trails rejoin. Ahead, you top out near chilly, unseen Tsuga Lake, just west of the trail, and then descend past a lower pair of Snow Lakes, which have a scenic but chilly backdrop. About 200 yards beyond them, you could initiate a westward slog through huckleberries to shallow Wind Lake, though only the most determined angler will put up with its usual horde of mosquitoes. The descent ends at nearby, waist-deep Martin Lake, and then you traverse 0.4 mile to a junction with Nannie Creek Trail 3707 (6060–1.3), a 4.2-mile trail that is popular on summer weekends.

Back to the PCT on the Sky Lakes-Snow Lakes Trail. Northeastward, you're climbing on what is now called Snow Lakes Trail 3739, which makes an exhausting start that abates where it turns southwest (6320–0.4). Ahead lies an abandoned segment of the defunct Oregon Skyline Trail, a possible route back to the PCT (below). Your Snow Lakes Trail switchbacks up a ridge before switchbacking up to the top of a cliff. On it lie the upper Snow Lakes, which offer scenic, relatively mosquito-free camps. Just 0.2 mile past the southwest lake, your lake-blessed alternate route rejoins the PCT (6670–1.4–7.8).

Back to the PCT on an abandoned segment of the defunct Oregon Skyline Trail. Where Snow Lakes Trail 3739 turns southwest, look ahead for an abandoned but sometimes used segment of the defunct Oregon Skyline Trail. This segment climbs rather steeply 1.5 miles to the Devils Peak/Lee Peak saddle—your second route (and the most direct one) back to the PCT.

With the official PCT and the alternate routes rejoined except for the abandoned segment of the defunct Oregon Skyline Trail, above, you climb again, snaking up a ridge, and then obtain views of Mt. McLoughlin to the south as you round the west slopes of Shale Butte (7367). ▮ *Not shale or even slate, it is really a highly fractured andesite-lava flow.* ▮ Next, the trail traverses the east slope of Lucifer (7481) to a long saddle, on which you meet Devils Peak Trail 984 (7210–1.7).

Side route (from official PCT only). This traverses 1.5 miles northwest to Seven Lakes Trail 981, on which you can go 2.7 miles, first descending past South, Cliff, Middle, and Grass lakes and then climbing briefly back to the PCT. On summer weekends, the Seven Lakes Basin receives heavy use, and it should be avoided then.

Just 100 yards after you leave the saddle's northeast end, you'll spot an abandoned segment of the Devils Peak Trail (7190–0.2).

Side route (from official PCT only). The abandoned trail segment makes a ½-mile, no-nonsense climb to the summit, from which you can make an even steeper 300-yard descent to the Devils Peak/Lee Peak saddle. ▮ *Like Luther Mountain, Devils Peak is the remnant of an old volcano, and its summit views are well worth the effort. To the north, summit views include some of the Seven Lakes plus a good chunk of the Middle Fork canyon, including Boston Bluff. On the northern horizon is pointed Union Peak, which, like Devils Peak and Luther Mountain (2½ miles south of you) is the resistant plug of an eroded volcano. Immediately west of Union Peak, you see Mt. Bailey (8363), which, like pointed Mt. Thielsen (9182), is a hefty 36 miles away. Mt. Scott (8926) is the easternmost and highest of the Crater Lake environs peaks. On most days, you also see Mt. Shasta (14,162), 85 miles due south. Mt. McLoughlin (9495) is the dominating stratovolcano 15 miles to the south-southwest. Try to imagine this landscape, say, 20,000 years ago, when all but the major summits and ridges lay buried under glacier ice, and the glaciers extended east down canyons to the edge of the Klamath Lake basin.* ▮

Those who don't visit the summit have a leisurely climb up to the Devils Peak/Lee Peak saddle (7320–0.5), where they meet hikers who climbed Devils Peak as well as those who took the alternate route and then returned to the PCT on the abandoned segment of the Oregon Skyline Trail

With *all* routes finally rejoined, the descent from the saddle is often a snowy one, and it can be impassable to pack and saddle

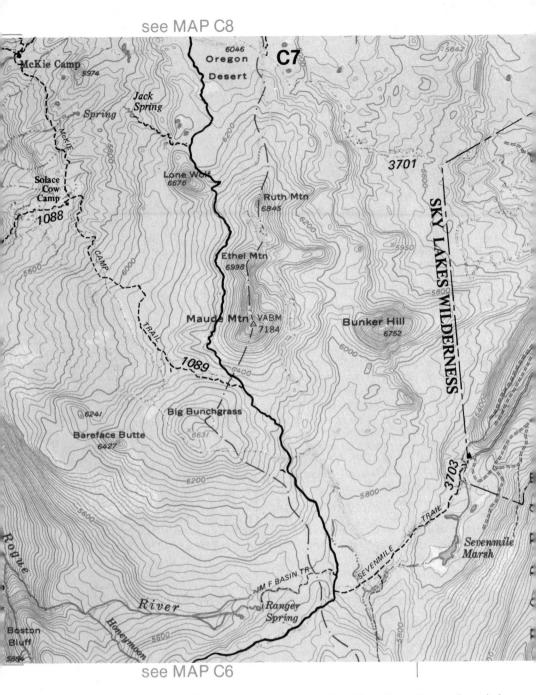

see MAP C8

see MAP C6

stock even as late as August. Early-summer backpackers generally slide or run down the snowpack until they locate the trail in the mountain-hemlock forest below. Those ascending this north slope on foot will find the climb strenuous but safe. The PCT northbound switchbacks down this slope, crosses a cascading, bubbling creek, and then in ¼ mile passes by a meadow. Cross its outlet creek, switchback downward, recross that creek plus the earlier, cascading creek, and soon arrive at a junction (6250–2.4).

Side route. Southwest, a trail traverses 0.3 mile over to Seven Lakes Trail 981, along which you can walk

See map C6

0.1 mile to Cliff Lake. A trail along the lake's east shore leads to a group of very popular campsites (the lake should be avoided on weekends). At the west end of this camping zone, by the edge of a large talus slope, you'll find a small, bedrock cliff that makes a perfect platform for high diving into the lake. No other lake in the wilderness can boast of such a feature.

Beyond the Cliff Lake lateral, you head northeast, quickly cross a creek, and then make a steepening descent to a junction with Sevenmile Trail 3703 (6130–0.7).

Side route. Southwestward, this trail drops to overused Grass Lake, with its multitude of campsites. If you feel compelled to camp near this lake, try sites along its south shore.

Northeastward, the PCT (a.k.a. Sevenmile Trail) rambles down to a couple of inferior campsites by usually flowing Honeymoon Creek (5980–0.5). Past it, you rollercoaster across generally viewless slopes and hear Ranger Springs, unseen below, as you approach a junction where you leave the Sevenmile Trail (5760–2.1).

Side route. This trail goes an easy 1.8 miles northeast down to diminutive Sevenmile Marsh Campground, at the end of Road 3334. On weekends the trailhead can be packed.

The PCT descends quickly to a flat, broad saddle, where it meets the Middle Fork Basin Trail (5750–0.2), which winds southwest 0.9 mile gradually down to the sonorous, tumultuous Ranger Springs. Northbound, water is scarce, so tank up at these pristine springs unless you plan to visit out-of-the-way Stuart Falls. If you don't visit remote Jack Spring and don't take the alternate route to Stuart Falls, you then have about an 18-mile trek to Annie Spring (along the alternate Crater Lake route) or a 19.2-mile trek to Dutton Creek (along the PCT).

Bound for Crater Lake, you first cross a dry flat and then make an ascent up to a junction with Big Bunchgrass Trail 1089A (6020–1.0); you may not see this trail, since it is officially abandoned. ▮ *In the past it wound 2.0 miles around Big Bunchgrass—a relatively youthful volcano—to a junction with Trail 1089.* ▮

On the PCT, you reach McKie Camp Trail 1089 (6380–0.9) as you approach a meadowy saddle.

Side route. This trail goes 3.1 miles down to a junction with Halifax Trail 1088. Solace Cow Camp lies about 90 yards down that trail. Just north from the Halifax Trail junction is a usually flowing creek with an adjacent hikers' camp. Northbound on the McKie Camp trail, you reach the McKie Camp environs in 1.6 miles, and it, too, has a usually flowing creek. You can then take the trail 1.9 miles northeast up to the Stuart Falls Trail, reaching it just under ½ mile northwest of the PCT. Hikers would take this described route only if they really needed water, for it is quite a bit out of the way. However, the route may appeal to equestrians, since Solace and McKie camps are popular horse camps.

From the saddle between Big Bunchgrass and Maude Mountain, the PCT climbs to the latter's west spur, from which it traverses north along west slopes past Ethel and Ruth mountains to a saddle just east of Lone Wolf. Now the trail starts east but quickly switchbacks northwest and descends ½ mile through a snow-harboring fir-and-hemlock forest before curving north to a flat. Here, where others have camped, you spy the Jack Spring spur trail (6190–2.7).

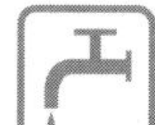

Water access. This trail heads west to a low saddle from which it drops steeply ½ mile northwest to Jack Spring. Due to the steepness of this descent, plus the difficulty some folks have finding bucket-size Jack Spring, you should take this trail only if you *really* need water.

Your route now winds gently down to the Oregon Desert. ▮ *The Oregon Desert holds a reservoir of water, all of it underground. The landscape has been buried in pumice and ash deposited from the final eruptions of Mt. Mazama about 5700 B.C., eruptions that led to the stratovolcano's collapse and the subsequent formation of Crater Lake in the resulting depression. Most of the area's streams were*

see MAP C9 | see MAP C10

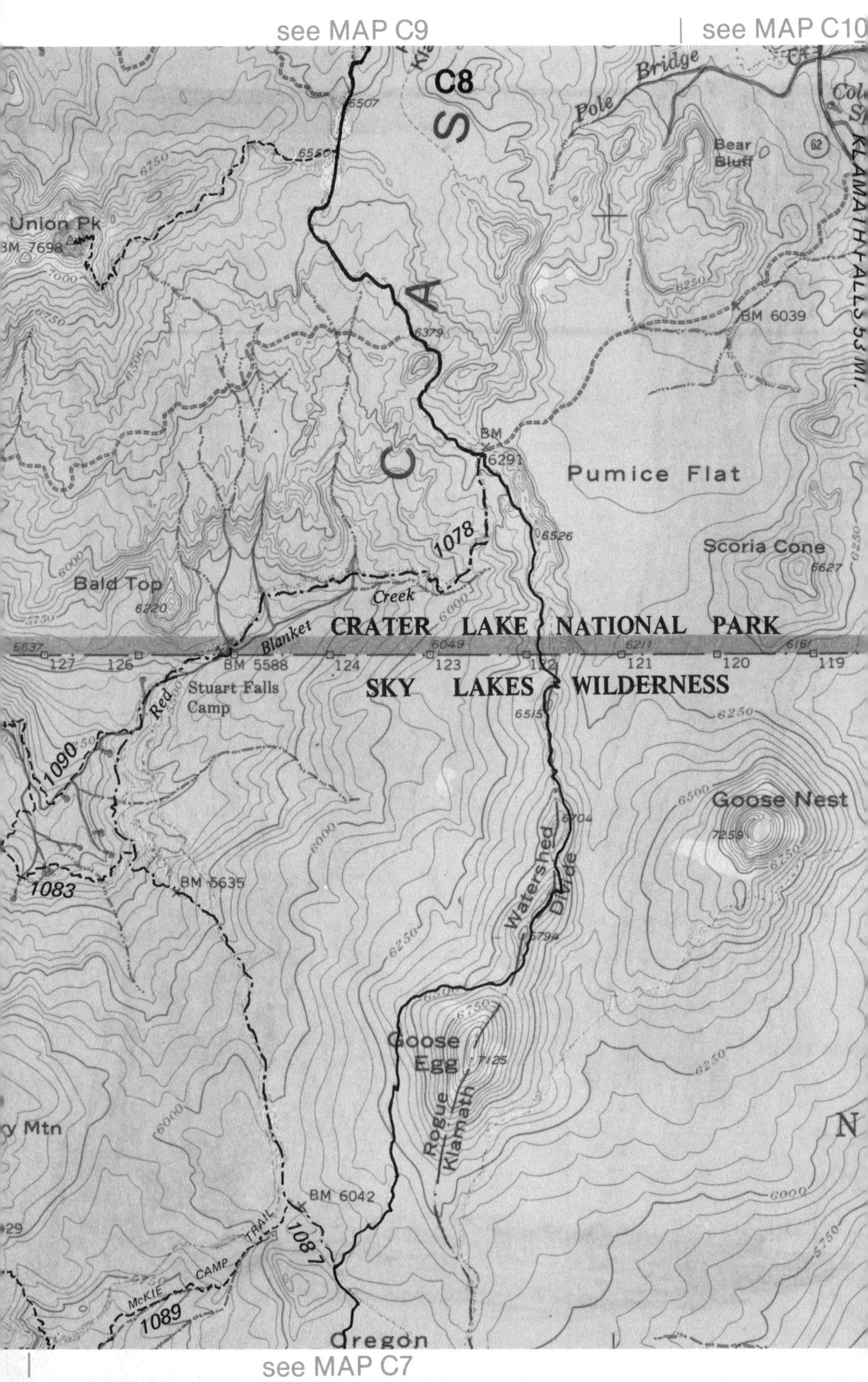

see MAP C7

buried under ash and pumice, and the trekker faces water-shortage problems all the way to Thielsen Creek in Section D, some 47 trail miles away. ▮ You traverse the west edge of the "desert," which in reality is an open lodgepole-forest flat, and pass a wisp of a trail heading east about ⅓ mile before you may see abandoned Dry Creek Trail 3701 (6040–2.4) striking southeast. Leaving the "desert" behind, you top a low, adjacent saddle and then meet the south end of Stuart Falls Trail 1087 (6050–0.2). Once the snow melts, you won't find any water on or near the PCT all the way north to Highway 62, some 10.8 miles away. And from there you'll have to walk almost a mile east to Annie Spring or ½ mile farther to Mazama Campground. Unless you've got enough water to make this stretch, you are going to have to take the Stuart Falls Trail, which is given as an alternate route, below.

Official PCT route. Meanwhile, from the south end of the Stuart Falls Trail, PCT devotees start northeast from the fork. The PCT heads toward the crest, once again thwarting your hopes for water. It climbs north across the lower slopes of the Goose Egg, reaches the crest just beyond that peak, and then stays very close to the crest as it descends to a crossing of an old, closed road only a few yards before the trail tread ends at a second old, closed road (6290–5.6) where the alternate route rejoins it.

Side route (from official PCT only). Southwest, the first road descends 2.5 miles to Stuart Falls Camp, reversing the last leg of the alternate route, below. Northeast, it traverses, as the Pumice Flat Trail, 2.8 monotonous miles to Highway 62.

Alternate route. In just under ½ mile, the Stuart Falls Trail meets the north end of McKie Camp Trail 1089, which was briefly described earlier. Next, walk an easy 1¼ miles north and then descend moderately northwest to a junction with Lucky Camp Trail 1083 (5420–2.3). Westward, this trail passes at least a half dozen springs as it rolls in and out of gullies 1.0 mile over to Red Blanket Falls Trail. That trail, in turn, drops 0.6 mile to Upper Red Blanket Trail 1090, reaching it just above the brink of two-tiered Red Blanket Falls. Trail 1090 then guides the hydrophilic adventurer 0.8 mile back up to the Stuart Falls Trail.

From the Lucky Camp Trail junction, the Stuart Falls Trail passes three creeks of various staying powers before it crosses always reliable Red Blanket Creek to reach the upper end of the Upper Red Blanket Trail (5360–0.7). (This trail is called *Upper* because it is now just the upper 3.8-mile part of the formerly much longer Red Blanket Trail. A first-rate road,

See maps C7, C8

Wizard Island in Crater Lake, from Rim Village

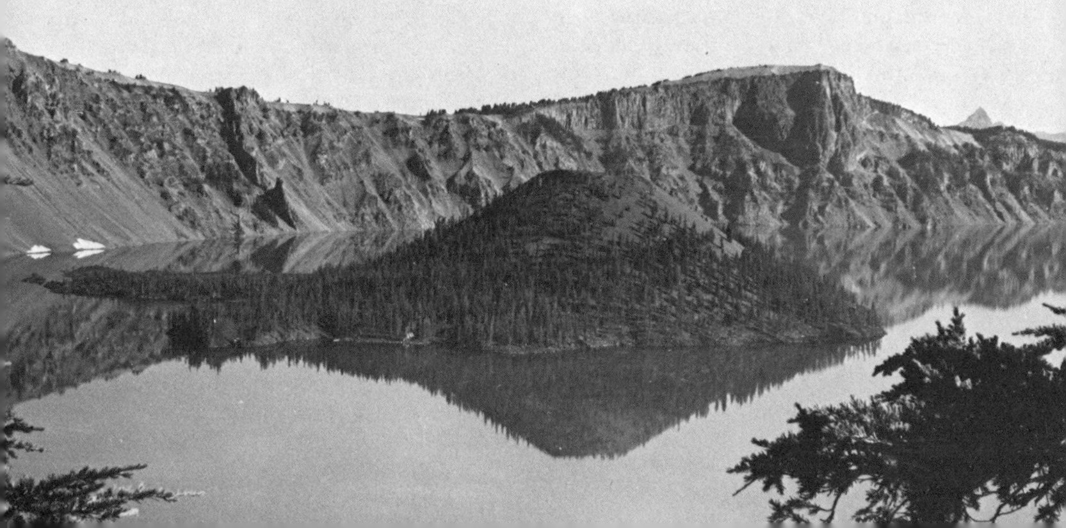

6205, has supplanted the trail, whisking wilderness travelers to the popular trailhead.

Now you stroll up along Red Blanket Creek to a spur trail which takes you momentarily to Stuart Falls Camp (5450–0.4). This large, flat area near the base of Stuart Falls is for humans only. If you've got stock animals, you must picket them immediately north of the Stuart Falls Trail, not down at the camp. Stuart Falls provides rhapsodic music for campers, a feature that few other southern Cascade campsites have. Next day, tank up on water and start up the Stuart Falls Trail. In about ⅓ mile, you enter Crater Lake National Park near a gully with a seasonal creek. From it, your route is an old, abandoned road, which faithfully guides you back to the PCT (6290–2.5–5.9).

Official PCT route and alternate route rejoined. Already a solid mile within Crater Lake National Park, you head deeper inland, progressing along the second old, closed road. In one mile, you may see an abandoned road branching west from yours, but only those with keen orienting abilities will notice it. Ramble onward, gaining slightly in elevation, enter an oval, open flat, and then top out at the south end of a long but narrow, open flat (6550–2.4).

Side route. From this end another closed road—the Union Peak Trail—meanders 1⅔ miles west over to the start of a steep summit trail. Weather permitting, you should not pass up the opportunity to scale this prominent landmark. Drop your heavy pack at the end of the old road and scramble, sometimes using your hands, up to Union Peak's tiny summit.

Onward, the PCT traverses the narrow, open flat and then takes you down through a dense, viewless forest that contains some of the finest specimens of mountain hemlocks you'll find anywhere. Before mid-July, this shady stretch can be quite snowbound. Finally, you come to a small trailhead parking area along the south side of Highway 62 (6108–2.8). Ahead, your next on-trail water will be from the Castle Creek headwaters tributaries, at least 1¾ miles away.

Three options await you across Highway 62. *The first* is the official PCT route, which begins as a trail on the other side of the highway, makes a long arc around Crater Lake's west rim, generally staying 2 to 3 miles away from it and 1000 to 2500 feet below it. Equestrians must take the official PCT. You have no resupply options on the official PCT, because it bypasses the Park's post office. *The second* starts on the official PCT but branches off in 2.1 miles. In the 1990s, the Park Service constructed a hiker-only PCT rim route that branches off at the Dutton Creek Trail. This "hiker's PCT" also bypasses the Park's post office, but it does go through Rim Village (lodgings, cafeteria, gift store; no grocery store). We also describe this alternate "hiker's PCT." *The third* is the one for long-distance hikers who need to resupply. It's the "Alternate route/resupply access from Highway 62" that we describe below. This route passes near Mazama Village (campground, store, inn, gas station, and coin-operated showers and laundry), visits park headquarters, where you'll find the post office, and goes through the facilities at Rim Village before linking up with the "hiker's PCT." ▮ *The official PCT avoids the lake's rim because one of the criteria for the PCT is that it bypass heavily traveled routes—and the Rim Drive surely is one of them. However, another good reason to route the trail low is that the rim accumulates a lot of snow, which can last well into July, and sometimes into August, and equestrians wouldn't be able to use it until then.* ▮

Official PCT route from Highway 62—hikers and equestrians. The Pacific Crest Trail from Highway 62 over to the north-rim access road is about 1½ miles longer than the just-described alternate route via Mazama Village and Rim Village. However, it involves a lot less climbing and therefore less effort. This entirely viewless section begins by climbing, part of it up a fault-line gully. Then it descends momentarily east to the head of a second fault-line gully (6310–0.8). Southward, the Annie Spring Cutoff Trail heads down it, ending in a flat just west of Annie Spring. The PCT now descends to a closed road (6130–0.6) on which we'll hike 16.9 miles over to the park's north-rim access road. Start northeast and soon pass three seasonal tributaries of Castle Creek before turning west and passing a fourth, which is year-round in some years. About 2 minutes past it, you reach very reliable Dutton Creek (6080–0.7), with a spur trail southwest down to some close-by campsites. These comprise the first of three official camping areas

See maps C8, C9

along the park's PCT. The two others are at Bybee Creek and Red Cone Spring, the latter being your last source of water until well into Section D. Here you'll also find the Dutton Creek Trail, on which you can connect with the alternate route called the "hiker's PCT," described below; no stock animals are allowed on the "hiker's PCT" route.

Alternate route—"hiker's PCT." This route climbs 2.4 fairly hard miles on the Dutton Creek Trail to the vicinity of Crater Lake's Rim Village junction. ▮ *If you take this route or the "Alternate route/resupply access from Highway 62," you'll reach about 7700 feet elevation as you round The Watchman, and this locale then will be your highest PCT elevation in Oregon and Washington. For those on the official PCT, the highest PCT elevation will be near Tipsoo Peak, north of pointed Mt. Thielsen, in the southern part of Section D.* ▮ Pick up the rest of this "hiker's PCT" route at "To resume your journey" in "Alternate route/resupply access from Highway 62," below.

Staying on the official PCT. The PCT descends 1¼ miles to two-forked Trapper Creek, passing two seasonal creeks on the way. Trapper Creek flows most of the summer, but later on you'll have to go downstream to find it flowing. Ahead, you ramble about 1¼ miles over to a divide and then make a noticeable descent north to four forks of South Fork Bybee Creek. The first two flow most of the summer and have potential camps; the third flows just as long but is campless; the fourth is vernal. Past the fourth, the road briefly rises and then descends ½ mile to lasting Bybee Creek (5860–4.4). Immediately beyond it, an old road, the Lightning Springs Trail, begins a 4.1-mile climb to the Rim Drive. You can camp just north of the trail junction, or you can wind on down to another junction (5610–1.1) from which an old, closed spur road descends ⅓ mile west to camps along a tributary of Bybee Creek. If the tributary is dry, look for water just downstream.

Beyond the spur road, the PCT soon turns west and then descends ½ mile to a very abandoned road, which starts west in a small, grassy area. Your route turns north and soon crosses the fairly reliable South (5470–0.9) and Middle (5470–0.2) forks of Copeland Creek. Open, lodgepole-punctuated meadows stretch ¼ mile beyond the Middle Fork, and these, like the meadows north of them, are favorite browsing spots for elk. From the second set of meadows and an adjacent, westbound, abandoned road, you climb 2⅔ miles to a ridge, follow it briefly east, and then continue one mile east up gentle slopes to a junction with another abandoned road (6085–4.7).

Side route (from official PCT only). This is now the Crater Springs Trail, which descends moderately a full 3 miles west to the springs, which are at the head of Sphagnum Bog. That area is an interesting one for naturalists, but it is too far off the beaten track for most PCT hikers. No camping is permitted within ½ mile of the bog.

Next, you climb to a very important junction (6240–1.0) from which a spur trail heads 150 yards east-southeast to Red Cone Spring and several adjacent camps. If you plan to avoid any side trips to the Diamond Lake Recreation Area, your next on-trail water will be at Thielsen Creek, about 21 miles away. And if you plan to visit the recreation area, you will have similar water problems. Obviously, you don't drop to Diamond Lake to get water, since you could reach Thielsen Creek just as fast. Rather, you visit it to resupply and/or enjoy its amenities. Prepare yourself for a long, dry day, unless you are hiking before mid-July, in which case you're likely to encounter trailside snow patches.

If you find the thought of a long, waterless stretch too distressing, you do have a water-blessed option. And you have to hike a total of only about 14 miles to reach Broken Arrow Campground, above the south shore of Diamond Lake. To take this route, first continue north on the PCT like other trekkers, down to a junction with the Boundary Springs Trail (6128–0.6), where you can continue on the official PCT or take an alternate route to Boundary Springs and Diamond Lake.

Official PCT route. PCT adherents ignore the Boundary Springs alternate route, below, and make a generally uphill, usually easy traverse. Most of it is through an open lodgepole-pine forest, and you'll round avalanche-prone Red Cone about 1½ miles before you reach a small trailhead parking area alongside the north-rim access road (6510–3.3). You begin

See maps C9, C10, C11, C12

see MAP C11

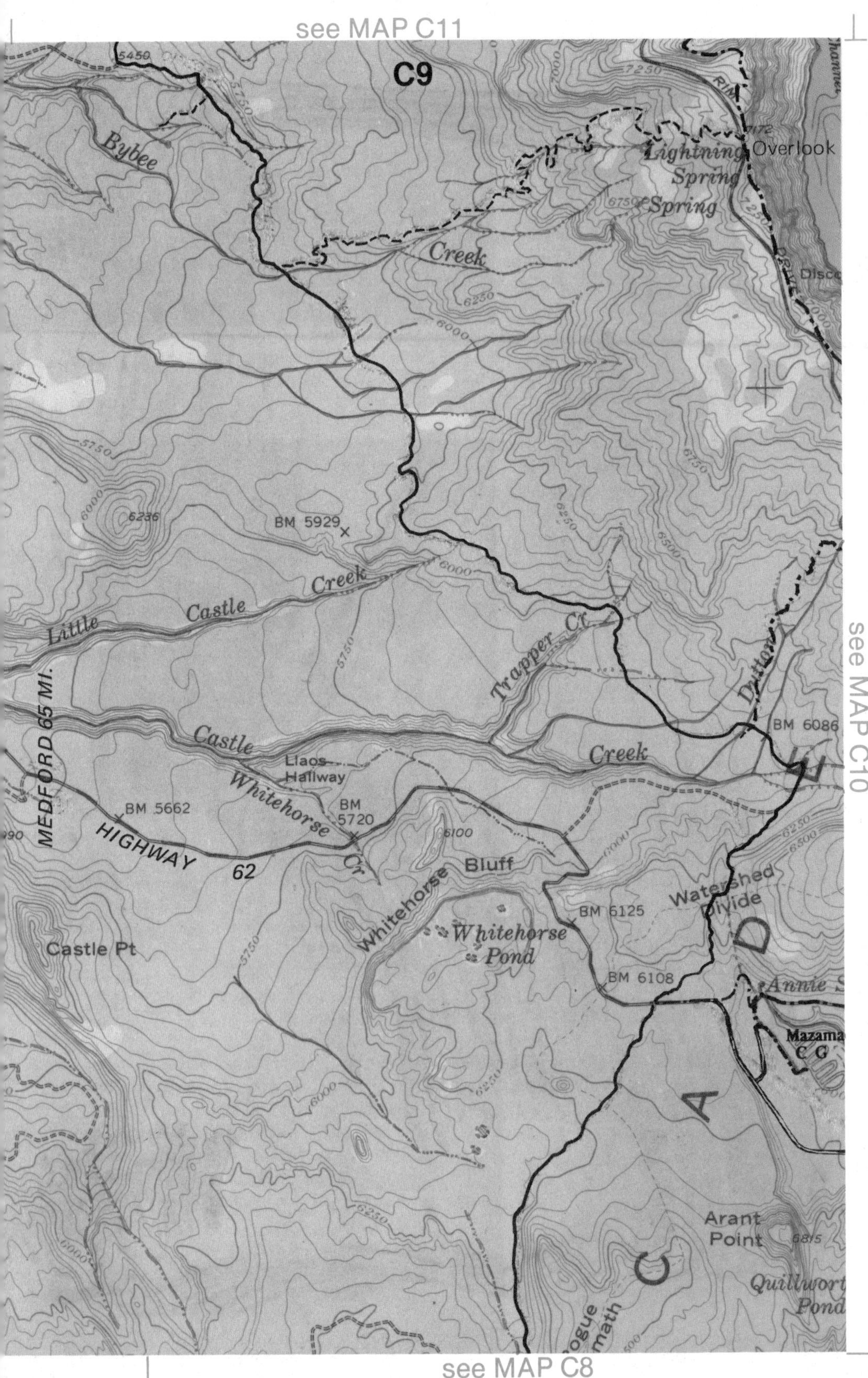

see MAP C10

see MAP C8

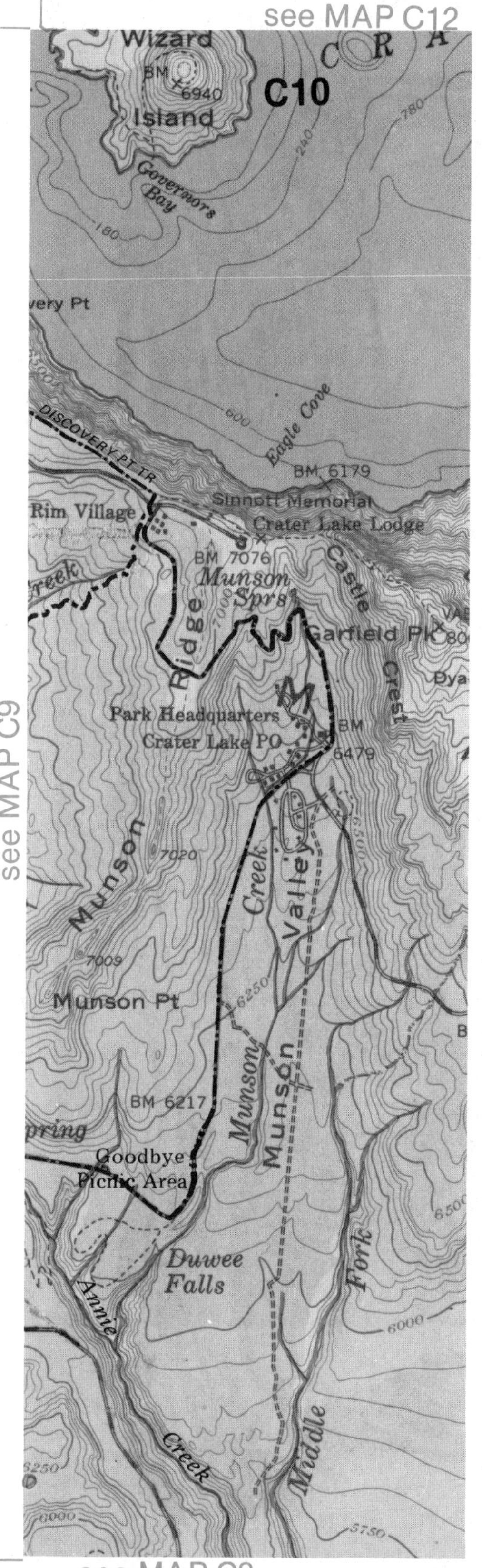

your viewless, waterless trek by walking east over to the nearby base of Grouse Hill. ▌*This huge mass of rhyodacite lava congealed just before Mt. Mazama erupted and collapsed to create the Crater Lake caldera. Its eruptions, occurring about 7700 years ago, "sandblasted" the top of Grouse Hill.* ▌Here, near where the PCT turns north (6510–0.1), the hikers' PCT, descending north from the Crater Lake rim, meets the older route, now the authors' recommended "Alternate route/resupply access from Highway 62," below following the "Alternate route to Boundary Springs and Diamond Lake."

SECTION C

Alternate route to Boundary Springs and Diamond Lake (to official PCT only). On this alternate route, you leave the eastbound PCT adherents as you descend a dry, viewless, monotonous trail north to a junction with the westbound Oasis Butte Trail (5635–4.1). Continue north, then northwest, down to Boundary Springs (5250–1.9), which are so voluminous that you could start, immediately below them, a raft trip down the Rogue River (though fallen trees make such a trip impractical). ▌*For many years, Crater Lake National Park's north boundary crossed this vicinity.* ▌No camping is allowed within ½ mile of the springs, so continue north down the Rogue River canyon, leaving the park in about ¾ mile and then presently reaching a junction (5080–1.2). From it, your Boundary Springs Trail 1057 heads 100 yards north to Road 760, while Rogue River Trail 1034 heads northeast along the river to the road (5070–0.2). If you want to do some camping, take the former trail to Road 760 and follow it west 0.4 mile over to Lake West, which caters to car campers.

If you're bound for Diamond Lake, take Rogue River Trail 1034, reach Road 760, and immediately bridge the Rogue River. On 760, you head east, then northeast, to a junction (5390–2.9) from which a short road winds 0.3 mile northwest to busy Highway 230. Northeast, you continue on an abandoned road whose end is blocked off by a newer section of Highway 230 (5240–2.3). Cross the highway, relocate the abandoned road, and follow it north to the *old* Highway 230 section (5210–0.3). Southbound hikers: note that this

See maps C11, C12, C14, C15

see MAP C14

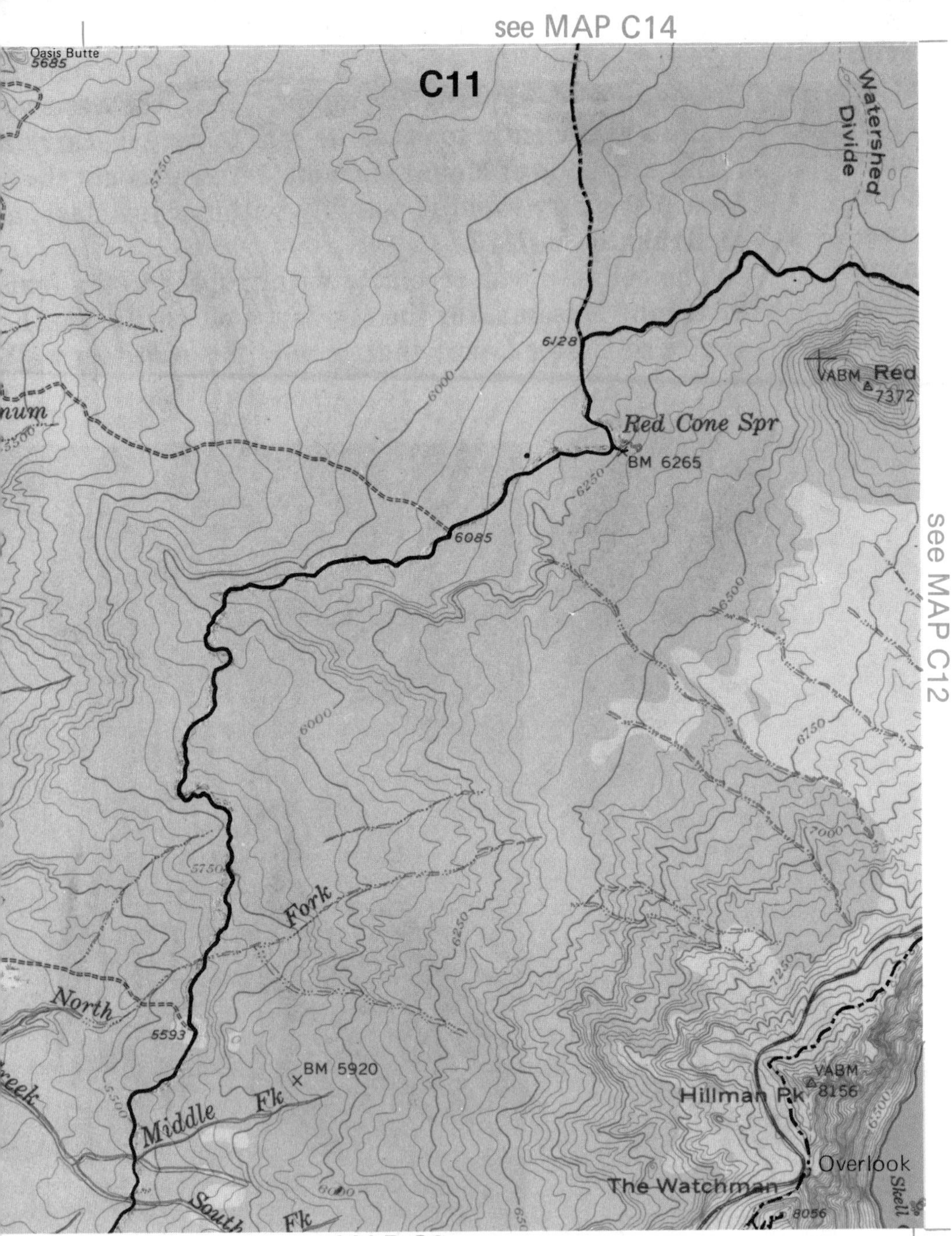

see MAP C12

see MAP C9

road begins about 100 yards east of Horse Lake; if you reach that lake, you've walked a bit too far. On old Highway 230—Road 100 today—head northeast to its end at Road 6592 (5210–0.8). Anywhere along this stretch, you can head north over to adjacent, giant Broken Arrow Campground. On Road 6592, you head briefly north to a junction with Road 4795 (5205–0.3), which circles Diamond Lake. Starting on a northbound segment of Road 4795, you walk briefly over to a day-use parking area to the west and the old Mt. Thielsen Trail to the east (5190–0.1–14.1). From the parking area, you can take a path briefly south-

See maps C15, D2

see MAP C13

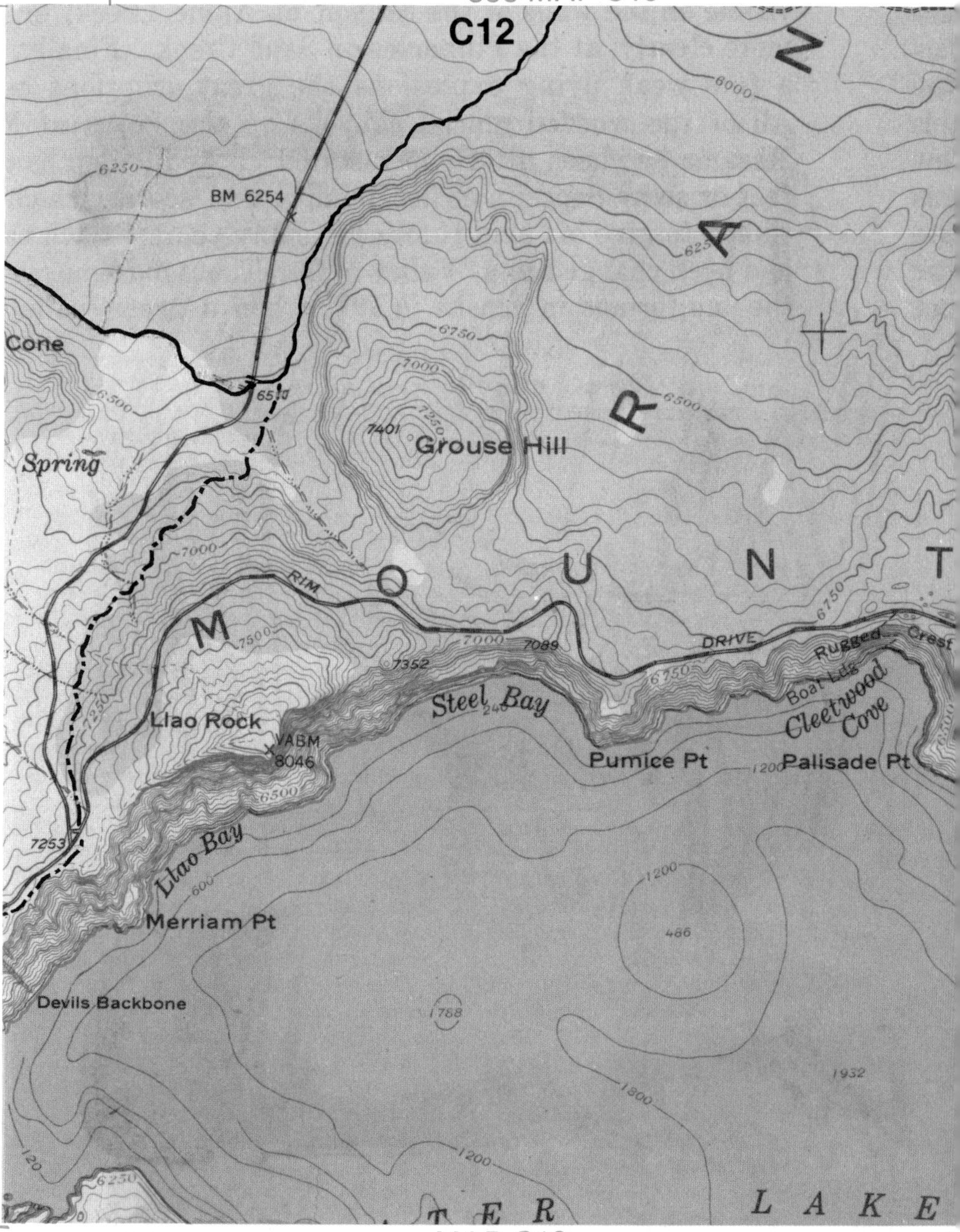

C12

BM 6254
Cone
Spring
Grouse Hill
7401
M O U N T
R
A
N
RIM DRIVE
Llao Rock
VABM 8046
7352
7089
Steel Bay
Pumice Pt
Rugged Crest
Boat Ldg
Cleetwood Cove
Palisade Pt
Llao Bay
7253
Merriam Pt
Devils Backbone
466
1788
1932
L A K E

see MAP C11

see MAP C10

west over to a bikers' and hikers' camp, with five sites, tap water, and flush toilets (!). Just above the southeast corner of Diamond Lake, this is the ideal place to spend the night.

For further instructions, see Section D's first alternate route, which continues north from this vicinity.

Alternate route/resupply access from Highway 62. From where the PCT crosses Highway 62 at a level stretch 0.8 mile west of the highway's junction with the park's south-rim access road, you start east along the highway. In ⅓ mile, the highway bends southeast, and you leave it, descending ¼ mile northeast on the old highway's abandoned roadbed. This ends at the base of a gully, up which the Annie Spring Cutoff Trail climbs ½ mile north back to the PCT. Your route heads south-southeast about 300 yards over to the Crater Lake south-rim access road (6010-0.7). This is about midway between Annie Spring and the entrance to Mazama Campground.

Since you won't have a legal camping opportunity anywhere along the park's roads, you might as well head 250 yards south to the campground's entrance road and then 0.4 mile on it to the campground proper. If you've started your day's hike from Stuart Falls by 7 A.M., you'll reach the campground by 3 P.M., even if you've taken in the side trip to Union Peak. By 5 P.M., the campground is often full, though on weekends it can fill much earlier. The campground is in Mazama Village, which also includes a store, inn, gas station, and coin-operated showers and laundry.

Next morning, retrace your steps to where you first met the south-rim access road and curve 0.1 mile along the road and over to a bridge that spans Annie Creek (6010–1.1). You'll see copious Annie Spring—the source of the creek—just upstream from the bridge. Eastbound, you pass Goodbye Creek Picnic Area (6010–0.8), with water, and then soon reach a curve north (6040–0.4). From it, the Godfrey Glen Trail makes a one-mile loop out to vertical-walled Annie Creek canyon and back. North, you have almost an hour's trek up Munson Valley along the viewless access road, and you pass ranger residences before reaching Crater Lake's Rim Drive (6460–2.2). Still well below the rim, you start north, only to meet park headquarters and its post office (6479–0.1). Pick up whatever packages you've mailed to yourself. You can also get information on weather, naturalist programs, wildflower conditions, and the like. Here, too, you can get a wilderness permit, should you wish to camp in the park's backcountry (such as at Lightning Springs or Red Cone Spring). And you can buy books and pamphlets about the park and the Cascade Range.

From the park headquarters, head north up the Rim Drive, which in ⅔ mile bends south. You wind in and out of a couple of gullies and, upon reaching the westernmost one, you have the option of hiking ⅓ mile due north up it to Crater Lake Lodge. Otherwise, head southwest on the Rim Drive up to Munson Ridge and then north ¾ mile to the Rim Village junction (7090–2.7). Just 60 yards before this junction, you'll see the top end of the Dutton Creek Trail. This alternate-route's distance to here, including a 1-mile detour to Mazama Village, is 8.0 miles. Those taking the alternate hiker's PCT will meet you here, and this route's description comes after a discussion of Crater Lake's formation and a brief description of the amenities at Rim Village.

■ *Your reaction to your first view of this 1932-foot-deep lake, like that to your first view of the Grand Canyon, may be disbelief, as your memory tries to recollect a similar feature. As the deepest lake in the United States and the seventh deepest in the world, Crater Lake is a pristine ultramarine blue on a sunny day, and the 900-foot height of this Rim Village vantage point deepens the color. The lake is also one of the world's youngest, having begun to fill just after the demise of Mt. Mazama and reaching its present level by around 5000 B.C. Mt. Mazama was a large volcano that was born about ½ million years ago. Over several hundred thousand years, it grew, via periodic eruptions, to a large Cascade Range stratovolcano. Fairly late in the Ice Age, perhaps 100,000 years ago, it may have reached an elevation of 11,000–12,000 feet. In size it was larger than Mt. Hood and perhaps close to the size of Mt. Adams. During glacial times, glaciers extended as far as 17 miles from the mountain's summit. But you know how rapidly a volcano can be destroyed in a cataclysmic eruption, such as the one that decapitated Mt. St. Helens in minutes on May 18, 1980. Mt. Mazama self-destructed about 5700 B.C., only its eruption was about 40 times more voluminous than that of Mt. St. Helens. The immediate landscape was buried under tens of feet of ash and pumice; Mt. Rainier, 280 miles to the north, was mantled with 3 inches of it, while southern British Columbia and Alberta received trace amounts. The eruption took place at night, according to an ancient Klamath Indian legend, and morning's light revealed a huge gaping hole—a caldera—where the mountain had stood. The mountain had died, but there was still enough magma in the bowels of the earth to construct a small volcano, Wizard Island, within perhaps months or years after the catastrophe. A smaller*

See maps C9, C10

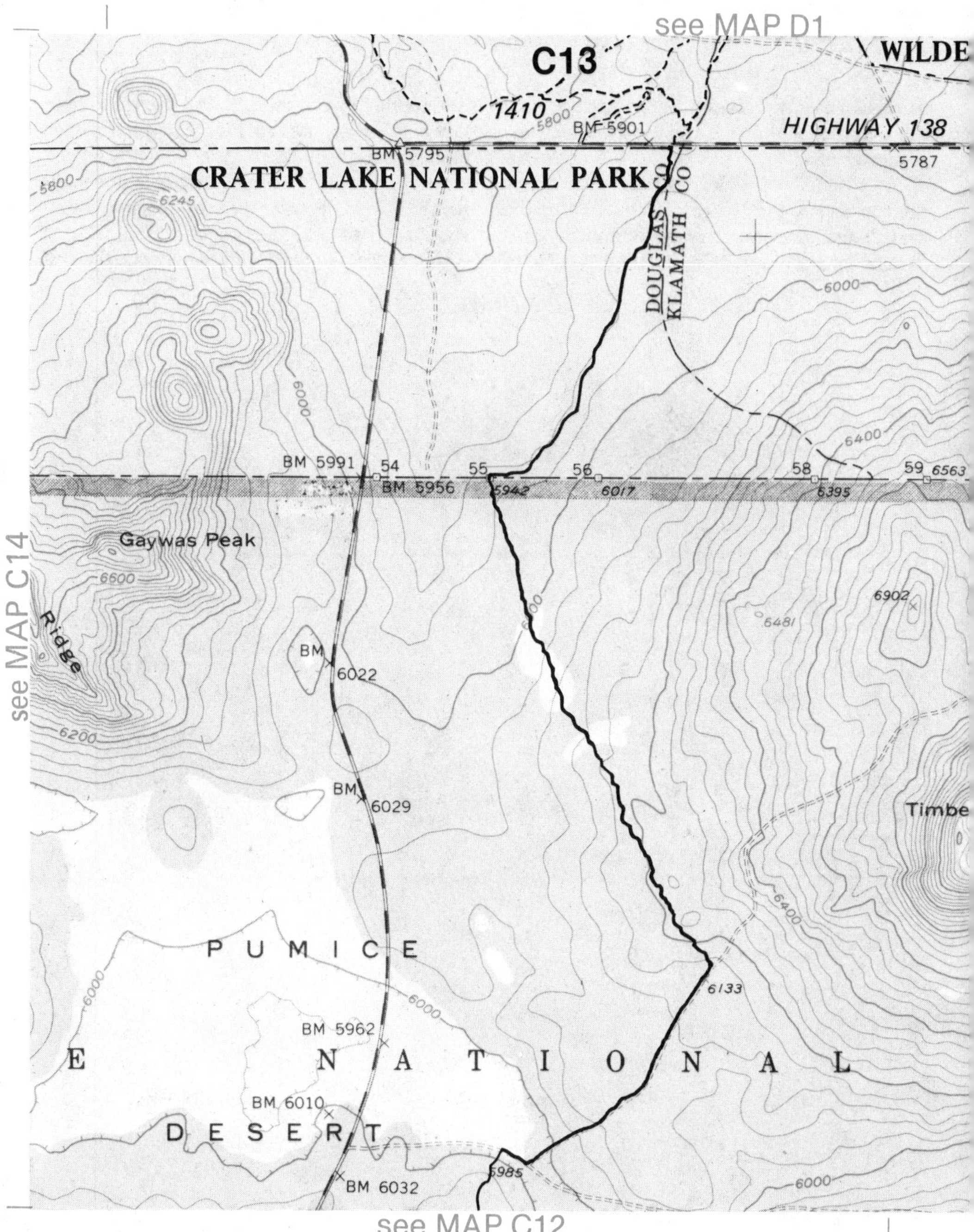

volcano known as Merriam Cone also formed, but 500 to 1000 years of precipitation filled the caldera to its present volume, about 4 cubic miles, and in doing so it buried the top of Merriam Cone under 500 feet of water. ▮

From the Rim Village junction, you can walk east through the "village," which has a complex with a gift shop, a cafeteria, and a restaurant. Behind this complex are rustic cabins for rent, usually on a daily basis. Just past the complex is a small visitor center, from which stairs drop to the Sinnott Memorial, which provides one of the best views of the lake. Crater Lake Lodge, open only during summer, looms above the end of the Rim Village road, and from it the

See map C10

Garfield Peak Trail climbs 1.7 miles to what author Schaffer thinks is the most scenic view of Crater Lake.

To resume your journey, start just above the top end of the Dutton Creek Trail, at the Rim Village junction. If snow abounds, you'll have to take the paved Rim Drive 5.8 miles to the north-rim access road and then 2.6 miles down it to the signed PCT's small trailhead parking area. The hikers' PCT is slightly longer.

From the Rim Village junction (alternate-route mile 8.0) take the rim-hugging, often snow-patched Discovery Point Trail northwest, reaching signed Discovery Point (the real

See map C10

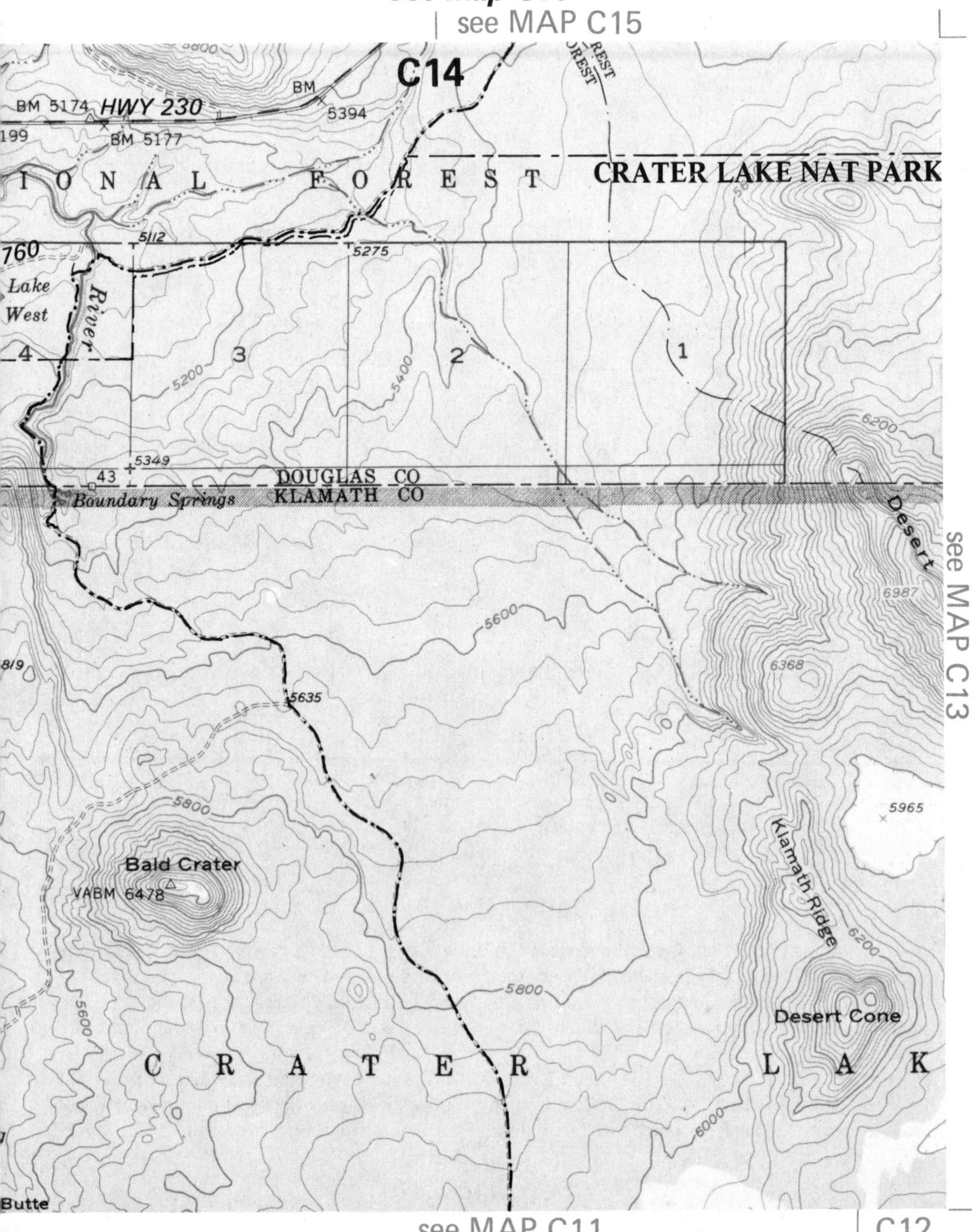

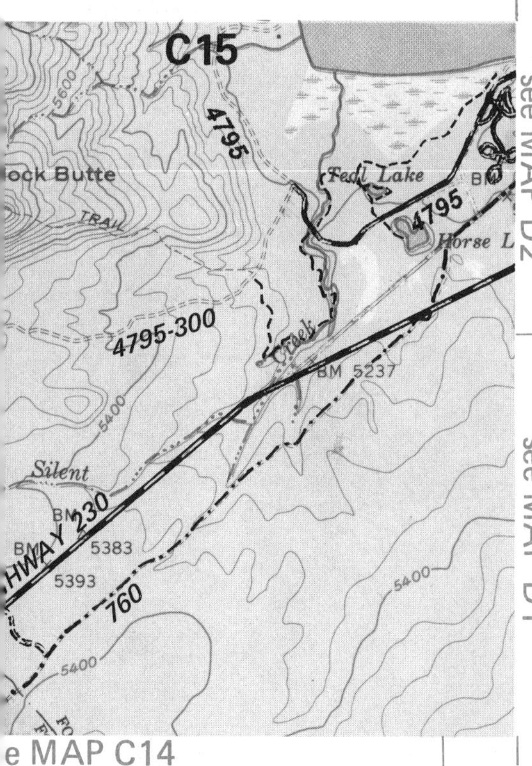

point of discovery is uncertain) at the second saddle. You then climb up and down to the third saddle, which has the top end of the Lightning Springs Trail (7172–2.3). At each of the viewful saddles, there's parking for tourists taking the Rim Drive, as is true with saddles ahead. About ¾ mile down the 4.1-mile Lightning Springs Trail is a short spur trail heading south to campsites among the two Lightning Springs.

The hikers' PCT leaves this saddle climbing north toward The Watchman, a lava flow that formed on Mt. Mazama's flank about 50,000 years ago. When slopes get too steep, your trail veers west, crosses The Watchman's west ridge, and then descends northeast to a prominent saddle with ample parking, the Wizard Island overlook (7600–1.4). This descent is across often snowy slopes, which can bury the route. About ½ mile before the overlook, the Watchman Lookout Trail starts a 0-4 mile climb to the summit. If you've got the time and energy, don't pass up the opportunity to take in the commanding views.

Beyond the Wizard Island overlook, the hikers' PCT starts north toward Hillman Peak and then, as before, the trail rounds the peak's west slopes and descends northeast to the Crater Lake rim. For about a mile, you have a true crest experience as you descend to the Rim Drive's junction with the north-rim access road. Just northeast past this junction, you angle left and immediately cross the Rim Drive (7260–2.4). Now you make an increasingly forested descent in and out of minor gullies down to the official (equestrians') PCT, just east of the access road (6510–2.7). The total mileage of your alternate route, starting from Highway 62, is 16.8 miles. If you joined the alternate route via the Dutton Creek Trail, then it is 11.2 miles.

SECTION C

With the official PCT route and the Alternate route/resupply access rejoined, hikers and equestrians tread north between road and flow, the latter two gradually diverging before you reach a short stretch of former road, once part of the South Timber Crater Trail. On it, you walk 260 yards east to a turn northeast (5985–2.9). On a former road, you climb gently up toward Timber Crater, and where the former road becomes steeper, you angle left (6150–1.3). You climb but ¼ mile northwest before continuing in that direction on a long, viewless, snaking descent to the pre-1980 north boundary of Crater Lake National Park (5942–2.7).

Heading toward Highway 138, the PCT first strikes east along the old boundary and then traverses north-northeast to reach the new boundary immediately before Highway 138 (5920–1.9). This the PCT crosses just 70 yards west of a broad, low crest pass of the Cascade Range. You won't find any parking here, so continue 230 yards from the highway to a junction, from which North Crater Trail 1410 descends ¼ mile northwest to a well-developed trailhead parking area.

See maps C9, C10, C11, C12, C13

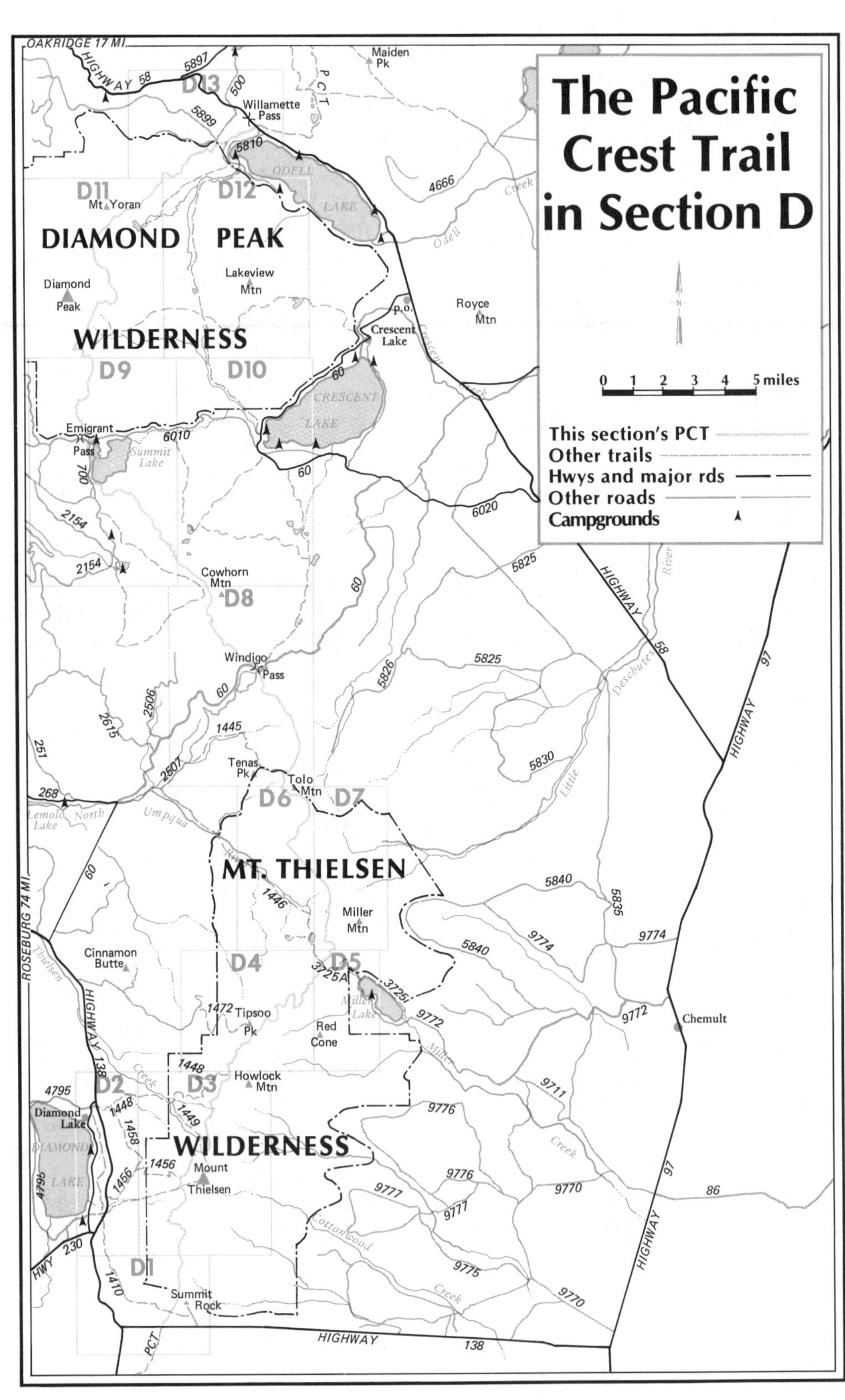
The Pacific Crest Trail in Section D
0 1 2 3 4 5 miles
This section's PCT
Other trails
Hwys and major rds
Other roads
Campgrounds
DIAMOND PEAK WILDERNESS
MT. THIELSEN WILDERNESS
OAKRIDGE 17 MI.
HIGHWAY 58
ROSEBURG 74 MI.
HIGHWAY 138
HWY 230
HIGHWAY 97
Maiden Pk
Willamette Pass
Odell Lake
Mt Yoran
Diamond Peak
Lakeview Mtn
Royce Mtn
Crescent Lake
Emigrant Pass
Summit Lake
Cowhorn Mtn
Windigo Pass
Tenas Pk
Tolo Mtn
Lemolo Lake
Miller Mtn
Cinnamon Butte
Tipsoo Pk
Red Cone
Miller Lake
Howlock Mtn
Diamond Lake
Mount Thielsen
Summit Rock
Chemult
D1
D2
D3
D4
D5
D6
D7
D8
D9
D10
D11
D12
D13

Section D:
Highway 138 near the Cascade crest to Highway 58 near Willamette Pass

Introduction: Needle-pointed Mt. Thielsen, approached early on this hike, is this section's star attraction; its terrain is even more spectacular than that seen along the PCT through this section's Diamond Peak Wilderness. Unfortunately, when the PCT was finally completed through this section around 1977, its route proved to be inferior in esthetics compared with its predecessor, the Oregon Skyline Trail. That trail touched on enjoyable Diamond Lake, which most long-distance PCT hikers visit anyway. It also took you past Maidu Lake, which was one of this section's best camping areas when mosquitoes weren't biting. The lake was an important water source; now it is almost one mile out of the way. Furthermore, the old trail went past a series of lakes, but this route has been replaced with a nearly lakeless route that remains more faithful to the crest. This new route tends to be snowbound about a month longer than the older route, Finally, whereas the Oregon Skyline Trail came to within ½ mile of the Cascade Summit store and post office at Odell Lake, the PCT comes only to within 1½ miles of it. Consequently, we will describe the old route as well as the new one.

Despite the foregoing criticism lodged against this section's PCT, it is still a good experience. The trail is well-graded and it has interesting, if not dramatic, views of Mt. Thielsen, Sawtooth Ridge, Cowhorn Mountain, Diamond Peak, and Mt. Yoran. All are easily accessible to peakbaggers, but Mt. Yoran should be left for experienced mountaineers. The only *significant* lake along the official PCT route, Summit Lake, is, like Diamond Lake, a worthy place to spend a layover day.

Declination: 18°E

Points on Route	S→N	Mi. Btwn. Pts.	N→S
Highway 138 near the Cascade crest	0.0		61.3
Mt. Thielsen Trail	6.2	6.2	55.1
Thielsen Creek Trail	8.4	2.2	52.9
Howlock Mountain Trail	11.5	3.1	49.8
Maidu Lake Trail	18.3	6.8	43.0
Tolo Camp	24.5	6.2	36.8
Windigo Pass	30.4	5.9	30.9
Stagnant pond (6380′)	37.4	7.0	23.9
Road 6010 near Summit Lake Campground	43.1	5.7	18.2
Unnamed lake (6030′)	55.1	12.0	6.2
Midnight Lake	58.2	3.1	3.1
Pengra Pass	59.7	1.5	1.6
Highway 58 near Willamette Pass	61.3	1.6	0.0

Supplies: Since there are no on-route supply points, most long-distance PCT hikers take one of our alternate routes down to a walk north along Diamond Lake. The store at

Diamond Lake Lodge is one of the best to be found anywhere near the PCT. This spacious resort also has a post office (97731), and it serves good meals at reasonable prices.

Near Section D's north end, you can leave the PCT at Pengra Pass and descend 1.5 miles to Shelter Cove Resort. The resort does accept mailed packages but can only hold them for about 2 weeks. Send them via UPS only to: Shelter Cove Resort, West Odell Lake Road, Highway 58, Crescent Lake, OR 97425.

Maps:

Pumice Desert East, OR	*Tolo Mountain, OR*
Mount Thielsen, OR	*Cowhorn Mountain, OR*
Diamond Lake, OR (alternate route)	*Emigrant Butte, OR*
Miller Lake, OR	*Diamond Peak, OR*
Burn Butte, OR	*Willamette Pass, OR*

THE ROUTE

This section's hike begins at Highway 138 (5920) just 70 yards west of the almost flat watershed divide in this locale of the Cascade Range. Trailhead parking is available just north of Highway 138 and west of the PCT. The short road that goes northeast to the trailhead starts from Highway 138 just 0.5 mile west of the Cascade divide and 0.8 mile east of Crater Lake's north-rim access road.

From Highway 138, the PCT heads northeast 230 yards to a junction with the south end of North Crater Trail 1410 (5910–0.1). Just 3 minutes into the hike, you're faced with a decision—the first of several routes leaving the

See map D1

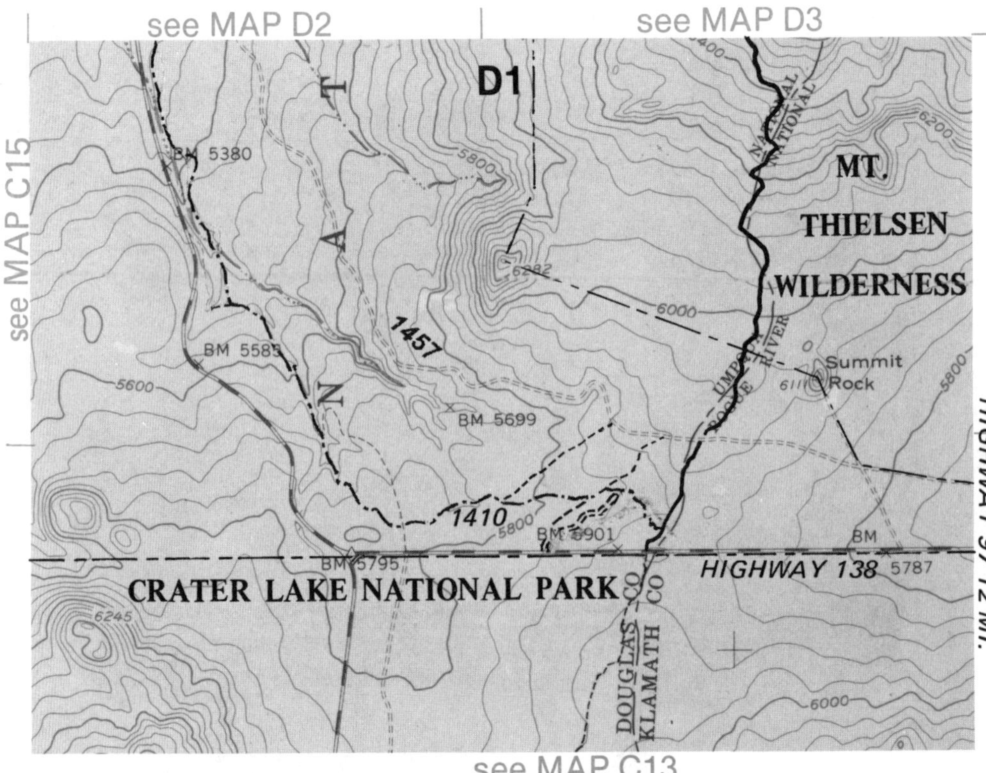

PCT for the Diamond Lake environs. The North Crater Trail doesn't go to any crater; rather, it descends toward Diamond Lake, runs north above its east shore, and then in 9.3 miles ends at the Diamond Lake Corrals, which are situated about ½ mile northeast of Diamond Lake Resort. If you want the quickest, easiest route to Diamond Lake, start along this trail

Resupply access. North Crater Trail 1410 reaches the trailhead parking area in 1/4 mile and then continues onward. In 60 yards, it reaches an old southwest-descending road that dies out in both directions. Go just 200 yards down this road and then fork right onto a broad path that descends to a gully. From here, a snowmobile route climbs northeast, leading eastbound hikers astray. Westward, you cross, in 0.5 mile, an old road, which was referred to at the end of Section C. Just 0.6 mile later, the trail tread joins that road again, where it loops into a gully (5640–1.9). Follow the road 3/4 mile down to where it curves west and flattens out. Leave the road and take a trail that starts north along a crest between two gullies. Your route ahead should now be obvious, and you parallel Highway 138 until it diagonals across your path (5275–2.5). Dash across the busy highway and follow a short trail segment over to Highway 230 (5245–0.2). You could continue north along the North Crater Trail, but since that route is largely viewless, you might miss a number of lakeside attractions. Therefore, walk 100 yards west on Highway 230 to a junction with east-shore Road 6592. Just under 1/2 mile north on it, you meet a straight, southwest-heading road—the old Highway 230, today's Road 100—along which Section C's Boundary Springs Trail alternate route joins your route (5220–0.5). As in that route, you head 1/4 mile north to a junction with Diamond Lake's loop Road 4795. Anywhere along this last stretch, you could have walked west to the east side of nearby Broken Arrow Campground. Also, a momentary walk west on the road takes you to a path that goes 100 yards north to a bikers' and hikers' camp, with five sites, tap water, and flush toilets—an ideal place to spend the night. From it a path goes north momentarily to another path on which you can walk about a minute northeast over to Road 4795.

See maps D1, D2

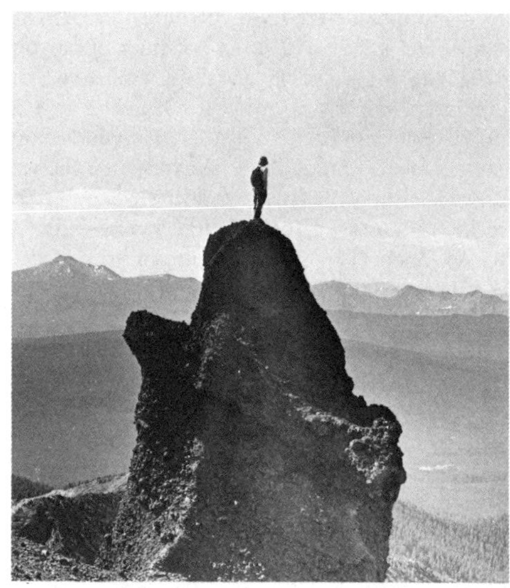

A Mt. Thielsen pinnacle and distant rim of Crater Lake

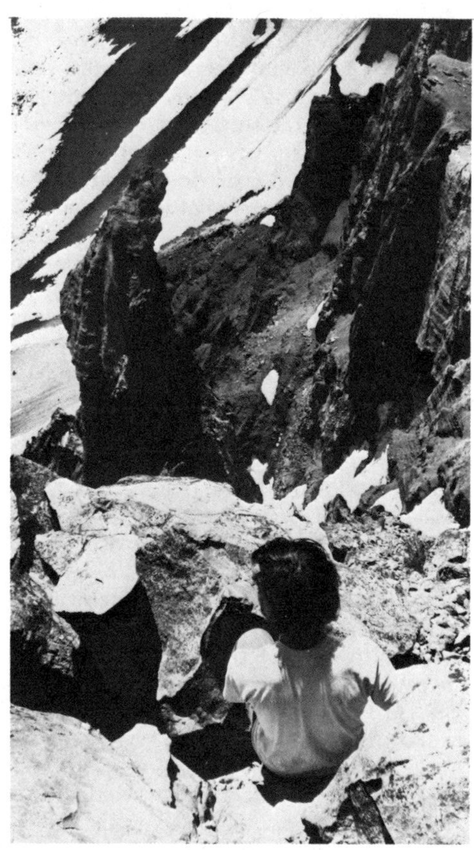

View south-southeast from Thielsen's summit

If you didn't head over to the camp, then at the Roads 4795/6592 junction, start north on 4795 and momentarily pass the trail over to the camp, starting southwest. Opposite it is a short trail east back to Trail 1410, which you recently left. Immediately ahead, you reach a private campground on your right and then soon arrive at South Store (5190–0.5). If you've been living for days out of your pack, you'll certainly welcome this store and its café. Just north of the store is the south end of 2-mile-long Diamond Lake Campground, which is sandwiched between the lake and Road 4795. You can drop to it any time you desire. Midway along the lake's east side, you reach an intersection (5236–1.4) with the campground's entrance to the west and the Diamond Lake Information Center to the east. From that center, a spur trail goes to the North Crater Trail. Onward, you pass more of the campground; then, from its north end, you can hop onto a trail that parallels your road and the lakeshore over to Diamond Lake Resort's entrance road (5200–1.2). Head over to the complex (5200–0.3), resupply at its well-stocked general store, pick up your mailed parcels at the post office, and/or enjoy a hearty meal at the restaurant. If you're well-funded, rent a fishing boat and catch a rainbow trout or two, which grow considerably larger here than in the lakes of Sky Lakes Wilderness. Some long-distance hikers may even be desperate enough for civilization's amenities to stay at the resort's lodge.

After your stay, however brief or long, start north up the road immediately east of the gas station. This road climbs up to Road 271, reaching it only a minute's walk west of a junction with Road 4795 (5340–0.5). Also at this junction is the entrance road to Diamond Lake Corrals. Walk east to the road's far end, and beside it you'll find a tread (5340–0.1–9.1). Northward, Howlock Mountain Trail 1448 swings east, spinning off Spruce Ridge Trail 1458 (which goes over to Mt. Thielsen Trail 1456) and Thielsen Creek Trail 1449. All take you back to the PCT and will be described in the pages to come. Southward, North Crater Trail 1410 snakes 9.3 miles to the PCT, ending just north of Section D's start, Highway 138.

Official PCT route. From the North Crater Trail 1410 junction, those taking the mostly viewless, waterless PCT route have an easy climb up to the old, abandoned Summit Rock Road (5935–0.5).

See maps D1, D2

See map D1

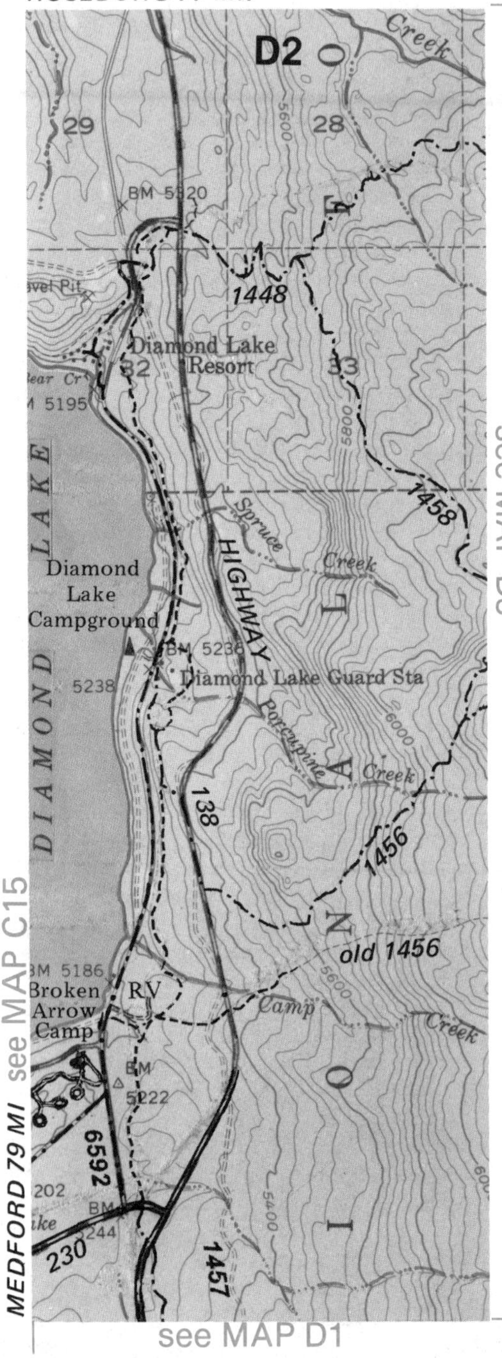

Side route. This road (Trail 1457), which is a ski route in winter, also provides one with a route—albeit inferior—to Diamond Lake. The road curves 4.2 miles over to the new Highway 138, along whose shoulder you walk 0.4 mile and then follow the defunct Mt. Thielsen Trail 0.5 mile west over to Road 4795, at the lake's southeast corner.

See map D1

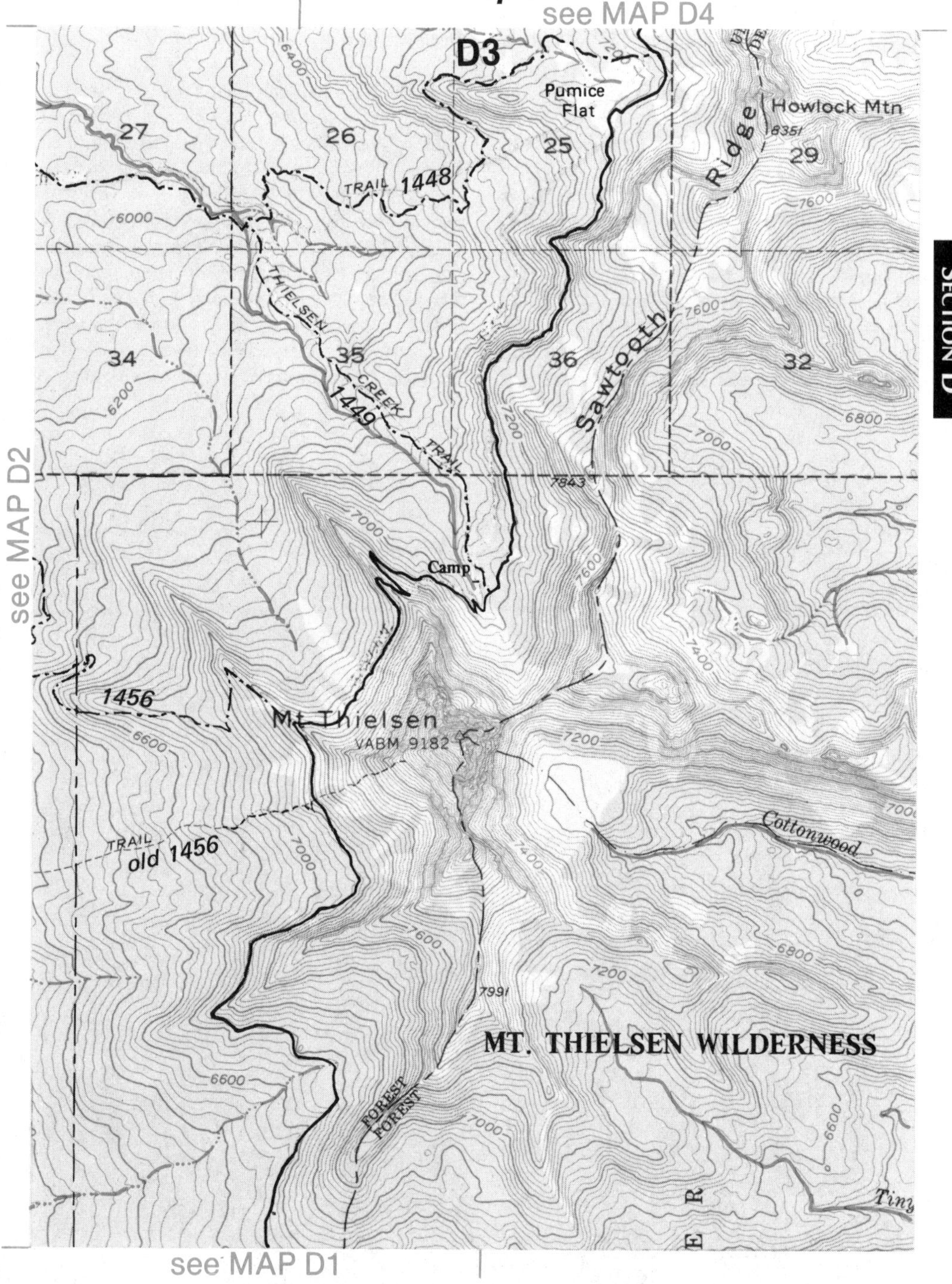

see MAP D4

see MAP D2

see MAP D1

Onward, the PCT climbs gently north for a mile; then the gradient steepens, and the trail makes a few open switchbacks up a ridge before it curves northwest around the ridge. Now you make a long but comfortable ascent, rounding Mt. Thielsen's southwest ridge before traversing across a glaciated bowl to a trail junction on the peak's west flank. Here you meet the top part of the *old* Mt. Thielsen Trail (7260–5.3), which will now be described east up to the summit.

Side route. The summit of Mt. Thielsen (9182), sometimes called the "Lightning Rod" of the Cascades, is easily accessible and should not be bypassed. When you ascend it, however, leave your pack behind; Mt. Thielsen has probably one of the steepest trails in existence —more of a climb than a hike. The trail quickly exits above treeline and then climbs up increasingly loose pumice slopes toward a cleaver, where it seems to veer right (south) around the cleaver. This scree slope is the *descent* route. Rather than fight your way up this unstable slope, climb up solid rock along the left (north) side of the cleaver and continue up toward the 80-foot-high summit pinnacle, which can be climbed unroped only from its southeast ridge. The near-vertical north and east faces make these last few feet off-limits to those with acrophobia.

The view from the summit area is both spectacular and instructive. You can see north 107 miles to Mt. Jefferson (10,497), and south 120 miles to Mt. Shasta (14,162). You can see from the dips, or inclinations, of the strata that Mt. Thielsen's summit once lay to the east, and about 1000 feet higher, above what is now a deeply glaciated canyon. Here is a vulcanologist's natural observatory, for the mountain's anatomy is stripped bare. After downclimbing the summit pinnacle, head south a short way along the ridge and pass some enormous pinnacles clinging to the

See maps D1, D3

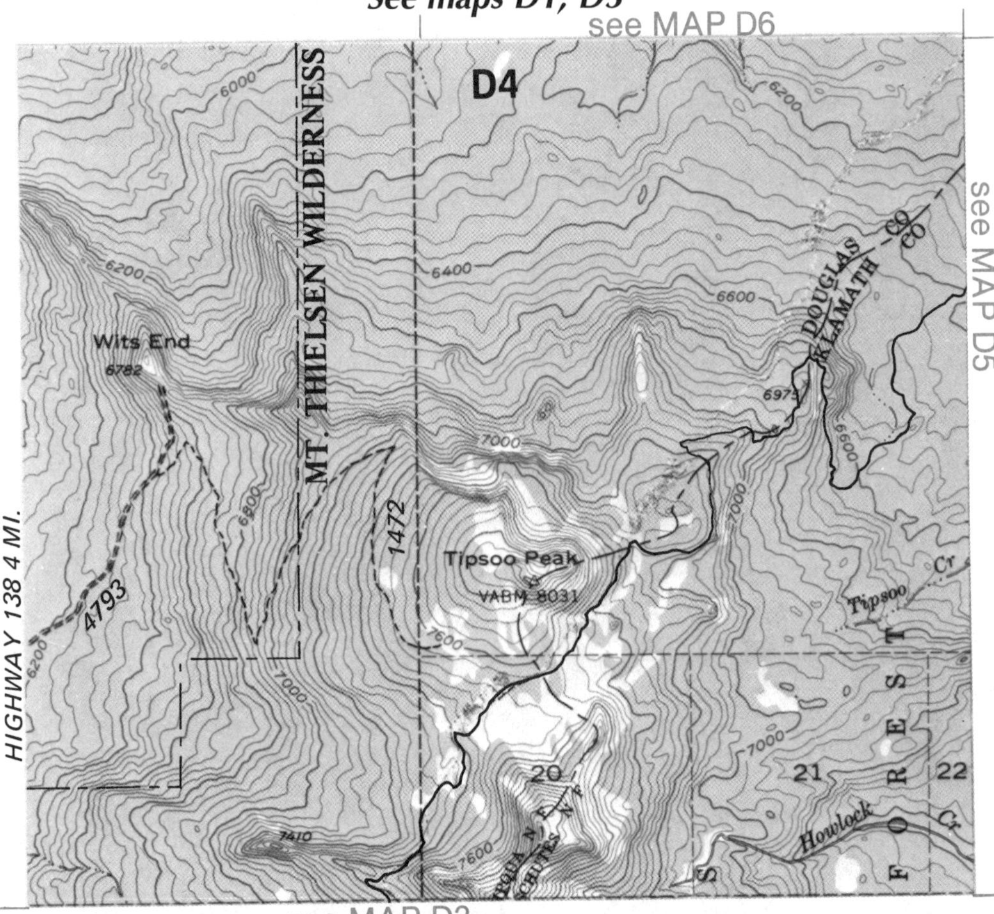

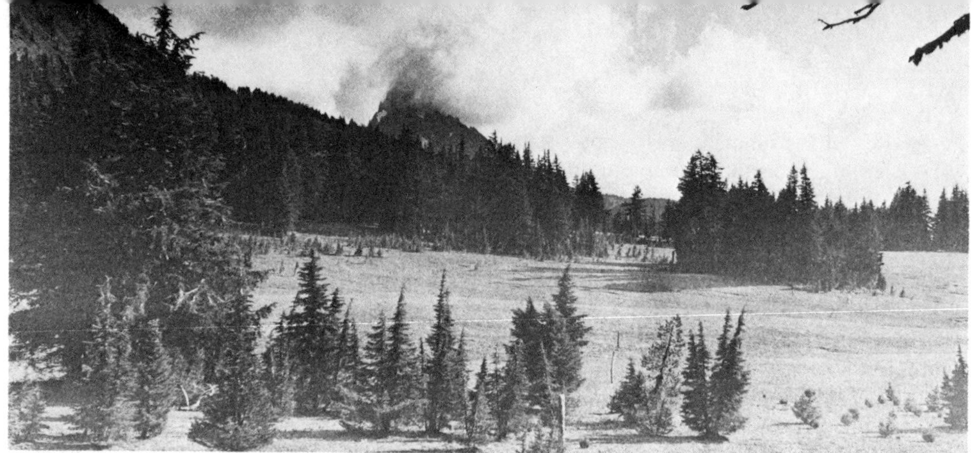

Cloud-capped Mt. Thielsen, from near Tipsoo Trail junction with PCT

east wall. Soon you come to an obvious spot, not too far from an isolated, scrubby whitebark pine, where nearly everyone begins to descend the scree slope to the trail.

From Mt. Thielsen's summit trail, the PCT traverses north to the peak's west ridge, on which it meets the newer Mt. Thielsen Trail 1456 (7330–0.3), on which you can make a side trip to Diamond Lake.

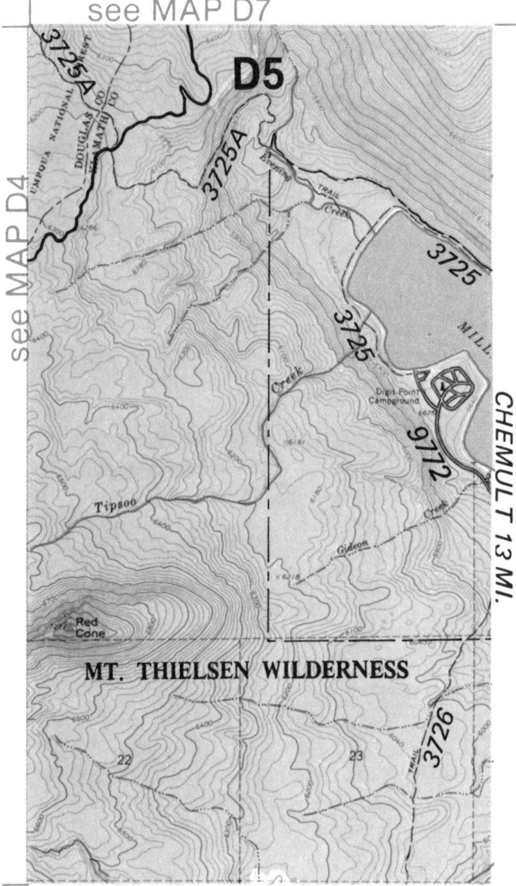

  **Side/alternate route.** If you want to drop to Diamond Lake for recreation or supplies, start down the Mt. Thielsen Trail. This descends at an average gradient of 9¼%, versus 13% for the old Mt. Thielsen Trail. ▮ *Since the PCT is not supposed to exceed 15%, the old Mt. Thielsen Trail fell within acceptable limits of steepness, and it is unfortunate that the newer, 1¼-mile-longer trail was built.* ▮ But the new trail's gradient does make for an easy descent, and in under an hour you arrive at a junction with Spruce Ridge Trail 1458 (6240–2.3). You can take either route down to Diamond Lake, but to maximize scenery, why not make a loop?

On the waterless Mt. Thielsen Trail, descend to a trailhead on Highway 138 (5360–1.7). Unfortunately, the trail doesn't continue west to the lakeshore road, as the old trail did, so hike ½ mile north on 138 to where it begins to curve northeast. Drop west about 200 yards cross-country to North Crater Trail 1410. Walk ¼ mile north on it to where a trail heads west over to a USFS information center. You continue westward and quickly reach east-shore Road 4795, which is opposite the entrance to Diamond Lake Campground (5236–1.1). Now follow the previous side route 1.2 miles north to Diamond Lake Resort's entrance road, 0.3 mile over to the resort, 0.5 mile up a minor road to Road 271 and momentarily east to nearby Road 4795, and then 0.1 mile east through Diamond Lake Corrals to the Howlock Mountain trailhead (5340–2.1–7.2).

Howlock Mountain Trail 1448 heads northeast, joining another trail from the corrals immediately before passing through a horse tunnel under Highway 138 (5360–0.2). From

See maps D2, D3

the far side of the tunnel, a trail heads northward, but you climb southeast up the slopes of a lateral moraine. ▌*The glacier that carried this morainal debris originated on the north slopes of Mt. Mazama, a towering volcano that collapsed about 7700 years ago at the site now occupied by Crater Lake.* ▌Immediately beyond the crest of the moraine, you meet a second minor trail, which heads north down a gully. You then switchback to the crest of a higher moraine and on it meet Spruce Ridge Trail 1458 (5680–1.0), which is the first of three options back to the PCT:

1. Spruce Ridge Trail option. If you went to Diamond Lake as a side trip, take this return option if you don't want to miss a foot of the PCT. The waterless Spruce Ridge Trail 1458 starts along a minor ridge and makes an easy, spruce-free, generally viewless ascent south to the Mt. Thielsen Trail (6240–2.6). Up it, retrace your steps to where you left the PCT, on the west ridge of Mt. Thielsen (7330–2.3–6.1 miles from Diamond Lake Corrals).

2. Thielsen Creek Trail option. Continue east on the Howlock Mountain Trail, passing in ⅓ mile the seasonal west fork of Thielsen Creek, later skirting Timothy Meadow, and then ½ mile beyond it reaching Thielsen Creek and adjacent Thielsen Creek Trail 1449 (6040–2.4). Take this moderately climbing trail, which parallels its namesake, back up to the PCT (6960–2.3–5.9). You'll pass a short spur trail over to Thielsen Creek Camp just 100 yards before this junction.

3. Howlock Mountain Trail option. From the lower end of the Thielsen Creek Trail, continue east up Howlock Mountain Trail 1448, which can have snow patches in mid-July but can be waterless by early August. You'll see Howlock Mountain, rising 1000 feet above you, just before you reach the PCT (7320–3.6–7.2).

If you began your alternate route from the southern end of North Crater Trail 1410, your total mileages for these three return routes will be 15.2, 15.0, and 16.3 miles, respectively. If you began your alternate route from the upper end of Mt. Thielsen Trail 1456, your total mileages will be 13.3, 13.1, and 14.4 miles, respectively.

Staying on the PCT instead of going to Diamond Lake. From the Mt. Thielsen Trail 1456 junction, the PCT crosses the open, view-packed northwest slopes of Mt. Thielsen to the peak's northwest ridge (7370–1.0). From here you see your next major peak—bulky, snowy Diamond Peak The trail now makes long switchbacks down from the ridge; then it descends southeast to Thielsen Creek (6930–1.1). Over this last mile of trail, snow sometimes lingers through late July. Thielsen Creek is your first source of permanent water since Red Cone Spring, 21 miles back. Your next on-route *permanent* source of water is at Summit Lake, a whopping 33 miles ahead, so many hikers stop at out-of-the-way Maidu Lake, a good camping area only 10.8 miles ahead. Just past the Thielsen Creek crossing, you reach Thielsen Creek Trail 1449 (6960–0.1), where you meet the Thielsen Creek Trail return option from Diamond Lake.

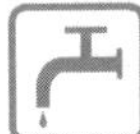

Water access. You can descend about 100 yards on Thielsen Creek Trail 1449 to a spur trail that leads 100 yards west down to Thielsen Creek Camp. Since this is the first PCT campsite with water since Red Cone Spring, it can be overcrowded.

Leaving the Thielsen Creek area, the PCT makes a winding contour 2.7 miles north to an open bowl, Pumice Flat, through which the Oregon Skyline Trail once traversed northeast. The PCT heads east just above it into a stand of mountain hemlocks. If you are hiking through this area in early season, you might want to camp under a cluster of hemlocks and lodgepoles near the low summit ¼ mile west of you. Early-season water is obtained from the seasonal creek just north of it or from nearby snow patches.

After the PCT heads east into the hemlocks, it quickly starts an ascending, counterclockwise traverse around the bowl. Just past a meadow where the trail turns from north to northwest, you'll reach a junction (7320–3.1) with well-used Howlock Mountain Trail 1448. The last Diamond Lake side/alternate route, described earlier, ends here.

With the official PCT and all side/alternate routes rejoined, the PCT, which can be vague in spots over the last half mile, now makes an obvious climb to a crest saddle (7435–0.4) that lies on a western spur of the ragged, severely glaciated Sawtooth Ridge.

See maps D2, D3, D4

see MAP D8

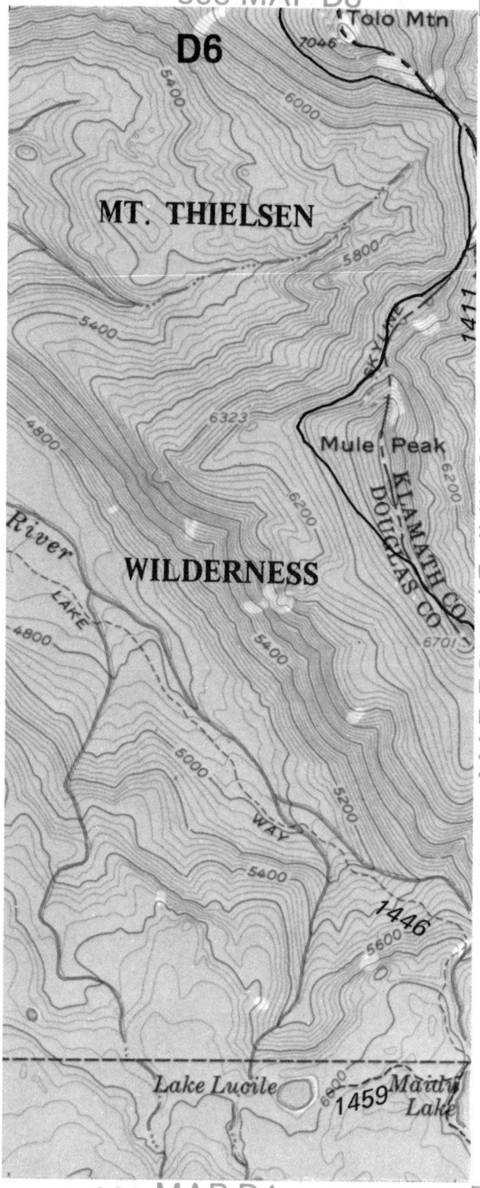

D6

D7

see MAP D7
see MAP D6
see MAP D4 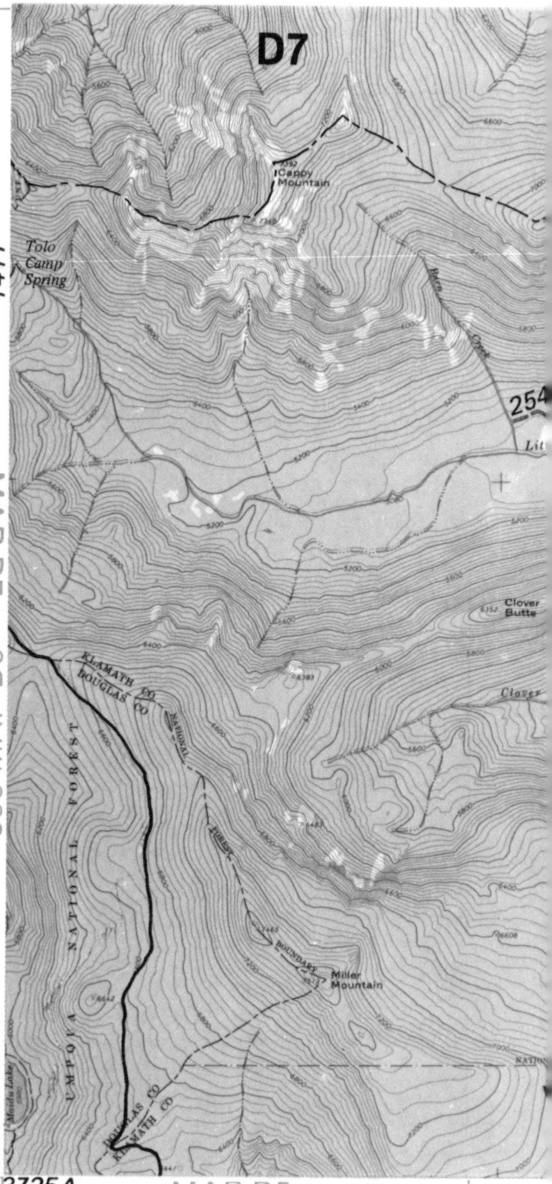
see MAP D5

Leaving the crest saddle, you may encounter lingering snowbanks before you reach your first meadow. The meadows usually have posts through them to help PCT hikers keep on track. On this stretch, you reach the high point—in elevation—of the Oregon-Washington PCT (7560–1.3).

Side route. Tipsoo Peak, due north, is an easy 20-minute climb for peak-baggers, and its summit views are second only to Thielsen's for providing an overview of this region.

On the lower south slopes of Tipsoo Peak, just north of a broad saddle, the PCT starts a descent northeast. About halfway to a saddle, the trail bends north across an open gully and then hugs the forested lower slopes of Tipsoo Peak as it continues northeast to that saddle (7300–0.8). Here you can inspect the severely glaciated north face of red-black Tipsoo Peak.

See map D4

D9
see MAP D10

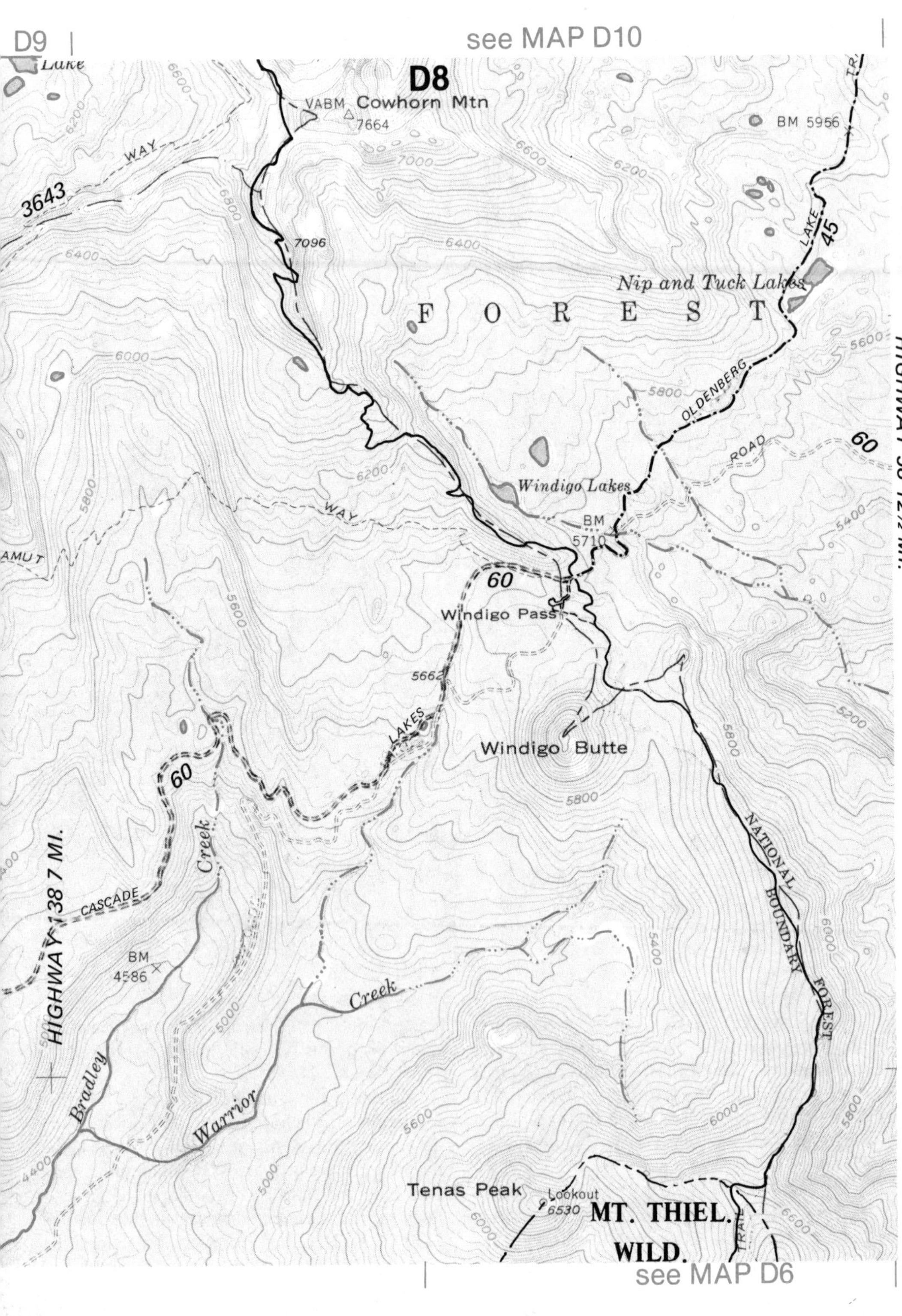

see MAP D6

From this saddle, hikers used to zip northeast straight down to Maidu Lake, but the route has been changed so that you now make a long, counterclockwise traverse around a flat, volcanic summit. This traverse provides three scenic viewpoints that reveal Red Cone and Miller Lake; then the trail veers northeast across the county-line crest to a switchback. The trail then makes a long, winding, viewless descent to the west end of a broad saddle on which you cross Maidu Lake Trail 3725A (6190–4.3).

Water access. Here the Maidu Lake Trail starts north, proceeds to cross the county-line saddle, and then descends a gully to the south shore of shallow, semi-clear Maidu Lake. Most hikers will want to make the 0.9-mile trek down to this lake's relatively warm waters, for the next PCT campsite with near-water access is the sometimes-overcrowded Tolo Camp, 6.2 miles farther. The lake's shore has abundant space for camping, though until early August a tent is necessary to provide refuge from the myriad of mosquitoes.

From the PCT's crossing of the Maidu Lake Trail, you can also start south on this trail, which winds 2.0 miles down to Miller Lake Trail 3725, which you can then follow 0.8 mile south over to the Digit Point Campground. Few hikers will want to make this longer excursion.

The PCT leaves the Maidu Lake Trail, quickly crosses that trail's former tread, and then climbs to a spur-ridge view of Miller Lake. After getting several views of the lake, cross the spur ridge and follow it north to a crossing of the main, county-line ridge (6490—1.3). Beyond it you climb gently up to an auxiliary saddle; then, with an equal climb, you top out at a junction from which the abandoned Oregon Skyline Trail once descended southwest to Maidu Lake. The PCT now contours for ¼ mile and then begins a gradually steepening descent to a crest saddle (6470–2.3).

The trail now climbs up to the long Mule Peak crest, crosses it, diagonals northwest down the peak's west slopes, and then diagonals northeast to a saddle (6300–1.9). Contin-

See maps D4, D5, D7

Shallow arm between Nip and Tuck Lakes

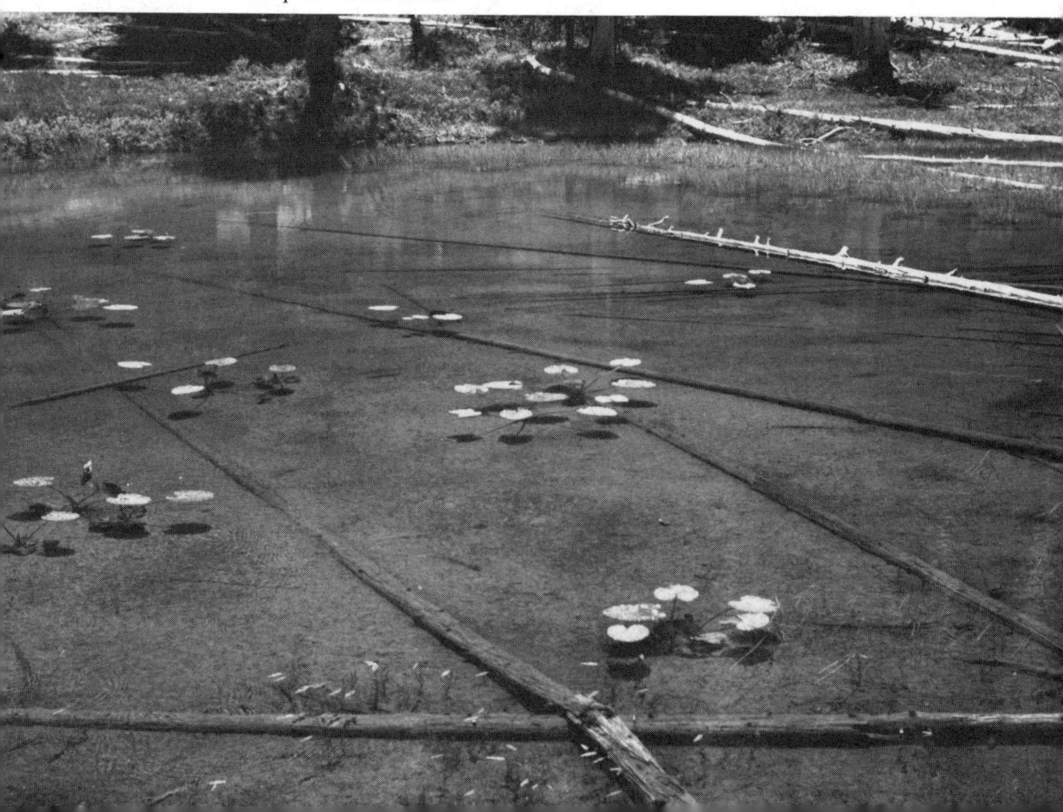

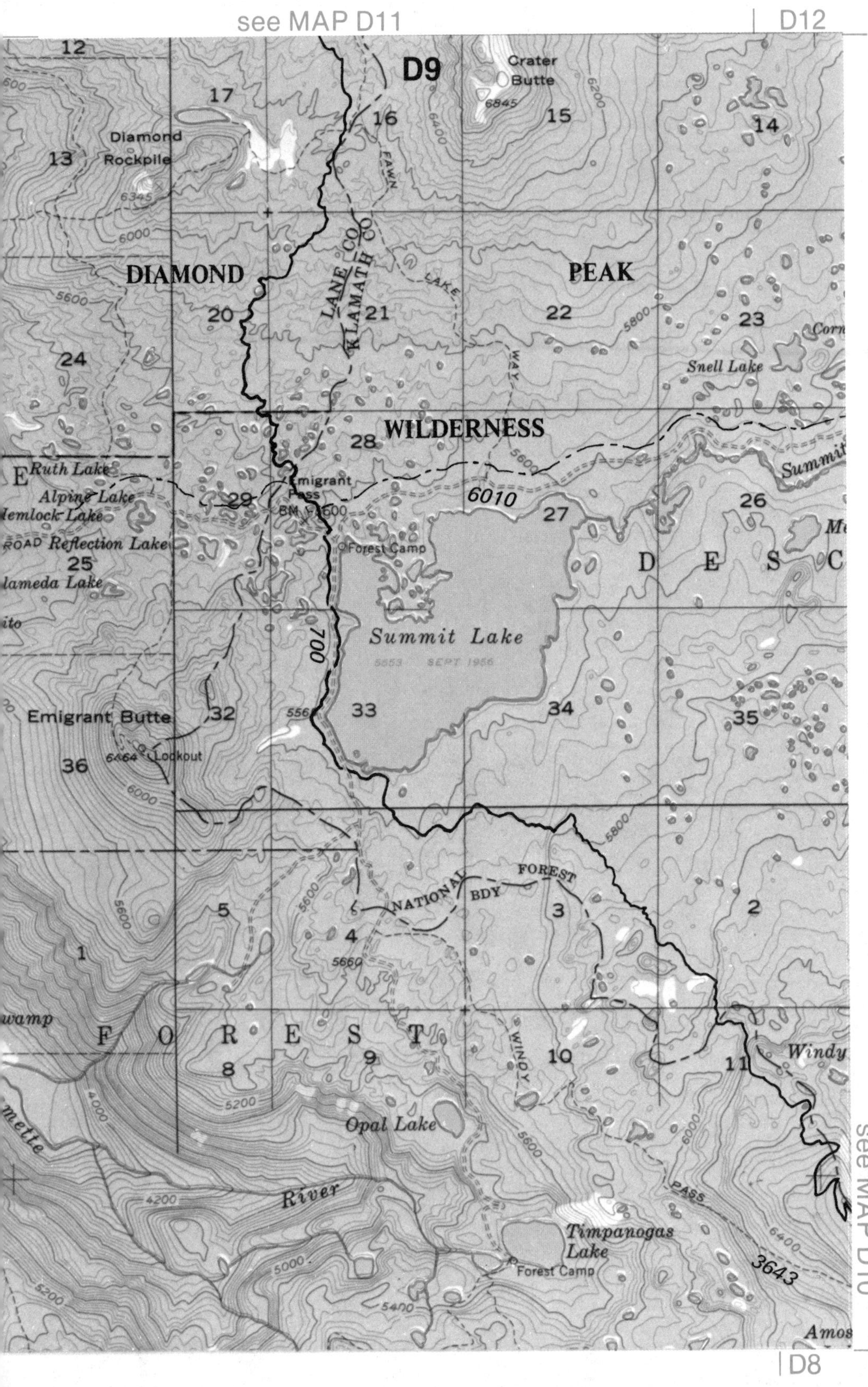
see MAP D11
D12
D9
Crater Butte
6845
Diamond Rockpile
6345
DIAMOND
PEAK
WILDERNESS
LANE CO
KLAMATH CO
FAWN
LAKE
WAY
Snell Lake
Ruth Lake
Alpine Lake
Hemlock Lake
ROAD
Reflection Lake
Alameda Lake
Emigrant Pass
BM 5600
6010
Forest Camp
Summit Lake
5553 SEPT 1956
700
Summit
D E S C
Emigrant Butte
6464
Lookout
NATIONAL
FOREST
BDY
F O R E S T
Windy
WINDY
Opal Lake
River
PASS
3643
Timpanogas Lake
Forest Camp
Amos
see MAP D10
D8

see MAP D12

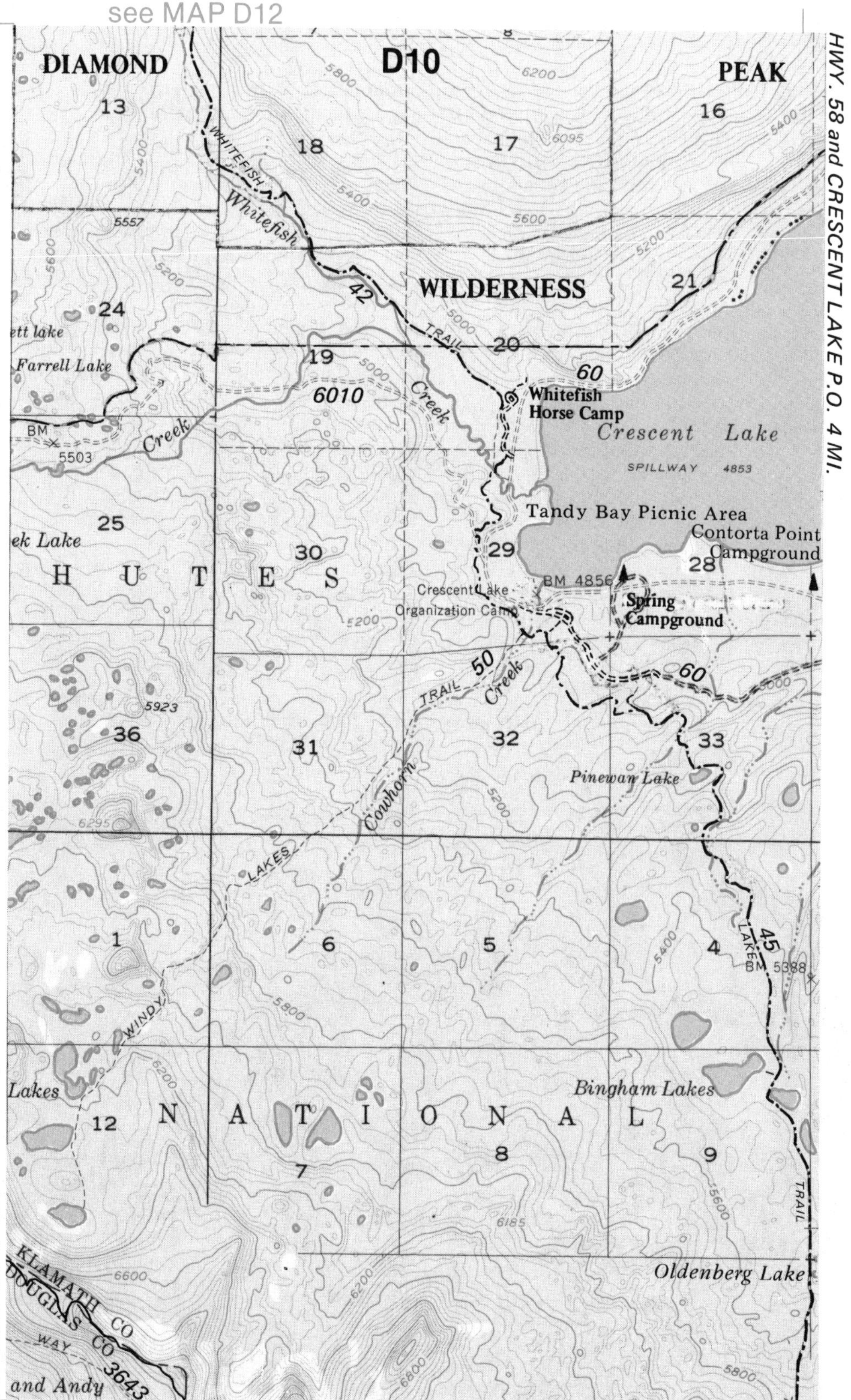

HWY. 58 and CRESCENT LAKE P.O. 4 MI.

see MAP D8

uing this crest route, you descend to a second saddle, where lies Tolo Camp (6190–0.7), which has camping space for about six hikers. From the camp, Trail 1411 switchbacks eastward ⅓ mile down to Six Horse Spring, which has no available camping space. From Tolo Camp, there will be no reliable water until Summit Lake, 17.0 miles farther. However, near-trail water and campsites are found at several places north of Windigo Pass.

From the Tolo Camp saddle, traverse over to another saddle (6325–0.6) and then traverse across the south and west slopes of Tolo Mountain to Tenas Trail 1445 (6610–1.3), which starts west down a ridge to the old Cascade Lakes Road. Now outside Mt. Thielsen Wilderness, the trail turns east, descends to the ridgecrest, and then follows it for over 2½ miles before swinging west across a broad, low saddle to the lower north slopes of a pyroclastic cone called Windigo Butte (6420). Now descend less than ¼ mile along the butte's north spur and then curve northwest over to a junction with a spur trail (5845–3.7) that goes 250 yards west to a trailhead parking area immediately west of the old Cascade Lakes Road.

Starting north from the junction, the PCT quickly drops into a gully, climbs over a low ridge, and reaches the new Cascade Lakes Road 60 (5820–0.3) only 140 yards east of Windigo Pass. The old road, which starts by the trail's west side, takes you ¼ mile southwest to the Windigo Pass trailhead parking area, used by north- and southbound hikers alike. From this junction with Cascade Lakes Road 60, you have the choice of staying on the official PCT, described first, or taking an alternate route, the old Oregon Skyline Trail, described below. The authors recommend the alternate route.

Official PCT route. From Windigo Pass on the Cascade Lakes Road, the PCT begins a 7-mile-longer route to Willamette Pass. It climbs ½ mile to a crest crossing from which you could head due north ¼ mile, staying east of the crest as you descend to the southwestern Windigo Lake, about 130 feet below you. Avoiding water, the PCT closely follows the crest for about one mile and then climbs 400 vertical feet on a winding course to a minor crest saddle (6620–2.3).

See maps D6, D8

Diamond View Lake reflecting Diamond Peak

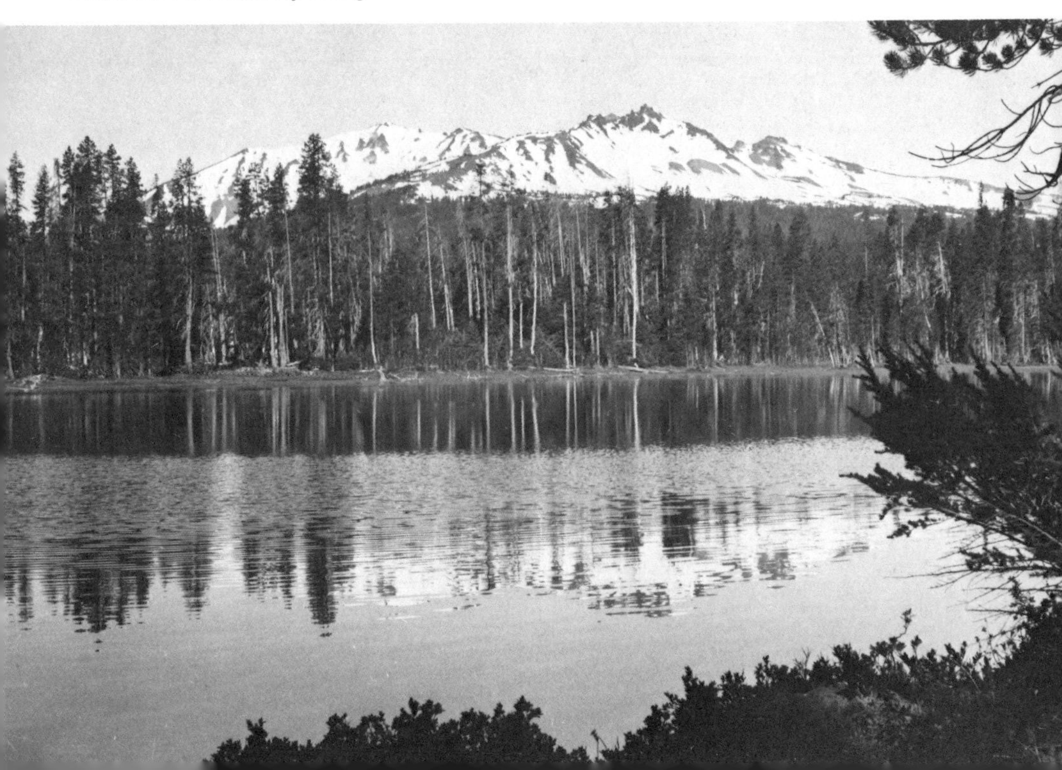

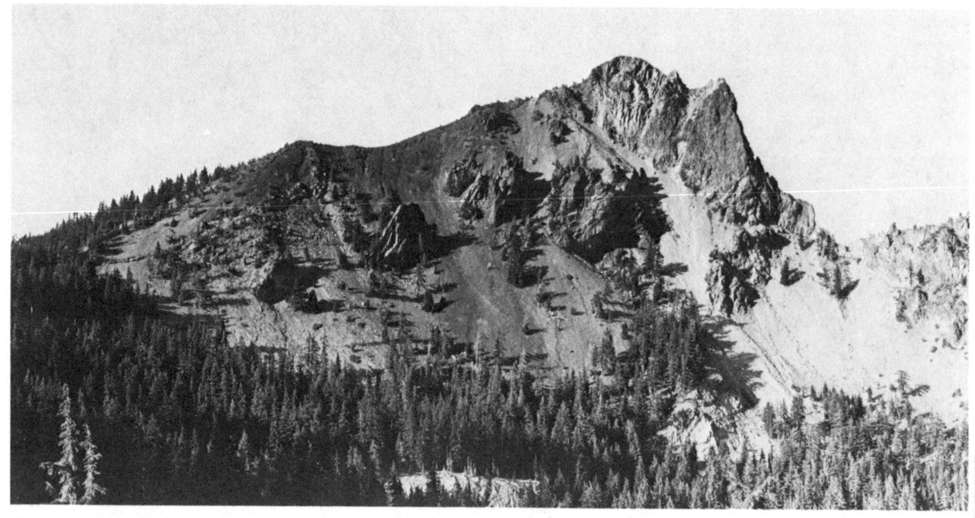

Asymmetrical Cowhorn Mountain, viewed from the southwest

Water access (from official PCT only). From here you can traverse 200 yards northwest across relatively flat terrain to an unseen lakelet with acceptable water and a possible campsite.

Beyond the unseen lakelet, the PCT climbs the crest over to a saddle (7100–1.6) by the southwest ridge of pointed Cowhorn Mountain.

Side route (from official PCT only). The short, rewarding climb to the top of this miniature Mt. Thielsen is an obvious though steep one.

The trail now descends northwest along the crest, eventually switchbacking down to the edge of a forested bowl that contains a small, somewhat stagnant pond (6380–3.1). This, unfortunately, is the only *permanent* trailside water between Summit Lake, 3.8 miles ahead, and Thielsen Creek, 29 miles behind! It's too bad that PCT hikers must go out of their way to get water or to camp. This section of the PCT could have easily been routed past springs, creeks, and lakes.

Water access (from official PCT only). From the stagnant pond you can head cross-country over the low crest and drop ¼ to ½ mile into the Windy Lakes basin for water and a campsite.

About ½ mile beyond the pond, you start a diagonal descent across a considerable escarpment and soon reach an amorphous terrain on which you cross an imperceptible crest. A little over 3 miles of viewless meandering brings you close to Summit Lake's south shore (5560–4.1), and a short traverse west brings you to Road 700 (5570–0.2), at the lake's southwest corner. Cross this road three times as you follow the PCT north along it to a crossing of Road 6010 (5590–1.4).

Side route (from official PCT only). From here you can head 200 yards over to Summit Lake Campground, above the lake's northwest corner. This lake is a good one for a layover day, for, like *large* Cascade Range lakes, it has clear water and relatively few mosquitoes.

From Road 6010, the trail starts northeast, and you enter Diamond Peak Wilderness as the trail winds northwest past a series of seven ponds and lakelets shown on the map and even more smaller, unmapped ones. After leaving the west shore of the last mapped one (5670–1.1), the trail winds north up a relatively dry stretch to a slope above the south shore of one of the few accessible lakes you'll see (5860–0.9), near which adequate camps can be established. The trail curves down to the lake's east shore and then, in ⅓ mile, crosses a

See maps D8, D9, D10

see MAP D13

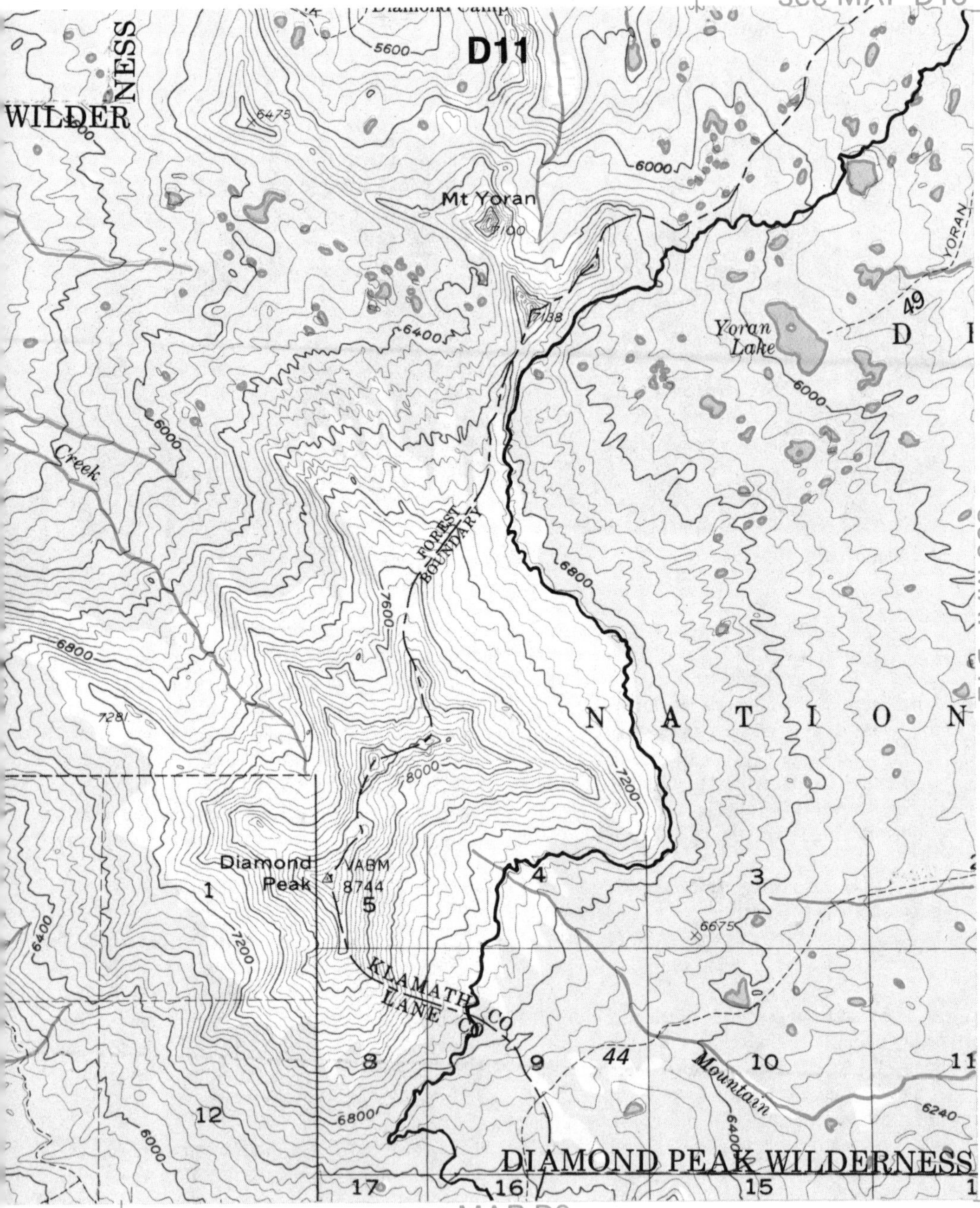

D11

WILDERNESS

Mt Yoran

Yoran Lake

FOREST BOUNDARY

N A T I O N

Diamond Peak

VABM 8744

KLAMATH CO

LANE CO

Creek

Mountain

DIAMOND PEAK WILDERNESS

see MAP D12

see MAP D9

"spring" from an unseen pond only 30 yards from the trail. Continuing north, you wind up to a forested flat across which the Fawn Lake Trail once traversed. Beyond it, you climb north and then northwest easily up to a switchback (6560–2.8) from which you get one of several forthcoming views of stunning, steep-sided Mt. Thielsen. The trail northeast climbs gently-to-moderately across the imperceptible Lane/Klamath county line and levels off in a glaciated bowl just east of Diamond Peak.

Side route (from official PCT only). Hikers wishing to climb this peak can scramble west from here up Class-2 rubble slopes.

see MAP D13

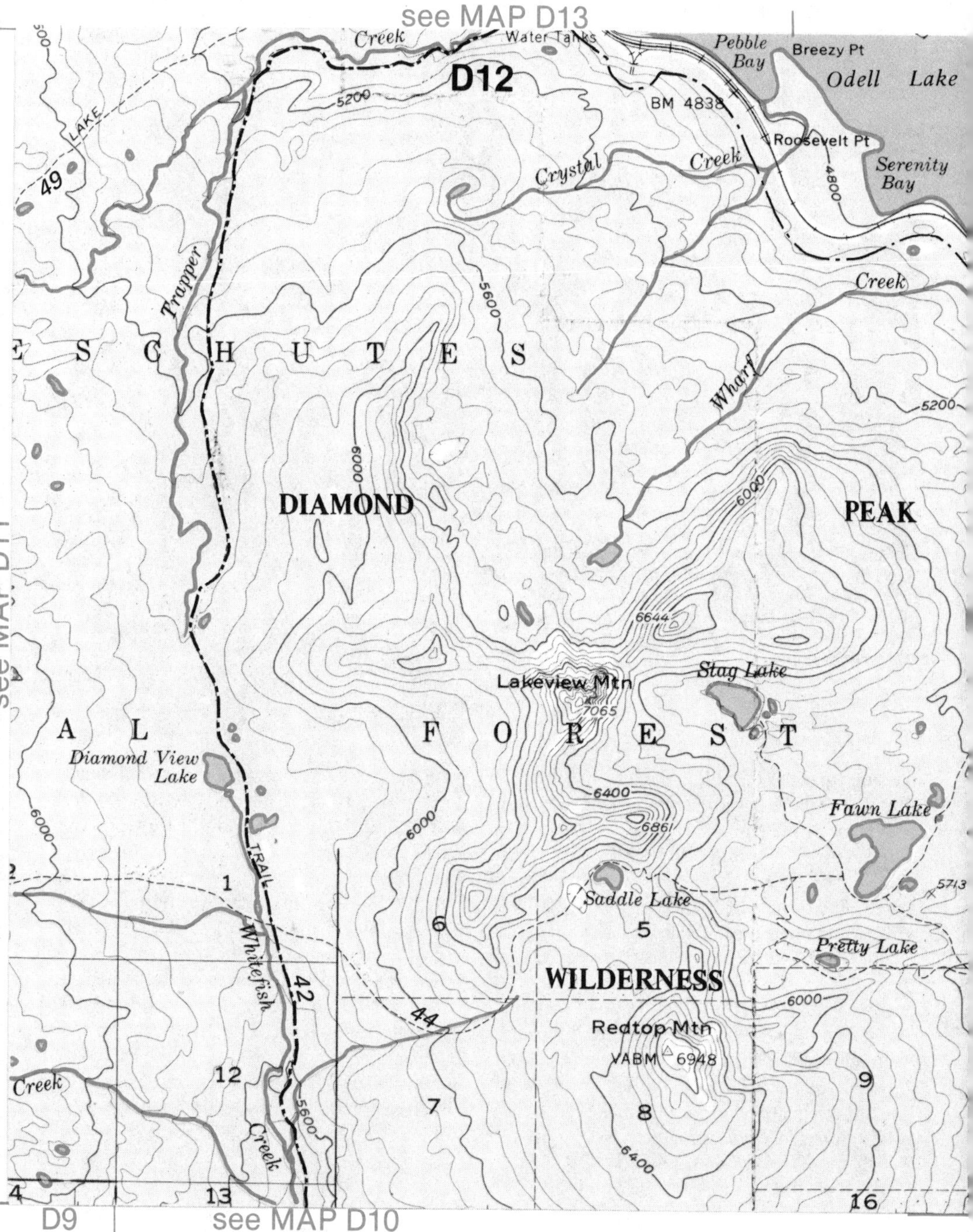

see MAP D10

Leaving the bowl, you traverse east and catch a view in the south of Crater Lake's rim framed between Mt. Thielsen (9182) on the left and Mt. Bailey (8363) on the right. Closer, in the southeast, is large Crescent Lake. You round the curving, northeast ridge of Diamond Peak and soon exchange southern views for northern ones. ▮ *In open breaks in the mountain-hemlock forest, you may see—if weather permits—South Sister (10,358), Middle Sister (10,047), Mt. Washington (7794), and very distant Mt. Jefferson (10,497). Closer by stand two imposing monoliths, Mt. Yoran (7100) and Peak 7138; you'll traverse below the latter.* ▮ Before that northeast traverse, however, the winding course makes a broad arc northward,

See map D11

see MAP E1

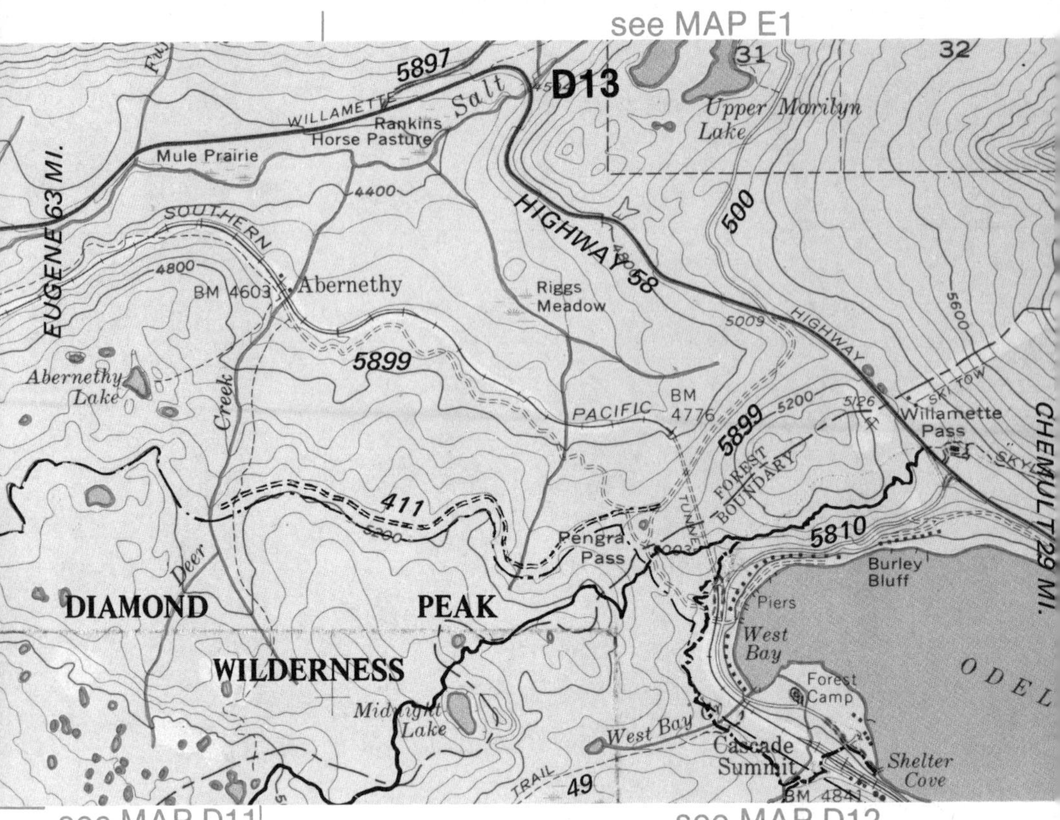

see MAP D11

see MAP D12

passing by some reliable creeklets and then by tiny tarns before commencing a steady descent past Peak 7138.

Leaving the ridge slopes behind, you descend to lake-and-pond-dotted slopes and arrive above the north shore (6030–7.2) of a green, unnamed lake near which you could camp. All the lakes and ponds between it and the Rosary Lakes, north of State Highway 58, are less attractive. Not too far beyond the lake, you see an even larger lake to the east through the trees, and the trail descends to within about 100 feet of its northwest corner (5840–0.6). Lack of adequate level ground makes camping at this corner of the lake undesirable, but more-distant shores offer better potential.

Beyond this lake, you descend for 1¼ miles past shallow, mosquito-infested ponds before angling southeast and descending to a broad flat of silver fir, mountain hemlock, and western white pine. A bend northward takes you up to a low saddle from which you descend to within 70 yards (5370–2.5) of fairly well-hidden Midnight Lake, which has poor camping potential. You may wish to stop for water here or at a nearby pond ¼ mile farther along the route. Beyond both bodies of water, you cross a saddle and then descend steadily to a closed road at Pengra Pass (5003—1.5), just 80 yards southeast of its junction with Road 5899.

Resupply access (from official PCT only). To get food or mailed packages at Shelter Cove Resort (mentioned in the alternate route), follow this road ½ mile southeast down to Road 5810 and then follow that road southeast one mile over to the resort. To return to the PCT, either backtrack or else follow the last part of the alternate route—a maintained section of the defunct Oregon Skyline Trail.

At Pengra Pass, you leave the wilderness and contour east to a junction with the old Oregon Skyline Trail (5040–0.5), at which the alternate route ends. Here you'll also find an old trail that descends steeply south ¼ mile to Road 5810.

Alternate route. Many hikers still prefer to take the old Oregon Skyline Trail, which closely approaches Odell Lake and which certainly has more lakes at which you can camp. These lakes, of course, have mosquito problems, at least before August, so before then you can choose between mosquitoes on the Oregon Skyline Trail and snow patches on the PCT. If you decide to hike the Oregon Skyline Trail, then hike northeast down the Cascade Lakes Road to a trailhead (5710–0.7), just 15 yards past a seasonal but obvious creek.

The trail's name has been changed to Oldenberg Lake Trail 45, and on it you start northeast up the old Oregon Skyline Trail, contour across gentle slopes of manzanita and sparse forest cover, and then descend slightly to the Nip and Tuck Lakes spur trail (5715–1.7). This heads east-southeast for a level 200 yards to the two lakes, which are only one lake in early summer. The peninsula that juts between the two lobes makes an excellent campsite, and the warm, shallow lake water is very inviting. The OST heads north-northwest and climbs gently at first, but then it makes a short, somewhat sunny, moderate-to-steep climb up to a ridge (5956–1.0), providing you with only one reward—a view south of Mt. Thielsen. The trail ahead is now downhill almost all the way to Crescent Lake.

Now you start moderately down and head north to the west shore of Oldenberg Lake (5475–1.3) and then north past two of the Bingham Lakes to a junction (5450–1.1) with a west-northwest trail to the third. This third Bingham Lake, at the end of the hundred-yard spur trail, is the largest and perhaps the clearest of all the shallow lakes between Maidu Lake and Crescent Lake. Continuing north along the route, you pass through an "Oregon desert" of sparse lodgepoles and then descend gradually and cross a seasonal creek whose luxuriant green vegetation contrasts vividly with the surrounding sparsely needled lodgepoles. The trail rounds a low ridge and then reaches the northeast end of murky, manmade Pinewan Lake (5180–2.0), which has a habit of drying up in late summer. Here, and for a short distance west, the trail follows the immigrant road built and used by the Elliot Wagon Train in October 1853.

Go about 100 yards before the trail forks right (northwest) from the road and winds ¼ mile down to a gully. Ahead, it wraps around a minor ridge and then descends ¼ mile to a junction with an abandoned trail (5010–0.7). Ahead, the old Oregon Skyline Trail once wove its way northwest down to an organization camp at Crescent Lake's southwest corner. Today, it goes but 80 yards northwest to a gully and then turns northeast, dying out before reaching close-by Road 60. If you'd walk ¼ mile west on that road, you'd reach Road 260, which descends ½ mile to Crescent Lake's Spring Campground.

From the junction, you head west on the Metolius-Windigo Horse Trail. It rapidly reaches the gully, curves around a minor ridge, and then weaves northwest down to a junction (5030–0.9). Northeastward, a spur trail heads 150 yards over to Road 60 and then continues just beyond it to a trailhead parking area for the Oldenberg Lake and Windy Lakes trails. Just ¼ mile southeast up Road 60, you'd find Spring Campground's Road 260. Westward, go about 220 yards before meeting southwest-climbing Windy Lakes Trail 50. Anyone who abandons the high and dry PCT and descends about 4 miles down this trail will join you here.

Onward, the Metolius-Windigo Horse Trail almost touches Road 60 as it traverses from northwest to north over to Summit Lake Road 6010. Cross it, parallel it 100 yards north, walk 100 feet up the road, and find the trail starting from the road's east side. In ½ mile you wind down to the boggy environs of Whitefish Creek and then, 200 yards past it, reach Road 220 (4870–1.4) only 60 yards west of its junction with Road 60. Follow this road north through Whitefish Horse Camp and in ⅓ mile reach a campground loop. This has piped water, which for late season trekkers could be their last reliable water until Diamond View Lake, 5½ miles away. Branch left and locate the Whitefish Creek Trail 42 trailhead along the northwest part of the loop. From the loop's north part, the Metolius-Windigo Horse Trail heads northeast.

You start northwest on Trail 42, enter Diamond Lake Wilderness in about ½ mile, and then climb rather gently to a fairly reliable tributary of Whitefish Creek (5080–1.6). The trail remains within hearing distance of Whitefish Creek—when it's running—as you climb northwest and then north up to a flat and a linear pond at an intersection with Crater Butte Trail 44 (5770–3.1), 4 miles due east of Diamond Peak (8744).

See maps D8, D10

From the junction, your trail heads north past several shallow, somewhat stagnant ponds before arriving at large but shallow Diamond View Lake (5780–0.7). Photographs are best when the peak is snow-clad, which, unfortunately, is when the lake is mosquito-clad. You pass campsites and then leave the lake behind as you make tracks north through swampy lodgepole flatlands to the headwaters of Trapper Creek. This creek remains unseen and unheard for 2 miles until the trail reaches slopes above the creek where the latter cascades north down toward a marsh. In the third mile, the trail reaches the creek, more or less follows it to the marsh, and then goes east through a shady mountain-hemlock forest. In order to avoid the creekside's wet ground, the trail generally stays on the lower slopes just south of the creek. Follow the creek as it meanders east past tempting campsites and then cascades northeast down past a small, breached dam. Almost immediately after sighting this concrete structure, you reach a trail junction (4870–4.9–21.1) where an access trail continues northeast but your trail turns north.

The access trail descends 240 yards to the Southern Pacific railroad tracks and crosses them 20 yards west-northwest of a huge, steel overhead signal. Head east across the tracks and under the overhead signal to a dirt road that descends 150 yards to Road 5810 along the west shore of Odell Lake (4788). ▮ *This lake was named for William Holden Odell who, with B.J. Pengra, surveyed the military wagon road up the Middle Fork of the Willamette in 1865. On July 26th, Odell climbed a butte and discovered this lake; both butte and lake now bear his name.* ▮ If you walk ¼ mile northwest on Road 5810, you'll reach the entrance to Trapper Creek Campground. If you walk 250 yards southeast on Road 5810, you'll reach the Shelter Cove Resort, which has a small store, coin-operated showers, and for PCT hikers, a relatively inexpensive campsite fee. As was mentioned at the beginning of this chapter, the resort holds parcels mailed by UPS.

After backtracking to the Trail 42 junction (mile 21.1), you curve west 150 yards down to a bridge that crosses Trapper Creek only 35 yards below the breached dam. Leaving this creek behind, contour the slopes and reach an intersection with Yoran Lake Trail 49 (4900–0.5). This trail goes northeast moderately to steeply 250 yards down to the railroad tracks, from which you follow a dirt road 70 yards to Road 5810. You can follow this road a quarter mile east to the Trapper Creek Campground and then 0.4 mile farther to the Shelter Cove Resort.

North of the trail intersection, the trail parallels the railroad tracks below and passes seasonal creeklets before reaching a spur road (4850–0.7) that climbs northwest 0.4 mile to Pengra Pass. Start along this road from a point 70 yards west of the tracks and follow it up 80 yards around a bend to a resumption of the trail, which branches right and ascends 130 yards northwest to a small creek under the shade of a Douglas-fir forest. ▮ *Here you find shooting stars, bluebells, bunchberries, and Oregon grapes, which are typically associated with this type of forest.* ▮ The trail now climbs gently northeast and reaches a junction with the PCT (5040–0.5–22.8). Midway up this short ascent, you meet the upper end of a shorter, steeper trail (an alternate route) that starts where the railroad tracks enter a tunnel.

With the official PCT and the alternate route rejoined, the PCT now climbs a short ⅓ mile to a small bluff, where the Eagle Rock Overlook provides the only good view of Odell Lake along the route. The trail climbs a few yards beyond the viewpoint, contours over to a pond on the right and then makes a short, switchbacking descent to Highway 58 (5090–1.1), which you reach ¼ mile southeast of Willamette Pass.

See maps D10, D12, D13

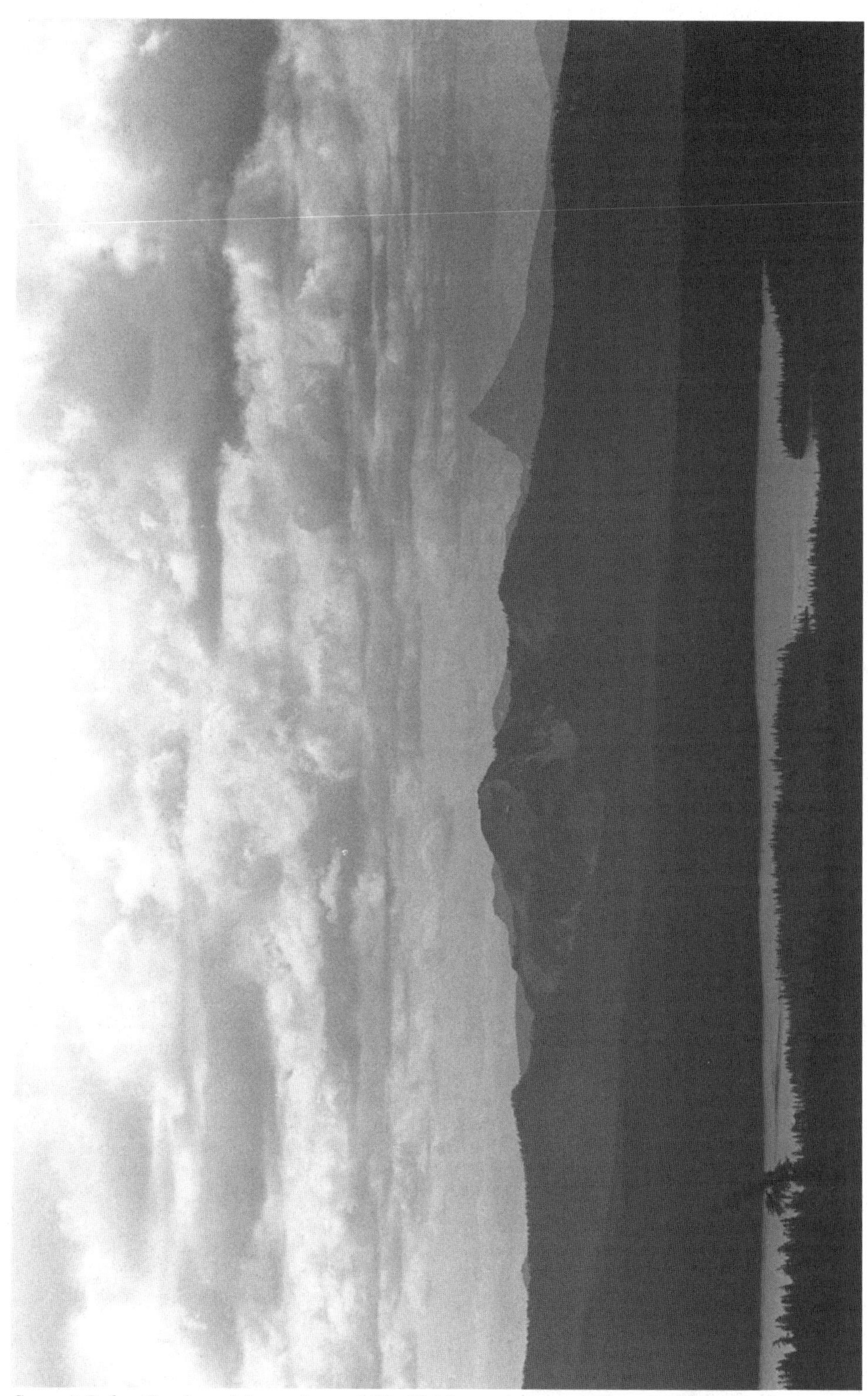

Summit Lake, Cowhorn Mountain, and Mt. Thielsen, view south from Diamond Peak Wilderness

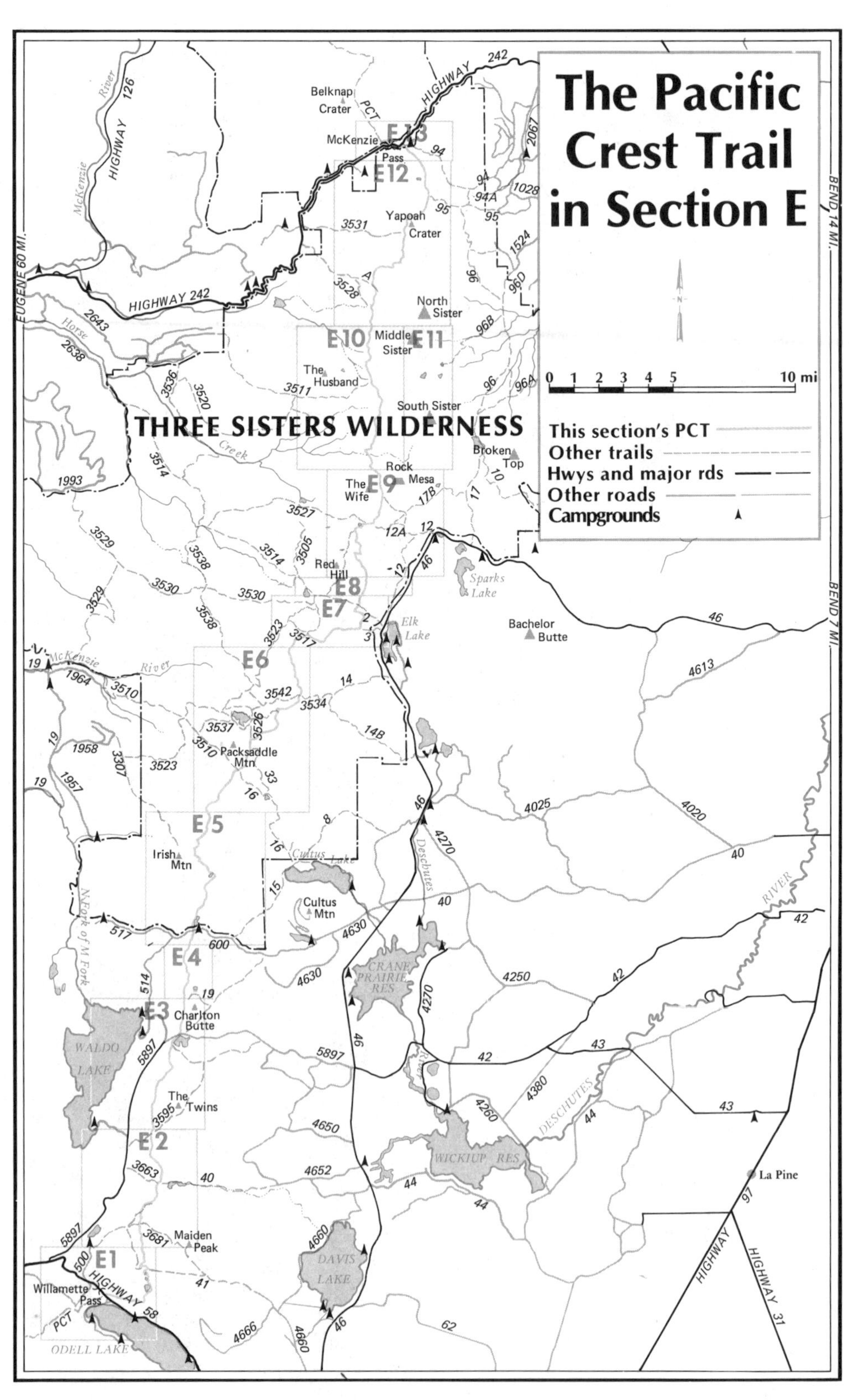

The Pacific Crest Trail in Section E
0 1 2 3 4 5 10 mi
This section's PCT
Other trails
Hwys and major rds
Other roads
Campgrounds
THREE SISTERS WILDERNESS
Belknap Crater
McKenzie Pass
Yapoah Crater
North Sister
Middle Sister
The Husband
South Sister
Broken Top
Rock Mesa
The Wife
Red Hill
Sparks Lake
Elk Lake
Bachelor Butte
Packsaddle Mtn
Irish Mtn
Cultus Lake
Cultus Mtn
Charlton Butte
Waldo Lake
The Twins
Crane Prairie Res
Wickiup Res
Davis Lake
La Pine
Maiden Peak
Willamette Pass
Odell Lake
HIGHWAY 242
HIGHWAY 126
HIGHWAY 58
HIGHWAY 97
HIGHWAY 31
EUGENE 60 MI.
BEND 14 MI.
BEND 7 MI.
McKenzie River
Deschutes River
N Fork of M Fork
Horse Creek
PCT

Section E: Highway 58 near Willamette Pass to Highway 242 at McKenzie Pass

Introduction: In Section E, the PCT traverses three types of terrain. The first third of this section's PCT traverses slopes deficient in both views and lakes. On the middle third, which starts at Irish Lake, the trail traverses flatter land that is still generally viewless but that is peppered with very enjoyable lakes (once the mosquito population dwindles). On the northern third, the trail skirts the Three Sisters, and views abound of glacier-draped peaks and spreading, sinister lava flows. Like Section C's Sky Lakes Wilderness, this section's Three Sisters Wilderness, which dominates most of the section, is flooded with weekend hikers. And for good reason—it is very scenic and readily accessible.

Declination: 18¼°E

Points on Route	S➣N	Mi. Btwn. Pts.	N➣S
Highway 58 near Willamette Pass	0.0		76.0
Lower Rosary Lake	2.2	2.2	73.8
Moore Creek Trail to Bobby Lake	9.0	6.8	67.0
Charlton Lake Trail	16.6	7.6	59.4
Road 600 at Irish Lake	22.2	5.6	53.8
Cliff Lake Trail	35.6	13.4	40.4
Island Meadow Trail to Elk Lake	44.5	8.9	31.5
Camelot Lake	50.4	5.9	25.6
North fork of Mesa Creek	54.9	4.5	21.1
Glacier Way Trail	65.2	10.3	10.8
Minnie Scott Spring	68.3	3.1	7.7
South Matthieu Lake	71.7	3.4	4.3
Trail to Lava Camp Lake	74.6	2.9	1.4
Highway 242 at McKenzie Pass	76.0	1.4	0.0

Supplies: No on-route supplies are available, but you can make a 1¼-mile detour to Elk Lake Resort, which has a café and a small store that caters to anglers. The resort also holds PCT packages (address: Elk Lake Resort, P.O. Box 789, Bend, OR 97709). Before mailing packages, contact the resort to verify that it still offers this free service.

Problems: Long-distance PCT hikers seem to agree that the trail's worst concentrations of mosquitoes are found either in Sky Lakes Wilderness in Section C or in the lake-and-pond-dotted south half of Three Sisters Wilderness. Therefore, bring a tent and plenty of mosquito repellent if you are hiking through this section before August.

Maps:

Willamette Pass, OR
Waldo Lake, OR
The Twins, OR
Irish Mountain, OR
Packsaddle Mountain, OR
Elk Lake, OR
South Sister, OR
North Sister, OR
Mt. Washington, OR

SECTION E

THE ROUTE

Where southeast-northwest Highway 58 reaches broad Willamette Pass, you'll find a Visitor Information Center and ski area immediately north of it. About 0.4 mile southeast on Highway 58, you'll reach West Odell Lake Road, branching southwest, and just 100 yards before it is a short spur road branching northeast and then quickly turning east. At its end is trailhead parking, and from there an 80-yard spur trail goes north to the PCT, which crosses Highway 58 about 0.1 mile northwest of the trailhead's road.

Starting from Highway 58 (5090), follow the PCT as it curves east behind the Highway Commission's long cinder-storage building and then meet the trailhead-parking spur trail (5130–0.2) immediately past it.

The PCT now climbs steadily east through a forest of Douglas-fir, western white pine, and mountain hemlock to a saddle and then curves north to pass a hundred-foot-high rock jumble before reaching the ridge above South Rosary Lake (5730–2.0). This clear lake is deep in early summer, and in this it contrasts strongly with the other lakes its size that you've seen so far along the entire route. By late summer, however, the lake level can fall more than twenty feet due to seepage through the porous volcanic rocks, leaving its eastward drainage channel high and dry. You quickly encounter a very good ridgetop campsite and then curve northward, cross the lake's outlet, and reach an equally good campsite. Now climb northwest to a campsite near the southwest corner of deep, blue-green Middle Rosary Lake (5830–0.6), which is even more impressive than the south lake because it lies at the base of 400-foot-high Rosary Rock. ▮ *On a weekend, you're likely to see climbers scaling this rock.* ▮ Walk alongside the lake and then pass the low dividing ridge between the middle and north lakes, on which is an excellent campsite. You reach shallower North Rosary Lake (5830–0.3) and then follow the trail as it climbs west above the lake's north shore before switchbacking east-northeast up to a junction with Maiden Lake Trail 41 (6060–0.6), which descends east-southeast before contouring east toward that lake.

SECTION E

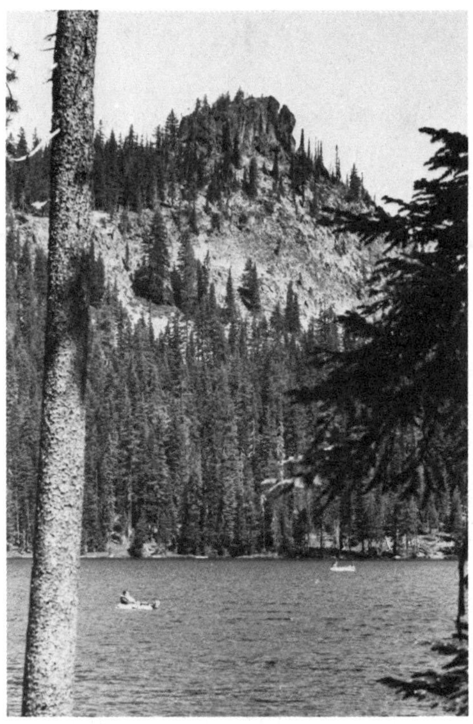

South (Lower) Rosary Lake

Continue east for 130 yards and then switchback west up to a saddle (6170–0.5), but not before getting one last glance back at Rosary Rock and the Rosary Lakes, and in the distance, Odell Lake, Odell Butte, and Crescent Lake—all lakes owing their existence to glacial excavation. ▮ *Until the late 1980s, the PCT followed the original Oregon Skyline Trail, descending northwest along, appropriately, Skyline Creek. Doing so, it passed three camps: T-M-R, Bark Table, and Waithere. The newer stretch, unfortunately, avoids both camps and water and hugs the crest as a crest trail is supposed to do. Still, the lack of camps will be missed by some old-time hikers and equestrians, and will only add to the camping pressure at the Rosary Lakes. Plan accordingly.* ▮

After heading north along the east-facing slopes of a linear ridge, a stretch that offers Maiden Peak views, the newer stretch crosses the ridge at a minor saddle (6070–1.3) and then

See maps E1, E2

see MAP E2

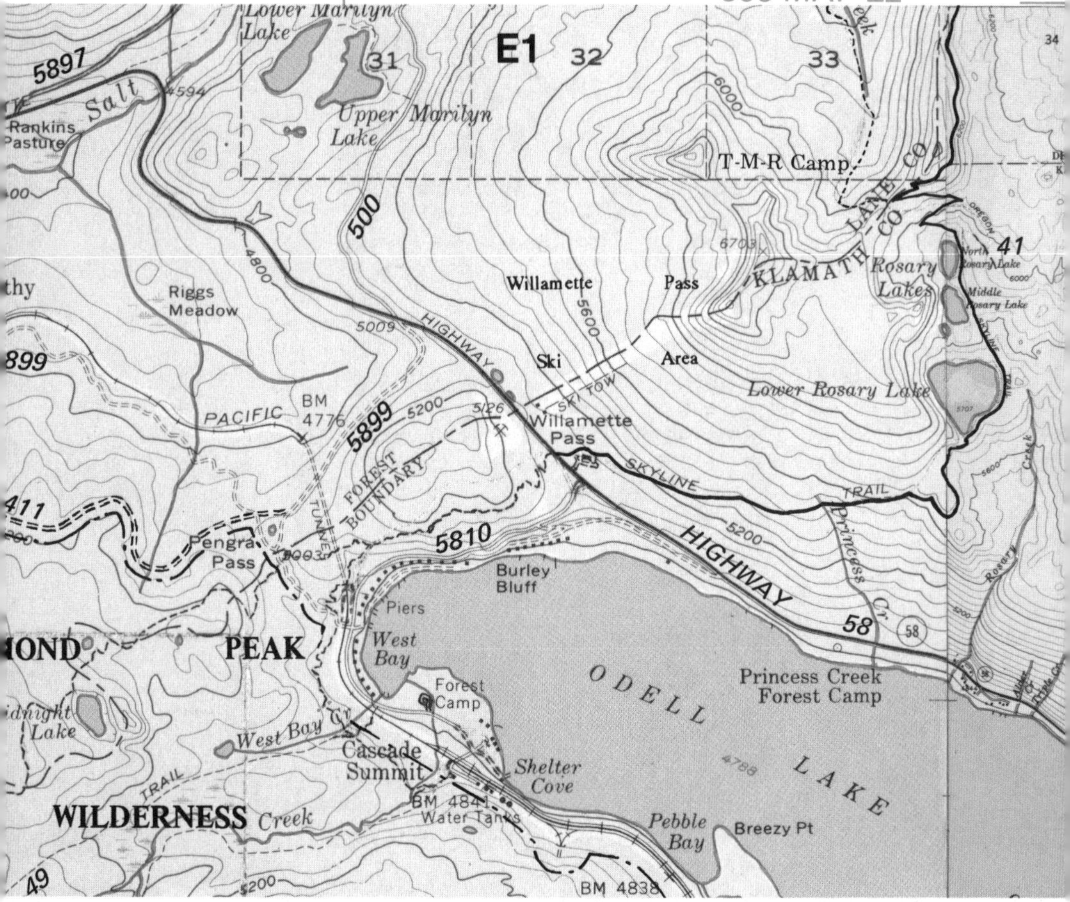

see MAP D12

soon descends moderately to an intersection of Maiden Peak Trail (5800–1.1).

Side route. West, this trail descends ¾ mile to Waithere Camp, situated just south of the trail's junction with the old, creekside Oregon Skyline Trail route.

The PCT continues north, first dropping moderately for ¾ mile and then traversing north about a mile before curving north across wet meadows up to a junction with Bobby Lake Trail 3663 (5440–2.2); west, it traverses 2 miles to paved Road 5897, the Waldo Lake Road.

Turn right (northeast) and start up the trail as it curves quickly up to a triangular junction where two forks of Moore Creek Trail 40 (5470–0.2) branch off from the PCT and merge just east of it.

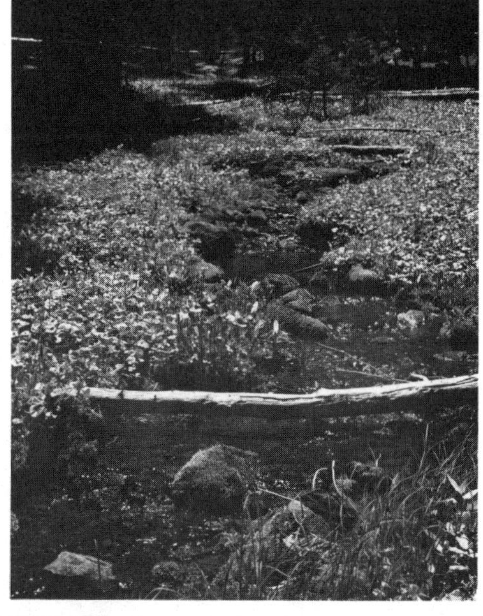

Skyline Creek

See map E2

see MAP E3

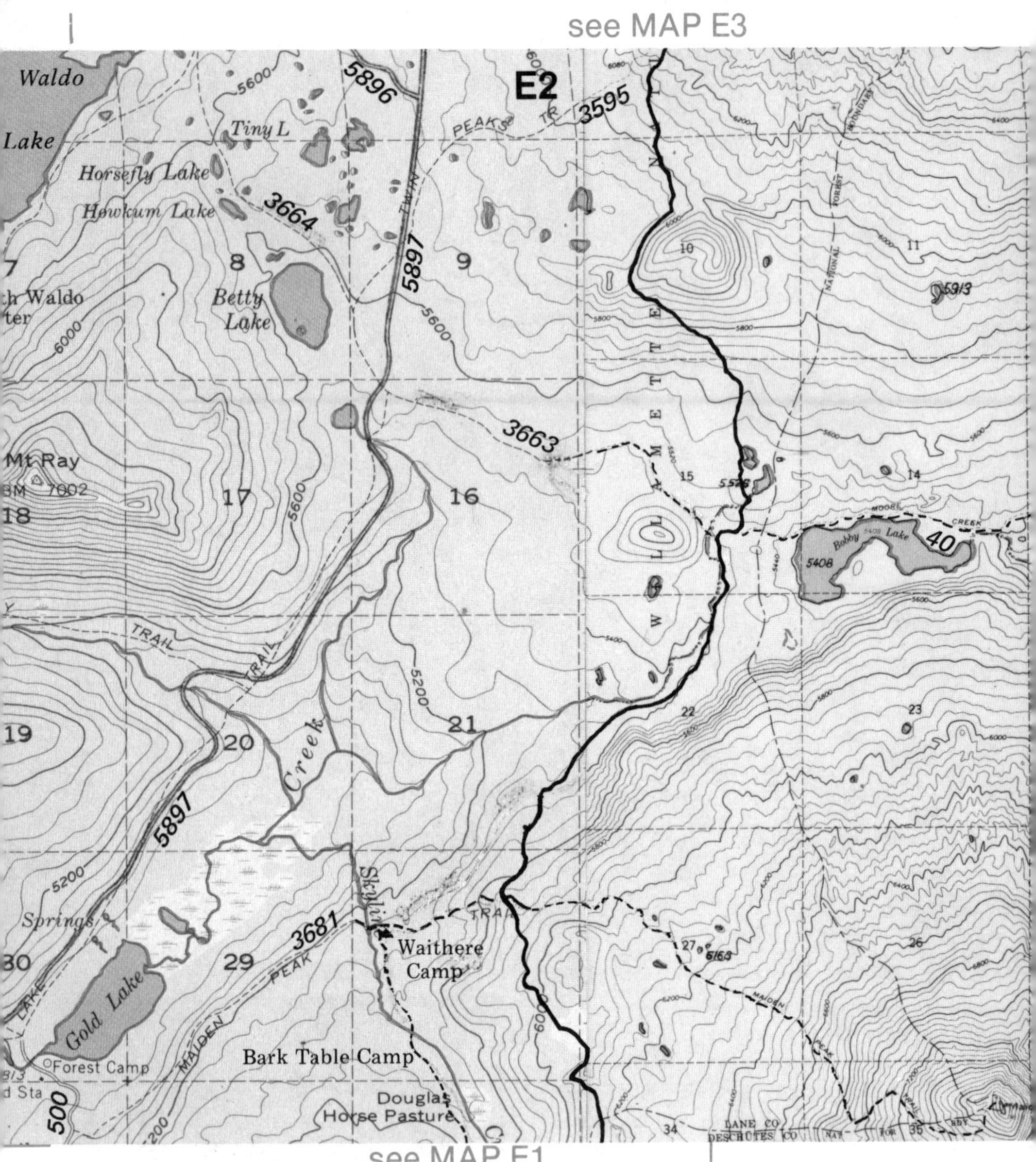

see MAP E1

Water access. It's best now to head east ¼ mile down this trail to a nice campsite at the west end of large, clear Bobby Lake (5408), for the next reliable source of water is Charlton Lake, about 7⅔ miles farther. *It seems ironic that as one progresses north into ever thicker, wetter forests, the water sources become spaced farther apart. You expect drought over the miles of pumice-covered lands around Crater Lake and Mt. Thielsen, but it can be frustrating to be in a dense forest during a drizzling rain and yet to have to hike miles to find running water to drink. In such areas, groundwater percolating through the volcanic-rock structures certainly is the major form of water transport.*

Back on the PCT, head north past two large ponds, climb northwest to a saddle (5980–1.4), curve northeast gently down from it, and then climb to an intersection with Twin Peaks Trail 3595 (6220–1.3). About a mile north from this junction, you can walk 70 yards west across rock slabs and obtain an unobstructed view westward, from Diamond Peak north to Waldo Lake.

Next, the trail shortly starts a gentle descent and begins to cross gullies one after another. You eventually pass above a small pond and

See maps E2, E3

see MAP E4

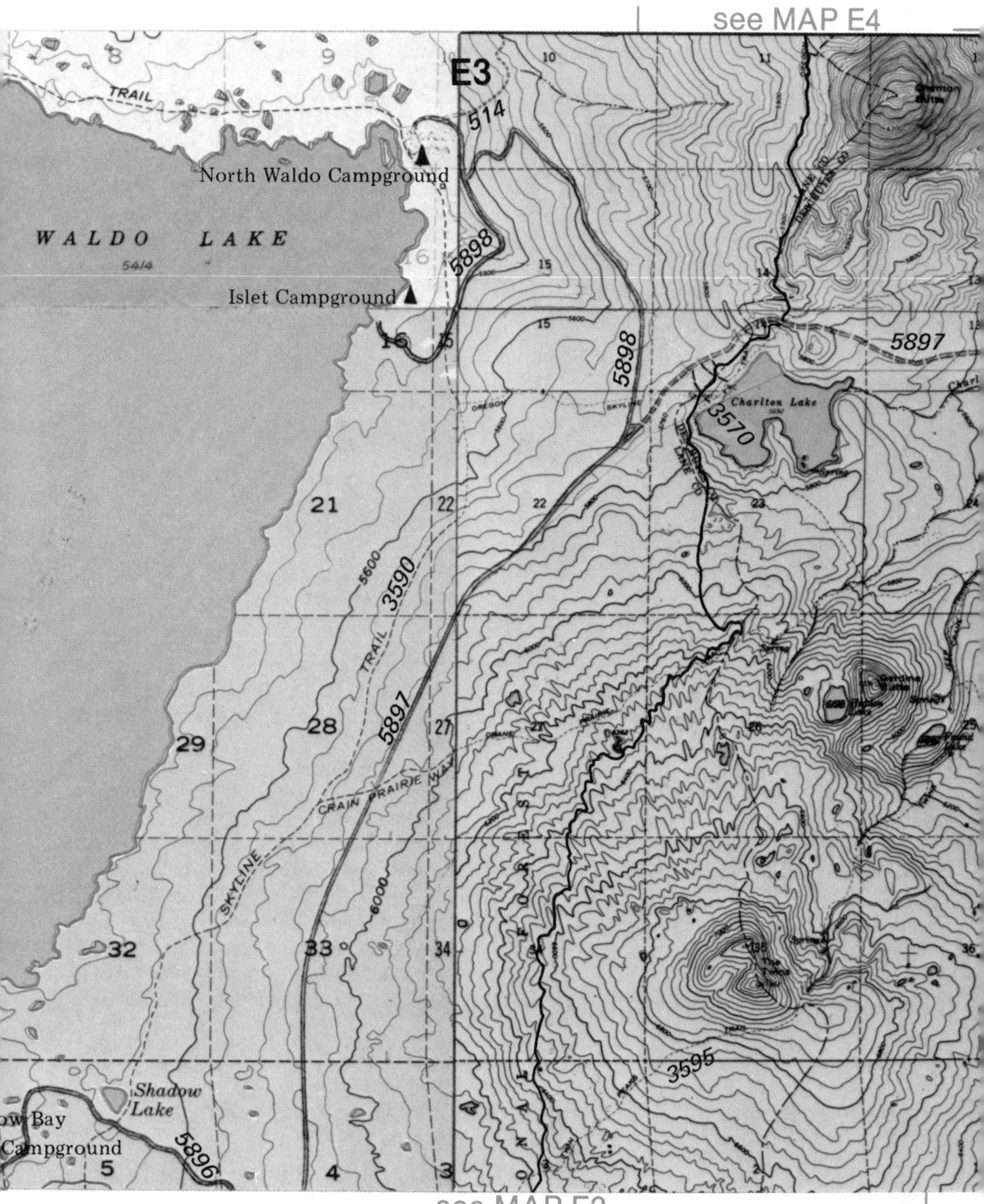

see MAP E2

then quickly reach a cluster of three ponds (6320–2.4) grouped around the small knob identified on the map as 6362. The route now descends northeast across gullies, reaches the watershed divide by a small pond, and then descends west a short distance before curving north toward gentler slopes above Charlton Lake (5692). Head north through a forested flat area, reach the slopes above the lake, and descend to an intersection with Charlton Lake Trail 3570 (5725–2.5) about a hundred yards north of a small pond. The lakeshore is 100 yards southeast; Road 5897 is 150 yards northwest, just beyond a pond. By heading northeast for 0.1 mile, you reach a closed spur road heading southeast to the lake from Road 5897. Then you diagonal north across the road to a broad trail that you follow north about 45 yards to

See map E3

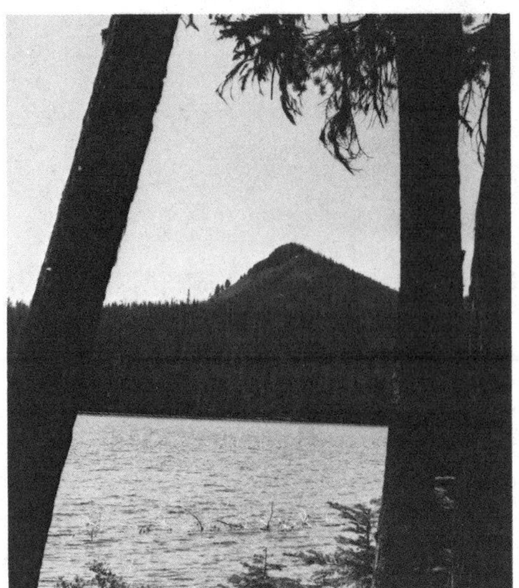

Charlton Lake and Gerdine Butte

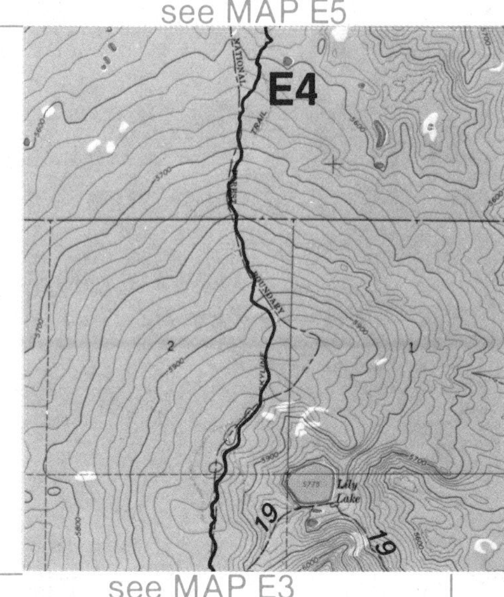

where it bends northwest 40 yards to a roadside parking area. From this bend, the PCT heads east-northeast and climbs gently up the divide to a diagonal crossing of Road 5897 (5840–0.6) at a 20° bearing.

The trail starts north, climbs northwest to the low watershed divide, and then contours north past small ponds and Charlton Butte to a junction on the right (east) with Lily Lake Trail 19 (5965–1.4), which descends about ¾ mile to that isolated lake. Continuing north, you keep following the divide down a north slope to a small flat and then climb over two low mounds before reaching the southwest arm of shallow Taylor Lake (5550–3.3). The trail immediately angles away from the lake, heads north past a pond on the left (west), and then reaches Road 600 at Irish Lake (5549–0.3). Popular Irish Lake Campground is ¼ mile east on the road.

To pick up the trail again, go west 25 yards on the road and then north 50 yards along a spur road to the trailhead. You enter Three Sisters Wilderness as the route heads north above the west shore of Irish Lake and then passes west of shallow but clear Riffle Lake (5575–0.8), which has an adequate campsite on its west shore. Now you climb a low ridge and descend slightly to a flat with two large lily-pad ponds before climbing up to a higher

See maps E3, E4, E5

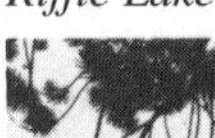

Riffle Lake

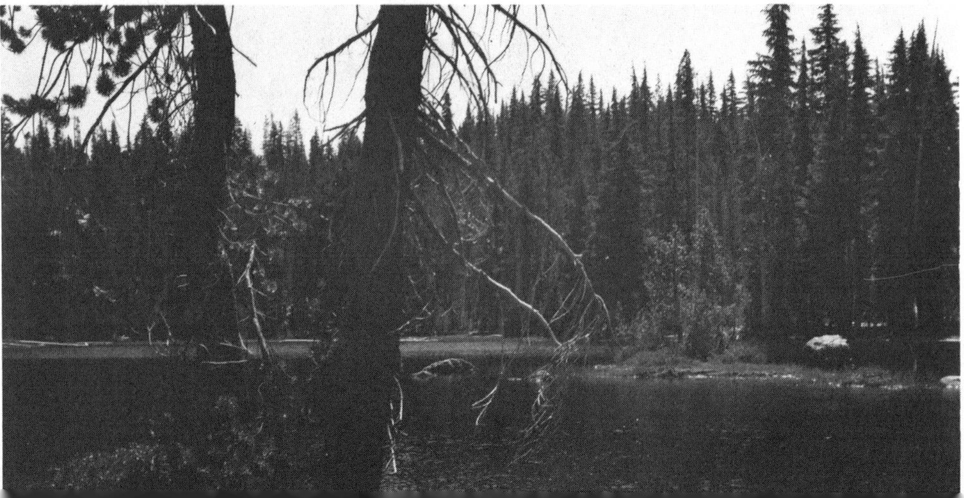

ridge (5730–1.2). The lakes and ponds of this area are shallow, and, like those in the Sky Lakes region, they support a superabundant mosquito population from late spring through mid-July.

Passing a number of stagnant ponds and small lakes in rapid succession, you descend to a nice campsite on the east shore of Brahma Lake (5657–0.6), which is distinguished by a forested island. The route continues north along the lake's shore, contours west, and then climbs moderately up slopes and through a miniature gorge before reaching the northeast corner of clear Jezebel Lake (5855–1.1). A

See map E5

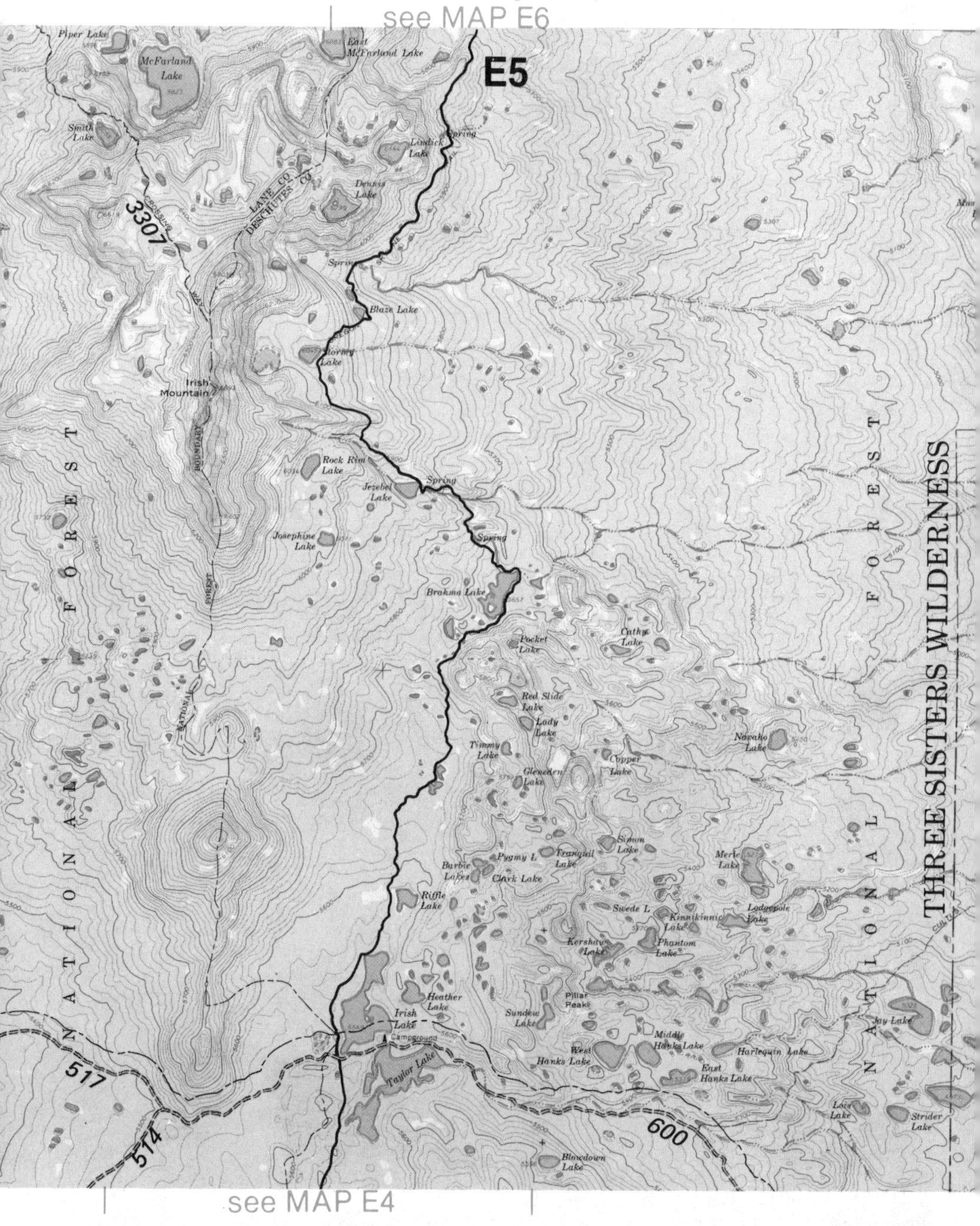

see MAP E7

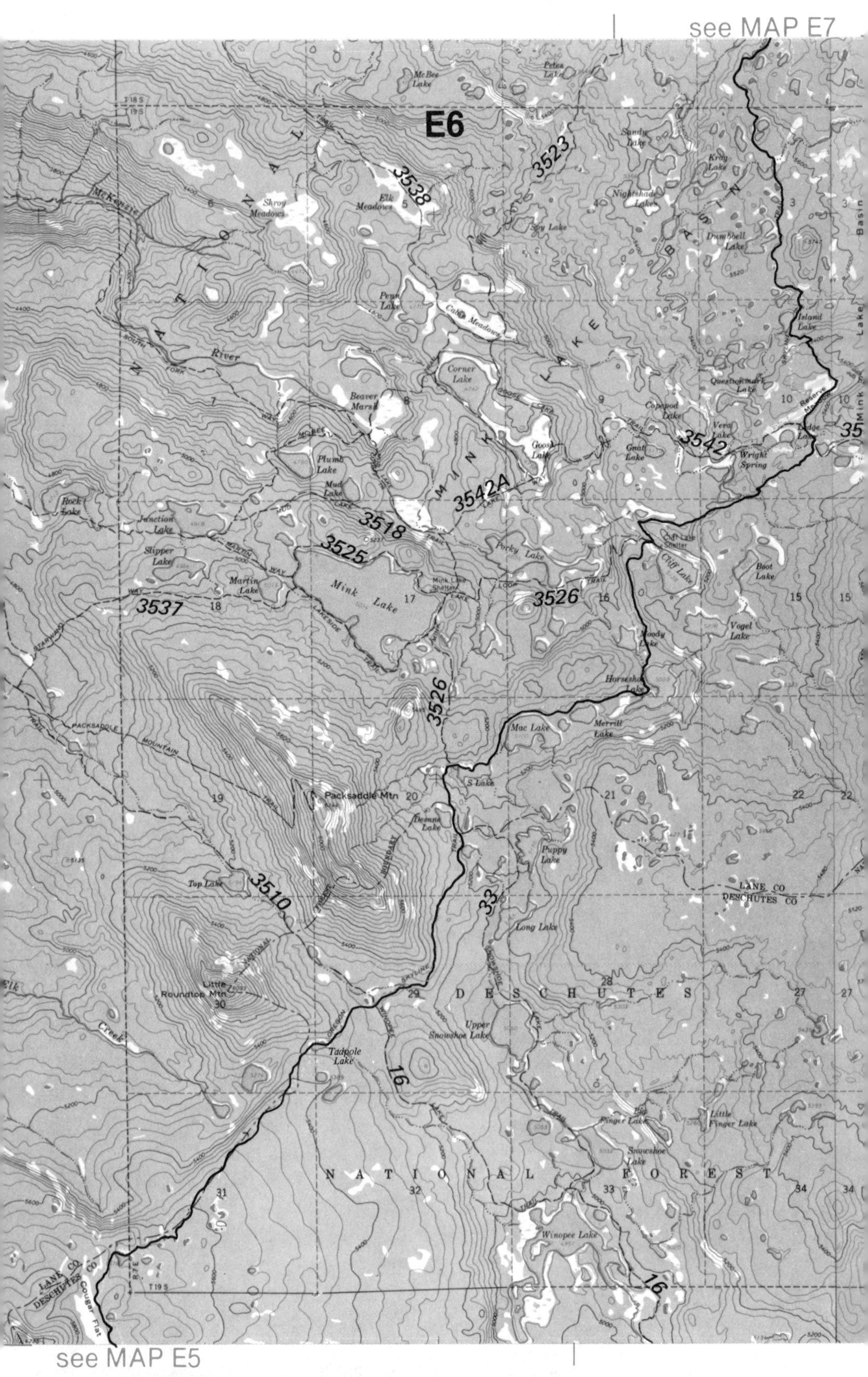

see MAP E5

Irish Mountain above Stormy Lake

campsite is perched on the low ridge north of this corner. Climbing northwest above the lake, you reach a shady glen from which a trail once climbed ¼ mile west-southwest to Rock Rim Lake. Your trail rounds a linear ridge descending east, climbs west along its north slope, and then angles north to a good campsite beside the outlet of Stormy Lake (6045–1.0). The sight of the towering cliffs of Irish Mountain over this lake will leave you with a vivid memory of this choice spot.

Leaving this lake behind, you descend to smaller, slightly cloudy Blaze Lake (5950–0.3) and then contour northward past an abundance of ponds before the trail descends a ridge to a low divide just east of open Cougar Flat (5750–2.1). Your route winds down to Lake 5678 and then passes smaller water bodies as it follows the ridge northeast down to Tadpole Lake (5340–2.0), perched on a forested saddle. Traverse the lake's grassy north shore and then descend north to a grassy pond and a junction with the Elk Creek (#3510) and Winopee Lake (#16) trails (5250–0.4).

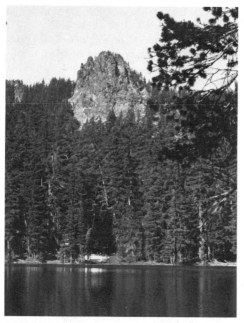

Side route. The Elk Creek Trail climbs northwest over a low saddle and descends into the Elk Creek drainage; the Winopee Lake Trail curves south around a knoll before descending to Winopee Lake.

Continue northeast across the lower slopes of Packsaddle Mountain (6144), walk north past a polluted lake to the east, and arrive at a junction with Snowshoe Lake Trail 33 (5250–1.2), which descends east. Now you hike north past Desane Lake and enter Willamette National Forest again as you cross a flat divide and descend into the Mink Lake Basin, where you meet a junction with Mink Lake Loop Trail 3526 (5160–0.4).

Side route. This 2.7-mile loop climbs northwest up a low, broad ridge before descending north to

See map E6

A bedrock peninsula cuts deep into Dumbbell Lake

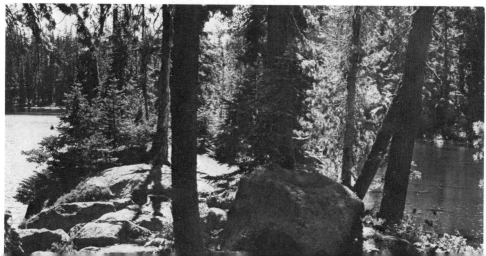

Mink Lake, stocked with eastern brook and rainbow trout. From there, the loop winds east, dropping to Porky Lake, with more eastern brook, and then climbs back to the PCT at the Cliff Lake outlet creek.

The PCT follows a string of sparkling lakes that make an appropriate necklace for South Sister. In rapid succession you encounter S Lake (5150), Mac Lake (5100), with rainbow, Merrill Lake (5080), and Horseshoe Lake (5039), a very shallow lake with both rainbow and eastern brook. The trail curves around to the north shore of this lake and then reaches a spur trail (5040–1.5) that bears 0.2 mile north to Moody Lake (5020). You cross the usually dry outlet of Horseshoe Lake and then continue north gently up and around a band of cliffs to a reunion with Mink Lake Loop Trail 3526 (5130–0.8) beside the Cliff Lake outlet creek.

Just 130 yards southeast up a spur trail beside this creek is deep, green, rock-and-alder-lined Cliff Lake (5138). The best campsites are atop the cliff along this popular lake's northwest shore, but should you be caught in foul weather, you can camp in comfort in the Cliff Lake shelter. ▮ *Good eastern-brook-trout fishing justifies a stop at this lake, as do good diving rocks near large aspens along the northeast shore. Backtracking from these, you pass beargrass blooming between boulders, and, near the shelter, avoid stepping on delicate bunchberries and shooting stars that grow on the moist, shady forest floor.* ▮

Back at the loop-trail junction, you cross Cliff Lake's outlet creek, walk northwest, and then round a pile of large boulders and climb gently to a seasonal creek (5225–0.8). Cross it, hike up a switchback, and then work up northeast to a junction with the Goose Rock (#3542) and Senoj Lake (#3534) trails (5330–0.6).

Side routes. The Goose Rock Trail starts northwest down toward a meadow and then heads west and down to Goose Lake. The 5.6-mile Senoj Lake Trail starts southeast to an unnamed lake, heads east to the divide and then continues as Trail 14 east down to Cascade Lakes Highway 46.

See map E6

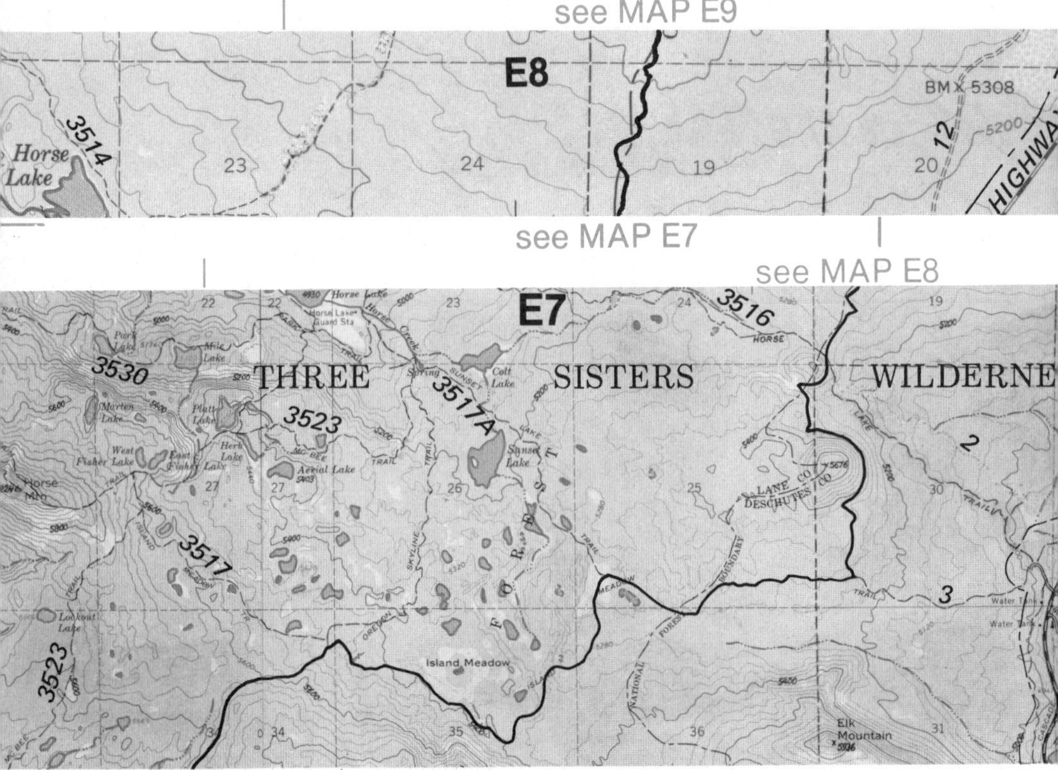

Start north, quickly descend to Reserve Meadow, and head northeast along its edge before curving northwest away from its large, east-end campsite (5320–0.4). The PCT then climbs up to relatively deep Island Lake (5438–0.5), which has a patch of grass in its center. From this lake, you climb up the trail to a rockpile, contour west past two stagnant ponds, and then hike north until you are just above a 50-yard-long peninsula that juts southwest into Dumbbell Lake (5502–0.7). From this rocky spur, you can fish or dive in the lake's warm, clear waters. The trail now gradually climbs north past many ponds to a low divide (5660–2.2) and then descends to a junction with the old Oregon Skyline Trail (5460–0.5), which heads 6.3 miles to Camelot Lake via popular Horse Lake.

From this junction 1½ miles south of Horse Lake, the PCT branches east. After a few minutes' hiking, you reach an obvious spring seeping from the ground only 10 yards downslope from the trail. This is a good place to obtain water, for the route beyond may be dry until Camelot Lake, 8.8 miles farther. Continuing east, you descend toward Island Meadow but stay within the forest's edge as you hike southeast along its southern border. You soon reach a bridge across a small creek and find a fair trailside campsite above its east bank, 70 yards south of the meadow. The trail strikes southeast again but shortly turns and follows a wandering route northeast before descending north to a mile-high meadow across which you traverse north-northeast to a junction with Sunset Lake Trail 3517A (5235–1.9), which passes that lake midway in its descent to the Oregon Skyline Trail. Now go east-southeast on the PCT, enter forest, pass a large seasonal pond 50 yards south, and then snake east over an undetected drainage divide before descending to a junction where the PCT leaves Island Meadow Trail 3/3517 (5250–1.3) and angles north.

Side route. The Island Meadow Trail makes a southeast descent 0.9 mile to a trailhead parking area, from which a road descends 270 yards to Cascade

See maps E6, E7

South Sister, from Koosah Mountain (left) and from Wickiup Plain (right)

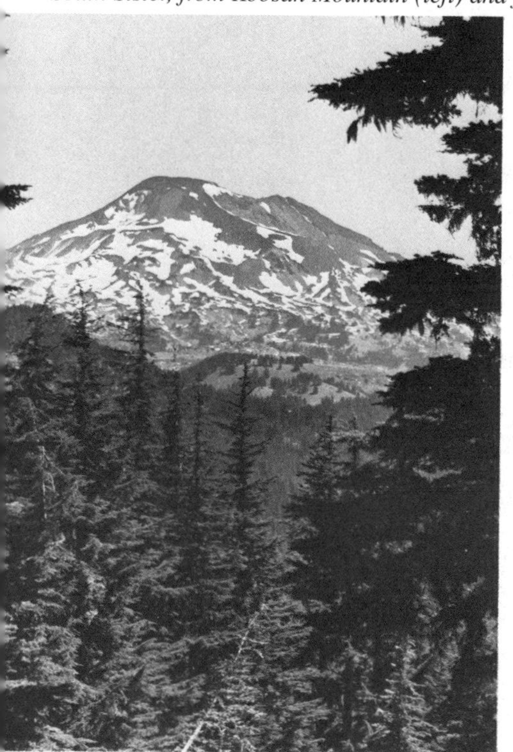

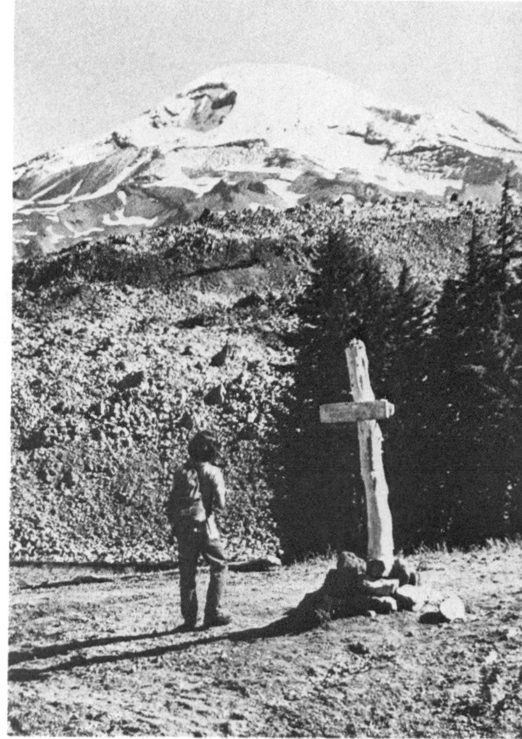

Lakes Highway 46. On this you can head south 70 yards to the Elk Lake Resort entrance. Down at the lakeside resort, you can obtain meals plus limited supplies. ▌ *If you visit the resort by early July, you'll likely see barn swallows nesting in the rafters above its entrance.* ▌ Large, 57-foot-deep Elk Lake (4884) offers very good trout fishing and is a nice place for a layover day at Elk Lake Campground, just south of the resort. ▌ *Although the lake has no outlet and no permanent inlets, its water stays quite clear because fresh groundwater continues to seep into the lake at about the same rate that groundwater leaves it.* ▌ Rather than backtrack up the Island Meadows Trail, you can head north on the road 0.2 mile past its trailhead and start up Horse Lake Trail 2, which takes you 1.6 miles northwest up to the PCT.

Back where the PCT leaves the Island Meadow Trail, the PCT climbs north toward a cinder cone (5676), rounds its eastern half and then heads north to a lesser summit before reaching an intersection on a saddle with Horse Lake Trail 2/3516 (5300–1.3). Trail 2 southeastward descends to the same trailhead parking area but takes 1.5 miles to reach it. Following the divide, the PCT climbs gently north at first but steepens as it curves over to the western slope of Koosah Mountain (6520).

See maps E7, E8, E9

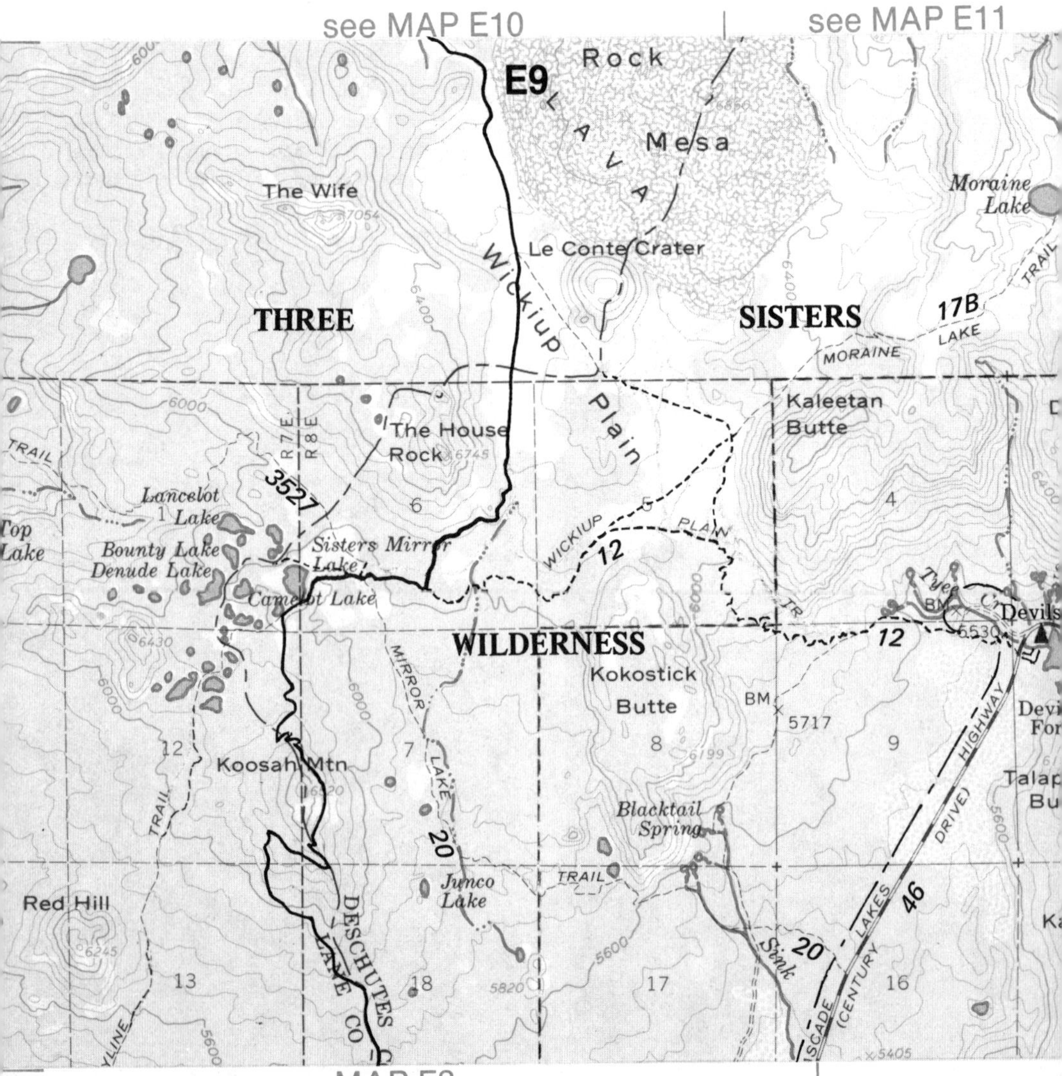

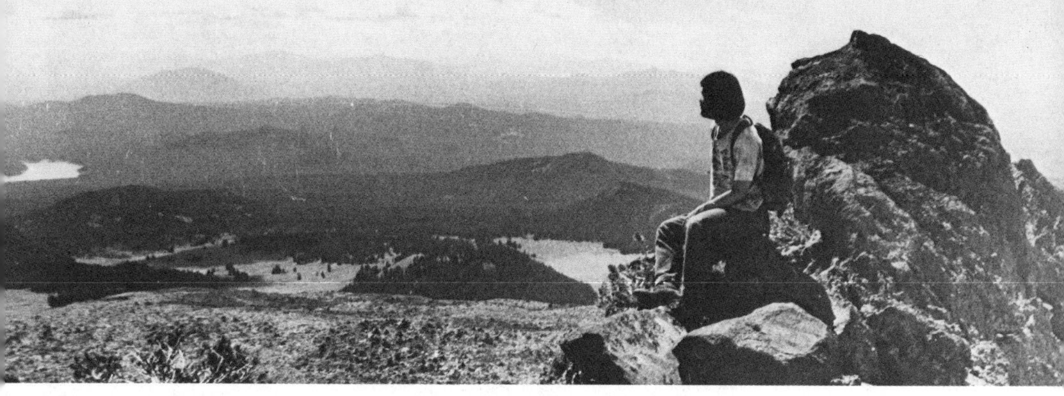

Rock Mesa and Elk Lake, viewed from south slopes of South Sister

Here, the PCT makes a long switchback up to the ridge and then contours to its east slope, where, by stepping a few yards east, you can absorb an eastern panorama from Elk and Hosmer lakes north past conical Bachelor Butte (9065) and deeply glaciated Broken Top (9175) to South Sister (10,358). ▮ *Although you can't see the Cascade Lakes Highway below, you can hear the rumble of logging trucks on it.* ▮

Hiking northwest, you encounter switchbacks down the north slope and then reach a flat and continue north to a junction at the south shore of placid, shallow Camelot Lake (5980–4.6). Here, the Oregon Skyline Trail route heads southwest along the Red Hill Trail. After a brief hike northeast on the PCT, you reach the south edge of Sisters Mirror Lake (5980–0.1), from which you'll see South Sister mirrored in the lake when the water is calm. From here you can head along the west shore to some good camps on a rocky bluff along its northwest shore. ▮ *Some camps in this general vicinity may be closed, due to previous camper impact, and the Forest Service urges visitors to camp at the lakes lying west of Camelot and Sisters Mirror lakes.* ▮ On the rocky bluff you'll see a use trail that heads west toward some of these lakes.

The PCT heads north along Sisters Mirror Lake's east shore, and along this short stretch you can climb up to a low bench that offers small campsites. Next, the trail turns east from the lake, and in about 300 yards it reaches a junction with the use trail heading westward across a meadow toward the lake's rocky bluff. ▮ *The Forest Service may attempt to obliterate this trail, so don't be too concerned if you don't see it.* ▮ Near the east end of the meadow, about 130 yards past the junction, you'll come to a junction (5990–0.4) with two official trails, Nash Lake and Mirror Lake trails.

Side route. Nash Lake Trail 3527 starts north before turning northwest, while Mirror Lake Trail 20 makes a long, mostly gentle descent south-southeast, eventually reaching Cascade Lakes Highway in about 3.5 miles.

Now the route climbs slightly in a traverse east to an important junction (6030–0.3).

Side route. From here, the well-graded Wickiup Plain Trail first rambles about 1¼ miles east across a fairly youthful lava flow to a junction with the southwest end of the Moraine Lake Trail. Then the Wickiup Plain Trail heads ½ mile east along the south edge of the Wickiup Plain to another junction. From it, a narrow trail goes 0.5 mile north to an intersection of the Moraine Lake Trail and then continues 1.3 miles northwest over to the PCT. The Wickiup Plain Trail leaves its namesake for a well-graded 2.2-mile descent to the Devils Lake area, with camping, picnicking, and fishing (this spring-fed lake is too cold for comfortable swimming). A large trailhead parking area lies just south of Tyee Creek, between the highway and the lake, and is quite heavily used by Bend's residents and visitors. This city, the largest Oregon city east of the Cascades, lies about a half-hour drive away.

From the west end of the Wickiup Plain Trail, the PCT heads north along a minor ridge to the south base of House Rock and then traverses along its wooded lower slopes up to an arm of the Wickiup Plain. The trail climbs

See map E9

see MAP E12

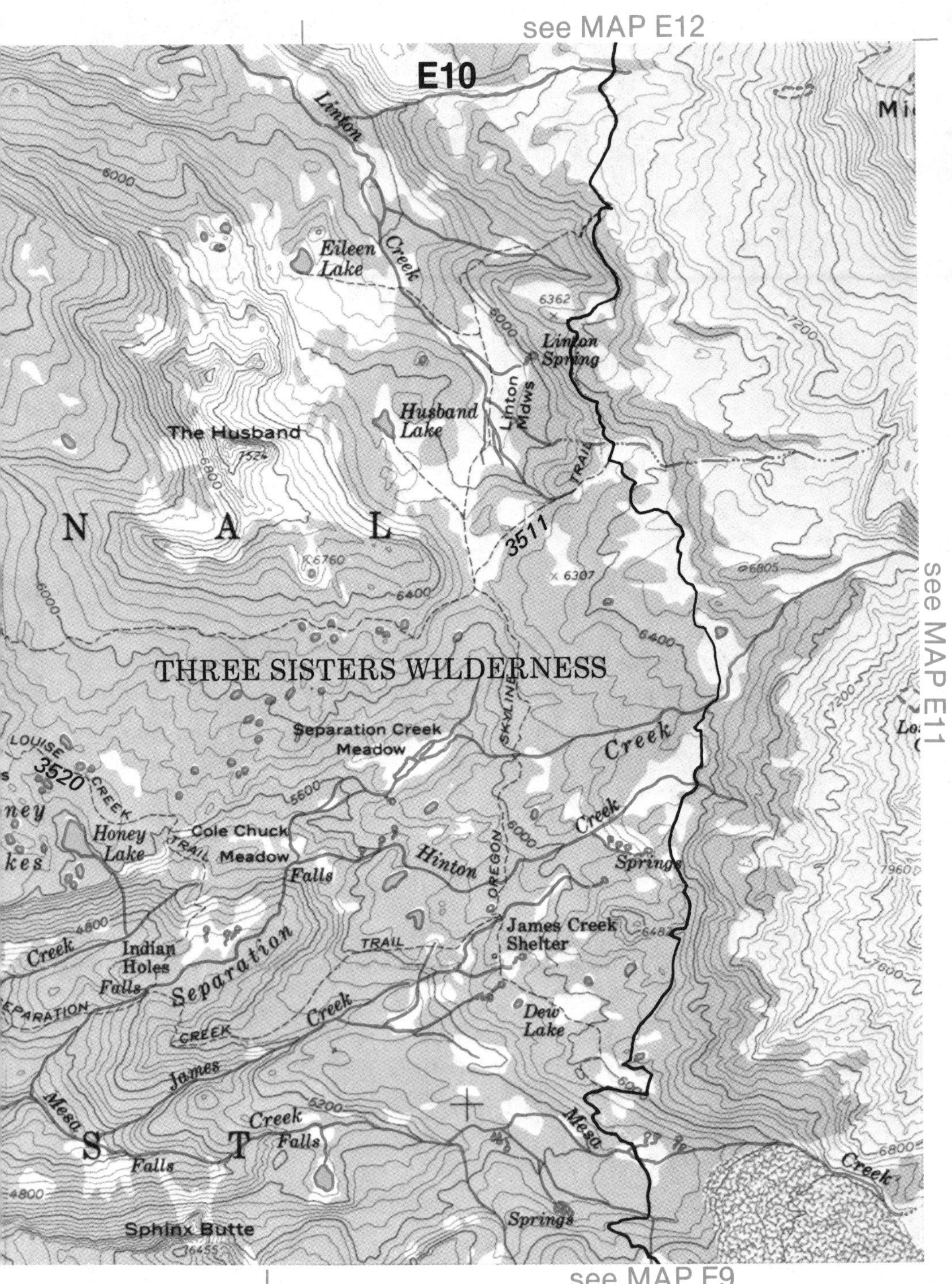

see MAP E11

see MAP E9

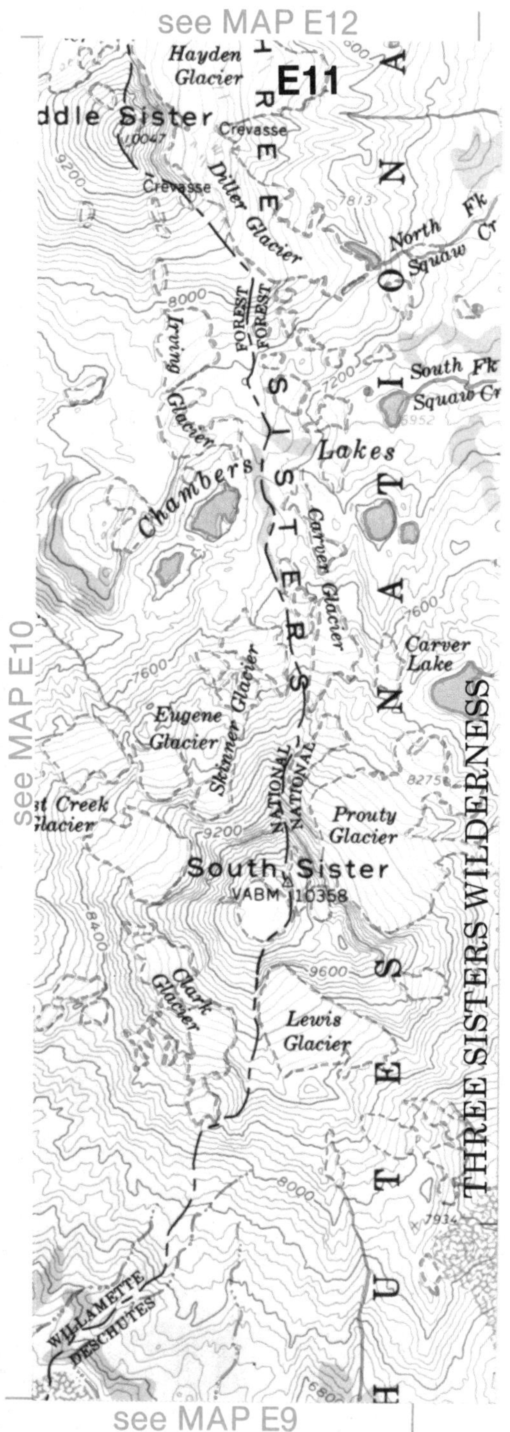

north gently up this partly forested plain and after ½ mile crosses the broad county-line divide (6210–1.2).

▮ *As you approach Le Conte Crater, a low cinder cone to the northeast, you begin to picture a sequence of events that molded this volcanic landscape. The thick stand of mountain hemlock on the northern half of Le Conte Crater indicates that this cone is at least several thousand years old. An educated guess, based upon comparisons with cones of known ages, is that an eruption took place 6000 to 8000 years ago and built up the cinder cone. Immediately following this eruption came outpourings of fluid, basaltic lava that breached the cone's south rim and flowed south down the gently sloping Wickiup Plain. You see this flow today as the forested, undulating surface south of the cone and off to your right (east). The section of the Wickiup Plain over which the trail passes is probably no more than 20,000 years old, for it shows little sign of erosion. You can be quite sure its age is greater than 10,000 years, since it was in existence when the last great Pleistocene glaciers marched down from South Sister and deposited their debris on its eastern side; a conspicuous moraine ends on top of the plain roughly 1½ miles due east of the cones.* ▮

Due west from the crater's north base, you meet a previously mentioned trail (6160–0.5) that goes 1.8 miles southeast to the Wickiup Plain Trail; starting near Devils Lake, that trail provides the fastest way in to the South Sister vicinity. Just north of Le Conte Crater, you see a vast, desolate, steep-sided chaotic jumble appropriately called Rock Mesa. ▮ *The high point near its east side marks the location of the vent from which rhyodacite lava was extruded over 2000 years ago. Because the lava was so viscous, the flow not only solidified before reaching Le Conte Crater, it also solidified halfway down the relatively steep slopes of the Mesa Creek drainage just north of you. It did succeed, however, in covering up any trace of a conduit that might have given rise to the older flows of the Wickiup Plain.* ▮

By now you've probably noticed The Wife (7054), a conspicuous summit off to the west, and you've probably observed that South Sister (10,358) is a redhead.

See map E9

see MAP E13

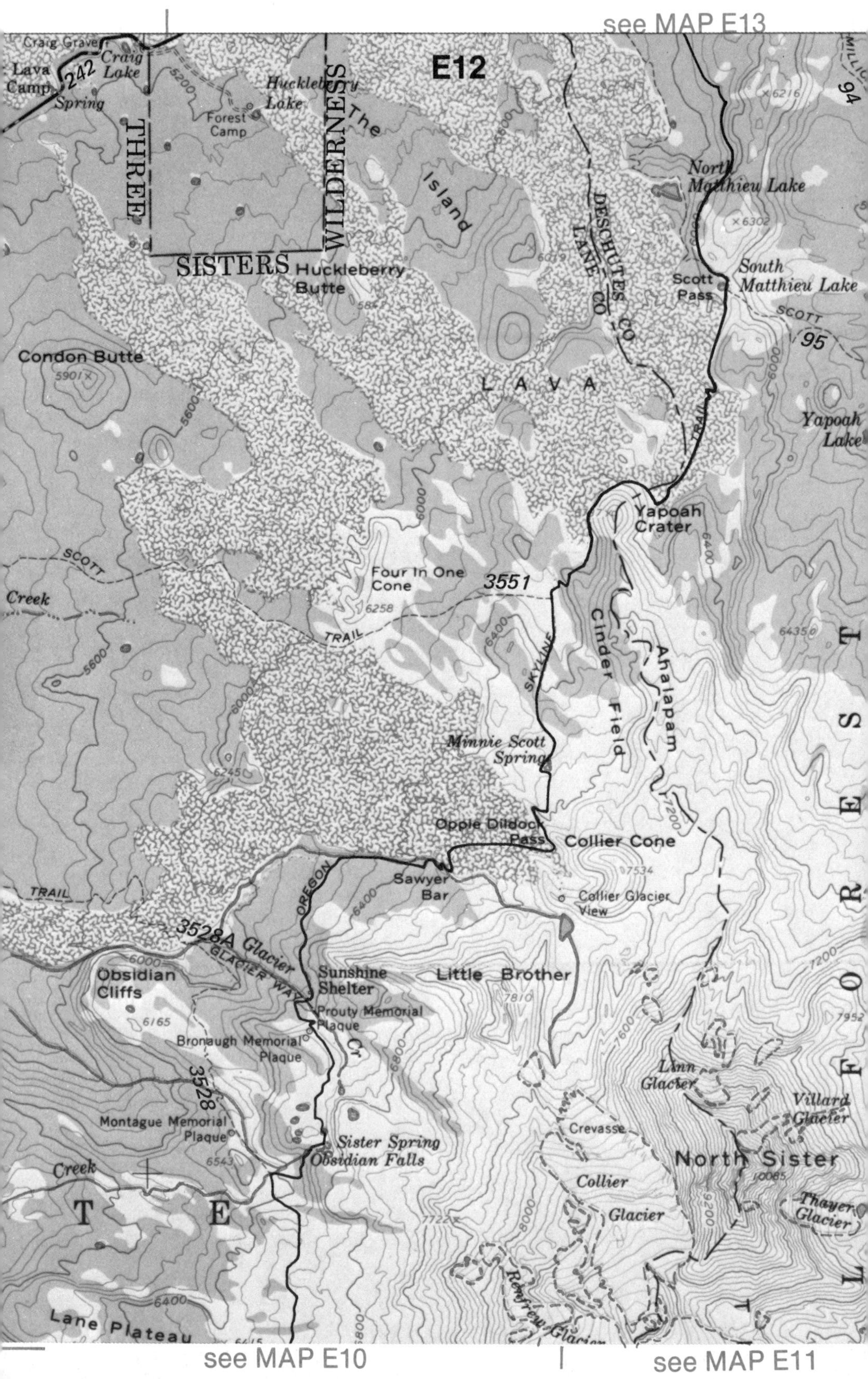
E12
Craig Lake
Lava Camp
Spring
242
Huckleberry Lake
Forest Camp
THREE SISTERS WILDERNESS
The Island
North Matthieu Lake
DESCHUTES CO
LANE CO
Huckleberry Butte
Scott Pass
South Matthieu Lake
SCOTT
95
Condon Butte
LAVA
Yapoah Lake
TRAIL
Yapoah Crater
Four In One Cone
3551
Creek
TRAIL
SKYLINE
Cinder Field
Ahalapam
Minnie Scott Spring
Opple Dildock Pass
Collier Cone
Sawyer Bar
OREGON
Collier Glacier View
TRAIL
3528A Glacier
GLACIER WAY
Obsidian Cliffs
Sunshine Shelter
Little Brother
Prouty Memorial Plaque
Bronaugh Memorial Plaque
3528
Linn Glacier
Villard Glacier
Montague Memorial Plaque
Crevasse
Sister Spring
Obsidian Falls
North Sister
Creek
Collier
Glacier
Thayer Glacier
Renfrew Glacier
Lane Plateau
FOREST

see MAP E10 see MAP E11

Side route. Should you wish to climb to its summit, strike east from a point just south of Le Conte Crater and then head northeast along the east margin of Rock Mesa. When you reach the peak's lower slope, climb north directly up it and pass between the Clark and Lewis glaciers as you near the summit cone. When you top its rim, you'll find it crowned with a snow-clad lake (10,200) that occupies a crater which may have been active in the last few thousand years. ▮ *South Sister, with at least three major periods of eruptions, is a geologically complete volcano; its slopes contain over two dozen types of volcanic rocks. This sister is the youngest of the three, and it still retains much of its symmetry because it has been exposed only to late-Pleistocene and Recent glaciation. The latest eruption in the Three Sisters area occurred within the last 200 years.* ▮

By the time you finish reading the above discussions, you could have been well on your way to the north end of Wickiup Plain. ▮ *Newberry knotweed and scattered grass attest to the dryness of the pumice soil, but plentiful gopher mounds indicate that at least one mammal thrives here.* ▮ At the north edge of the plain, the trail curves northwest over a low saddle and then descends to a creek (6010–1.2) which passes through a large meadow. ▮ *In early July this meadow is a continuous field of yellow cinquefoil that contrasts sharply with the wintry chill of deep snow patches on the surrounding forested slopes.* ▮ You leave this island of sunshine behind and press onward northwest into the forest and down alongside a small gully. The trail makes a switchback east and leads down to the south fork of Mesa Creek. Step across it, hike north into a large, grassy meadow, and then reach the north fork of Mesa Creek (5700–0.8). You'll find near-creek campsites both east and west of the meadow. Past the north fork, you reach a tributary in 100 yards—a scenic lunch spot.

Leaving the meadow and its sparkling creeks behind, you turn your back on the frozen "tidal wave" of Rock Mesa and climb northwest up to a junction with the James Creek Trail (5920–0.6), which makes a gentle ascent west before curving north along the old Oregon Skyline Trail route. Ascend east, curve north, and then round a murky lakelet just to the east. Continuing to climb north, the route tends to follow the break in the slope between the foot of South Sister to the east and the Separation Creek headwaters to the west. Along the course, you pass through numerous small meadows and beside a fine, six-foot-diameter mountain hemlock before you descend slightly to cross Hinton Creek (6320–2.1). After hiking to the other side of the low divide, you descend past a cliff of a high-density, parallel-fractured, shalelike flow. Here you cross Separation Creek (6400–0.5), whose flow, like that of Hinton Creek, has usually sunk beneath the pumice by mid-August.

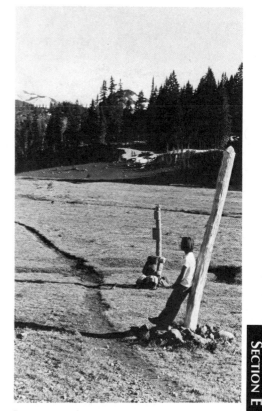

Rest stop at Scott Trail junction

Now you come face-to-face with Middle Sister (10,047), which can be easily climbed up its south or west slope. Continuing north, you follow posts and rock piles across a pumice flat and reach a shallow, clear lakelet (6460–0.4), beside which good campsites can be found. The fragile timberline ecosystem here is very

SECTION E

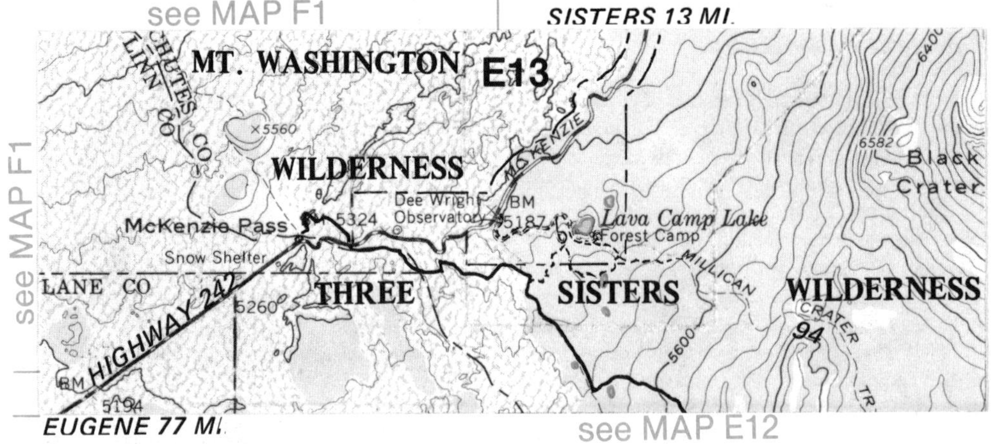

sensitive to human impact, so treat it gently. ▮ *Beyond, the trail crosses a level bedrock that has a previous glacier's signature etched upon it in the form of striations. The glacier also left souvenirs of its visit: erratic boulders.* ▮

The route north now crosses half a dozen seasonal, step-across creeks as it descends toward Linton Creek and finally bends west down to a meadow at whose north end you meet Foley Ridge Trail 3511 (6270–1.3), which leads south-southwest down a slope. About 25 yards west, at a forested flat, is a justifiably popular campsite. ▮ *The Husband (7524), off in the west, is the resistant plug of an ancient volcano that once reigned over this area before the Three Sisters matured.* ▮ Just after you start north again, you reach a tributary of Linton Creek and then 70 yards farther reach a second tributary.

From these seasonal creeks, the trail climbs gradually north through a hemlock forest to where it meets the Linton Meadows Trail (6440–1.7) descending steeply southwest. The PCT ascends moderately northeast to a spring and then angles north to a gentle slope from which you can look south and identify, from east to west, the Mt. Thielsen pinnacle (9182), the Mt. McLoughlin pyramid (9495), and the Diamond Peak massif (8744). Now follow an open, post-lined, undulating pathway north over loose slopes with trailside rose paintbrushes, yellow cinquefoils, pink heathers, and

See maps E10, E12

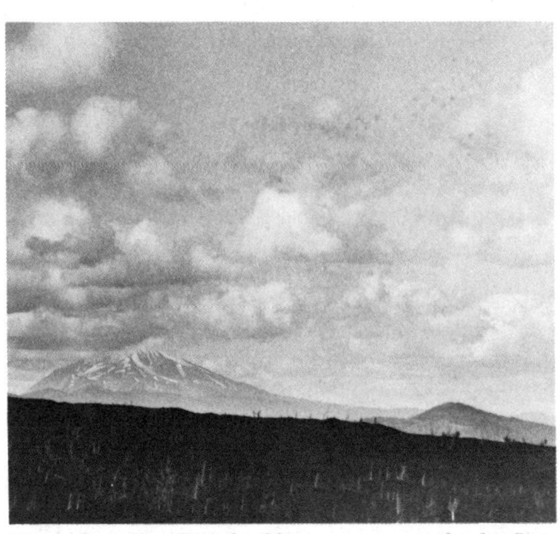

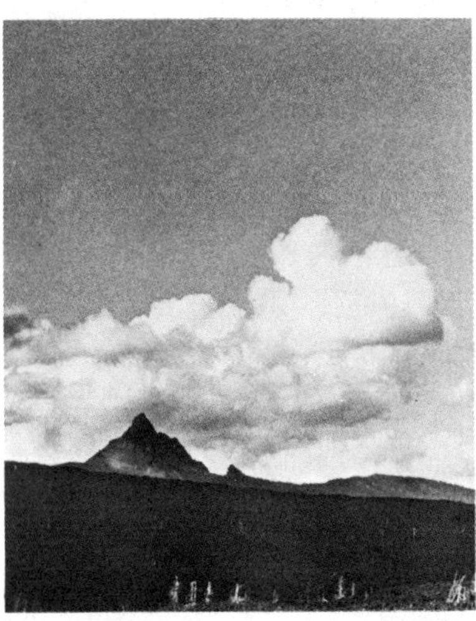

Views from Dee Wright Observatory: south, the Sisters; north, Mt. Washington and, just barely, Three Fingered Jack

See maps E1,

white pasqueflowers. Cross a rocky meadow and descend to a junction with Obsidian Trail 3528 (6380–2.1) just above Obsidian Creek.

Side route. This trail takes you down to Frog Campground by the McKenzie Highway.

Start hiking east moderately up to a slope and then go northeast up to trickling, 50-foot-high Obsidian Falls, from which you top a small shelf and cross Obsidian Creek. Now tread north on a trail that sounds and feels like glass. ▮ *It is. The black obsidian is nature's own glass.* ▮ The trail, which passes some outstanding camps past the last junction, soon leaves the shelf, descends a ridge, and then turns east and intersects Glacier Way Trail 3528A (6370–1.6).

Side route. This path descends moderately 0.7 mile to the Obsidian Trail, which can be followed 3.4 miles to Frog Campground. An efficient mountaineering party can follow this route up from the campground, climb North and Middle Sisters via the Collier Glacier col, and return to camp late the same day. From the col, Middle Sister (10,047) can be climbed via its north ridge without any special equipment. Likewise, North Sister (10,085) can be climbed via its southwest ridge to the south arête, but the climb north along this sharp crest requires a safety rope. The view from Middle Sister is particularly instructional, for from it you can compare the degree of glaciation on all Three Sisters. North Sister, the oldest of the three, has suffered repeated ravages from quite a number of glacial advances. South Sister (10,358), the youngest, retains her symmetry, for she hasn't lived long enough to feel the icy tongues cut deep into her body.

Twenty yards east of the Glacier Way intersection, you bridge Glacier Creek and then reach a pleasant, hemlock-shaded site where Sunshine Shelter once stood; you may find this area closed to camping. Climb briefly north over the western spur of Little Brother (7810) and then descend slightly to the steep south slope above White Branch Creek (6210–0.9). After climbing along this creek, which can go dry in August, you eventually cross it; here, you can camp above its north bank on a flat called Sawyer Bar.

The trail bears north 200 yards partway across a basalt flow and then angles east up a ridge of solidified lava to the breached Collier Cone—the obvious source of this flow. Here, mountaineers' paths take off south up to Collier Glacier. You turn north and work your way across several lava ridges before descending north to Minnie Scott Spring (6650–2.2), which is likely to be snowbound through mid-July; you can camp on the level ground west of the spring. The trail now makes a curving, counterclockwise descent almost to the Minnie Scott Springs creek, crosses a ridge, descends north to a large, grassy meadow, and shortly meets Scott Trail 3551 (6300–0.9).

Side route. Descending west to the McKenzie Highway in about five miles, this trail follows the narrow strip of land between the Four in One Cone (6258) basalt flow on its north side and the Collier Cone (7534) basalt flow on its south side. ▮ *The age of these flows, and of the Yapoah Crater (6737) basalt flow immediately north of you, is about 2600 years.* ▮

The PCT now follows the Scott Trail north as it curves northeast and switchbacks up a northwest spur of the Ahalapam Cinder Field. The trail then curves around the slopes of Yapoah Crater and enters Deschutes National Forest. ▮ *Yapoah Crater's lava flow—at least 400 years old—extends north to Highway 242 and beyond. Looking north, you can see a row of peaks: Mt. Washington (7794), Three Fingered Jack (7841), and the snowy Mts. Jefferson (10,497) and Hood (11,235).* ▮

Now the PCT winds along and around ridges of the Yapoah lava flow, and you're thankful that the rocky trail exists, even when it is covered with snow patches. A cross-country hike across this material would be very exhausting! Reaching the edge of the flow, you parallel it north on a blocky cinder trail to a junction from which Scott Trail 95 descends east-southeast toward Trout Creek. Just 70 yards north down from this junction is Scott Pass and adjacent, diminutive South Matthieu Lake (6040–2.5). ▮ *At this pass you get one of your best views eastward of central Oregon, which is drier than the west countryside*

See map E12

because of the rain shadow cast by the Cascade Range. ▮ Here, too, around the 70-yard-wide lake, you'll find several small campsites that can offer uplifting sunrise views. Just beyond a campsite above this lake's northwest corner, you come to a junction with the old Oregon Skyline Trail route (6070–0.1); you can stay on the official and waterless PCT, described below, or take an alternate route with water on the Oregon Skyline Trail, following that.

Official PCT route. From the junction near South Matthieu Lake, the PCT first crosses slopes of a fairly young cinder cone, which on a clear day offers you a far-ranging view of northern Oregon's higher Cascade Peaks: Mt. Washington, Three Fingered Jack, Mt. Jefferson, and Mt. Hood. Then comes a fairly long, viewless, though mostly well graded descent to another junction with the old Oregon Skyline Trail route (5450–2.1) where the alternate route rejoins the PCT.

Alternate route. The Oregon Skyline Trail descends to North Matthieu Lake, and this 2.1-mile stretch is a preferred route over the equally long stretch of waterless PCT. This alternate segment first winds ⅓ mile down to the southeast corner of appealing North Matthieu Lake and then in ¼ mile leaves it at its northwest corner. Along this near-shore traverse, you'll spot several campsites. From the lake, switchbacks guide you down steep slopes, and then you parallel the east edge of Yapoah Crater lava flow, passing a small pond on the east and then one on the west before rejoining the PCT.

Official PCT route and alternate route rejoined. Now you have a gentle descent northwest along the east edge of the Yapoah Crater lava flow, and soon you come to a junction (5310–0.7) with an important lateral trail.

Water access. This lateral trail snakes ¼ mile northeast to a fairly large trailhead parking area that lies along the south side of Road 900, a State Highway 242 spur road that goes over to Lava Camp Lake. Since your next potential source of trailside water is at *sometimes dry* Coldwater Spring, 11.2 miles distant, you should consider camping over at the lake's campground. You'll find the lake just northeast of the parking area, the two separated by a minor ridge. If the weather looks bad, look for a shelter above the southeast corner of the lake. The shallow lake's water is not pristine, so if you'd rather not treat it, you might get safe water from car campers. Should you need supplies, walk out to nearby State Highway 242 and hitchhike 15 miles east to Sisters, a prosperous, upscale tourist town.

From the lateral-trail junction, the PCT makes a zigzag course west over the blocky lava field, and leaves Three Sisters Wilderness as you cross narrow McKenzie Highway (242) (5280–1.1) 500 yards west of the Dee Wright Observatory, a lookout tower well worth visiting for its views. Just 0.2 mile west down this highway is a parking area with a trailhead for those starting their hike north from McKenzie Pass. ▮ *This pass was named for the river that was explored in 1811 by Donald McKenzie, a member of John Jacob Astor's Pacific Fur Company. It was opened to travel in 1862 when Felix Scott, with a party of 250 men, chopped their way through the forest, building the road for their 106 ox-hauled wagons as they traveled. They crossed the divide by what is known as the Old Scott Trail, two or three miles south of the present road.* ▮

Having crossed the highway, you enter Mt. Washington Wilderness. Due to the jumbled nature of the lava flow, the trail must take a twisted route over to the small trailhead parking area (5210–0.3), where this section's hike ends.

See maps E12, E13

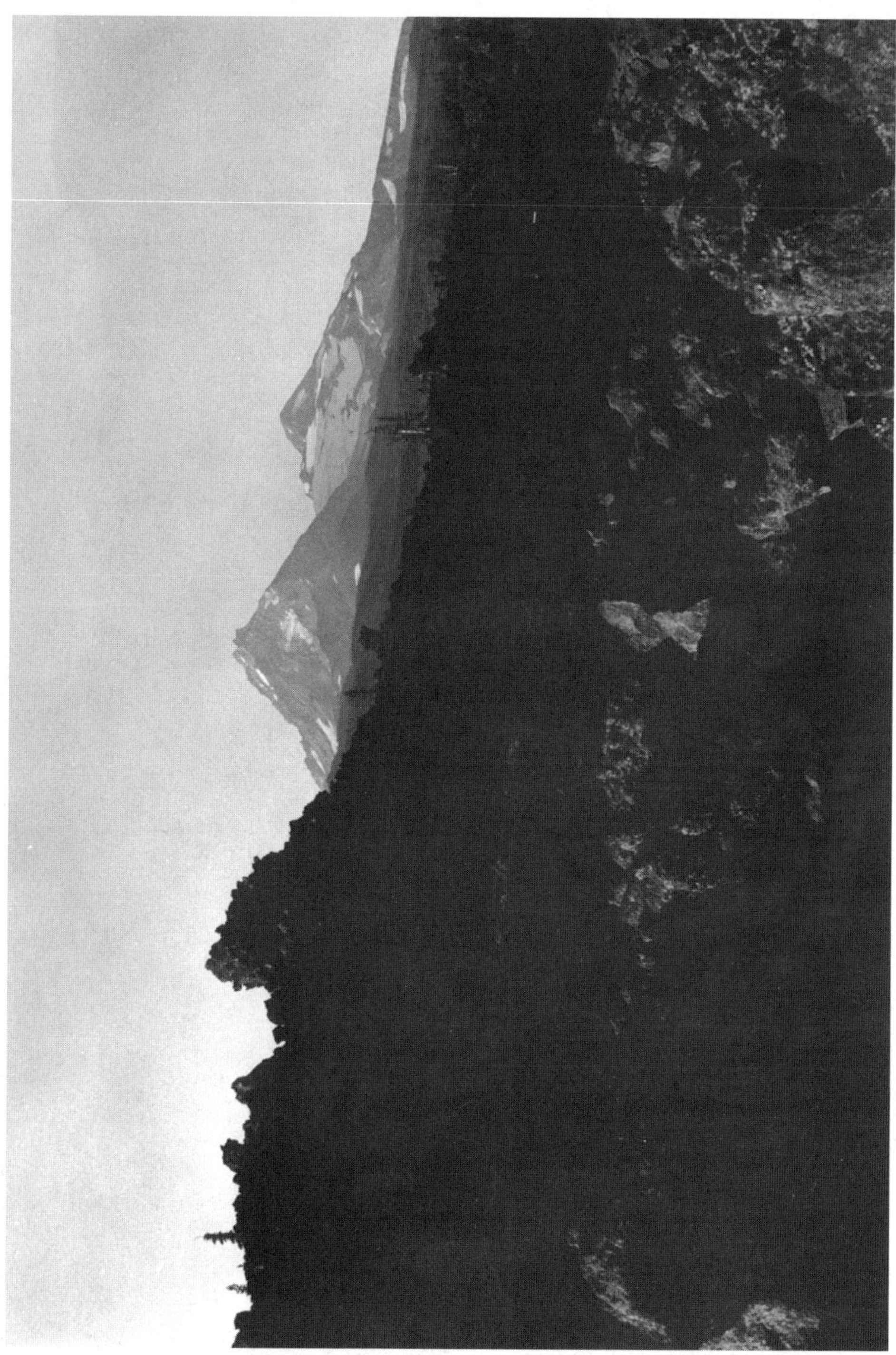

North and Middle Sisters, from McKenzie Pass

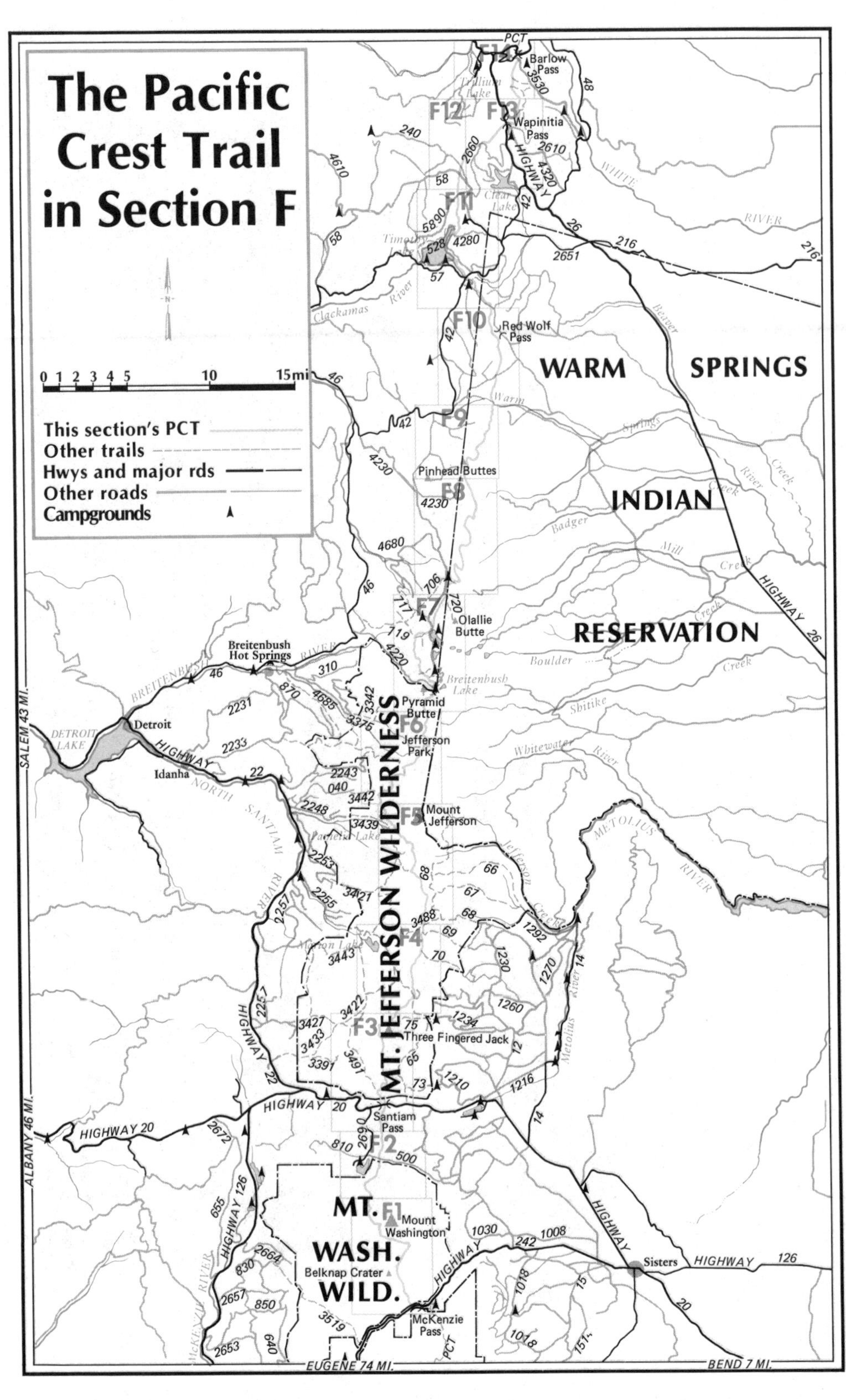

The Pacific Crest Trail in Section F
0 1 2 3 4 5 10 15mi
This section's PCT
Other trails
Hwys and major rds
Other roads
Campgrounds
WARM SPRINGS INDIAN RESERVATION
MT. JEFFERSON WILDERNESS
MT. WASH. WILD.
Barlow Pass
Wapinitia Pass
Timothy Lake
Clear Lake
Red Wolf Pass
Pinhead Buttes
Olallie Butte
Breitenbush Hot Springs
Breitenbush Lake
Pyramid Butte
Jefferson Park
Detroit
Detroit Lake
Idanha
Mount Jefferson
Three Fingered Jack
Santiam Pass
Mount Washington
Belknap Crater
McKenzie Pass
Sisters
SALEM 43 MI.
ALBANY 46 MI.
EUGENE 74 MI.
BEND 7 MI.

Section F:
Highway 242 at McKenzie Pass to Highway 35 near Barlow Pass

Introduction: The terrain crossed in Section F is an approximate mirror image of that crossed in Section E. Starting from Highway 242, you head north across recent lava flows that also make up the last part of Section E. You then pass three major peaks—Mt. Washington, Three Fingered Jack, and Mt. Jefferson—just as you passed the Three Sisters. All six peaks are volcanoes in various stages of erosion. Mt. Jefferson, the northernmost, and South Sister, the southernmost, are the two youngest.

North of Mt. Jefferson, you hike through the lake-studded Breitenbush Lake-Olallie Lake area, which is a smaller version of the southern Three Sisters Wilderness. Finally, you hike a lengthy stretch across slopes that are deficient in both views and lakes, just as you did in the first third of Section E. Both sections, on the average, are fairly scenic, and it is difficult to say which is better. For many, however, Jefferson Park is the scenic high point of the Oregon PCT. But on this spectacular plain, you'll find a backpacking crowd to match or exceed that on any other part of the tri-state PCT.

Declination: 18½°E

Points on Route	S➛N	Mi. Btwn. Pts.	N➛S
Highway 242 at McKenzie Pass	0.0		112.5
Washington Ponds spur trail	7.3	7.3	105.2
Coldwater Spring	9.7	2.4	102.8
Highway 20 at Santiam Pass	17.1	7.4	95.4
Minto Pass	27.3	10.2	85.2
Rockpile Lake	31.0	3.7	81.5
Start of Pamelia Lake alternate route	37.9	6.9	74.6
Shale Lake	39.7	1.8	72.8
End of Pamelia Lake alternate route	44.2	4.5	68.3
Trail north to Scout Lake	50.3	6.1	62.2
Skyline Road 4220 near Breitenbush Lake	56.9	6.6	55.6
Skyline Road 4220 near Olallie Lake Guard Station	63.4	6.5	49.1
Jude Lake	67.1	3.7	45.4
Lemiti Creek	73.1	6.0	39.4
Warm Springs River	84.2	11.1	28.3
Miller Trail to Clackamas Lake Cmpgrnd.	92.7	8.5	19.8
Little Crater Lake Trail	99.5	6.8	13.0
Highway 26 at Wapinitia Pass	107.5	8.0	5.0
Highway 35 near Barlow Pass	112.5	5.0	0.0

Supplies: Just 11.1 miles north into this section, at a junction 1.4 miles north of Coldwater Spring, you can descend a broad trail 0.7 mile to the grounds of the Seventh

Day Adventists' Big Lake Youth Camp. This camp accepts PCT trekkers' packages. Mail them to: Big Lake Youth Camp, Highway 20, Box 13100, Sisters, OR 97759.

Not far beyond this section's halfway point, you reach the Olallie Lake Guard Station and, just east of it, Olallie Lake Resort. The resort has a fair selection of food, but more important, it holds your parcels. Send them to the Clackamas River Ranger District, which weekly takes them up to the resort. The district's address is: 595 N.W. Industrial Way, Estacada, OR 97023.

At the end of this section, you could hike several miles out of your way, down to the settlement of Government Camp, which has a post office and a moderately well-stocked store.

Maps:

Mt. Washington, OR
Three Fingered Jack, OR
Marion Lake, OR
Mount Jefferson, OR
Olallie Butte, OR
Boulder Lake, OR
Fort Butte, OR
Pinhead Buttes, OR
Mount Wilson, OR
Timothy Lake, OR
Wolf Peak, OR
Wapinitia Pass, OR
Mount Hood South, OR

THE ROUTE

This section's PCT begins at a small trailhead parking area just west of ill-defined McKenzie Pass. This trailhead is very easy to find, for it is at a bend in Highway 242 from which the road to the east is very curving but that to the southwest is as straight as an arrow.

SECTION F

From this trailhead at the south boundary of Mt. Washington Wilderness, make an ascent northwest up the Belknap Crater basalt flows and pass between two forested islands of older, glaciated basalt that stand in a sea of younger basalt. ▮ *The desolate young basalt flows look as if they had cooled only a few years ago, yet those emanating from Little Belknap (6305) are 2900 years old. The flows seen today on Belknap Crater (6872) and its flanks are mostly 1500–3000 years old. All the flows between North Sister and Mt. Washington compose a 65-square-mile field that represents the Cascades' greatest post-Pleistocene outpouring of lava. Belknap Crater is an excellent example of a shield volcano and is quite simi-*

See map F1

Hiking up the Belknap lava field toward Mt. Washington

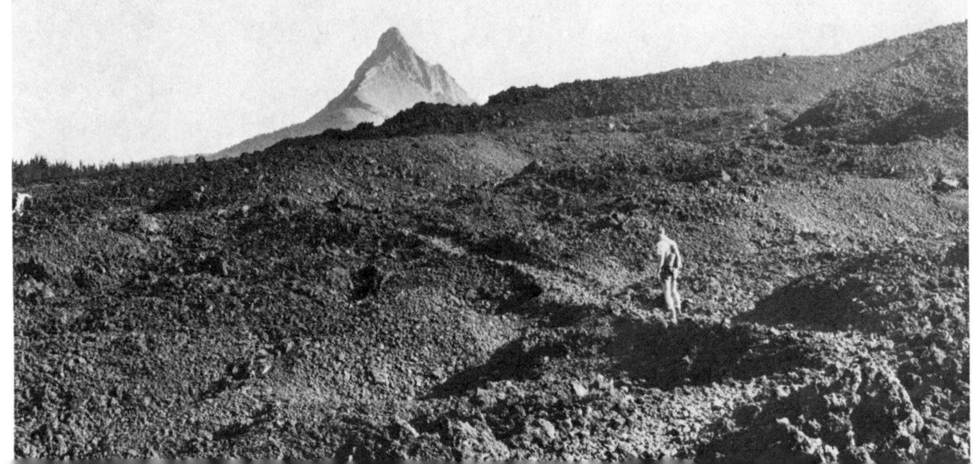

see MAP F2

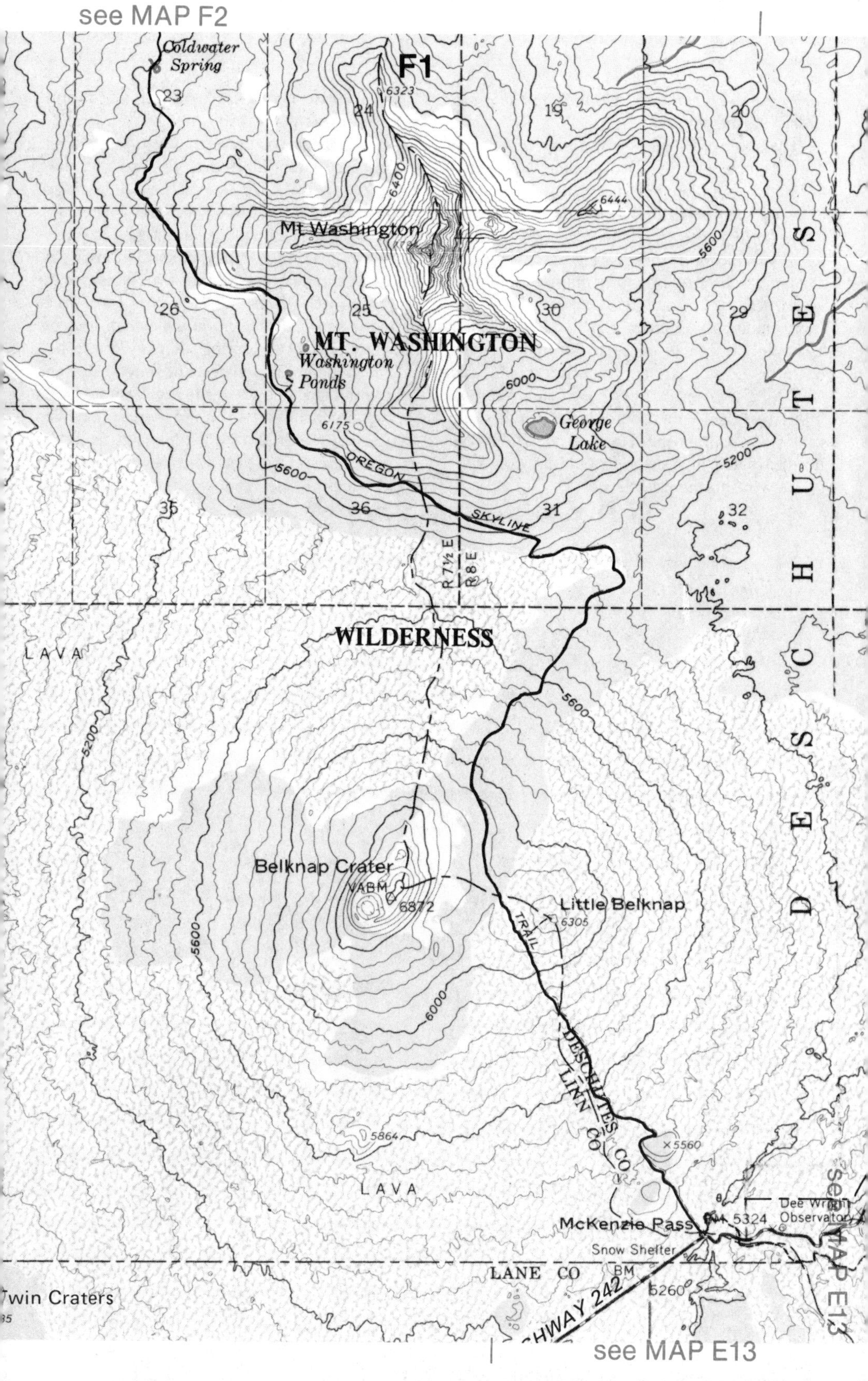

see MAP E13

see MAP E13

lar to the shields that the Three Sisters and Mt. Thielsen grew upon. ▮

The route now takes you up to a junction with a spur trail (6120–2.3) that leads east-northeast up to the summit of Little Belknap. ▮ *This area you're in looks quite lifeless, yet up here among the rocks you might spot a whistling marmot scurrying for its hole or, even more astounding, you might discover a western toad.* ▮ Mountain chickadees sing out their name as you enter a strip of forest near Belknap Crater and descend through it to the eastern edge of a fresh-looking flow (5320–2.5). First head north and then west, up along its edge, which borders the south slope of Mt. Washington. The trail switchbacks northeast and in a couple of minutes switchbacks west-northwest.

Side route. From this second switchback, you can climb due north rather steeply up fairly open slopes and across minor ridges over to George Lake. If you're on track, you'll reach a steep ridge immediately south of the lake. Some hikers try to avoid unnecessary elevation gain to this ridge by heading north-northeast, hoping to arrive at the east end of the lake. However, if they are just 200 yards east of the lake, they may not see it at all and could waste lots of time and energy wandering aimlessly. You, however, have been forewarned, and will do better. Follow the ridge down to the lake's east shore, by which you'll find a campsite. Better ones lie above the north shore. Camping at George Lake is superior to that at lower Washington Pond, which in turn is superior to that at rusty,

See map F1

see MAP F3

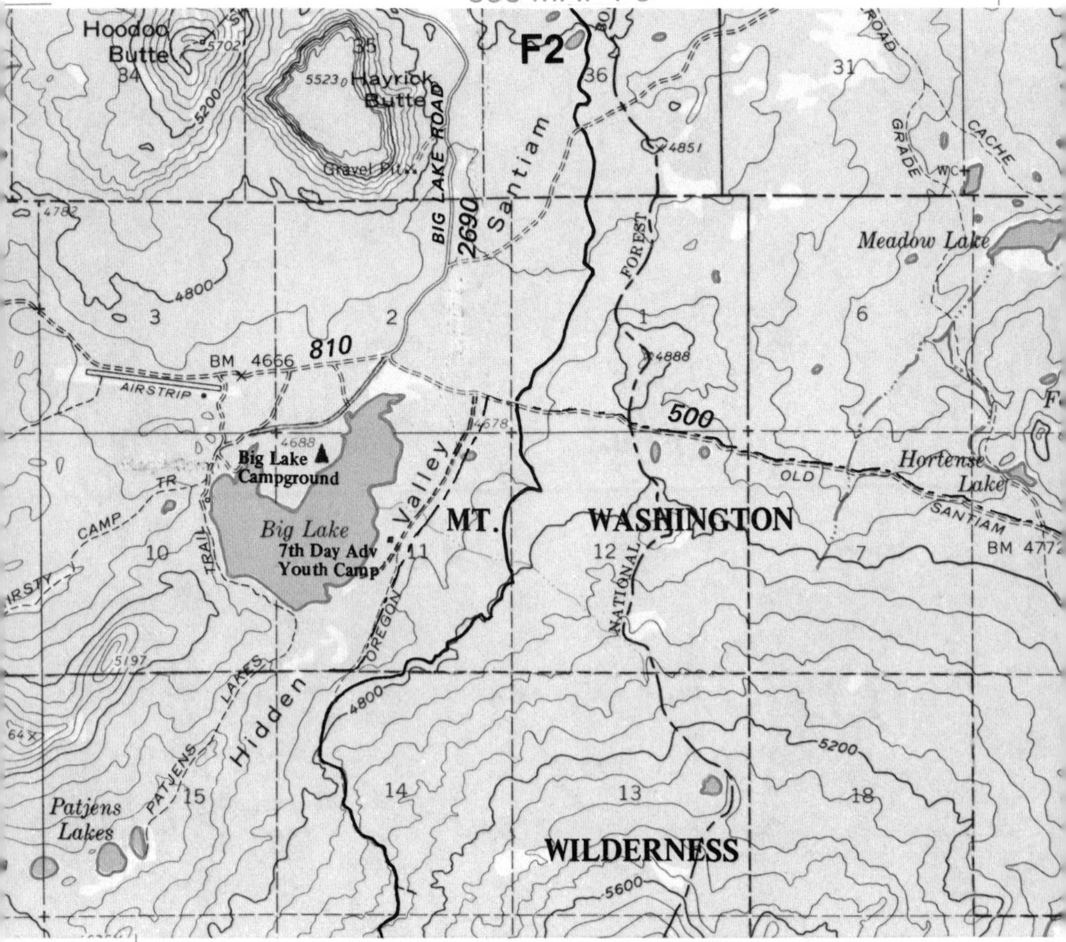

see MAP F1

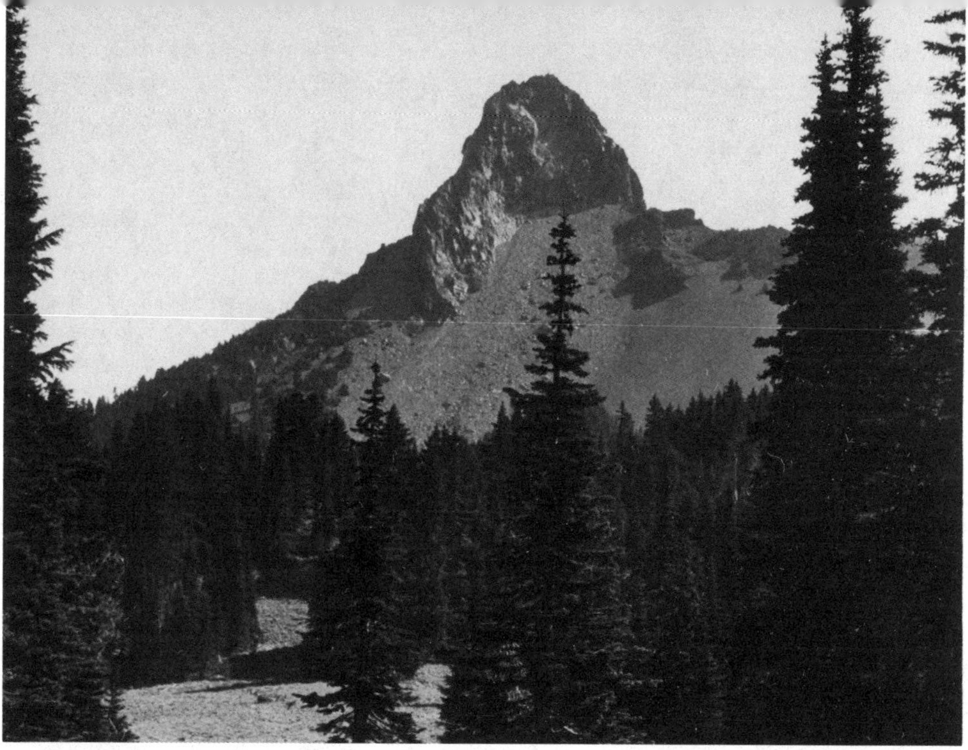

Mt. Washington, from the southwest

horse-urine-tainted, seasonally dry Coldwater Spring. When you are ready to return to the PCT (George Lake is good for a layover day), head due south from the east shore, attain a low ridge, and then diagonal south-southwest across undulating slopes to the PCT.

From the point where the trail switchbacks west-northwest, you climb steadily to the Cascade divide, where the PCT levels off. Now traverse northwest for about ¾ mile before curving north for a ⅓-mile stint to a gully in which the easily missed Washington Ponds spur trail starts northeast (5710–2.5).

Side route. In 200 yards, this spur trail curves over to shallow, 25-yard-wide lower Washington Pond, beside whose semiclear water desperate hikers have been known to camp.

Beyond this unmarked junction, you climb slightly higher through a meadow that affords an excellent view of the basalt plug that makes up the steep-walled summit block of Mt. Washington (7794).

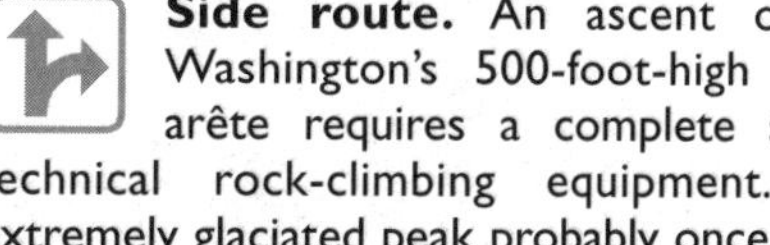

Side route. An ascent of Mt. Washington's 500-foot-high south arête requires a complete set of technical rock-climbing equipment. This extremely glaciated peak probably once stood as high as North Sister at a time when that peak was still undergoing its growing pains.

Your route arcs west and descends moderately alongside the west spur and then descends northward around it to an overused meadow that contains an obvious well (18-inch-diameter pipe) known as Coldwater Spring (5200–2.4). It is the last fresh water on-route until Rockpile Lake, about 21.5 miles farther. Less desirable ponds and lakes exist near the trail, and snow patches linger through mid-August on the northwest slope of Three Fingered Jack. ▮ *Since this meadow is the only trailside PCT campsite in Mt. Washington Wilderness that has "fresh" water, it has been overused, so much so that, in fact,* it sometimes dries up. *Be prepared. On weekends, as many as two dozen mountaineers will make this their base camp and then climb up the north spur to the 300-foot-high north arête of the summit*

See map F1

see MAP F4

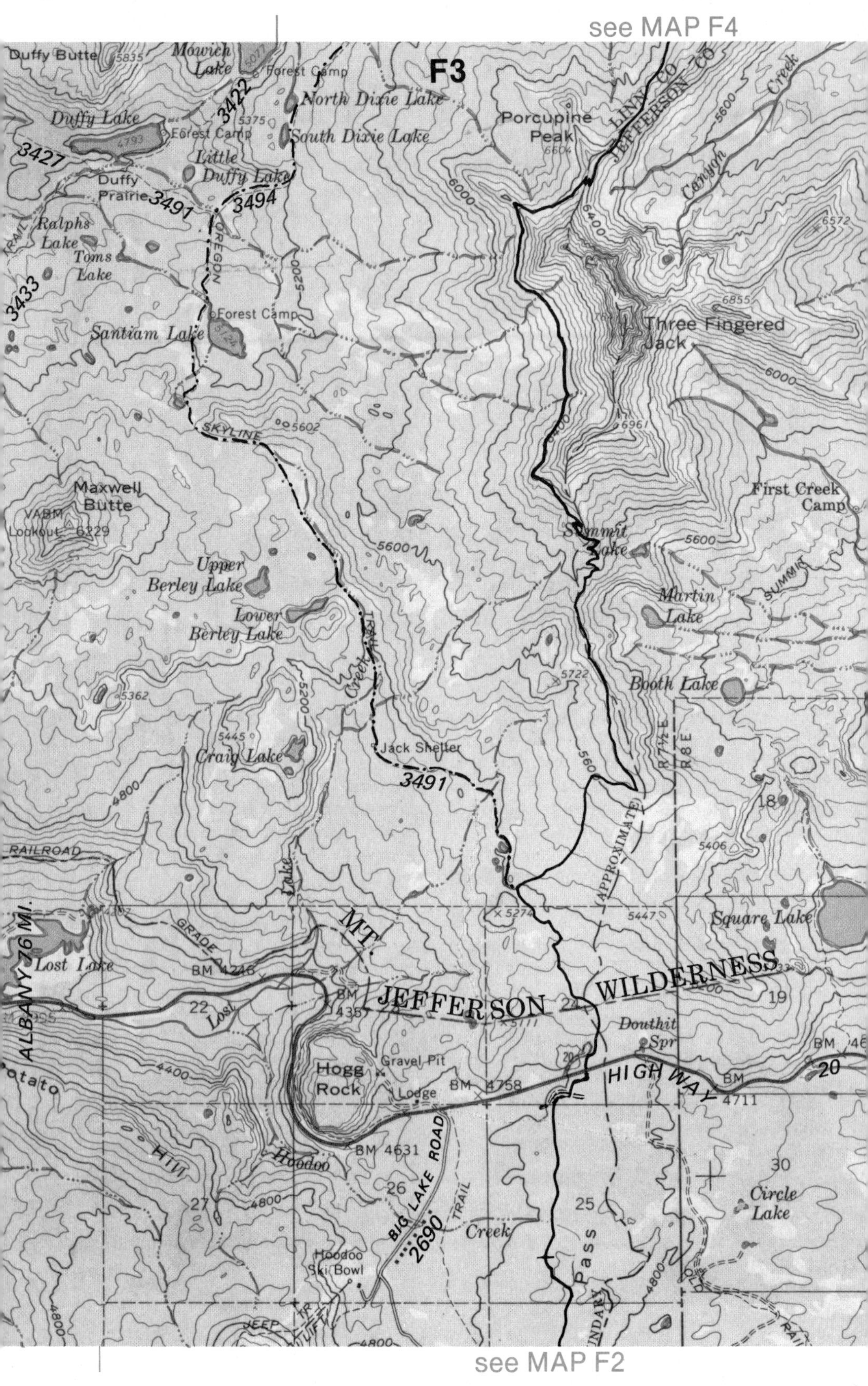

see MAP F2

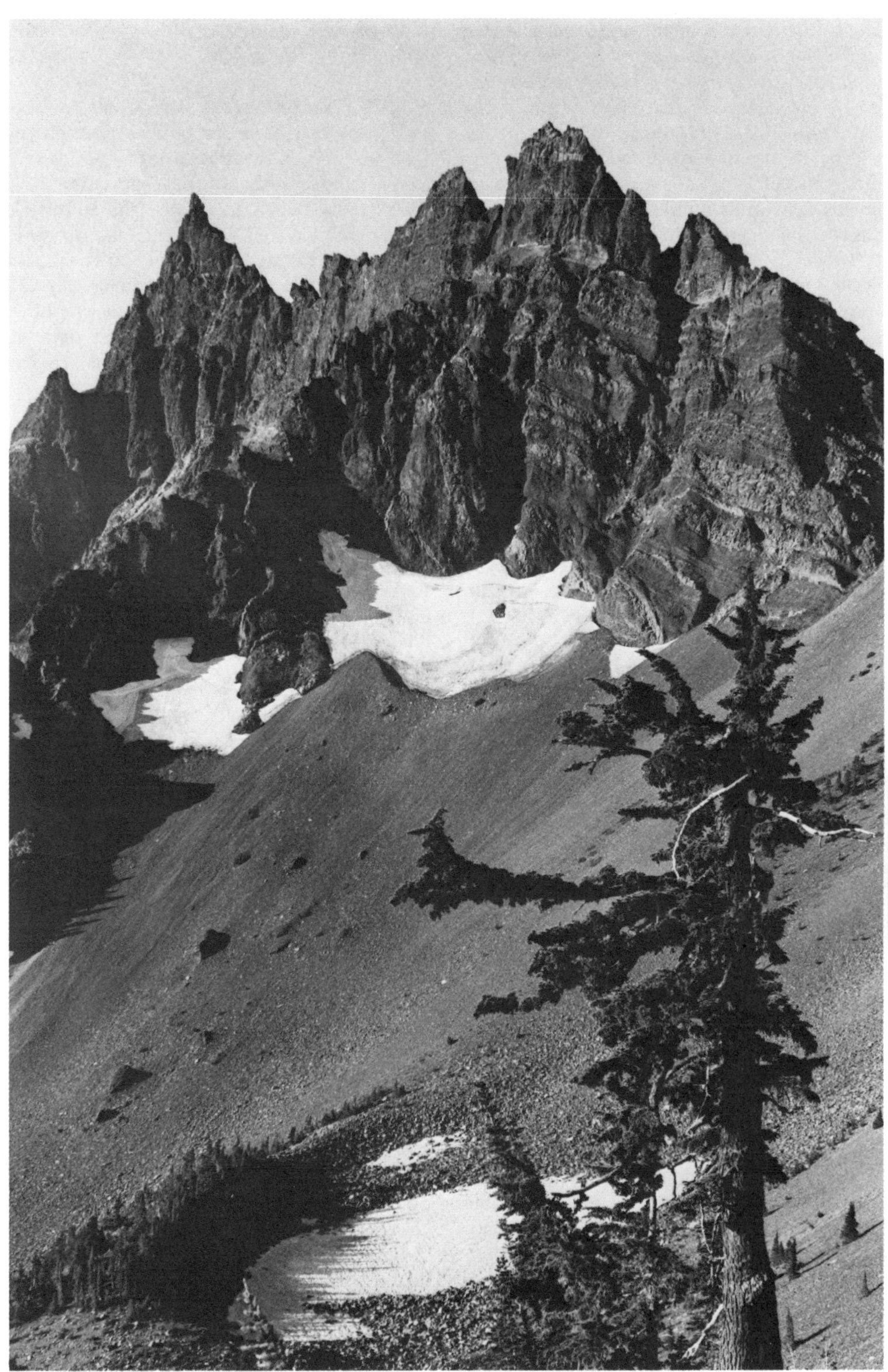

Three Fingered Jack, northeast face

block—the easiest summit route, but one that still requires ropes and other equipment. The organic evidence lying profusely around the grassy meadow says that horses use this site, too. As always, treat the water. ▮

The PCT continues its northward descent through a hemlock forest occupied by clicking juncos and drilling red-shafted flickers. You pass by an unmarked climbers' trail (5050–0.5) that ascends east-southeast toward the peak's north spur and then descend north to a fork with a broad trail (4760–0.9) that continues straight ahead.

Water access. If you sorely need water or want to pick up your mailed parcels, descend 0.7 mile on this old stretch of the former Oregon Skyline Trail to the Big Lake Youth Camp, operated by the Oregon Conference of Seventh Day Adventists. For water, look for a faucet about 60 yards east, by their horse corral. From the grounds you can continue north ¾ mile to Old Santiam Road and then 250 yards east over to the PCT.

Onward, the PCT veers right (northeast) and traverses slopes that are waterless once the snow patches disappear. Leave Mt. Washington Wilderness just before reaching the old Santiam Wagon Road (4680–2.0). ▮ *This waterless spot is very popular with car campers on summer weekends and during hunting season.* ▮

From the old Santiam Wagon Road, the PCT heads northeast past abandoned logging roads on a route that gradually turns north and reaches a hundred-yard-long lily-pad pond (4790–2.0), just west of the trail. This stretch you have just passed through is easy to follow, despite old roads. Southbound along it, the hiker at least has open if not scenic views of Mt. Washington. Just north of the pond, you climb over a low saddle and into a mature forest once again, and about ⅔ mile through it, you intersect the North Loop Trail, a cross-country ski route. Now the route is quite steadily north for ¾ mile; then it turns northeast, quickly crosses a minor road, and in 0.3 mile reaches Santiam Highway (US Highway 20) (4810–2.0) about 200 yards west of the national forest boundary at Santiam Pass. ▮ *This pass was first crossed in 1859 by Andrew Wiley. He explored an old Indian trail up the Santiam River and worked his way farther east each year on his hunting expeditions from the Willamette Valley.* ▮

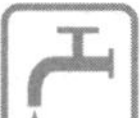

Water access. If you are low on water, head east on Santiam Highway toward Douthit Spring, which can be a bit hard to find. About ¼ mile east of the PCT, the highway begins to curve right, and you'll soon see a mile "81" highway sign. Just 30 yards east of it is a minor road, on your right, and just opposite that, on your left, is a small gully. Go up the gully 50 yards to usually seeping Douthit Spring. Be warned, however, that at times it dries up. You can camp nearby and then return to the PCT's crossing of Santiam Highway.

Just 240 yards west of the highway crossing is a PCT access road that curves 0.2 mile northeast to a parking area at a popular trailhead. Cross the highway and, after 200 yards, spy the parking area immediately to the west. Your trail bears north, curves northwest, enters Mt. Jefferson Wilderness, and then climbs increasingly steep slopes, passing a few stagnant ponds just before a junction with Santiam Lake Trail 3491 (5200–1.4), which curves northwest around a prominent boulder pile.

Alternate route. Because most of the PCT through Mt. Jefferson Wilderness is rather lakeless, one hiker has suggested we mention an alternative, the old Oregon Skyline Trail. Since author Schaffer didn't map this route, he is basing the following description on USFS topographic maps and mileages.

Take Santiam Lake Trail 3491 2.1 miles northwest to Lower Berley Lake and then 1.9 miles farther to more attractive Santiam Lake. Just 0.6 mile north of it, you reach a junction where Santiam Trail 3491 turns west. Go northeast on Trail 3494, hike north past South and North Dixie lakes, and in 1.5 miles reach a junction with Trail 3422. Next, in 1.0 mile, you hike northeast past diminutive Alice Lake and average-sized Red Butte Lake to reach a junction by the south shore of fairly large Jorn Lake. Trail 3422 heads past the lake's west shore, but you head east on Trail 3492 about 0.7 mile to Bowerman Lake and then traverse 2.7 miles beyond it to a junction with Trail 3437, which climbs 2.7 miles southeast up to Minto Pass and the PCT.

See maps F1, F2, F3, F4

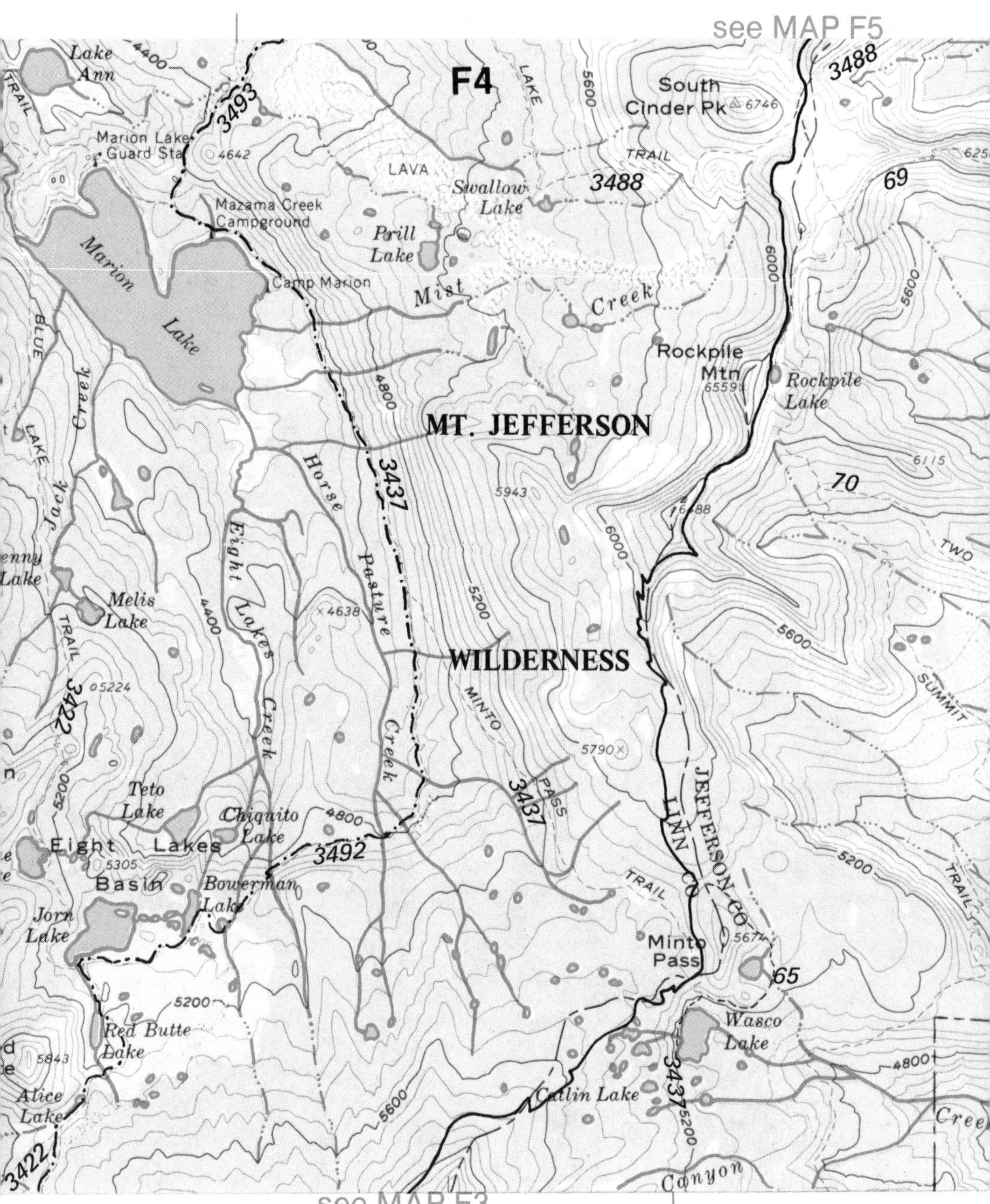

Next, you descend 2.0 easy miles on Trail 3437 to a junction on a descending ridge that juts into Marion Lake. Leaving the wilderness's largest lake, climb 1.6 miles up Trail 3493 to the John Swallow Grave. From this vicinity, Trail 3488 climbs 3.7 miles up to the PCT. Keeping to Trail 3493, you quickly pass aptly named Midget Lake, soon cross Whiskey Creek, find Lake of the Woods just beyond it, turn west at Puzzle Creek, and end your 2.7-mile stretch at a junction with Trail 3421 below the crest of Bingham Ridge (just off map F5). Northeastward, you soon cross the ridge as your Trail 3493 traverses 2.6 miles, passing pint-sized Papoose Lake before reaching a junction with a trail that climbs 1.8 miles southeast to the PCT, on a saddle near the south end of the Cathedral Rocks.

From this junction, you drop 1.4 miles to the Hunts Cove spur trail and then go 3.1

See maps F4 and F5

see MAP F6

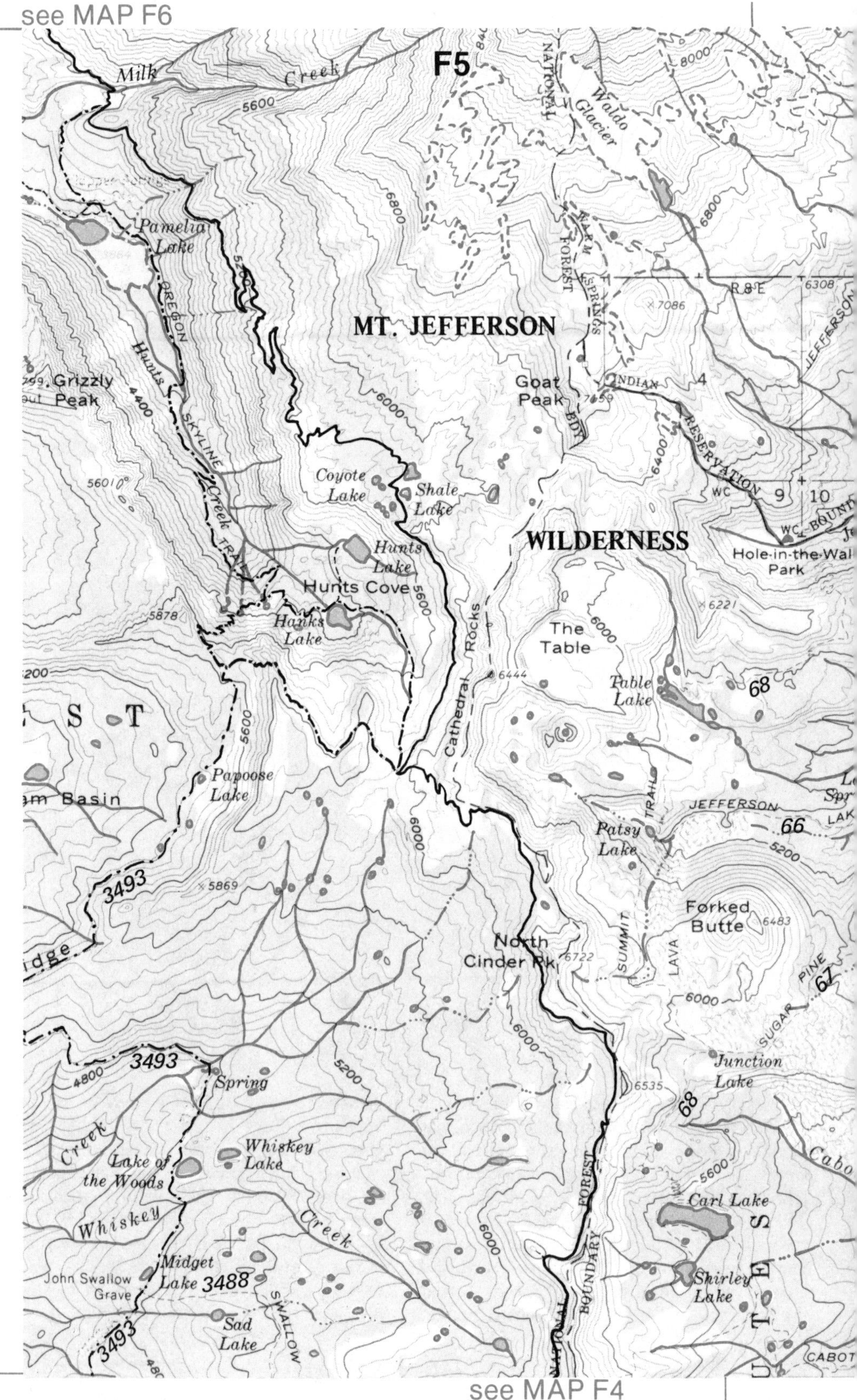

see MAP F4

miles to the north shore of Pamelia Lake, from which you climb 0.7 mile north back to the PCT. The total length of this route is 24.6 miles, more or less, versus 25.5 miles for the comparable stretch of PCT.

From the Santiam Lake Trail 3491 junction with the PCT just 1.4 trail miles north of Highway 20, you climb northeast up to a forested ridge and then follow it north-northwest toward Three Fingered Jack. The trail eventually leaves the ridge, curves northeast across a prominent cliff above Martin Lake, then heads up a small gully, and quickly curves north-northwest (6000–2.5).

Water access. If you are in desperate need of water, you can now head east cross-country, starting from an obvious flat atop the cliff and then follow markers 0.4 mile north down to sparkling Summit Lake (5800), a favorite among mountaineers.

Back on the PCT, follow the trail as it switchbacks up to the ridge again, crosses it, and traverses up the lower west slope of Three Fingered Jack (7841). ■ *Up close, this peak has a totally different appearance from the one you saw from a distance: here, "he" seems to have considerably more than three fingers.* ■

Side route. The easiest route to Three Fingered Jack's highest summit is a Class-3 ascent that starts on a faint trail up its southwest talus slope and then climbs its south ridge. Most of the routes up to the serrated crest require climbing equipment.

The PCT rounds the peak's northwest spur (6390–2.6), turns east toward a snow patch that lasts through mid-August, and then curves northeast up to a saddle (6500–0.5) along the Cascade divide. ■ *From this vantage point, you can observe the remaining structure of an ancient volcano that stands today as a crest called Three Fingered Jack. This peak is composed of remarkably uniform, thin, alternating beds of cinders and flows that dip west about 20°; their* regularity *over such a great thickness indicates a long period of minor eruptions. The reddish-brown, unsorted cinders consist of ash, lapilli, blocks, and bombs that contrast strongly with the brownish-gray andesite flows.* ■

Now the PCT descends several switchbacks, soon recrosses the divide, and then descends northeast along forested slopes to a smattering of stagnant ponds just southwest of

See maps F3, F4, F5

Mt. Jefferson, from escarpment north of North Cinder Peak

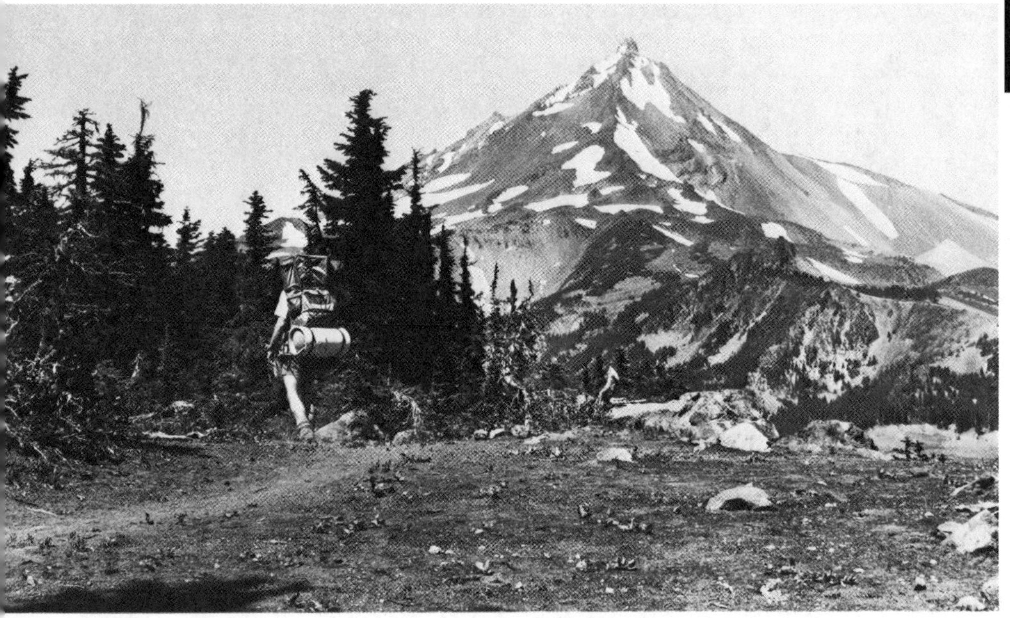

see MAP F7

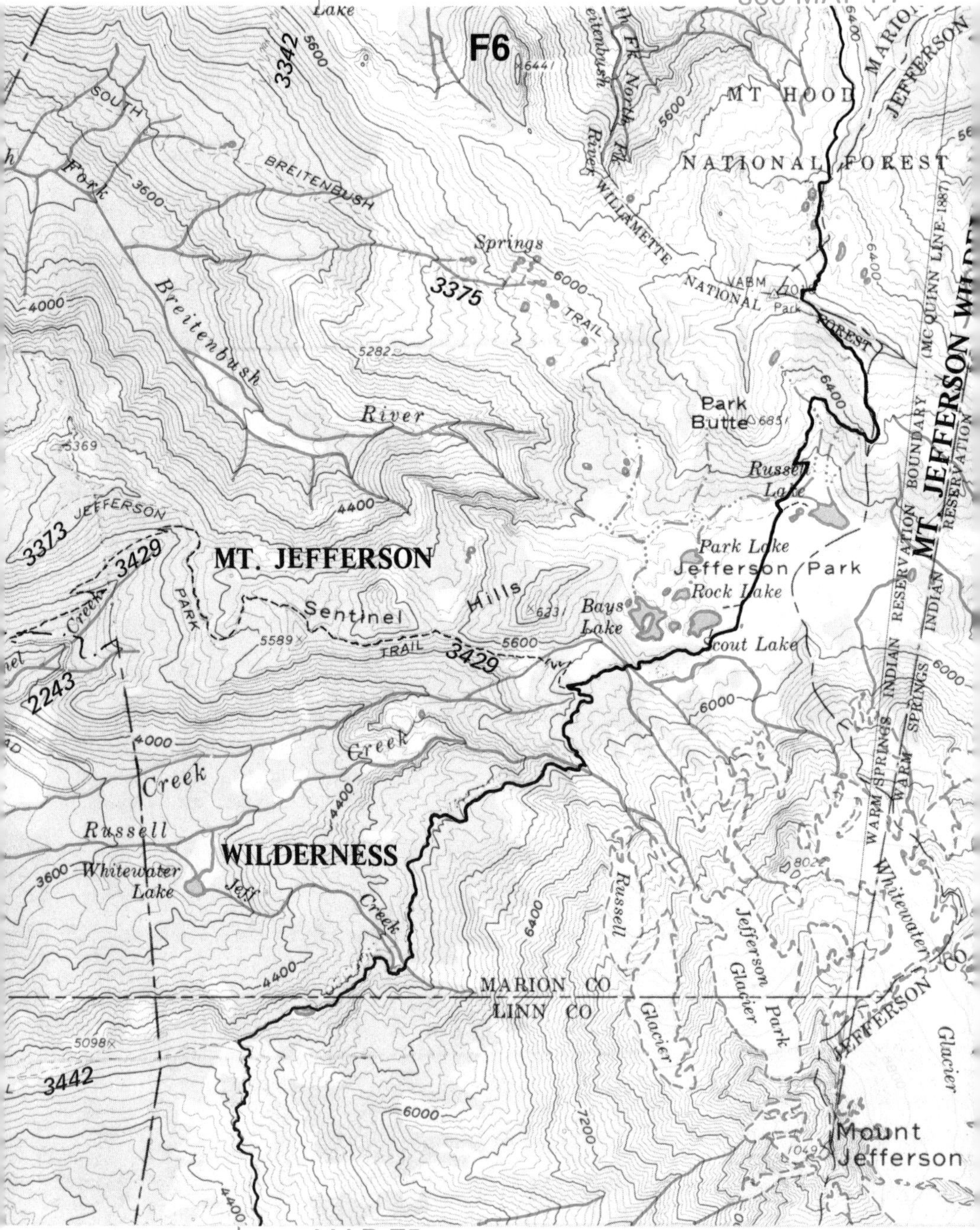

F6

see MAP F5

an intersection with Minto Pass Trail 3437 (5350–3.2) at Minto Pass.

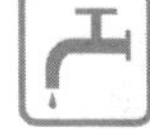

Water access. This trail descends south one-quarter mile to large, green, ten-foot-deep Wasco Lake, whose shores see a lot of campers in August once the mosquitoes have left.

The PCT quickly turns north, climbs to a saddle, and reaches the Wasco Lake loop trail (#65) (5430–0.5), which descends southeast

See map F4

half a mile to an unnamed lake before curving west to Wasco Lake. You continue north up the divide, switchback as it steepens, and then traverse to the southeast spur (6210–2.2) of Peak 6488, from which you can look south and see how Three Fingered Jack got its name. Continuing north, contour to a saddle and then contour across the east slope of Rockpile Mountain (6559), and pass Two Springs Trail 70, descending southeast, just before reaching a pond and beautiful Rockpile Lake (6250–1.0). This shallow but clear lake has an excellent campsite above its southeast shore and a very good one at its north end.

Your trail heads north on the rocky slope along the lake's west shore and then descends the divide to a saddle where a trail (6140–0.5) forks right and drops generally east—soon as Trail 69—toward roads near Abbot Butte. Your route stays west of the divide and climbs up to a level, open area just east of a breached cinder cone. ▮ *Although there are no lakes or ponds nearby, you may find that in midsummer this flat is crawling with one-inch toads.* ▮ Continuing north, you pass a second cone, South Cinder Peak (6746), which is of post-Pleistocene age, as is the first cone. Soon the trail reaches a saddle and an intersection with unmaintained Swallow Lake Trail 3488 (6300–1.0), which descends 2 miles southwest to Swallow Lake and 2 miles northeast to Carl Lake.

The PCT continues north along the west slope of the divide and reaches a saddle (6400–1.2) on a northwest ridge from which a spur trail climbs west-northwest to a small knoll with a good view of Mt. Jefferson, six miles north. Now the trail crosses a snow patch that lingers through late July, arcs eastward to the divide, and descends it to a level section that contains an adequate campsite beside a small, freshwater pond 50 yards east of the crest. Hiking a few minutes longer, you encounter an unsigned trail (6240–0.9) that descends southeast about a mile to large, emerald Carl Lake (5500), where camping is prohibited.

From this junction, hike once again up the ridge route and then contour across the forested west slopes of North Cinder Peak (6722) to a small, grassy meadow (6240–1.7) that has obviously been camped at, and for a good reason. A hidden, rock-lined pond lies on the

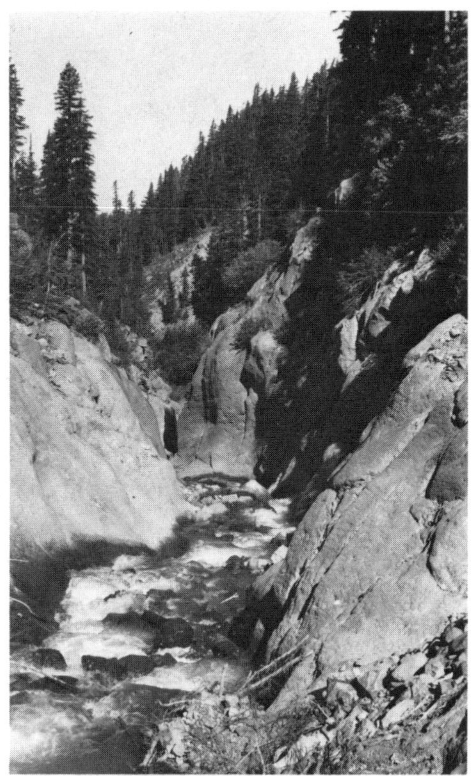

Russell Creek

other side of a low pile of rocks that borders the meadow. This is a good water hole to stop at if you are passing through late in the summer.

After a brief ascent north, you arrive at an escarpment (6340–0.4) where Mt. Jefferson (10,497) towers above in all its presidential glory. ▮ *On March 30, 1806, Lewis and Clark saw this snowy peak from the lower Willamette River, and they named it after their president. At the base of its south slope, below you, lies a bizarre glacio-volcanic landscape. During the last major glacial advance, glaciers cut a deep canyon on each side of the resistant Sugar Pine Ridge, seen in the east. After these glaciers disappeared, volcanic eruptions burst forth and constructed Forked Butte (6483) east of North Cinder Peak. This butte was subsequently breached by outpourings of fluid basaltic andesite that flowed east down the glaciated Jefferson Creek and Cabot Creek canyons. A smaller cone with a crater lake, north of here, also erupted about this time, but it was aborted*

See maps F4, F5

see MAP F8

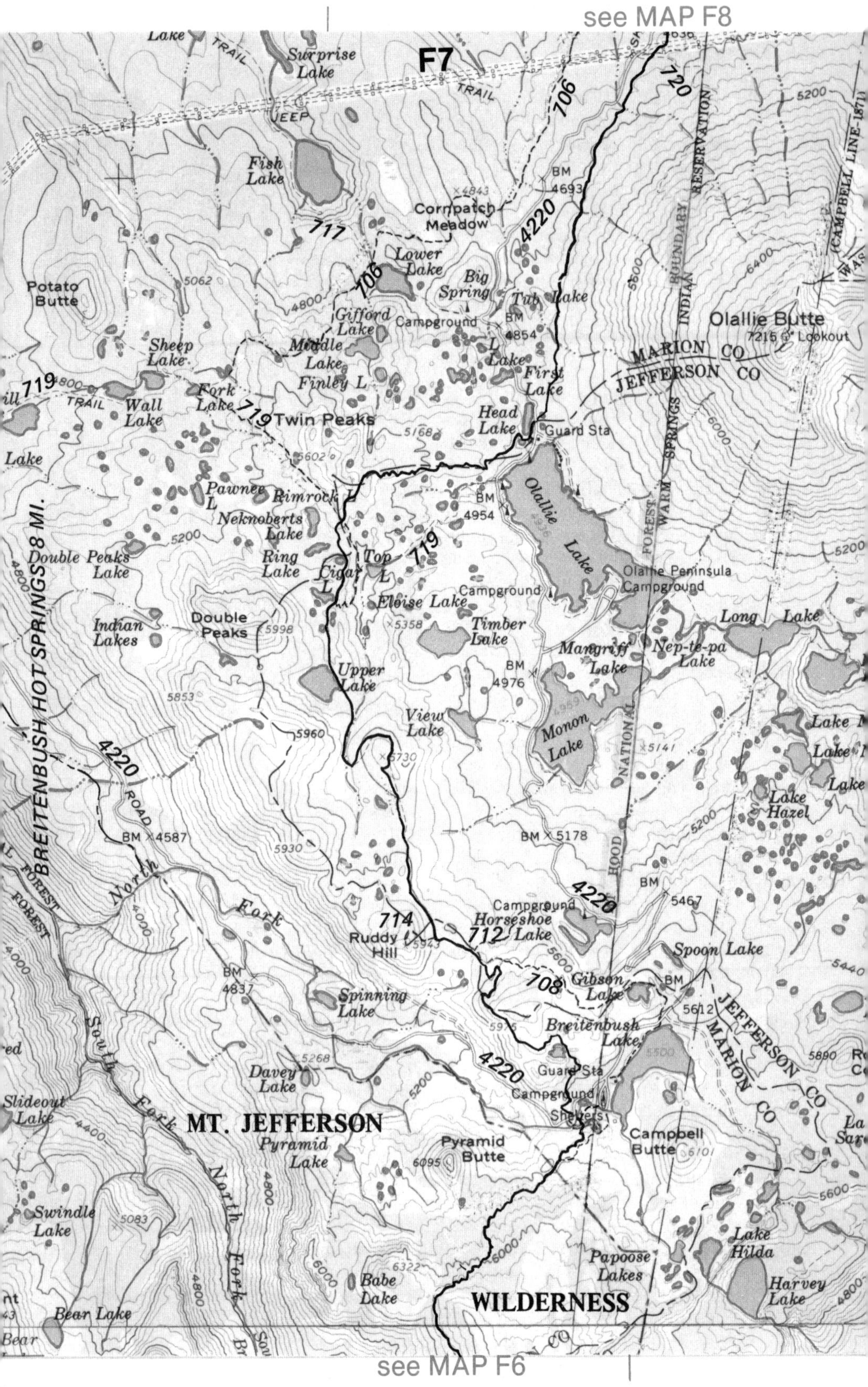

see MAP F6

by nature before any flows poured forth. To its north stands the flat Table, and between it and the ridge of Cathedral Rocks is a large, deep, enigmatic depression that may represent a collapsed flow ▮

Time, which allowed nature to sculpt this surrealistic artwork, now forces you to press onward. Descend northwest, still marveling at the configurations below, leave the ridge, and switchback down to a junction where a faint, unsigned trail (6130–0.7) climbs 100 yards back to the divide before descending into the marvelous basin. After more switchbacking down, you reach a saddle (5910–0.5) from which three variations of the PCT continue northward. We'll describe them in this order: the now-official newest route, the oldest route (now an alternate), and the newer route (also an alternate). We recommend one of the alternates.

Official PCT route. The *newest PCT route*, completed in the early 1970s, starts on a gentle descent north-northeast from the saddle and heads along the lower slopes of the inspiring Cathedral Rocks which, judging by their color, must have been constructed in the Dark Ages. The route curves northwest to the crest of a lateral moraine well above sparkling Hunts Lake, leaves this escarpment, and winds north to the west shore of placid Shale Lake (5910–1.8), which is a logical place to stop for the night. You might try camping on relatively flat ground east and northeast of Shale Lake. ▮ *The shale implied by the lake's name is actually basaltic andesite that has become highly fractured along many parallel planes.* ▮

Just north of this popular lake, you reach a shallow, seasonally larger lake that in late summer dwindles to a mudhole. Beyond it, the trail drops west to the glaciated escarpment and then oh-so-gently descends it before entering a Douglas-fir forest and reaching a junction with the Oregon Skyline Trail (old PCT) (4320–4.5) just south of Milk Creek. Those taking the second alternate route rejoin the official PCT route here.

Alternate route. The *oldest route* is now essentially cross-country, and it starts north steeply down the glaciated valley and curves west to shimmering, pure Hanks Lake (5144–1.2). Along its north shore, the Hunts Cove spur trail climbs north up to another gem, Hunts Lake (5236–0.4). It also descends west to a junction with a newer PCT route (5020–0.5–1.7).

Alternate route. The *newer route*, which was the standard one through 1972, starts on a contour northwest from the saddle, crosses a low ridge, and then makes a descent to the Trail 3493 junction (5640–1.8), near a saddle, before it switchbacks down to the Hunts Cove spur trail (5020–1.4). The oldest route joins this newer one here, continues a descent into the glaciated valley, and finally arrives at the southeast shore of shallow Pamelia Lake (3884). Paralleling the shore, the route curves west to a junction with Pamelia Lake Trail 3439 (3970–3.1), which takes you down to many campsites near the lake's deeper end. Early in the season, the lake is high and attractive, but by August, Pamelia is reduced to a putrid puddle dotted with hikers who climb the easy 2.4-mile trail to this lake. Leaving this potential eyesore behind, you ascend north and then northeast, toward Milk Creek and reach a junction (4320–0.7–7.0) with the newest PCT route.

Official PCT and alternate routes rejoined. Start up the gravelly, bouldery outwash deposits of Milk Creek canyon and pass a lavish display of wildflowers and shrubs before hiking north past a two-person campsite to a crossing of aptly named Milk Creek (4320–0.2). ▮ *Its silty color is caused by fine volcanic sediments that may in part be glacially ground to create "rock flour." You'll see many more creeks like it as you encounter glacier-clad volcanoes along this journey north.* ▮

Beyond this minor torrent, you now make tracks northwest across many small, deceptive ridges before reaching the real Woodpecker Ridge and a junction with lightly used Woodpecker Trail 3442 (5040–1.6), which descends west. Head east gently down from the ridge, soon passing a stagnant pond with a fair but illegal campsite at its west end. ▮ *The open forest here is quite choked with an understory of spiraea, corn lily, gooseberry, rhododendron, and the ubiquitous huckleberry. You'll easily identify Whitewater Lake, way below you, by its milky color, due to a high influx of fine sediments.* ▮

Not much farther along, you pass a small spring, enter a shady forest, and then cross a

see MAP F9

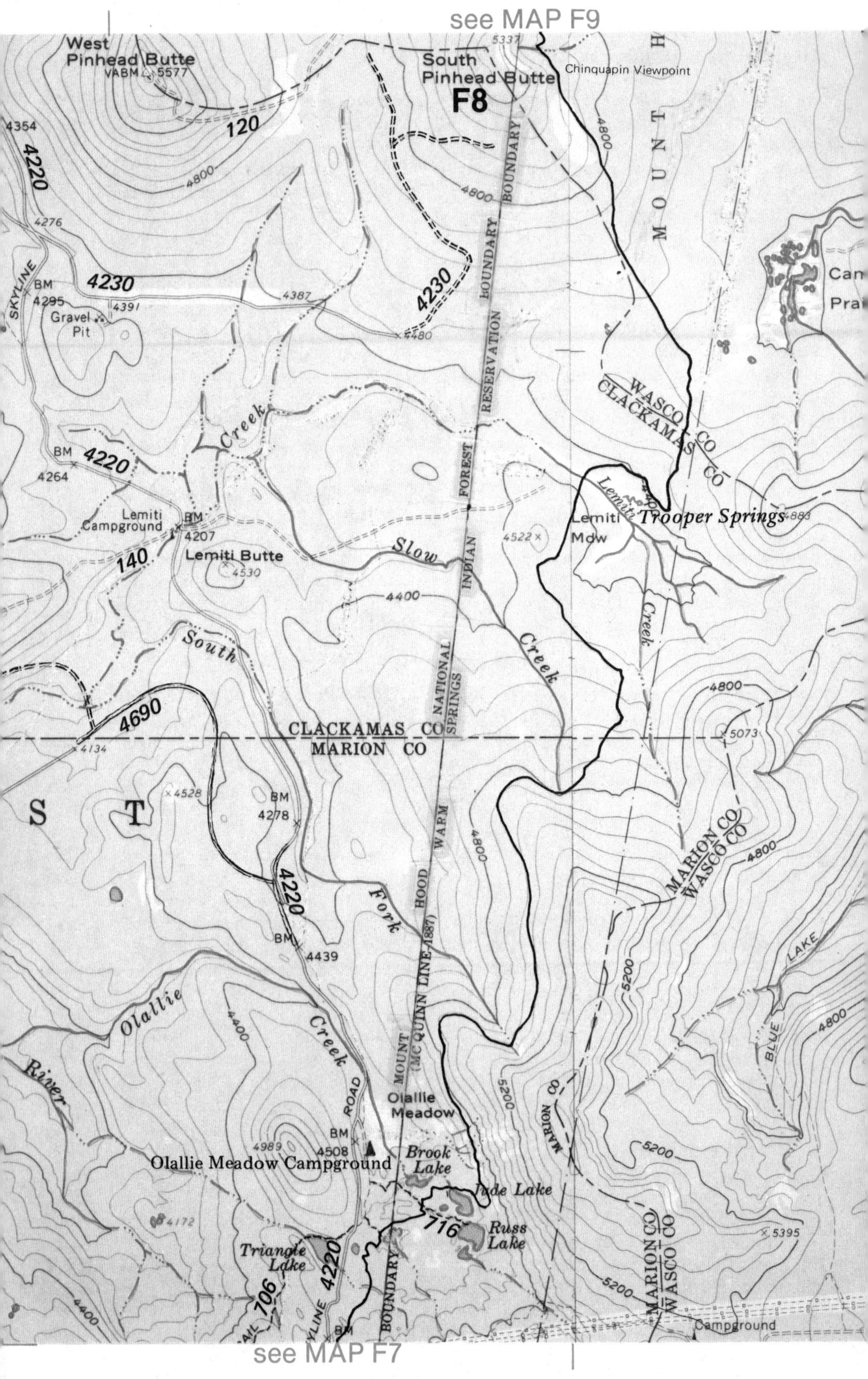

see MAP F7

creeklet whose gully is a channel for periodic avalanches. Two minutes past it, you cross Jeff Creek, cross a nearby two-person campsite, and see more evidence of avalanches. After ½ mile of gently ascending north, the trail ascends east, sometimes moderately, and then quickly drops to a ford of milky Russell Creek (5520–2.8). Plan to cross this creek *before 11 A.M.* The afternoon's warmer temperatures greatly increase the snowmelt from the Russell and Jefferson Park glaciers, and that increased flow has swept some hikers on a one-way trip down the gorge immediately below the ford. ▮ *This diurnal fluctuation is a second characteristic of the glacier-fed creeks that you'll encounter on future traverses around major Cascades peaks.* ▮ If the creek looks too brisk for safe crossing, look for a better spot about 70–100 yards upstream.

The trail now curves around a minor, westward-descending ridge with a poor campsite, soon makes a loop around a small, boggy area, and then briefly descends to cross the headwaters of a Whitewater Creek tributary. From its north bank, you make a minute's walk west to a junction with heavily traveled Jefferson Park Trail 3429 (5640–0.6). Starting from the end of Whitewater Road 1044, this trail—the shortest one into popular Jefferson Park—climbs 3.9 miles to the main branch of Whitewater Creek and then climbs an additional 0.4 mile to your junction.

From this point, the PCT/Jefferson Park Trail makes an easy climb east-northeast to ford that branch (5680–0.4). This crossing can be a wet one, but, unlike the ford of Russell Creek, it is always a safe one. Continue this easy ascent in the same general direction and then curve north for a momentary climb to the south rim of beautiful but overpopulated Jefferson Park.

The trail quickly curves northeast (5860–0.5), and at that point, a short spur trail descends to the nearby shore of cool, deep, green Scout Lake (5830). Camps rim the lake's shoreline, but like other lakeside camps in Jefferson Park, and in *every* wilderness, these are illegal. However, there is no other acceptable camping alternative.

▮ *If you enjoy crowds, camp at Scout Lake. Otherwise, try nearby Bays Lake, more-distant Park Lake, or some dry, nonmeadow spot in between. Beneath hemlocks on the north shore of Scout Lake, you get beautifully framed views across the reflective lake of stately Mt. Jefferson (10,497) with its ermine robe of glaciers. At this lake and the adjacent lakes of Jefferson Park, you might make a strange catch while fishing for trout: Pacific giant salamanders that inhabit these lakes' shady waters.* ▮

See map F6

Mt. Jefferson, from Olallie Lake Resort

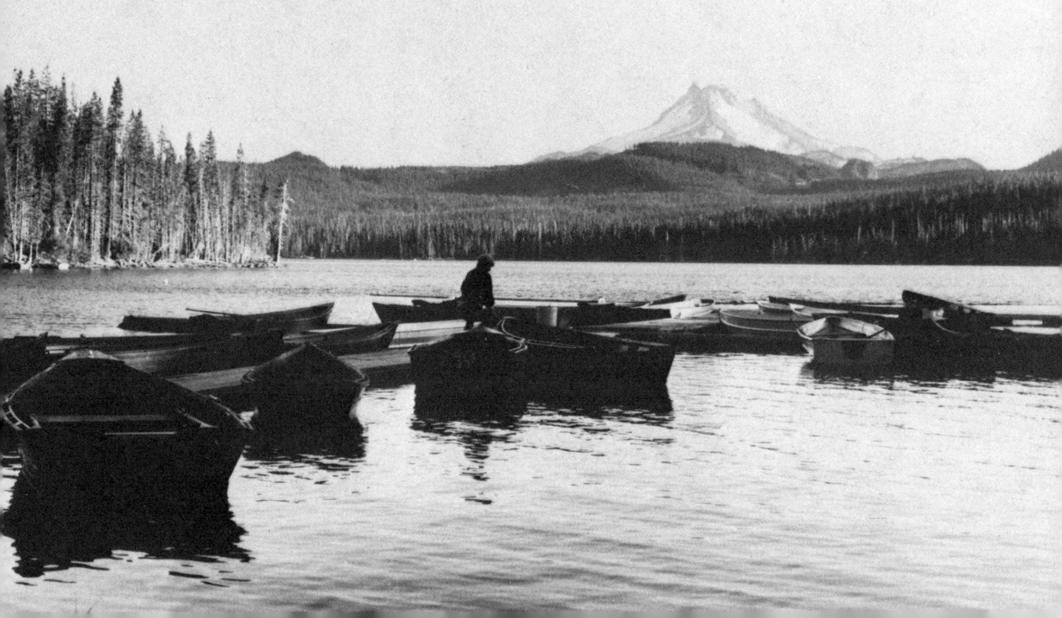

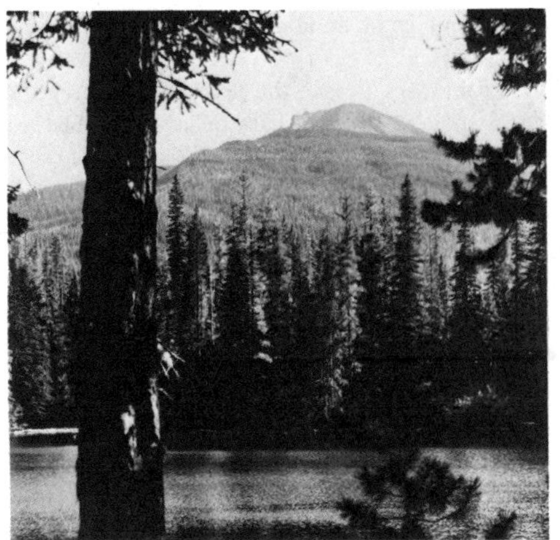

Olallie Butte, from Russ Lake

The PCT turns right (northeast) at the first spur-trail junction, follows blazes past radiating, narrow spur trails, curves north past a seasonal pond, and reaches a spur trail (5930–0.3) that heads west to Scout and Bays lakes. Now you hike north-northeast across the open flat of Jefferson Park and obtain impressive views back at the peak all the way to a junction with South Breitenbush Trail 3375 (5870–0.5), which starts west-southwest before descending northwest. Just 30 yards farther, a prominent spur trail branches northeast 250 yards to shallow Russell Lake (5856). Camping is prohibited at this lake, but you might consider camping in the vicinity at a fair distance from the lake. By late season, this lake may be fairly

See map F6

see MAP F10

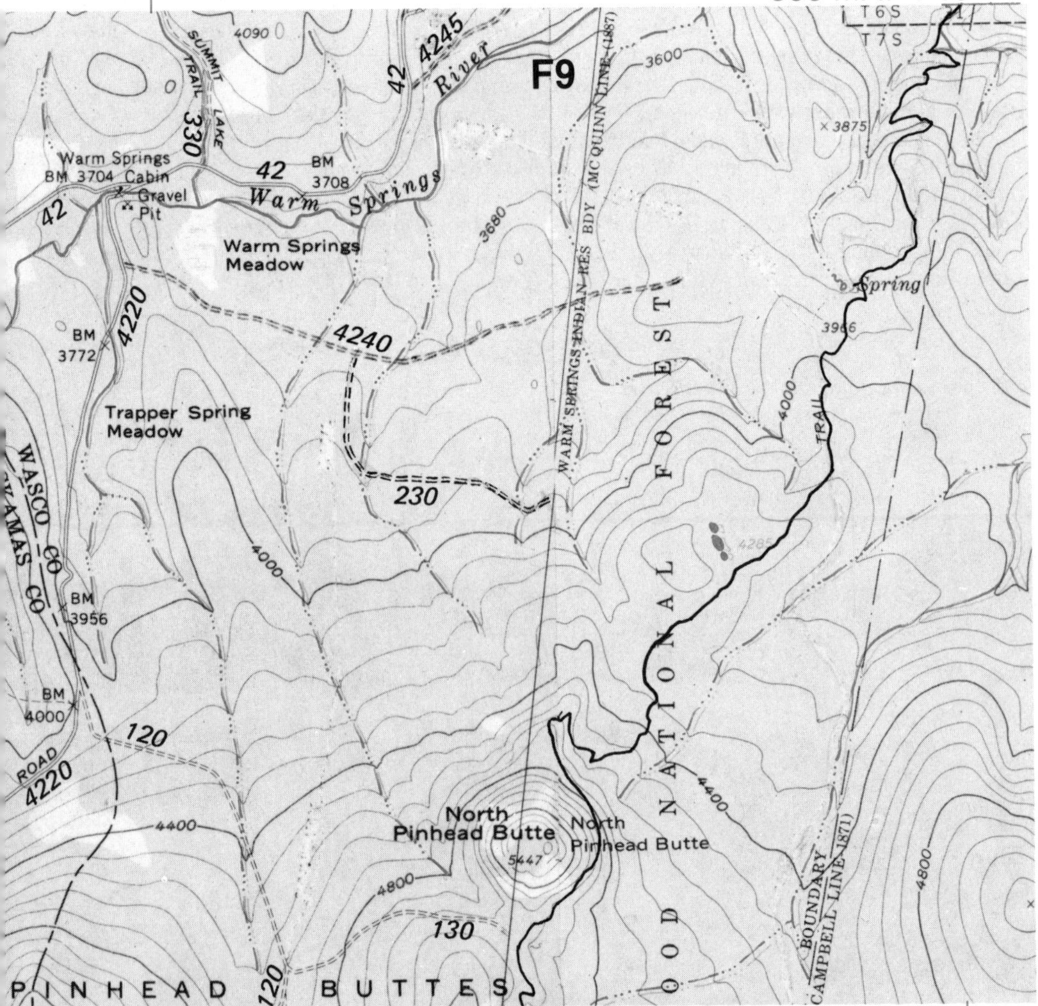

see MAP F8

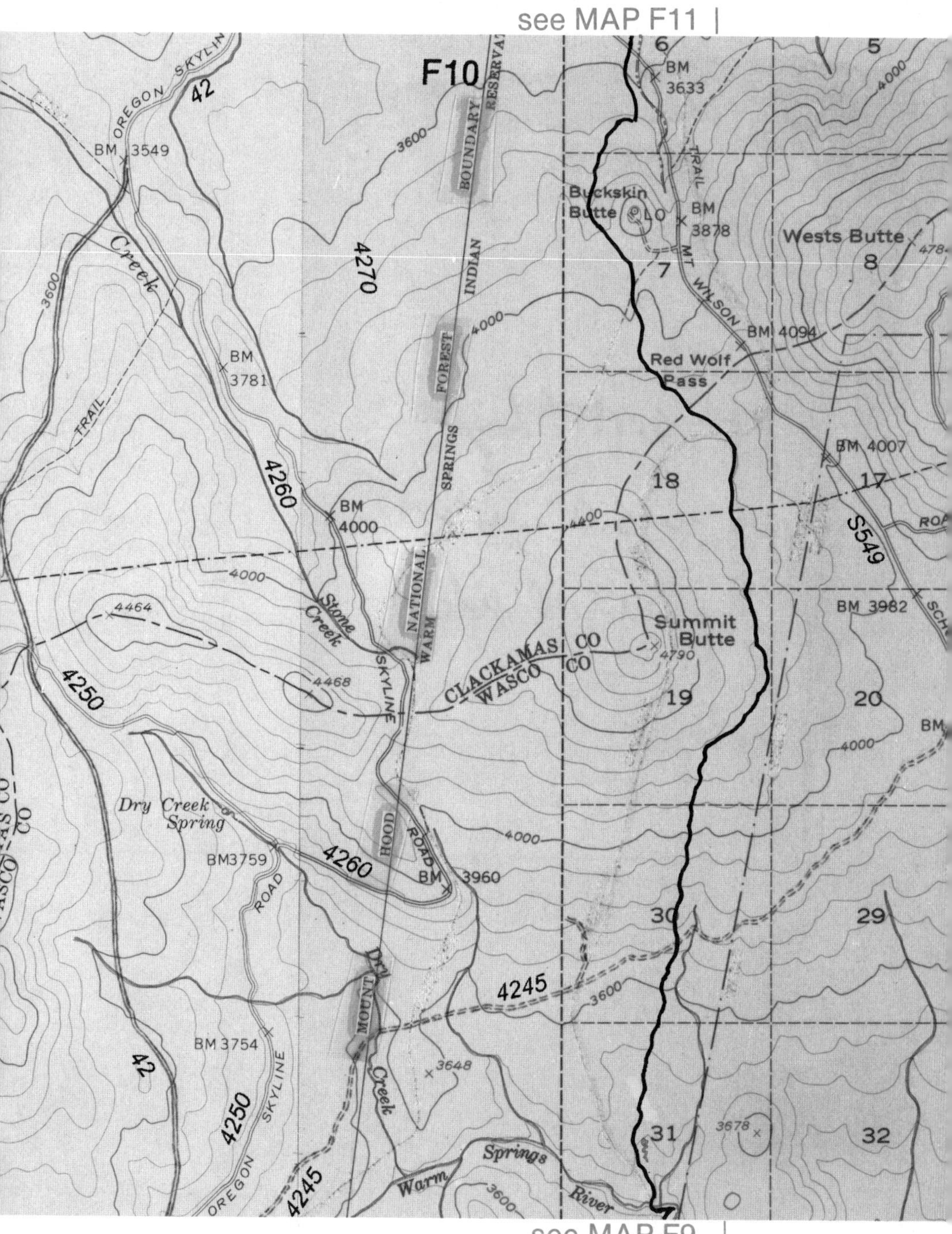

depleted and the others in the basin may be completely dry.

The PCT turns abruptly northwest at this junction and then quickly descends northeast to a step-across ford of South Fork Breitenbush River (5840–0.1). As you begin your ascent northeast, you can spot an excellent campsite 40 yards southeast just above the other side of the "river." The trail now climbs steeply up a slope and into a glacial cirque, where you again step across the river. Here, a steep shortcut northeast may look more like the trail than the trail itself does. ▮ *It developed, as so many shortcuts do, when early-season hikers chose*

See map F6

see MAP F12
see MAP F13

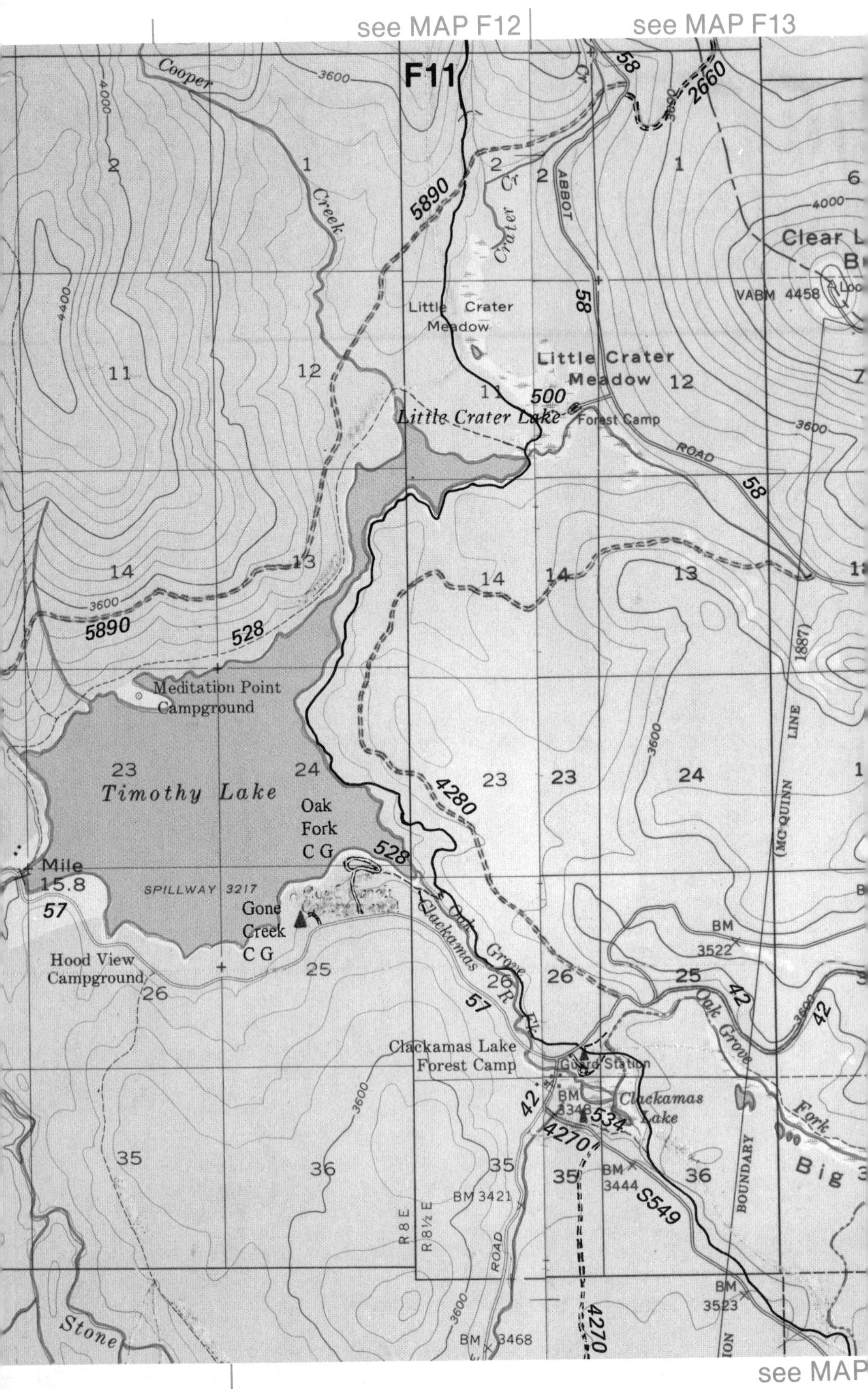

see MAP

to descend straight down the slope rather than follow the buried trail across snow patches. ▮ The real trail parallels the trickling river a short way north, curves, and then climbs moderately southeast to a spur on the Cascade divide. Climb this in an arc up to Park Ridge and then traverse 70 yards west to a viewpoint (6920–2.0), where you get a last look down at justifiably popular Jefferson Park.

Side route. A short trail climbs 200 yards west up to Peak 7018 for an even better view. In the distance, just east of north, towers magnificent Mt. Hood (11,235), and just to the west of north stands southern Washington's decapitated Mt. St. Helens (8364).

Now you descend the trail—or, rather, the semipermanent snowfield—toward small, shallow lakes and ponds. As the gradient eases, the trail becomes very obvious as it selects a pond-dotted route north out of the alpine realm and into the hemlock forest. The path momentarily takes you over a low saddle (6150–2.1) and then meanders northeast, giving views of locally dominating Pyramid Butte (6095) as it crosses many minor gullies and ridges. Views disappear, and soon the trail starts through a small flat with a low hill on your left. Here, you leave Mt. Jefferson Wilderness and immediately meet a conspicuous trail—the Old Oregon Skyline route—branching right.

The trail rambles onward for ⅓ mile, passing a small, volcanic butte of shalelike rocks before it meets Breitenbush Lake's outlet creek. Beside it is a spur road, which goes east to a large, nearby trailhead parking area, constructed in 1989. Immediately east of it is the Warm Springs Indian Reservation Boundary, and squeezed between that boundary and the southwest shore of Breitenbush Lake is the Breitenbush Lake Campground, which is administered by the Forest Service. On the PCT, walk a few paces past the spur road to Road 4220 (5500–1.6), crossing it just 30 yards northeast of the start of the spur road. In this locale is a trailhead parking area.

Keeping within Mt. Hood National Forest, you climb a winding trail up to the east shore (5750–0.5) of a shallow lake, curve around to its north shore, and then pass near a smaller, triangular lake. The trail then traverses the bouldery southwest slope of summit 5975 before winding down to a junction with the old Oregon Skyline Trail route (5510–1.0), now Gibson Trail 708. Starting northwest, you momentarily reach Horseshoe Saddle Trail 712 (5520–0.1)—logically atop a saddle above Horseshoe Lake.

Side route. You can follow this trail ¾ mile down to its trailhead by Road 4220's Horseshoe Lake Campground.

A short distance northwest along this ridge route, you encounter Ruddy Hill Trail 714 (5600–0.3), which climbs west. Now you contour northward through a thick forest and then climb up to a low knoll before descending slightly to Many Lakes Viewpoint (5660–1.2), which lives up to its description. ▮ *Mile-long Olallie Lake is the focal point of the basin, and andesitic Olallie Butte (7215) rules above it. ("Olallie" is what the native Indians called the huckleberries.) This volcano has been active in both glacial and postglacial times.* ▮

After hiking counterclockwise down the knoll's northern slopes, you reach a dry flat from which southbound hikers see the lofty crown of Mt. Jefferson beckoning them onward. Here the trail crosses a seasonal creek, descends north steeply alongside it, and veers northwest to a very good campsite at reposeful Upper Lake (5380–0.9). Continuing north, you pass several seasonal ponds and shallow, linear Cigar Lake (5350–0.4), from which a 0.6-mile trail first winds northeast down to Top Lake (5170), with a good west-shore campsite, and then climbs back to a mile-high crest junction with the PCT. Leaving Cigar Lake, the PCT takes an easier, more direct route to that crest junction (5280–0.4) from which Red Lake Trail 719 goes 1¼ miles northwest to Fork Lake.

The PCT contours north along the divide, curves northeast and crosses it, follows it east down past a small triangular, semiclear lake (5180–0.9), and arrives at the shore of deep, clear Head Lake (4950–0.7).

Resupply access. Here, a short spur trail curves eastward 60 yards to the Olallie Lake Forest Service Guard Station beside Skyline Road. For *northbound* hikers, this spur trail is the quickest way

See maps F6, F7

MAP F14

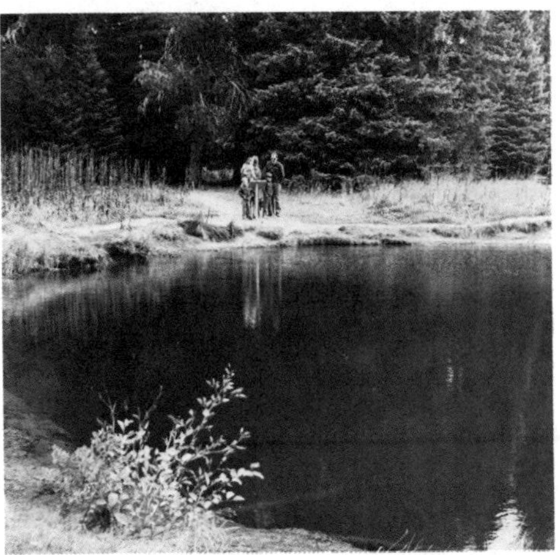

Little Crater Lake

to Olallie Lake Resort. Here you can pick up your mailed parcels, enjoy good food, and admire the view of Mt. Jefferson dominating the skyline south of the lake. Northward, you can look forward to good but expensive meals at Timberline Lodge, 54 miles distant. *Southbound* hikers: see "Resupply access," below.

From the spur trail, the PCT climbs above the southeast shore of Head Lake to pass a very good trailside campsite only 50 yards before reaching Skyline Road 4220 (4990–0.1) at a point 20 yards north of its signed 4991-foot divide.

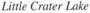

Resupply access. *Southbound* hikers can follow the road 100 yards south to a **Y** junction from which they can take a spur road 200 yards east to Olallie Lake Resort. It has a limited food selection, as did the store at Odell Lake's Shelter Cove Resort, about 143 miles back.

From the Skyline Road crossing, the PCT starts northeast and then makes a long, gentle descent north along the lower slopes of Olallie Butte (7215) to an intersection with Olallie Butte Trail 720 (4680–2.2), which descends 220 yards west alongside the southern powerline to Skyline Road. Cross under the three sets of powerlines and parallel the unseen road, going north-northeast until you observe a flat, bushy, open depression on the right (east). Then the trail veers northeast, but a blocked trail continues north. This trail (4570–1.0) is a 230-yard link between the PCT and the old Oregon Skyline Trail (now Lodgepole Trail 706). The PCT now enters Warm Springs Indian Reservation land and will remain on it almost to Clackamas Lake. ▮ *There is ongoing logging on the reservation, and the PCT crosses logging roads in various states of use. Not*

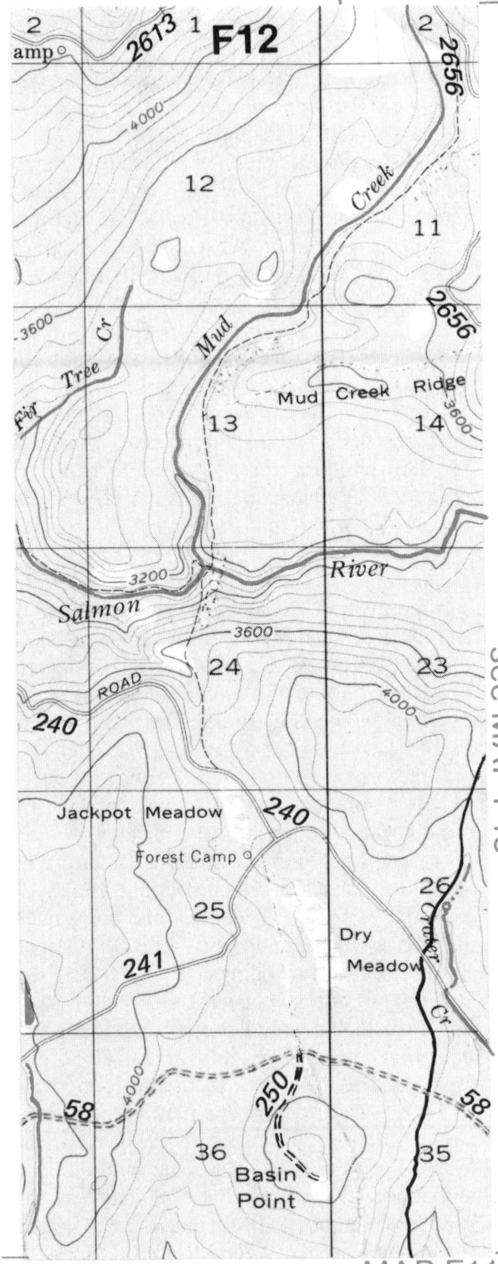

see MAP F13

see MAP F11

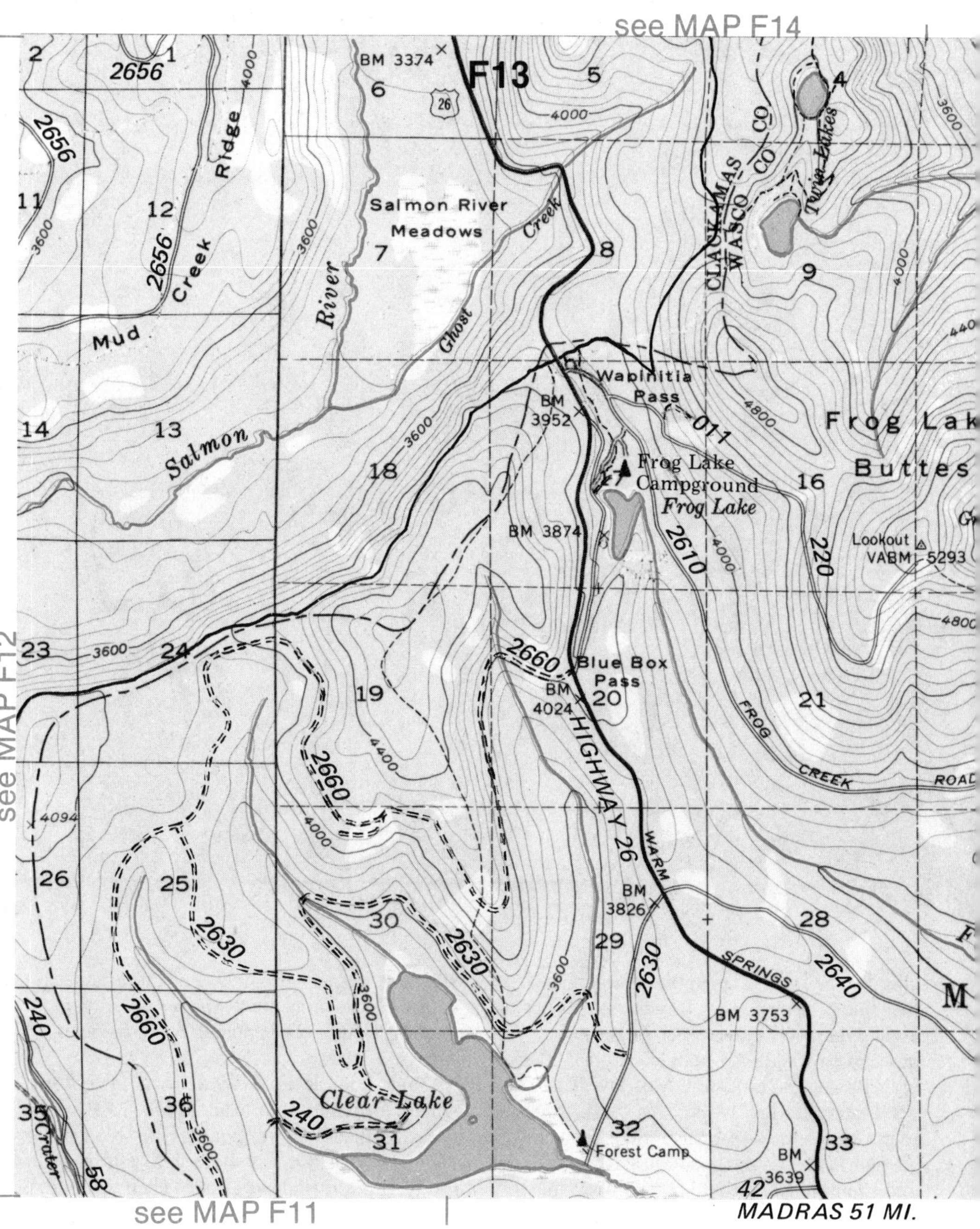

all are shown on the maps or are mentioned in the text. ▮ Continue northeast on a low ridge, angle north, and intersect Russ Lake Trail 716 (4550–0.3), ascending southeast from Olallie Meadow Campground; this trail continues 0.3 mile southeast past an adequate campsite at Jude Lake to a better one at deeper Russ Lake (4600).

Start north and then ramble northeast to shallow Jude Lake (4600–0.2), which has a good campsite on its northwest shore. Refill your water bottles here, for the spring 0.4 mile

See map F8

see MAP G1

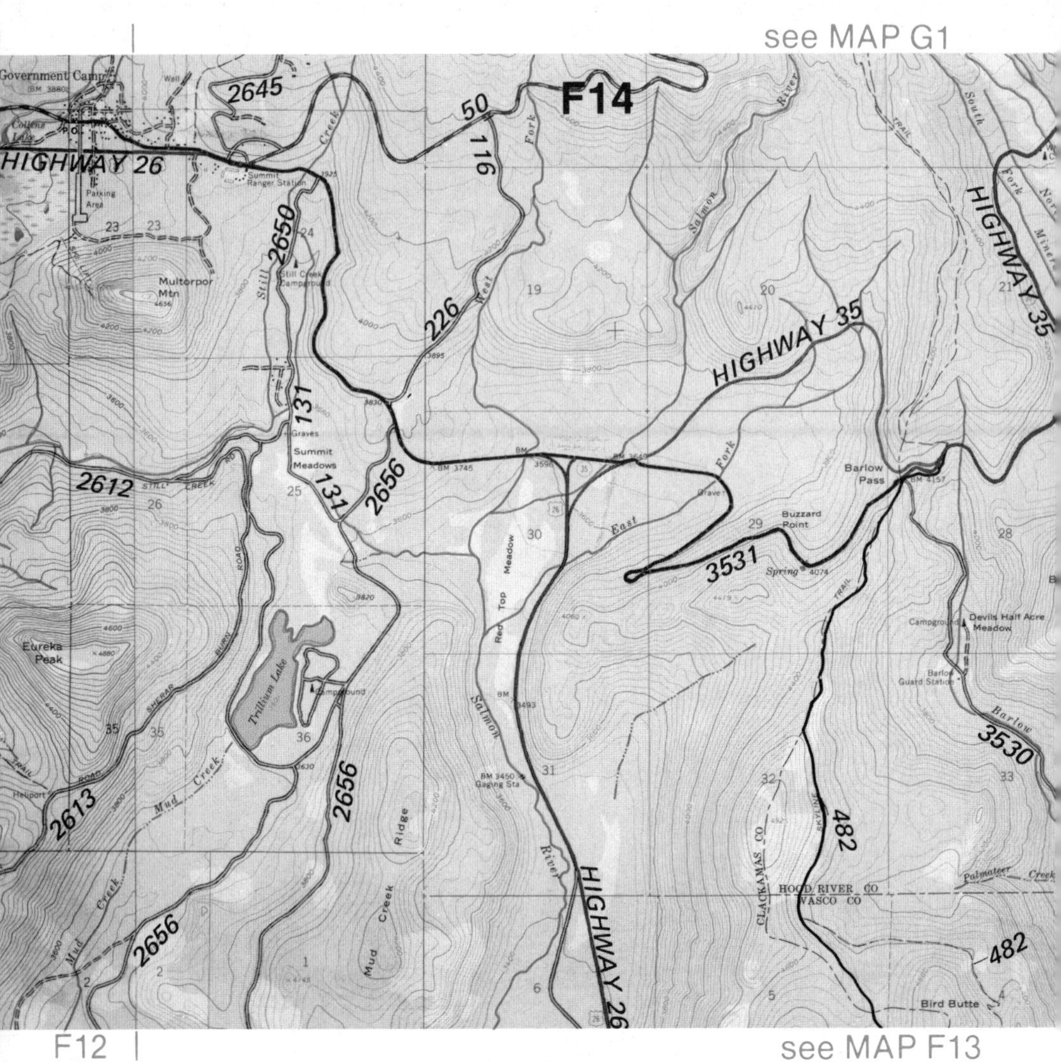

F12

see MAP F13

ahead sometimes dries up by mid-August. You then have a long, dry (though shady) walk around the lower ends of two ridges before you descend to trickling Lemiti Creek (4360–6.0) at the lower end of Lemiti Meadow. There is a good campsite just before this creek, superior to the campsite at Trooper Springs, just ahead.

The PCT continues southeast for 0.1 mile and then turns north to climb over the low Cascade divide. It more or less follows the divide north through a viewless forest, until South Pinhead Butte (5337), where you reach the trailside Chinquapin Viewpoint (5000–2.8) —rather disappointing, but at least it permits you to see over the forest. Better views are just ahead. Contour the butte's slopes northward, cross a saddle (4980–0.8) with an abandoned spur road going west, and then reach the southeast slope of North Pinhead Butte (5447), which is the youngest of the three andesite buttes. ▮ *Looking south, you see Mt. Jefferson once again and are reminded of the beauties of Jefferson Park.* ▮

Now you descend north to a lava flow, where a signed spur trail (4640–1.4) heads north-northeast 60 yards across it to an open view north of Mt. Hood (11,235) and east of the Warm Springs River basin. Then you make a switchback, descend back into the depths of the forest, and generally follow a gentle ridge route down to a junction with a spur trail (3860–3.3) that descends moderately west-southwest 70 yards to a seeping spring. The slopes steepen, and so does the route, which switchbacks down to a dry creek, contours northward, then turns west, and makes a crossing of Warm Springs River (3330–2.3), with a campsite nearby. ▮ *You've also just crossed the*

See maps F8, F9

45°N Latitude line and are midway between the Equator and the North Pole. If you hike the entire PCT, about 2600 miles long, you'll cover only 16½° of latitude, going from about 32½° at the Mexican border to about 49° in Manning Park. ▮

Climb north above a tributary gully and reach a flat, where you meet another signed spur trail (3450–0.4), which heads 70 yards east-southeast to a spring. Camp can be made almost anywhere in this open-forest area. Beyond the spring, you cross a northwest-trending linear meadow that is being invaded by lodgepoles and then climb gradually increasing slopes up to a junction with Road 4245 (3720–1.0); traveling southwest along this road, you would reach Skyline Road in 3.4 miles. Walk 17 yards northeast up Road 4245 to a resumption of the trail and follow it north up to the east slope (4230–1.7) of andesitic Summit Butte (4790). Next, you make a gentle descent north, pass under a six-cable powerline, cross northwest past unseen Red Wolf Pass (4120–1.4), and then reach a jeep road (3990–0.8) that diagonals northeast across the route.

The trail continues its northward descent and parallels a seasonal creek on the right (east) shortly before intersecting closed Road S549 (3580–1.3) which, like the PCT, heads toward the Clackamas Lake area. Cross this road and roughly parallel it northwest, leaving the Warm Springs Indian Reservation before reaching a junction with Miller Trail 534 (3400–1.9).

Water access. The Miller Trail makes a moderate descent northwest before contouring west to fairly large, well-maintained Clackamas Lake Campground, 0.3 mile distant. Why it is so popular is a mystery, for nearby Clackamas Lake appears to be little more than a polluted cattle pond, and campground vistas are virtually nonexistent. Could it be the campground's two old-fashioned, muscle-powered water pumps? Judge for yourself. Actually, the lake's water is better than you'd guess at first, for it is spring-fed.

The PCT turns north and proceeds through the forest bordering the meadow's edge to a usually dry crossing of Oak Grove Fork Clackamas River (3350–0.7) and, after 40 yards west, reach a spur trail that goes 280 yards southwest to Joe Graham Horse Camp. On the PCT, you go 300 yards west, meet Headwaters Trail 522 starting northeast toward the upper Oak Grove Fork Clackamas River and then in a few yards reach paved Skyline Road 42 (3370–0.2). The PCT crosses this road just 90 yards northeast of the entrance to Joe Graham Horse Camp, which in turn is 200 yards northeast of a junction with Road 57. Start west on the trail and soon see Oak Grove Fork Clackamas River below on the left (southwest). Momentarily, you descend to this creek, climb a little, and then pass a spring ⅓ mile before reaching Timothy Trail 528 (3320–1.4), which makes an eight-mile traverse around Timothy Lake (3217), passing campgrounds, picnic areas, and creeks before rejoining the PCT near the lake's northeast end.

You can see the lake from this junction, from which the PCT winds gradually down to the lake's unappealing east shore. The shoreline improves as you head north, where you are perhaps tempted to swim across the lake's narrow arm or make an adequate campsite beside it. Farther north, the arm enlarges to a shallow bay that in late summer becomes a swamp, and the trail contours northeast around it, passing several trailside springs, some of them seasonal, a few minutes before you reach a bridge over wide, clear Crater Creek (3220–4.3). Just north of this crossing, Timothy Trail 528 rejoins the PCT from the west.

About 250 yards beyond that junction, you reach Little Crater Lake Trail 500 (3230–0.2).

Side route. This trail strikes east 220 yards to 45-foot deep, extremely clear Little Crater Lake, which is an oversized artesian spring. Its purity is maintained by a fence that keeps out the cattle. You can camp either back near the trail junction or at pleasant Little Crater Lake Campground, which is just 200 yards east of the lake. Little Crater looks like the ideal swimming hole, but stick your arm down into it—brrrr!—as with most springs, its water stays an almost constant year-round 40°F. You re-enter forest and get back on the PCT.

The path north to Mt. Hood is now deficient in views, lakes, creeks, and hikers, but it is

See maps F10, F11

great if you like the solitude of a shady forest such as this one. ▮ *This forest has Douglas-fir; western and mountain hemlocks; western red and Alaska cedars; silver, noble, grand, and subalpine firs; and western white and lodgepole pines.* ▮ The trail starts northwest and then gradually curves north up to Road 5890 (3360–1.6), which gently descends northeast to a crossing of Crater Creek. Bear north for 30 yards on a diagonal across the road and then continue north up to Abbot Road 58 (3860–1.4), which would lead you back to Little Crater Campground and Skyline Road. Traversing through a forest of mountain hemlock and lodgepole, you next reach Linney Creek Road 240 (3880–0.8). Not far beyond it, you pass through a small campsite (3910–0.2) that has a seeping spring. This could be your last on-trail water until the upper Salmon River, 13.7 miles farther. However, water can be obtained ½ mile off the PCT at the Frog Lake Campground, about 4¾ miles away.

The PCT now climbs north to a saddle (4010–0.5) and then makes a long northeast traverse through a beautiful forest with rhododendrons to a junction with Blue Box Trail 483, which strikes south to Clear Lake (3500). In 50 yards you reach U.S. Highway 26 (3910–3.5) at Wapinitia Pass. We used to recommend that hikers follow this highway 7.7 miles to the post office and village store at Government Camp. While you can still take Highway 26 over to that settlement, you'll find the route noisy—in 1978 it was widened to four lanes to meet the demands of ever-increasing traffic. We now recommend another route that starts from Barlow Pass and is described at the end of this chapter.

Walking 70 yards closer to that pass, you reach a spur trail that goes 40 yards to the Wapinitia Pass PCT trailhead parking lot beside the busy highway.

Water access. From the parking lot, Road 2610 curves southeast and after ⅓ mile gives rise to Frog Lake Road 230, branching southwest. Starting on it, you'll come to the entrance to the new Frog Lake Campground, built in 1978. You might plan to camp here or at least get water at it.

Only 120 yards past the parking-lot trail, the PCT meets southbound Frog Lake Trail 530, which quickly crosses Road 2610, soon crosses Road 230, and then parallels 230 to the northwest lobe of Frog Lake. Leaving Trail 530, the PCT continues northeast through a solemn forest of western hemlock, curves southeast upward, and then makes a switchback north to a near-crest junction (4360–1.2). You can take the official PCT, below, or an alternate route, below, from this point. On the official PCT, no reliable water is found from this point until off-route sources near Barlow Pass.

Official PCT route. Beyond the near-crest junction, the PCT makes a shady, viewless traverse north to a broad saddle (4450–1.1) and then continues northwest to a reunion with the alternate-route loop trail (4500–0.5).

Alternate route. From here, the Twin Lakes trail immediately crosses a crest saddle, visits the two glistening orbs, and then, after a total length of 2¾ miles, rejoins the PCT. This lake loop used to be a part of the PCT, but the easily accessible Twin Lakes became overused, and the PCT was rerouted in the mid-1970s. Still, many PCT hikers prefer this longer route, if not for its aesthetics then at least for its water.

Official PCT and alternate route rejoined. From this junction, your route heads north, passes by southeast-descending Palmateer View Trail 482 (4550–0.5), and then soon hugs the crest for a 1.2-mile descent to an *old* section of Highway 35 at Barlow Pass (4157–1.5). You'll find a PCT trailhead parking area immediately west of here. Then, as you start to parallel the old highway northeast, you immediately cross Road 3530, descending south. Past it, the PCT soon becomes an abandoned road that takes you on a minute's walk to this section's end, a crossing of a new section of Highway 35 (4155–0.2). You should be able to find water in a gully about 130 yards east of this crossing. If not, and if you're desperate, then start down the following resupply access, which begins 0.2 mile back.

Resupply access. Most hikers will continue along Section G's PCT to Timberline Lodge, which serves good but expensive food and which also holds parcels mailed to it—for a fee (see Section G:

See maps F11, F12, F13, F14

Supplies). Long-distance PCT hikers on a shoestring budget may want to have their parcels mailed to Government Camp Post Office rather than to Timberline Lodge.

You can reach Government Camp by descending west along the old section of Highway 35, now Road 3531. Starting at Barlow Pass, this takes you down past an obvious roadside spring (4074–0.6) to a scenic hairpin turn and then down to a pioneer woman's grave, on your left, about 100 yards before crossing the East Fork Salmon River. Just ⅓ mile west of the crossing, Road 3531 ends at the new section of Highway 35 (3665–1.9).

Continuing west, you soon pass through the large, high-speed interchange of Highways 26 and 35 and then follow traffic over to the start of the Timberline Lodge road (3980–2.7), opposite the Summit Ranger Station. Just ¼ mile past it, you fork right and take the Government Camp road through town, reaching Government Camp Post Office (3840–0.8–6.0) just 250 yards past the moderately well-stocked village store.

Now backtrack to the Timberline Lodge road (3980–0.8), follow it up past the entrance to Alpine Campground (5450–4.5), and then go up to the road's end at giant Timberline Lodge (5940–2.2–13.5). At the north end of the large hikers' parking lot, below the lodge, register at a small hut. You'll find the PCT making an obvious slice across the slopes just above the lodge. Although you've bypassed part of the PCT by taking this alternate route, you can see from a distance the best part of what you've missed by scanning along the PCT for a long half-mile eastward to the White River Buried Forest Overlook, described in Section G.

See map F14

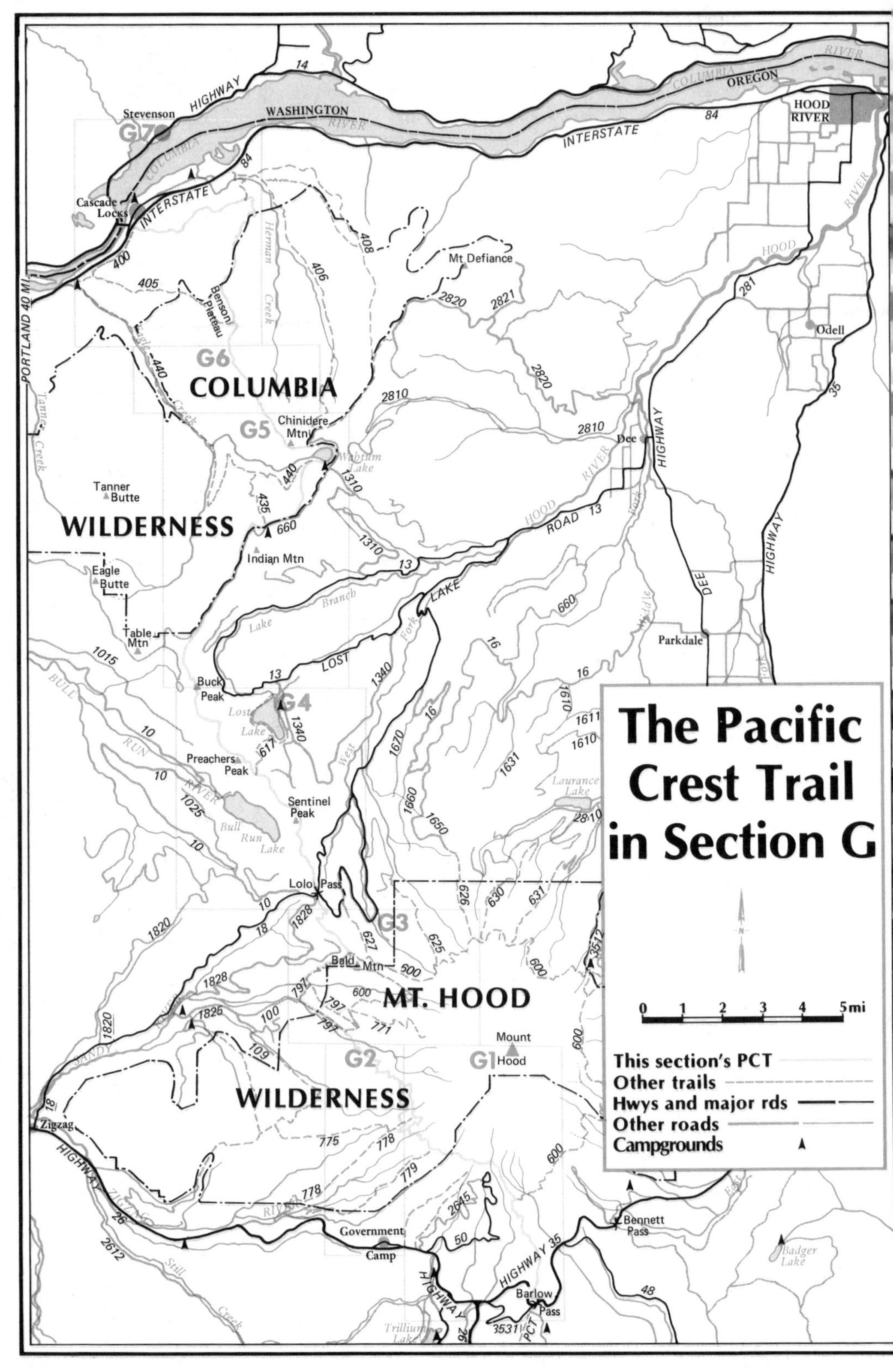
The Pacific Crest Trail in Section G
0 1 2 3 4 5mi
This section's PCT
Other trails
Hwys and major rds
Other roads
Campgrounds
COLUMBIA WILDERNESS
MT. HOOD WILDERNESS
WASHINGTON
OREGON
COLUMBIA RIVER
Stevenson
Cascade Locks
HOOD RIVER
Odell
Dee
Parkdale
Mt Defiance
Chinidere Mtn
Wahtum Lake
Tanner Butte
Indian Mtn
Eagle Butte
Table Mtn
Buck Peak
Lost Lake
Preachers Peak
Sentinel Peak
Bull Run Lake
Lolo Pass
Bald Mtn
Mount Hood
Laurance Lake
Zigzag
Government Camp
Trillium Lake
Barlow Pass
Bennett Pass
Badger Lake
PORTLAND 40 MI.
G1
G2
G3
G4
G5
G6
G7

Section G: Highway 35 near Barlow Pass to Interstate 84 at Bridge of the Gods

Introduction: In this short section, the hiker traverses around Oregon's highest and most popular peak, glacier-robed Mt. Hood. If you start your hike at Timberline Lodge, you can traverse around the peak in one long, though relatively easy, 18.7-mile day. However, hiking in the opposite direction requires considerable effort, for in that direction you have a *net* (not total) gain of 2520 feet instead of a net loss.

From Bald Mountain north past Lolo Pass to Wahtum Lake, the scenery is subdued—a typical, forested Oregon Cascades crest. North of Wahtum Lake, the PCT has the potential to be highly scenic if the route were only slightly relocated. As it now exists, it has a noticeable lack of views, particularly as you're descending into the spectacular Columbia River gorge. We therefore recommend the unusually beautiful, dramatic Eagle Creek Trail as an alternate route, for it abounds in waterfalls within a steep-walled canyon. This is a foot trail only; it is impassable for and prohibited to stock.

Declination: 18¾°E

Points on Route	S→N	Mi. Btwn. Pts.	N→S
Highway 35 near Barlow Pass	0.0		51.7
Join the Timberline Trail	3.6	3.6	48.1
Timberline Lodge	5.0	1.4	46.7
Paradise Park Trail	8.7	3.7	43.0
Reach Ramona Falls Loop Trail	13.8	5.1	37.9
Leave the Timberline Trail	18.2	4.4	33.5
Lolo Pass	21.0	2.8	30.7
Huckleberry Mountain Trail	25.3	4.3	26.4
Indian Springs Campground	33.5	8.2	18.2
Wahtum Lake at Eagle Creek Trail jnct.	36.1	2.6	15.6
Camp Smokey saddle	40.9	4.8	10.8
Teakettle Spring	44.6	3.7	7.1
Lateral trail to Herman Creek	47.6	3.0	4.1
Bridge of the Gods, east end	51.7	4.1	0.0

Supplies: This section is short enough that most hikers don't worry about supplies. However, long-distance hikers will certainly want to pick up packages they've mailed to Timberline Lodge, which lies only 5 miles into this section's route. Packages are held at the lodge's Wy'East Store, and in the past the store had a weekly charge for each package. Phone the store first for rates—(503) 272-3311—and if they are agreeable to you, then send your packages to: Timberline Lodge, Wy'East Store, Timberline, OR 97028. You can avoid a charge by mailing packages to the Government Camp post office (also 97028), a few miles off route. The settlement also has a small market and gas station. An alternate route at the end of Section F tells you how to reach this small settlement.

Timberline Lodge, like other premier mountain lodges, is expensive. Those who can afford it can get rooms, meals, and showers, plus the use of a hot pool and a sauna.

Halfway through your trek, you can take the Huckleberry Mountain Trail down to a small store at the north end of Lost Lake. However, few hikers do so. Finally, at trail's end in Cascade Locks (P.O.: 97014), you can find almost anything you need. If you can't, take the bus west into Portland or east to much closer Hood River.

Maps:

Mount Hood South, OR
Government Camp, OR
Bull Run Lake, OR
Wahtum Lake, OR
Carson, WA
Bonneville Dam, WA

THE ROUTE

Section G begins where the PCT diagonals across Highway 35 just east of Barlow Pass. This crossing is 90 yards northeast of a junction with the northeast end of Barlow Road 3531. Drive ¼ mile southwest down this road to find a PCT trailhead parking area—the start of Section F's alternate route that goes to Government Camp. If you must stock up on water, get it at an obvious roadside spring ½ mile southwest past the parking area or in a gully about 130 yards east of where the PCT crosses Highway 35.

From Highway 35 (4155), the PCT starts northeast, but it immediately angles west for a climb to the Cascade divide. Ascending north, it stays close to the crest of the divide, and you may see one or more cross-country ski routes, these marked by blue diamonds nailed on trees. For a short stretch, the PCT, when under snow, is part of a ski route. Eventually, the PCT curves northwest over to a gully (4870–2.7) with a campsite and with *usually* flowing water. From this cool forest retreat, your trail methodically climbs over to the slopes of the Salmon River canyon, where you can look west toward Alpine Campground and see a cliff below it of loose hornblende andesite debris. The trail then climbs northeast up to a junction with Timberline Trail 600 (5340–0.9), which starts a descent east to the White River. This trail, which stays near timberline as it circles Mt. Hood (11,235), offers an alternative 22.7-mile route if you take it counterclockwise to a reunion with the PCT near Bald Mountain. Clockwise, it coincides with the PCT, which starts northwest up a ridge of loose, gravelly debris.

▮ *If you look east at the cliff composed of unsorted volcanic debris that is above the White River, you'll get an idea of the type of sediments you're walking on. These deposits, which are on the south and southwest slopes of Hood, are remnants of a huge debris fan of hornblende andesite that was formed 1700–2000 years ago when a crater was blasted out near the mountain's summit, and a plug dome of viscous lava welled up, melting the surrounding ice field. The sudden release of frozen water created devastating mudflows that carried the volcanic debris down to these slopes that the PCT crosses today. Due north, you can identify Crater Rock (10,560), which is a remnant of that plug done. Just north of it, numerous fissures still emit steam and hydrogen-sulfide gas. On clear, windless days the gas emissions from these fumaroles are visible from as far away as Portland. Mt. Hood had minor eruptions during the last century, and you can be sure that it is still alive today.* ▮

Not too far ahead, you reach the White River Buried Forest Overlook (5790–0.8). ▮ *If you scrutinize the* lower *mudflow sediments in the canyon's wall opposite, you should be able to recognize a few buried snags. It was these snags that provided radiocarbon dates for eruptions mentioned above.* ▮

Leaving the overlook, the trail soon curves northwest away from the canyon views, crosses a dry creekbed, and then crosses the upper Salmon River (5900–0.3), which derives its

SECTION G

See map G1

see MAP G3

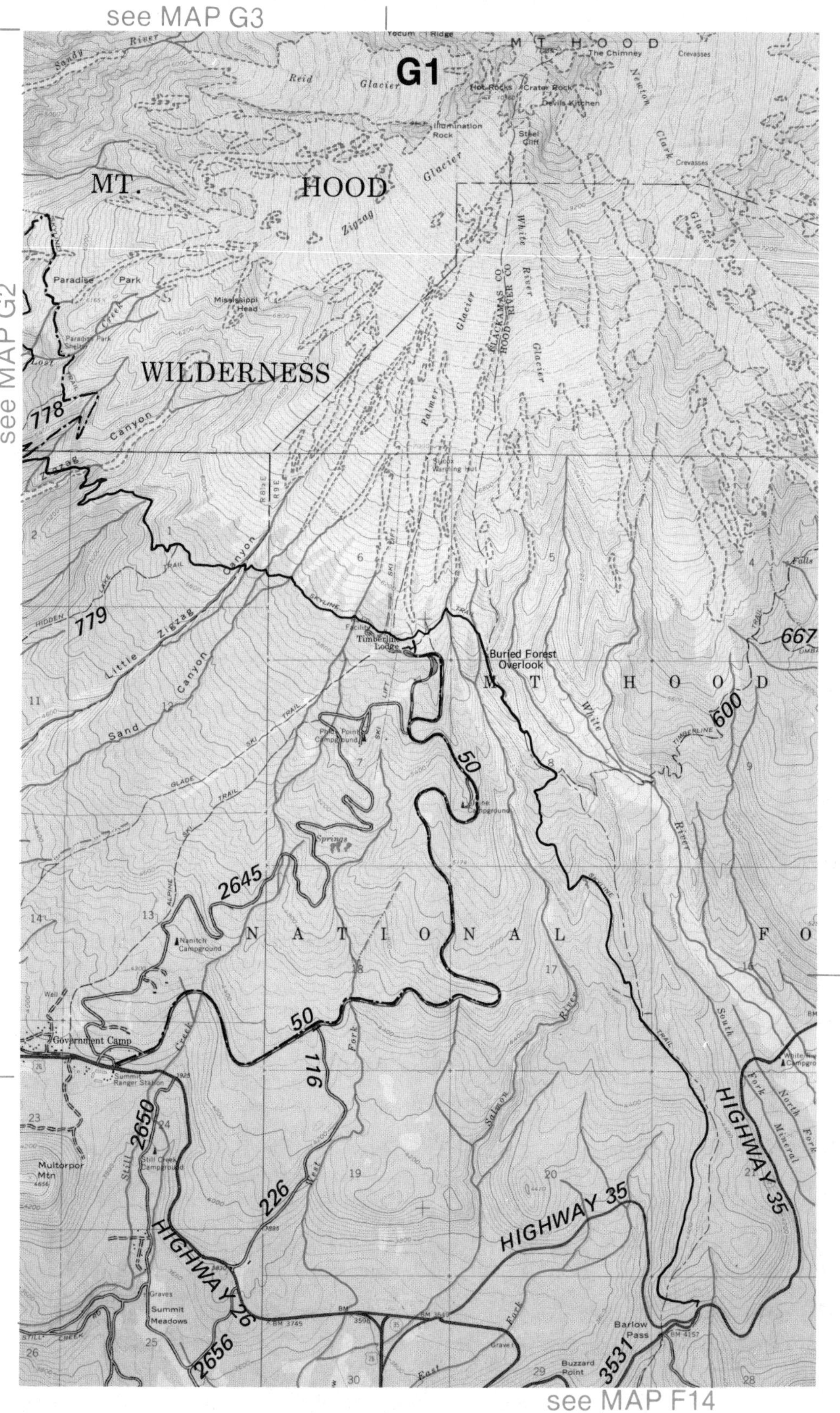

see MAP G2

see MAP F14

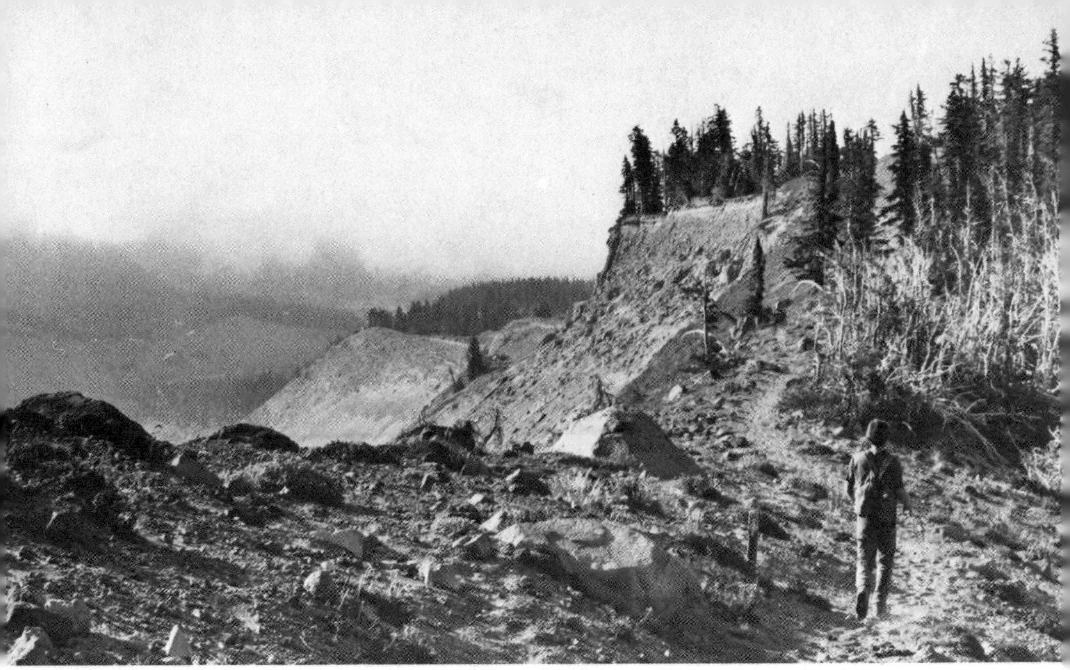

Southbound hiker near the White River Buried Forest Overlook

flow from an arm of the Palmer Glacier. This flow is the first reliable on-route water since a seeping spring just past Linney Creek Road, 13.7 trail miles south. The trail now contours southwest past an ascending dirt road and then quickly reaches a spur trail (5960–0.2)—one of many—that descends to the east side of gigantic Timberline Lodge.

Side route. No hiker should pass up the opportunity to inspect this grand structure, built by the Works Progress Administration in the late 1930s. Just east of and below the lodge's parking lot is an even larger lot for backpackers and mountaineers; at its north end is a small hut in which you should register if you plan to hike any farther or if you plan to climb Mt. Hood. Mountaineers who climb Mt. Hood often try to reach its summit by sunrise in order to avoid avalanche hazards generated by warming snow and ice. By early July rockfalls can become a real danger along south-slope routes. Don't attempt to climb the peak unless you are an experienced mountaineer and are familiar with Hood's routes and hazards.

After ascending one of the spur trails or roads from the lodge back to the PCT, hike west under the ski lift and past a microwave tower (5980–0.2) below and then gradually

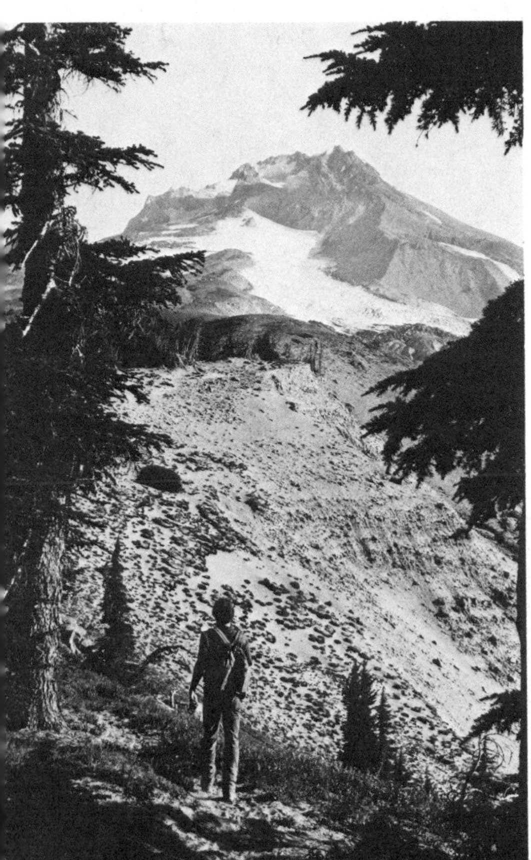

Mt. Hood's White River glacier

See map G1

descend westward with views south across a rolling topography to lofty Mt. Jefferson (10,497). You cross several seasonal creeks before making a three-yard boulder-hop across silty Little Zigzag creek (5760–0.9), entering Mt. Hood Wilderness, and continuing your descent to a junction with Hidden Lake Trail 779 (5680–0.4), which goes southwest down a morainal ridge to Hidden Lake. The PCT continues its rambling descent and then climbs to a narrow ridge from which you get a great view of Mt. Hood and glaciated Zigzag Canyon. Now switchback down the steep slope, jump across the silty Zigzag River (4890–1.3), and climb moderately into and out of a tributary canyon, up to a point where you have a choice of two routes: the newer, official PCT, following, and the older, more scenic ex-PCT route, given as an alternate below.

Official PCT route. The newer, official PCT, which equestrians *must* take, starts west-southwest and switchbacks up to a broad ridge where it intersects Paradise Park Trail 778 (5390–0.4), a footpath that climbs northeast. Your newer PCT ascends north across the ridge and passes a camping area below the trail just before it turns northeast to descend to splashing Lost Creek (5390–0.6), which cascades down a cliff just to the east. Cross it and its more reserved tributary and then pass another camping area below the trail as you climb west up to a ridge, top the ridge, and descend once again—this time to a crossing of Rushing Water Creek (5440–0.6) just below its narrow waterfall. After climbing steeply north out of this cliff-bound canyon, you follow a rather direct trail down to rejoin the older PCT route (5400–0.5).

Alternate route. Those on foot can take the older PCT route, a stretch of the old Oregon Skyline Trail that is by far the more scenic trail. It starts northeast and zigzags up the tributary canyon of Zigzag Canyon. ▮ *If you're wondering about the composition of the loose cliffs, yes, they are part of the debris-fan deposits that originated from the Crater Rock area.* ▮ The ascent finally eases just after gaining access to a ridge and meeting Paradise Park Trail 778 (5740–1.0), a footpath descending west-southwest through an alpine meadow. Now you hike over to Lost Creek (5720–0.2). ▮ *The banks of this creek are ablaze with common and Lewis monkeyflowers, lupine, bistort, corn lily, mariposa lily, yarrow, paintbrush, pasqueflower, aster, and eriogonum.* ▮

Remembering that campsites must be at least 100 feet from any creek or body of water, you push onward and quickly reach the Paradise Park Shelter (5730–0.1) in an open forest of dwarf hemlock. ▮ *This ten-foot-square*

See maps G1, G2

See map G1

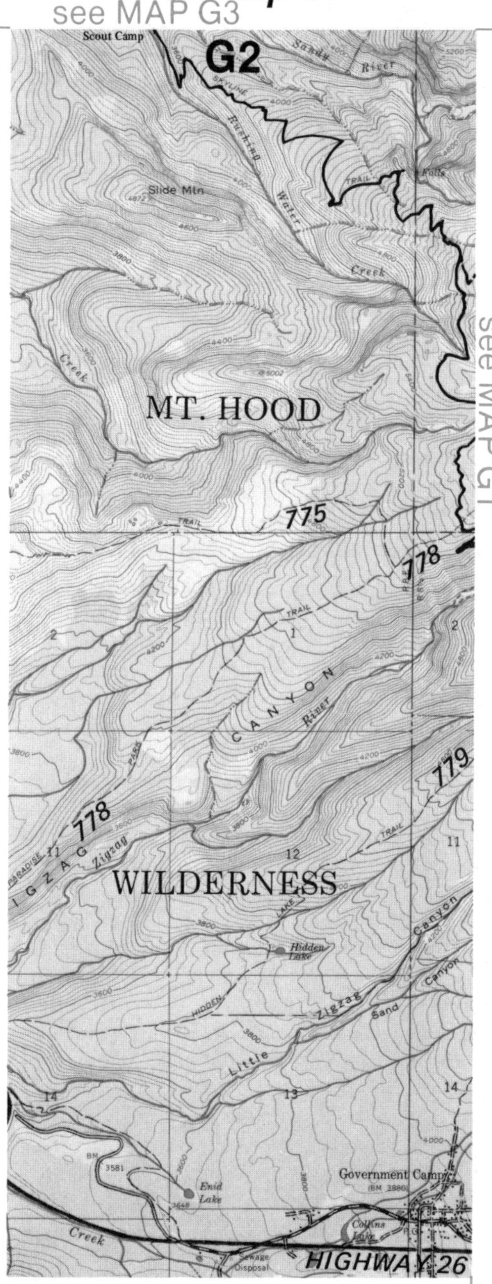

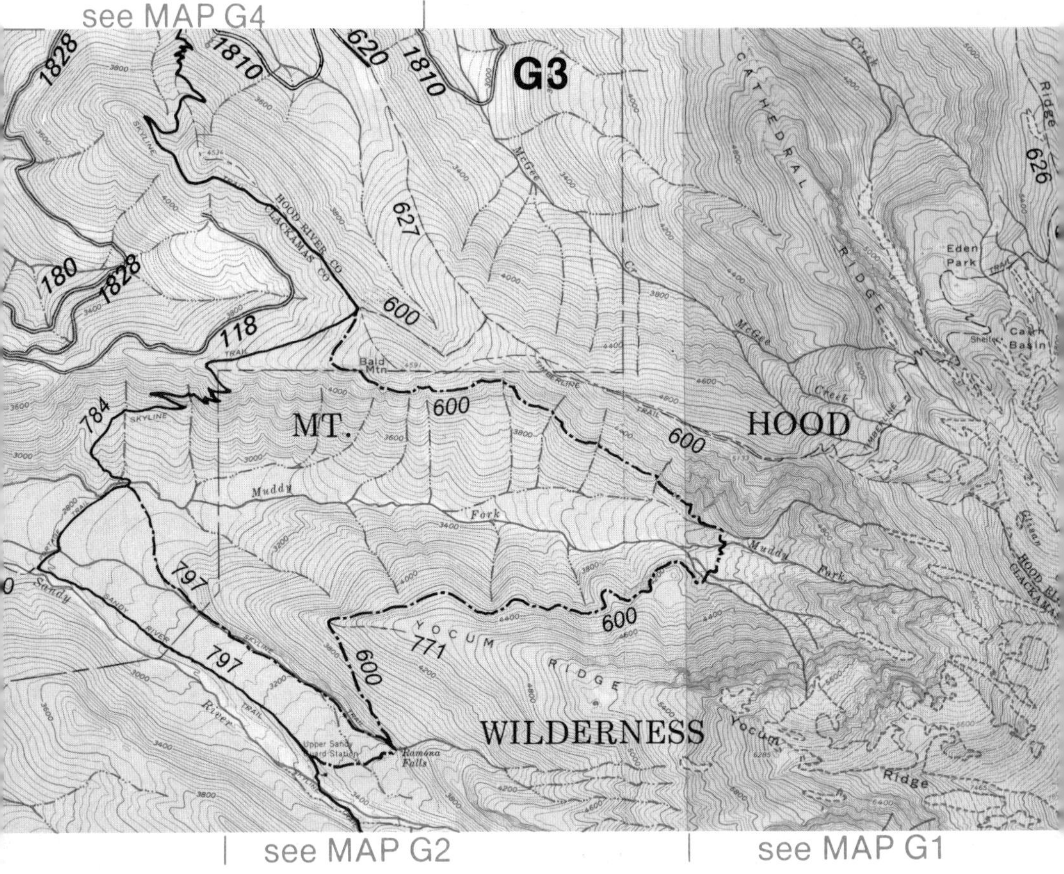

shelter, constructed with andesite blocks from the surrounding lava flow, once had an operable fireplace. ▌ There are a number of campsites nearby. Beyond the shelter, the trail makes a slight climb and then contours across more alpine meadows before it switchbacks down to a reunion with the PCT (5400–1.1–2.4).

Official PCT route and alternate route rejoined. Now you make a switchbacking descent and obtain two fantastic views: up toward the glacier-mantled summit above and down upon the mountain's anatomy below, exposed by the incising Sandy River. There's one more view, from a vertical-sided ridge at the end of a 50-yard spur trail, and it is the most revealing of all. ▌ *The cliffs of the Sandy River canyon and its tributary canyon are composed of andesite flows and interbedded pyroclastic deposits.* ▌ As if this flood of magnificent scenery were not enough to satisfy, the trail takes you down to the west side of the ridge where, from a viewpoint, you are saturated with the impressive, naked cliffs of Slide Mountain (4872) and of the Rushing Water Creek canyon all around you.

After such a scenic traverse, you may wish to stop and reminisce at large, flat Scout Camp (3400–3.0), which is beside Rushing Water Creek at the bottom of the switchbacks from the viewpoint. Beyond the camp, the PCT quickly reaches the bouldery, bushy bottom of the Sandy River canyon. During flood, the river can be wall-to-wall, up to 100 yards wide, and when it is, it can obliterate the trail. Generally, however, the river is only a few yards wide, and depending on what a past flood did to the trail, you'll hike down either one side of the river, the other side of it, or perhaps even between two parallel streams. After about a 300-yard ramble downstream among boulders and brush, you reach a low cliff of unsorted, poorly bedded sediments. The PCT makes a short climb up it and reaches a flat bench (3270–0.3) that is suitable for camping. From it, a steep path climbs about 50 yards east to Upper Sandy Guard Station, which is often locked and unmanned. From the bench, the PCT climbs north to reach

See maps G1, G2, G3

a junction with Ramona Falls Loop Trail 797 (3320–0.1).

Here, hikers have a choice of three routes: the official PCT route, which is the least scenic, and two more-scenic alternate routes. The authors highly recommend either of the alternate routes; their preferred route is the Ramona Falls Loop Trail-Timberline Trail alternate, below. Equestrians are restricted to the official PCT, although they can ride west to a stock fence near Ramona Falls and catch a glimpse of it.

Official PCT route. Least scenic is the official PCT route. From the junction just north of Upper Sandy Guard Station, the PCT heads northwest down the south arm of Ramona Falls Loop Trail 797, descending on a usually gentle grade as it parallels Sandy River at a distance. Midway along the route, you leave Mt. Hood Wilderness, and by the time you reach a junction (2780–1.5), the lodgepole forest has become quite open.

Side route (from official PCT route only). Should you need to exit toward civilization, you can take Trail 770 1¼ miles west from this junction to a popular trailhead and perhaps hitch a ride out. Also, from it, Road 1825-100 goes about ½ mile west down to a junction, from where you can head ⅓ mile south to Lost Creek Campground.

The PCT continues on the loop trail, traversing 250 yards northeast to the Ramona Falls branch of Sandy River before going ⅓ mile farther to a junction (2800–0.5); there's a nearby horse camp.

See map G3

Exposed sediments of Slide Mountain

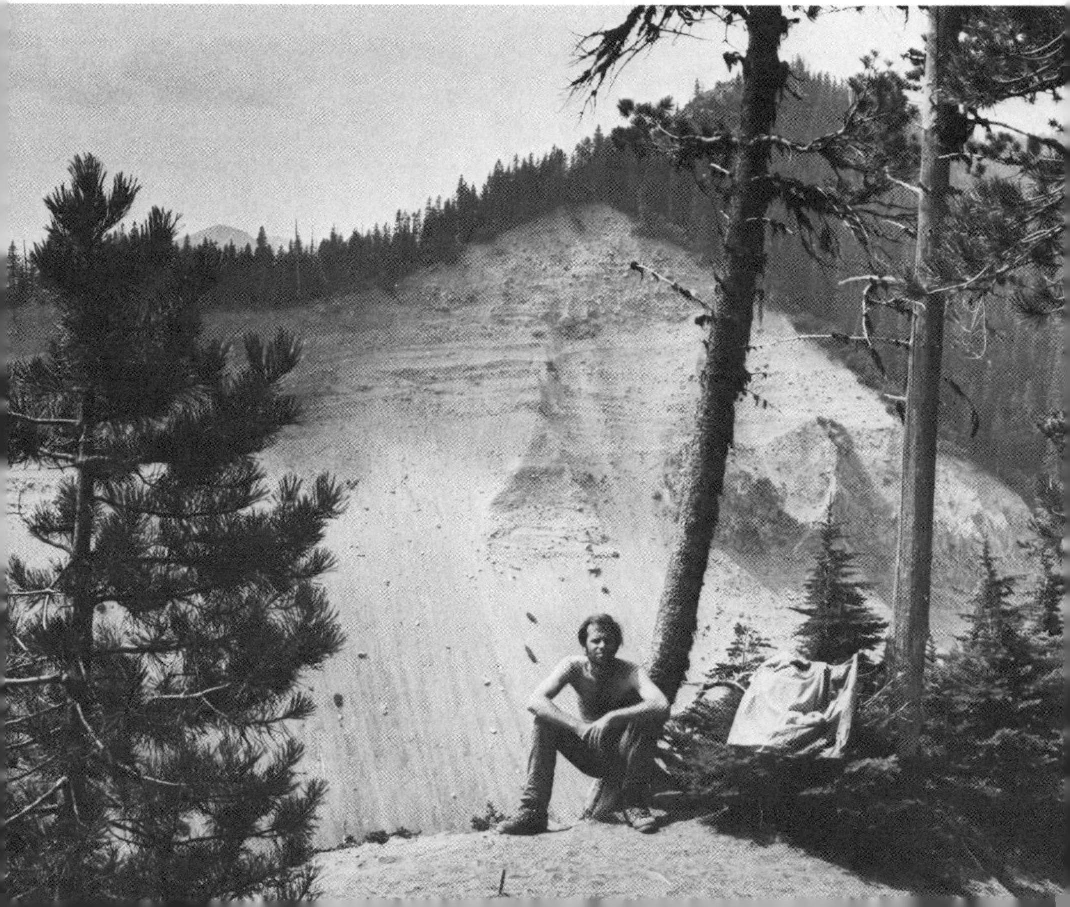

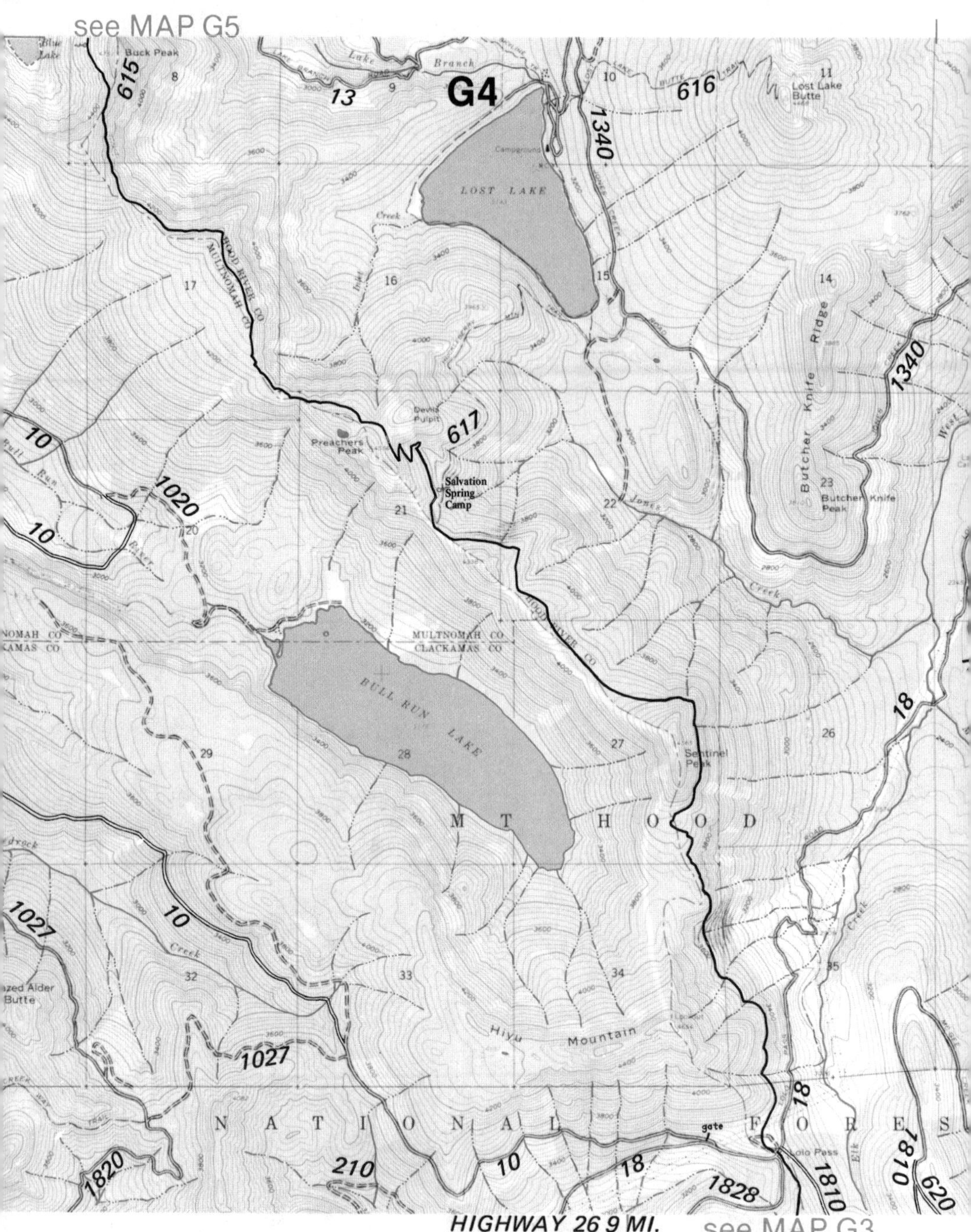

At this junction, the Ramona Falls Loop Trail alternate route, below, rejoins the official PCT. From this point, the loop trail starts northeast while you take the PCT north 70 yards to a bridge across broad, aptly named Muddy Fork. Now you make a moderate-to-steep, major, switchbacking ascent up Bald Mountain Trail 784 to a ridge (3910–1.7). From it you could head 100 yards north down to nearby Road 118. Ahead, you have an easier, merely moderate climb east to a junction just north of Bald Mountain (4270–0.7), where

See map G3

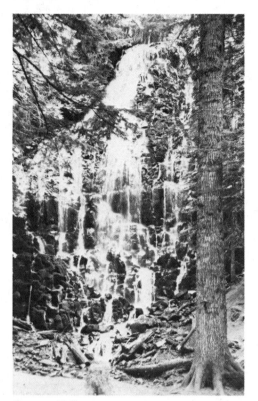

Ramona Falls

the Ramona Falls Loop Trail and Timberline Trail alternate route, following, rejoins the official PCT.

Alternate route, Ramona Falls Loop Trail—Timberline Trail. This is the most scenic alternate, and it is the authors' most preferred route. However, it is about 1⅓ miles longer than the PCT and the other alternate route. From the junction just north of Upper Sandy Guard Station, this alternate starts southeast on the east arm of Ramona Falls Loop Trail 797 and follows it east across a broad, corrugated terrace that sprouts a dry, open forest. Within earshot of the falls, you reach a stock fence. Equestrians must leave their animals here. East beyond the fence is a backpackers' camping area, and you can find sites above and below the trail. About a minute's walk ahead, descend to the base of Ramona Falls (3460–0.4), which splashes down moss-draped rocks. A few yards after the trail crosses the falls' creek, there is a junction. From here, go north-northwest on Timberline Trail 600. This leg starts with a serious, if relatively short, climb to a ridge junction with Yocum Ridge Trail 771 (4000–0.6), which climbs up to alpine slopes near the south edge of Sandy Glacier. The trail climbs more easily as it leaves this ridge trail, and then it levels and traverses in and out of gullies before dropping to a cluster of small campsites (4100–2.0) about 70 yards before the first glacier-fed tributary of Muddy Fork. You may have to wade across the first two tributaries, particularly if you are crossing them on a hot afternoon. Between the first and second fords, you get particularly impressive views up-canyon of a serrated, pinnacle-studded ridge that separates cascading creeks from spreading Sandy Glacier.

Beyond the second ford, you make a minute's stroll over to the jump-across third ford, which, unlike the others, is clear and flows beneath forest cover. Another minute down it, you come to a spur trail (4060–0.4) that immediately crosses the creek to a small, south-bank campsite. Just past it, Timberline Trail 600 leaves the canyon floor and, over the next ½ mile, makes a gentle ascent westward. Ascend past several creeklets before traversing Bald Mountain's south slopes. From these, there are unrestricted views—weather permitting—of towering Mt. Hood as well as views of forested Muddy Fork canyon and the upper canyon's glacier-fed cascades.

Views disappear as you curve north out of Mt. Hood Wilderness, enter forest cover, and make a ¼-mile easy descent to a shady, crest junction with the official PCT (4270–2.3–5.7), climbing from the west. Here, you leave Timberline Trail 600 to rejoin the official PCT route, while Timberline Trail 600 strikes east for a 22.7-mile loop of Mt. Hood's slopes.

Alternate route, Ramona Falls Loop Trail. This is the middle choice in terms of scenery. From the junction just north of Upper Sandy Guard Station, this alternate follows the Ramona Falls Loop Trail-Timberline Trail description, above, as far as the junction just beyond the crossing of Ramona Falls creek. From here, go northwest on the north arm of Ramona Falls Loop Trail 797, descend 1.0 mile northwest along Ramona Falls' creek, and then go another 0.7 mile north to a junction with the official PCT (2800–1.7–

See map G3

see MAP G6

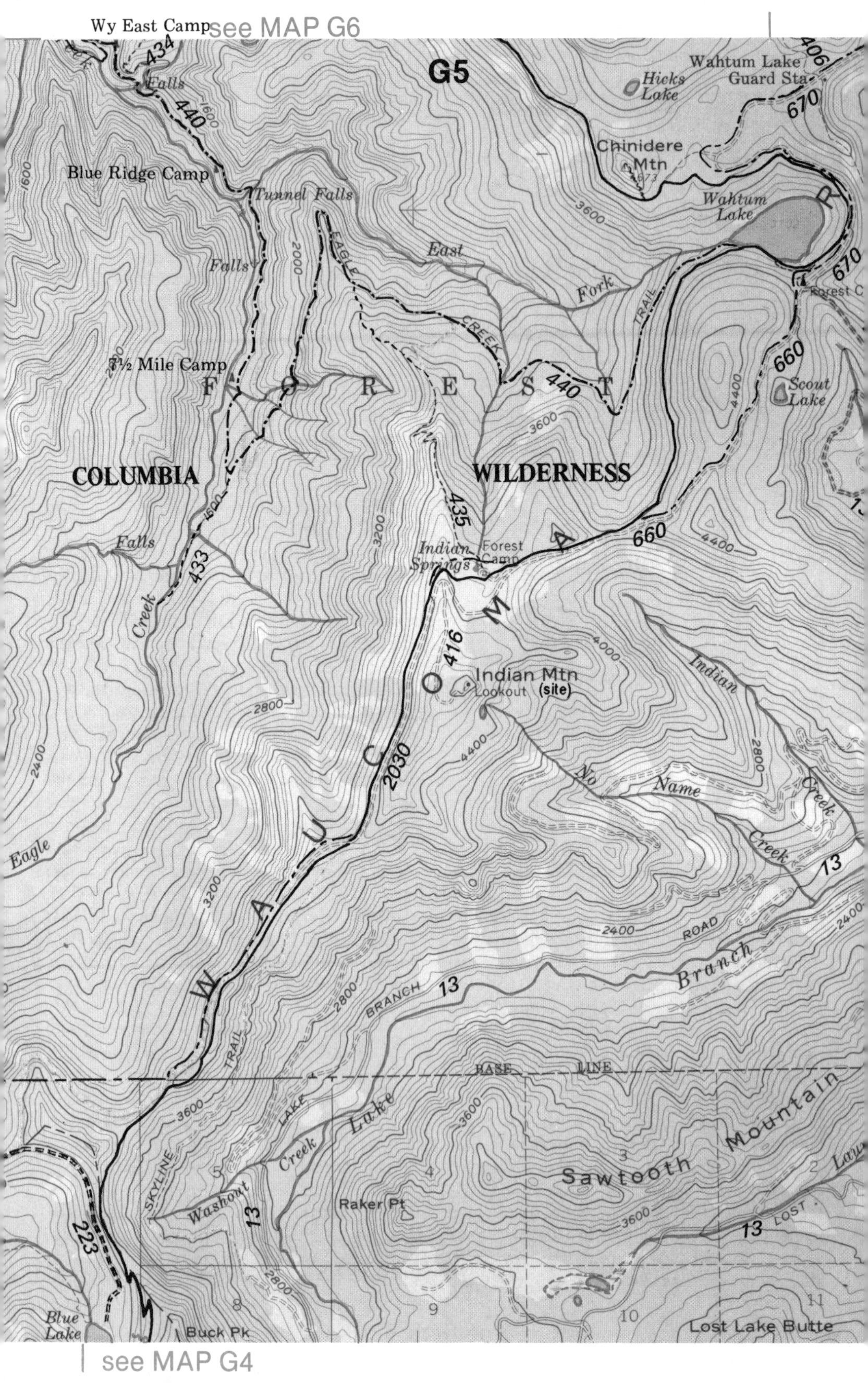

see MAP G4

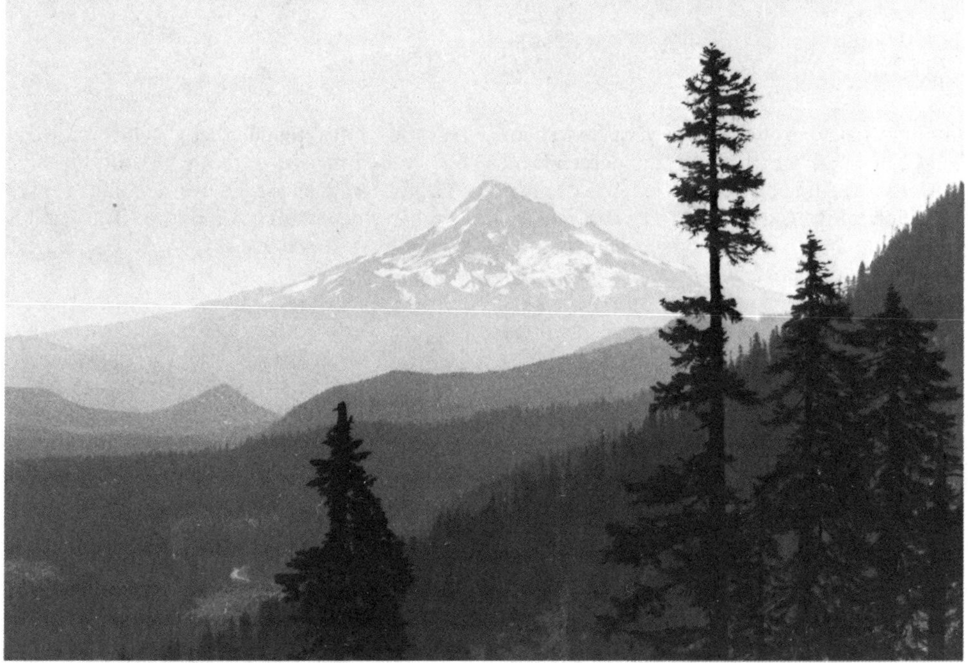

Mt. Hood, from one mile north of Buck Peak

2.1); there's a nearby horse camp. Continue in accordance with the official PCT description, above, from the paragraph beginning, "**At this junction, the Ramona Falls Loop Trail alternate route. . . .**"

With all three routes finally back together at this junction north of Bald Mountain, you begin the next leg of the PCT, whose route from here to the Columbia River is more down than up—and none of the "up" stretches are major.

Descending northwest 50 yards, you reach a junction with Top Spur Trail 785, which starts a westward descent toward Road 1828-118. Continue your forested route northwest to the crest's end (4200–1.4) and then start north down a series of switchbacks. The thorny gooseberries, thimbleberries, and giant Devil's clubs attest to the cool, moist slope of this forest, which you leave behind as you descend a drier north ridge to a flat clearing immediately south of Lolo Pass Road 18 (3420–1.4) at Lolo Pass.

Water access. A quarter mile west of here, you can find water running down to the road. Immediately east of the PCT, Road 1810 branches southeast from Road 18, going 0.4 mile to spring-fed water.

The northbound trailhead is about 20 yards southwest along paved Road 18 and 30 yards before this road's junction with paved Road 1828.

Start northwest from Lolo Pass, quickly cross north under four sets of buzzing power lines, and then glance back northeast at Mt. Hood's deeply glaciated north face. ▌ *Before the glaciers performed their cosmetic surgery, the peak's summit towered to about 12,000 feet.* ▌ You soon reach a gully with a trickling creek (3520–0.4) and then climb gradually north to the divide, and circle around the east slope of Sentinel Peak (4565). Rejoining the divide, the trail contours northwest past two low summits before arriving at a junction with Huckleberry Mountain Trail 617 (4020–3.9).

Side route. This descends slightly for 0.3 mile to a trickling creek in the gully below the Preachers Peak/Devils Pulpit saddle. If you descend this trail farther, you reach Lost Lake (3143–1.7), follow its east shore north to Lost Lake Campground (3160–0.8), and then finally reach a small store (3160–0.3–2.8) by the lake's north end. The Oregon Skyline Trail once followed this shoreline route, but the trail segment has since been abandoned.

See maps G3, G4

From the junction, contour 270 yards to a sharp bend in the trail, where a spur trail descends 50 yards to a trickling creek and a small flat called Salvation Spring Camp. Back on route, continue north to an obvious gully and then switchback up to the Preachers Peak/Devils Pulpit saddle (4340–0.9). Avoiding sermons from its two summits, you follow a huckleberry-lined path in a forest of hemlock and fir, descend to a saddle, climb north up the ridge above Lost Lake, and then descend west to a notch (4250–1.9). Now, a short, stiff climb north takes you to a saddle and a junction with Buck Peak Trail 615 (4500–0.5), which continues along the ridge up to Buck Peak (4751). Descend north across the west slope of this peak to discover a small spring (4340–0.4) a couple feet below the west edge of the trail. A little farther down the trail, you reach the ridge (4230–0.3) again and then switchback down to a long saddle from which you glimpse Blue Lake (3780) below to the southwest. As the trail arcs northeast, you leave Portland's Bull Run Watershed behind for good and with it the posted NO CAMPING signs that may have bothered you since Lolo Pass. Camping is prohibited in order to prevent forest fires.

Ahead, the PCT flirts with the southeast boundary of Columbia Wilderness for more than 7 miles, as both the PCT and the wilderness boundary parallel an old crestline road northeast. ▌ *Columbia Wilderness, about 61 square miles in size and containing about 125 miles of trail, was officially created in 1984. Before that date, the area had long been a* de facto *wilderness, spared the logger's ax. It's good to know that you won't see any clearcutting once you reach Wahtum Lake, but you'll certainly see enough of it to the east as you make the upcoming crestline traverse.* ▌

This next stretch follows a fairly level crest northeast, contours across the southeast slope of a low, triangular summit, and then finally climbs gently northeast to quickly reach Larch Mountain Road 2030 (4240–2.3), which is momentarily atop the ridge. Locate the trail on the northwest side of the road, parallel it north-northeast, and then round the narrow north spur (4400–1.6) of Indian Mountain (4890), from which you see Mts. St. Helens (8364), Rainier (14,410), and Adams (12,276). Descend eastward to Indian Springs Campground (4300–0.3), which has few car-campers because of the rough, rocky nature of Road 660, which is used to reach it. Unfortunately, this area had to be logged over to remove snags left by a devastating 1920 fire. The camp's spring is just beyond the west end of the camp's road loop.

Side route. Just beyond the spring, Indian Springs Trail 435 starts northwest toward Indian Mountain's north spur, follows it, and then steeply descends it 2 miles to Eagle Creek Trail 440. This is a great shortcut *down* to Wahtum Lake (3732), but parts are very steep, so it can be a hazard when wet. You wouldn't want to hike south *up* it with a full pack.

The PCT recommences at the east end of the campground's road loop and parallels the road, first below it and then above it, to a saddle, where it leaves the roadside and winds gently down a forested slope and then northeast down to a junction with Eagle Creek Trail 440 (3750–2.6) just above the southwest shore of Wahtum Lake (3732).

Here, you have a choice of the official PCT or a more-scenic alternate route. Eagle Creek Trail 440, described below, is a more-scenic alternative to the official PCT. The authors highly recommend the alternate route to non-acrophobic hikers only. However, sections of that trail are merely notches blasted into cliff walls to make passages suitable for non-acrophobic hikers but too low for riders and perhaps too exposed for acrophobic hikers. Therefore, equestrians are not allowed to use Eagle Creek Trail 440. Equestrians must, and acrophobic hikers should, take the official PCT, following.

The official PCT route, which is 0.8 mile shorter than the Eagle Creek route, starts a traverse east along Wahtum Lake's southwest shore. It then meets a lateral trail (3750–0.2).

Side routes (from official PCT only). This lateral trail climbs ⅓ mile up to the Wahtum Lake Campground, atop a saddle. From that saddle, Road 1310 descends southeast toward other roads that lead out to the city of Hood River, and crest-hugging Road 660, from Indian Springs Campground, crosses the saddle and traverses northeast high above Wahtum Lake.

SECTION G

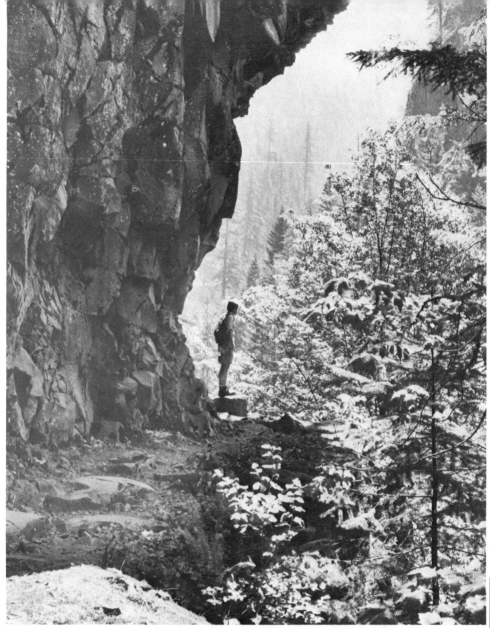

Along a part of the Eagle Creek Trail below Tunnel Falls

From the lateral-trail junction, the PCT, like nearby Road 670, circles Wahtum Lake, leaving its popular south-shore campsites behind. The trail's gentle, long, counterclockwise climb ends high above the lake at a junction with a ¼-mile-long spur trail that heads northeast to Road 670. In 200 yards, the now-level trail reaches a junction with the Chinidere Mountain Trail (4270–1.8).

Side route (from official PCT only). If you're having good weather, don't pass up this ⅓-mile-long, 400-foot ascent to Chinidere Mountain's superb, panoramic summit. From the summit, you can see decapitated Mt. St. Helens rising skyward above the north-northwest horizon, massive Mt. Adams lording it over the north-northeast horizon, and graceful Mt. Hood dominating the south-southeast horizon. You can also see the

See map G5

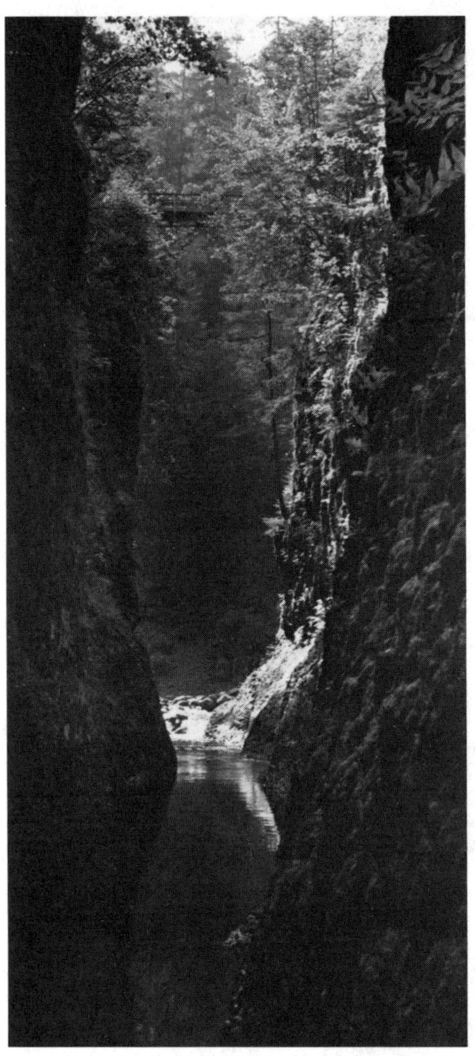

Eagle Creek gorge just above Loowit Falls

Columbia River and Wind River canyons, due north, while closer by, you're surrounded by deep, slightly glaciated canyons.

Leaving the Chinidere Mountain Trail junction, the PCT curves northwest around this miniature mountain to a saddle (4140–0.6) and then contours across the southwest slopes of summit 4380 to a crest viewpoint. It then drops to a second saddle (3830–1.4), and then traverses to a third saddle (3810–0.8), this one signed CAMP SMOKEY. ▌*Perhaps someone once smoked too much here, for these two saddles and the southwest-facing slopes between them were part of an area burned by a large forest fire.* ▌A small campsite is found at the Camp Smokey saddle, where there is a junction with the Eagle Benson Trail.

Side route (from official PCT only). A better campsite is found 180 yards down the Eagle Benson Trail. You'll find a refreshing spring just 50 yards past the campsite. Beyond the spring, the Eagle Benson Trail, descending to Eagle Creek, is usually unmaintained. Return to the official PCT from this point; the authors consider the Eagle Benson Trail too narrow and loose to be safely traveled with a heavy pack.

Pushing toward the deep Columbia Gorge, you leave the Camp Smokey saddle and climb up to the southeast edge of spreading Benson Plateau, which is a preglacial land surface that is being slowly devoured by back-cutting tributaries of Herman and Eagle creeks. In a gully on the plateau's southeast edge, you meet the *first*—and lightly used—Benson Way Trail

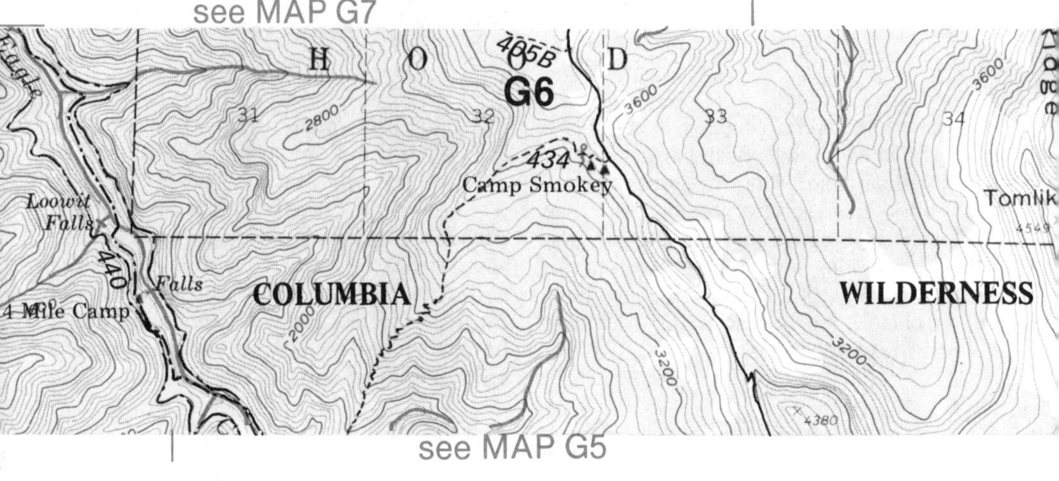

see MAP H1

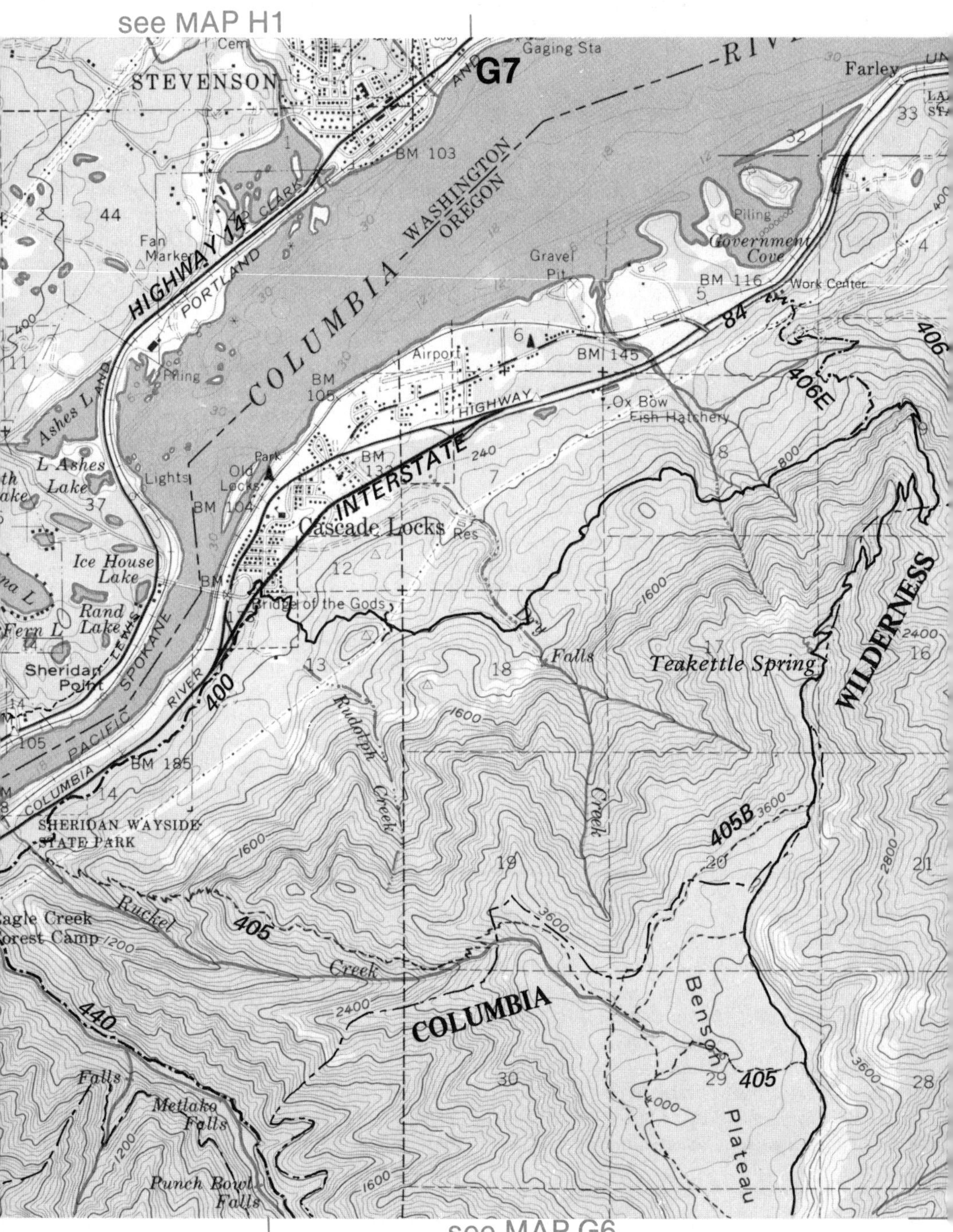

see MAP G6

405B (4100–0.5), which starts west but eventually curves north over to Ruckel Creek Trail 405.

Staying near the plateau's east edge, the PCT winds north to meet Ruckel Creek Trail 405 (4110–0.9).

Side route (from official PCT only). You can follow Ruckel Creek Trail 405 west ½ mile to a large campsite. This campsite is the only one between Wahtum Lake and Dry Creek that is suitable for equestrians, so don't be surprised if you find horses at it. Forty yards south of this

See maps G6, G7

campsite, you'll find a spring in a small meadow. From this campsite, you could continue about 4.8 miles down the trail to Gorge Trail 400, which is mentioned at the end of the alternate Eagle Creek Trail route, described above.

Beyond the Ruckel Creek Trail junction, the PCT descends gently northwest along the plateau's east edge, and it soon meets the abandoned-but-visible Benson Ruckel Trail (3980–0.7), which once traversed west-southwest one mile to Ruckel Creek Trail 405. Past this junction, the PCT curves northeast and leaves Benson Plateau by the time it arrives at a junction with the *second* Benson Way Trail 405B (3760–0.7). Here you'll find a waterless campsite that will accommodate four persons.

Now you hike north along a forested crest and pass another waterless campsite (3680–0.6) just before the trail curves east to begin a descent into the deep Columbia Gorge. Your moderately-to-steeply-dropping trail briefly descends the crest and then heads west to a switchback. Immediately past this turn is Teakettle Spring (3360–0.3), which you can easily miss when its sign is gone.

Past the spring, the trail switchbacks once again down to the crest, on which it reaches a barren area that gives you revealing views of the giant Columbia Gorge. ▮ *From here, you can identify the towns of Cascade Locks, Stevenson, and Carson. With the use of this book's maps, you can mentally sketch the winding route of the PCT up the gorge's north wall. You can also identify large landslides (see the beginning description of Section H). To the west, you see an impressive set of cliffs that are composed of the same kind of volcanic rocks that compose this barren area—pyroclastic rocks. These indicate that in pre-glacial times, a volcano may have existed at this site or close by.* ▮

From the barren area atop the crest, the trail starts west, turns north, soon crosses the crest, and then makes a fairly steep, viewless descent into the deep Columbia Gorge, recrossing the crest—now a ridge—near its lower end. From it, the PCT traverses ⅓ mile west to a junction (1120–3.0) with a 1.8-mile lateral trail that provides a fast way out to the highway, crossing Herman Creek and ending at the Columbia Gorge Work Center.

The hiker who intends to cross into Washington should continue along the westbound PCT. Departing from the lateral trail down to Herman Creek, the PCT continues its traverse across open talus slopes and then enters a cool, mossy forest of Douglas-fir and maple. You soon cross a creek (960–0.5), just beyond which you pass through a shallow saddle and then round a steep bowl. As the trail reaches a ridge and turns west to leave the bowl, a spur trail heads northwest steeply down the east side of a small gully. The PCT traverses southwest for about a mile, dropping slowly, turns south, and quickly descends to a bridge across perennial, misnamed Dry Creek (720–1.8). Camping is possible here and at other spots along this creek. Immediately beyond it, you encounter a dirt road.

Side route (from official PCT only). You can follow this road 0.2 mile up to its end, where you'll see an ideal shower: a 50-foot-high waterfall.

From the dirt-road junction, the PCT starts west and after a few yards passes a spur trail branching southeast. The PCT contours over toward a saddle and joins a powerline road (680–0.7) that climbs up and over that saddle. Head northwest down this road only 70 yards and then branch left on the trail. This segment rollercoasters west ½ mile around the north slopes of a low summit, turns north, and descends to Moody Avenue in the town of Cascade Locks. The Eagle Creek Trail alternate route ends here, opposite the PCT.

Alternate route. The hike from Wahtum Lake down to the Columbia River is far more scenic along the Eagle Creek Trail than along the PCT. We describe it here as a highly recommended alternate route.

From the Wahtum Lake outlet (3740–0.1), which is the East Fork of Eagle Creek, Eagle Creek Trail 440 begins as a typical trail, for it descends through a Douglas-fir forest with an understory that includes inconspicuous annuals such as coolwort, false Solomon's seal, queen's cup, bunchberry, and vanilla-leaf. In a north-draining canyon, you reach an adequate campsite beside a trickling creek (3300–1.2) and then arc westward gently down to a ford

See maps G5, G7

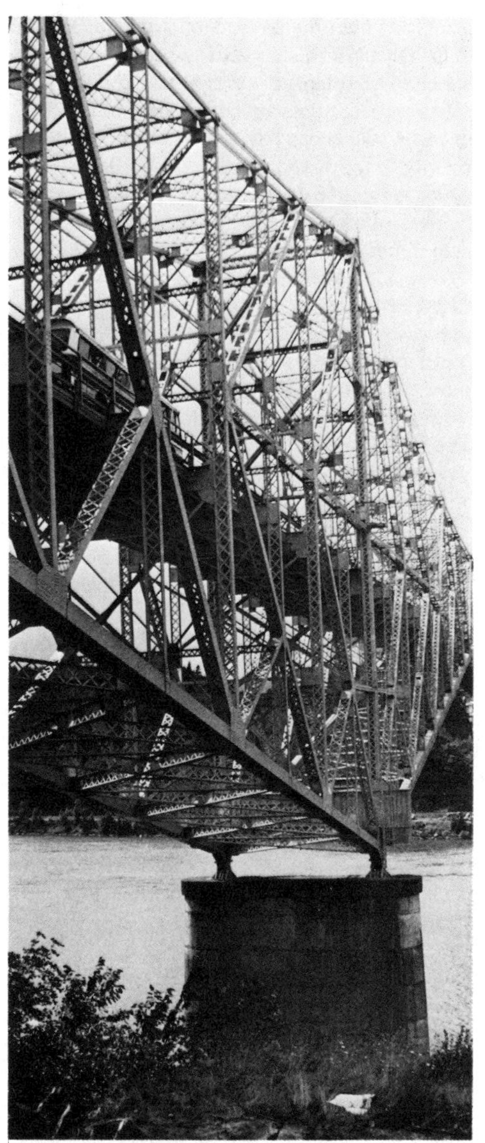

Bridge of the Gods

of the Indian Springs fork (3040–0.8) of Eagle Creek, which could be very tricky to cross in early summer. Along its banks is a very good campsite.

Now begin a descent northwest that takes you past rhododendron, gooseberry, red elderberry, thimbleberry, huckleberry, Devil's club, and Oregon grape. Along this cool descent, you may see Indian Springs Trail 435, which climbs two steep miles up to Indian Springs Campground. After reaching a viewpoint (2350–1.6) at the tip of a north spur, the trail turns south and descends past a campsite (1920–1.0) by a shallow gully, crosses seasonal creeklets, and then makes a switchback (1600–0.7) north. From here, Eagle-Tanner Trail 433 heads up-canyon.

The slope is now much gentler, and in the near distance you can hear Eagle Creek splashing merrily down its course. In a short distance you reach a rockbound creek (1440–0.5). ▮ *Don't be too surprised if a red-spotted garter snake is climbing a rock behind you; it needs water, too. It is not uncommon to encounter half a dozen of these beneficial snakes in a day's hike along this verdant route.* ▮ Just beyond this pleasant creek, you meet several trails that descend about 50 yards west to 7½ Mile Camp (1380–0.1), complete with a primitive shelter. If you intend to camp before reaching the trailhead, this certainly is a good place to stop. Before you lies the string of impressive waterfalls that make this last half of the trail so popular.

The trail gradually descends to the bank of Eagle Creek, and you see a 50-foot cascade—not too impressive, but a sample of what's to come. The creek enters a safe, very deep, crystal-clear pool (1120–0.3) that is extremely tempting for an afternoon swim, but the cool water will ensure that you won't stay in for long. Immediately beyond it is a two-stage, 100-foot-high waterfall, sliced into a narrow gorge, which you don't see until you round a vertical cliff where this exposed trail, blasted from the cliff, heads toward 150-foot-high Tunnel Falls (1120–0.3). This trail is definitely not for the faint-hearted, neither is its ceiling sufficient for those on horseback. The fall, in its grotto of vertical-walled basalt, is spectacular enough to make it the climax of this route, but your sensations of it are heightened even more as you head through a wet tunnel blasted behind the fall about midway up it. Exuberant from traversing behind this wall of water, you leave this grotto of the East Fork in expectation of more high adventure. Below you, Eagle Creek cascades 30 feet down to another layer of this Miocene Columbia River basalt.

The trail's exposure decreases considerably as you leave the falls' narrow gorge. Soon you reach pleasant Blue Ridge Camp (1120–0.3)

See map G5

and then continue on to a junction with must-miss Eagle Benson Trail 434 (1000–0.5), which climbs steeply up to the PCT. ▮ *This narrow footpath is not recommended by the authors, who believe it is too narrow to be safely climbed or descended with a heavy pack. In places it is quite easy to slip on loose gravel and then fall over a hundred-foot cliff.* ▮ Just around the corner from this junction, the trail enters another side canyon and bridges a murmuring tributary a hundred yards downstream from its slender, 80-foot-high fall.

Continuing northwest, you soon enter another side canyon, and this one provides you with Wy East Camp (960–0.5), which is just above the trail. Farther downstream, you reach a bridge (710–0.7) across Eagle Creek, 20 feet below. ▮ *A daredevil instinct may urge some to jump from the bridge into the tempting 8-foot-deep pool below, but better judgment takes hold, and you pass up the opportunity.* ▮

Now above the creek's west bank, you follow the singing creek down to the popular, excellent 4 Mile Camp (680–0.6), also known as the "Tenas Camp." ▮ *How many campsites do you know of that have a beautiful waterfall near them? You've just seen a few. This one has a two-step, 40-foot fall. Near it you'll find the dipper, or water ouzel, a gray, chunky, water-loving bird that tenaciously clings to the bottoms of swift streams in search of aquatic animal life. The name "dipper" refers to the bird's bobbing motions while standing on land. Taking "dipper" as a suggestion, you may decide to take a dip in the cold creek yourself. After a quick, invigorating frolic in the pools below the lower fall, you can stretch out in the afternoon sunlight to thaw out before hiking once again.* ▮

Back on the trail, you walk spiritedly north to a bridge (690 0.3) across a 90-foot-deep gorge that is only 30 feet wide. ▮ *A hundred yards downstream from this crossing, the swirling creek has cut, with the aid of churning boulders, deep potholes that would make superb swimming holes were it not for the cool temperature. The six-inch trout don't seem to mind it, though. Above the potholes, wispy Loowit Falls emerges from the vegetation to flow silently down the polished rock and into one of the pools.* ▮

Continuing downstream, you soon enter another side canyon, bridge a creek 50 feet above it, and then pass by massive, vertical-walled flows of Columbia River basalt. ▮ *The contact between two flows tends to be a weak point, and both the creek and its tributaries tend to flow along such contacts. The height of a waterfall often represents the thickness of a single flow.* ▮ The minutes pass by quickly, and before you know it, you cross Tish Creek and arrive at an overlook (500–1.4) above Punch Bowl Falls, which drops 40 feet into a churning cauldron below. ▮ *It's hard to judge just how deep this huge pool is, but right beneath the falls a depth of 20 feet wouldn't be much of an exaggeration.* ▮

Here the trail starts to climb high above the now-impassable gorge, and you soon see more reasons why horses aren't allowed on the trail. ▮ *At times, the overhanging walls seem to press you terribly close to the brink of the dead-vertical cliff below, and you are thankful that the trail crew installed cables along these stretches.* ▮ You now reach another overlook (520–0.7) where you can look 200 yards upstream to Metlako Falls, whose silvery course plummets another step down into the inaccessible gorge.

The route gradually begins to descend toward the trailhead, and you leave the threatening, moss-covered cliffs behind as you descend into the realm of a cedar-and-Douglas-fir forest. ▮ *Alder, maple, dogwood, ocean spray, blackberries, thimbleberries, moss, three species of ferns, and dozens of wildflowers harmonize with the conifers on these canyon slopes to create a symphony of nature at her best.* All too soon, the verdant route reaches the trailhead (150–1.5), which is by a bridge that spans Eagle Creek.

Side route (from alternate route only). On the creek's west side, you'll find a short, looping nature trail that splits off from climbing, 1.8-mile Wauna View Point Trail 402.

To reach Bridge of the Gods, take Gorge Trail 400, which starts from the parking area. This trail climbs through a picnic area, crosses the short road up to Eagle Creek Campground (200–0.1), passes between the campground and Interstate 84, and then quickly reaches a part of the abandoned, narrow Columbia River "highway." On this, you curve over to Ruckel Creek (230–0.6), where, on its east bank, Ruckel Creek Trail 405 makes a 5.3-mile climb to the PCT.

Your shady gorge trail continues northeast, and at times it almost touches Interstate 84. After traversing a few hundred yards across

See maps G5, G6, G7

grassy slopes—absolutely miserable in the rain—the trail ends at Moody Avenue opposite the PCT (280–2.9–16.3).

With both routes now rejoined, the PCT follows dirt Moody Avenue 70 yards to its junction with SE Undine Street (240–1.0), where it becomes paved. Moody Avenue immediately crosses under the freeway. Five yards west of the freeway's largest pillar, the PCT resumes. It curves 200 yards northwest over to the paved loop road that leads up to Bridge of the Gods (200–0.1) and a toll booth. Near this toll booth is a PCT trailhead parking area with flush toilets, covered picnic tables, and a lawn. Section G ends here, and Section H begins across the Columbia River at the bridge-road junction with Washington state's Highway 14, 0.5 mile distant. In 2000 it cost 50¢ to walk across Bridge of the Gods.

Resupply access. If you're a long-distance hiker, you'll want to resupply in Cascade Locks. Walk down to the town's nearby thoroughfare, old U.S. Highway 30, which here is known as Wa Na Pa Street. On it, you walk 0.2 mile northeast to the Cascade Locks Post Office, which is conveniently located opposite the Columbia Gorge Center, with a general store, a restaurant, and other stores. In another 0.3 mile, you reach a road that heads north to the Cascade Locks Marine Park. It has a campground and, nearby, in the visitors center, it has showers. One great feature of the park's campground is its roofed cooking area, with tables, under which you can keep dry on those all-too-often rainy days. ▮ *In this park, you can visit the shipping locks, built in 1896, which allowed ships to travel up-river beyond the Columbia River's Cascade Rapids. The town of Cascade Locks was spawned by the resulting commercial activity. The park's museum used to have an exhibit that said that Bridge of the Gods was a natural bridge that spanned the river. Not so. However, the river was likely dammed for a while by a huge landslide from the north, whence the Indian legend.*

▮ *If you are waiting for the weather to improve, you might spend some time at the city hall, on Wa Na Pa Street, 0.2 mile east of the park entrance. Most of this building is, surprisingly, occupied by an indoor basketball court, but there is also a neat little library tucked away in an upstairs room. Here you can catch up on all the gruesome news you've been missing while out on the trail.* ▮

See map G7

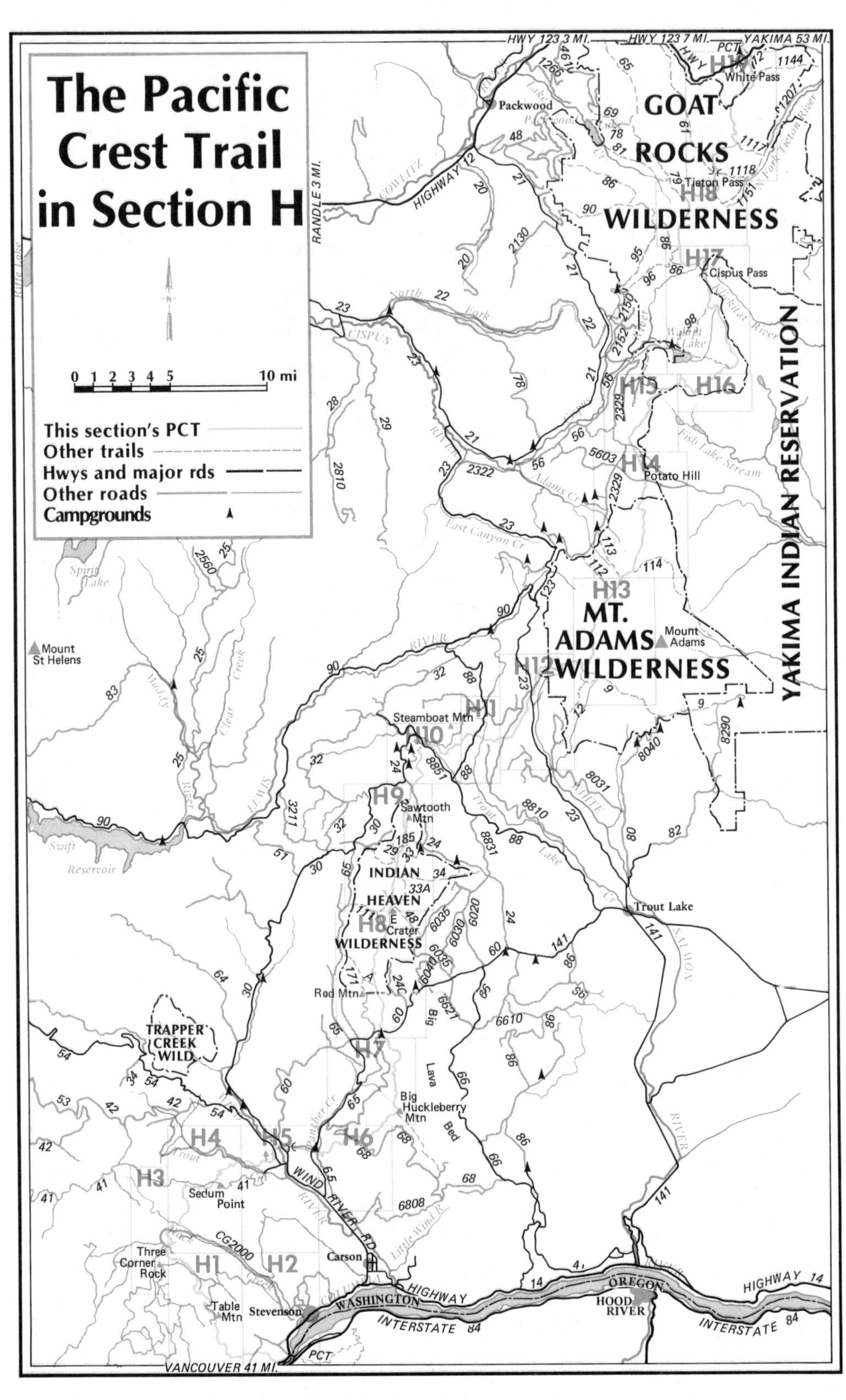

The Pacific Crest Trail in Section H
0 1 2 3 4 5 10 mi
This section's PCT
Other trails
Hwys and major rds
Other roads
Campgrounds
GOAT ROCKS WILDERNESS
MT. ADAMS WILDERNESS
INDIAN HEAVEN WILDERNESS
TRAPPER CREEK WILD
YAKIMA INDIAN RESERVATION
Packwood
White Pass
Tieton Pass
Cispus Pass
Walupt Lake
Potato Hill
Mount Adams
Mount St Helens
Spirit Lake
Steamboat Mtn
Sawtooth Mtn
E Crater
Red Mtn
Big Huckleberry Mtn
Big Lava Bed
Trout Lake
Sedum Point
Three Corner Rock
Table Mtn
Stevenson
Carson
HOOD RIVER
OREGON
WASHINGTON
HIGHWAY 14
INTERSTATE 84
WIND RIVER RD
Swift Reservoir
HWY 123 3 MI.
HWY 123 7 MI.
YAKIMA 53 MI.
RANDLE 3 MI.
VANCOUVER 41 MI.
PCT
H1
H2
H3
H4
H5
H6
H7
H8
H9
H10
H11
H12
H13
H14
H15
H16
H17
H18
H19

Section H:
Highway 14 at Bridge of the Gods to Highway 12 near White Pass

Introduction: Because this is the longest section and because it has the greatest elevation change, it is the most diverse. It starts near the west end of Bridge of the Gods, which at 180 feet elevation is one of the lowest points on the official PCT (the lowest point—140 feet—is met just one mile southwest from the start of this section). Near this section's end, the PCT climbs to 7080 feet elevation—its second-highest elevation in Washington—before it traverses the upper part of Packwood Glacier.

Between these two extremes, you pass through several environments. After starting in a lush, damp Columbia River forest, you climb usually viewless slopes; wind past an extensive, recent lava flow; traverse a lake-speckled, glaciated lava plateau; and climb to a subalpine forest. The trail then circles a major, periodically active volcano, Mt. Adams; traverses high on the walls of deep, glaciated canyons; and finally climbs up to an alpine landscape at Packwood Glacier. Along Washington's Section A, then, you pass through all of the landforms and vegetation belts that you see along the PCT from central Oregon to trail's end in southern British Columbia.

Declination: 19°E

Points on Route	S→N	Mi. Btwn. Pts.	N→S
Bridge of the Gods, west end	0.0		147.5
Gillette Lake	3.8	3.8	143.7
Spring near Table Mountain	9.7	5.9	137.8
Spur trail to Three Corner Rock water trough	15.3	5.6	132.2
Rock Creek	20.3	5.0	127.2
Sunset-Hemlock Road 41	26.1	5.8	121.4
Road 43 alongside Trout Creek	30.1	4.0	117.4
Road 65 near Panther Creek Campground	35.5	5.4	112.0
Big Huckleberry Mountain summit trail	44.1	8.6	103.4
Road 60 at Crest Campground	51.0	6.9	96.5
Blue Lake	58.4	7.4	89.1
Bear Lake	61.4	3.0	86.1
Road 24	67.7	6.3	79.8
Road 88	76.5	8.8	71.0
Road 23	82.3	5.8	65.2
Round the Mountain Trail	88.9	6.6	58.6
Killen Creek cascade	97.7	8.8	49.8
Lava Spring	102.7	5.0	44.8
East-west road near Midway site	106.3	3.6	41.2
Walupt Lake Trail	118.0	11.7	29.5
Sheep Lake near Nannie Ridge Trail	122.5	4.5	25.0
Trail 86 to Bypass Camp	127.0	4.5	20.5
Dana May Yelverton Shelter	129.1	2.1	18.4

Tieton Pass	136.0	6.9	11.5
White Pass Chair Lift spur trail	143.9	7.9	3.6
Highway 12 near White Pass	147.5	3.6	0.0

Supplies: When author Schaffer first mapped this section in 1973, it was 136½ miles long. You could pick up mailed parcels at Stevenson, early in the hike, and at Midway Guard Station, about two-thirds of the way through. Unfortunately for the long-distance hiker, the guard station burned down in 1976, and, with the completion of the last segment of trail in 1984, Stevenson no longer lies along the route. No supplies—mailed parcels or otherwise—can be found along this section, which today is 11 miles longer. If you aren't up to such a rigorous hike, you can bypass the first 35½ miles of the PCT, taking an alternate route on roads through the towns of Stevenson and Carson. Doing so will cut 21 miles off this section's length and will save you about a vertical mile of unnecessary climbing. In Stevenson, you should be able to purchase almost anything you'll need, but in Carson you'll find very little. Both towns have post offices (Stevenson, 98648; Carson, 98610), but the Carson Post Office is preferable because its being 4½ miles closer to White Pass shortens your walk with a full pack just a little. PCT adherents avoiding these towns will have to resupply at Cascade Locks (at the end of Oregon's Section G) and at White Pass (at the end of this section).

At White Pass, you can pick up mailed parcels (US mail or UPS) at the Kracker Barrel Store (48851 US Highway 12, Naches, WA 98937). The store has a gas station, hot fried food, snacks, an espresso bar, and a laundromat. For showers, treat yourself to a room at the adjacent Village Inn, which for most trekkers is too pricey. Most will opt for a tent at White Pass Campground and a quick, chilly dip in adjacent Leech Lake.

Special Restrictions: The Forest Service would like to see you camp at least 200 feet from the PCT when you are in an official wilderness area. Unfortunately, topographic and/or vegetative constrains often make this impossible. Nevertheless, try to choose a site that will have a minimal impact on the environment and on other trail users. Packers mustn't let their animals graze within 200 feet of lakes, and, if they pack in feed, it must be processed so as to prevent seed germination. All these rules apply to *all* of Washington's wilderness areas.

Maps:

Carson, WA (alternate route)
Bonneville Dam, WA
Beacon Rock, WA
Lookout Mountain, WA
Stabler, WA
Big Huckleberry Mountain, WA
Gifford Peak, WA
Lone Butte, WA
Little Huckleberry Mountain, WA
Sleeping Beauty, WA
Steamboat Mountain, WA
Mount Adams West, WA
Green Mountain, WA
Hamilton Buttes, WA
Walupt Lake, WA
Old Snowy Mountain, WA
White Pass, WA
Spiral Butte, WA (PCT barely enters map)

See maps H1,

THE ROUTE

The Cascade crest lies to the east, but the PCT begins westward, which makes for a very roundabout—and hilly—route. In general terms, this 35½-mile route climbs 3300 feet to a ridge, drops 2000 feet to Rock Creek, climbs 1700 to Sedum Ridge, drops 2200 feet to Trout Creek, and then climbs and drops hundreds of feet as it rolls east to Road 65 near Panther Creek Campground. Your net elevation gain from Bridge of the Gods is a mere 750 feet, and yet, with a fully laden backpack, you could take three days to do this arduous stretch. However, if you take the most direct route to Road 65, you can reach the PCT near Panther Creek Campground in a mere 14.7 miles. Furthermore, if you start with a light pack and wait until you reach the Carson post office to pick up your mailed parcels, then you have to hike with a full pack only 7.6 miles to reach the PCT. Following this plan, Panther Creek Campground is reached by a relatively easy one-day hike. We prefer this alternate route, which we'll describe after the official PCT route.

To take the official PCT from the west end of Bridge of the Gods toll road (180), head south on Highway 14 past Ice House Lake—an oversized pond—and just 80 yards beyond it to reach the PCT trailhead (150–0.2). You'll find limited parking space nearby, plus access for equestrians. The "trail" at first is along an old powerline road that parallels Highway 14, just below you. Because the roadbed is rather overgrown, the trail sticks to the road's outer edge, which in one short stretch is very exposed—one slip and you'll fall off a vertical cliff to almost-certain death. The short clifftop stretch soon gives way to safer slopes, and presently you reach a road that climbs briefly up to a nearby cistern, which is your first source of reliable water. Follow the road for 280 yards, angle right from it, and then, in 110 yards, cross a paved road (140–0.8), which climbs from Highway 14 to Wauna Lake.

Leaving civilization, you first climb to a ridge (250–0.4) from where Tamehnous Trail 25 starts southwest, meandering ¾ mile over to a large parking area opposite the Bonneville Locks and Dam North Shore Visitors Entrance. Ahead, the forested, often-fern-bordered PCT takes a convoluted, rolling route across a giant landslide.

Large and small landslides have descended from both walls of the Columbia Gorge. In part this is due to the steepness of the gorge's walls. However, it is also due to another factor. The volcanic flows and associated volcanic sediments composing the walls belong to two distinct time periods. The lower layers are about 25 million years old, while the upper ones are about 15 million years old. The surface of the lower layers thus had about 10 million years to deeply weather to clay in this area's warm, humid, preglacial climate before the clay was buried under a sea of younger deposits. This clay layer is the structurally weak element that causes overlying layers to give way, as in the landslides from Table Mountain and the Red Bluffs.

See map H1

View toward crest, from climb north up the west slopes of Table Mountain

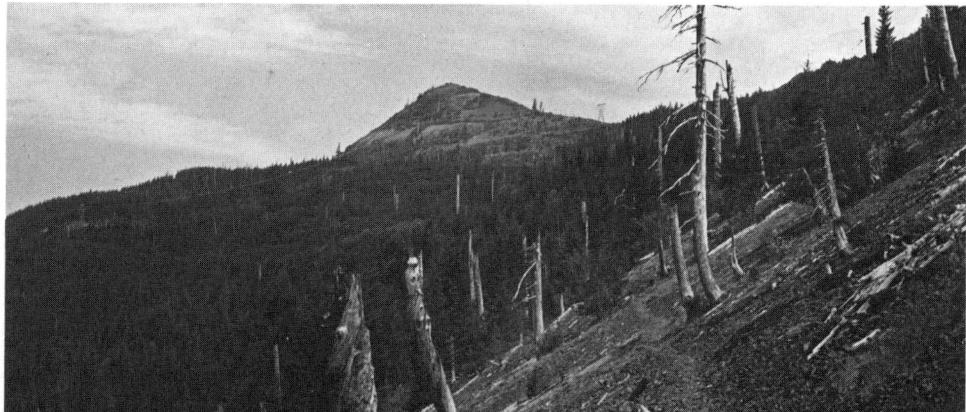

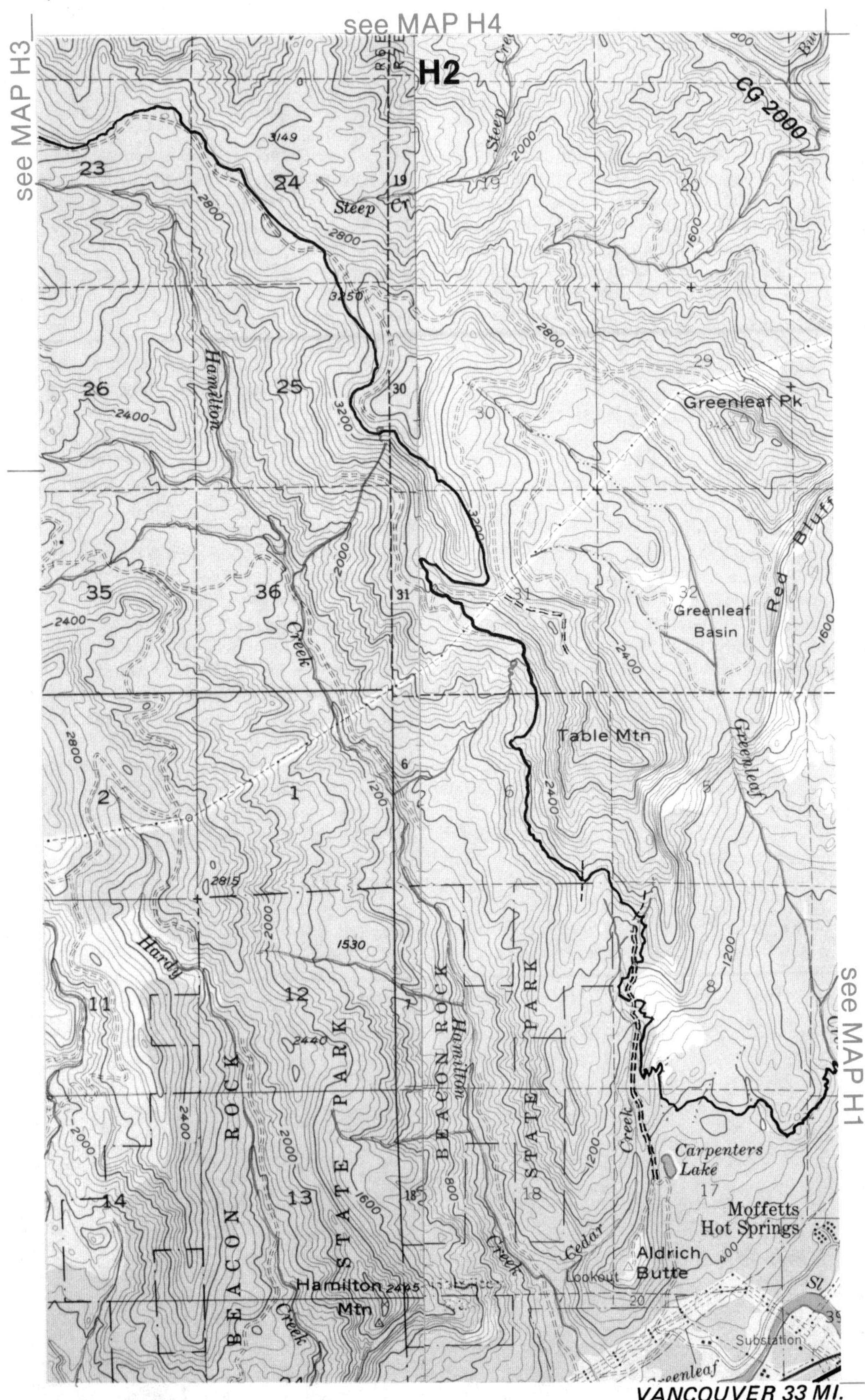

see MAP H4
H2
see MAP H3
see MAP H1
CG 2000
Steep Cr
Hamilton
Creek
Greenleaf Pk
Red Bluff
Greenleaf Basin
Table Mtn
Greenleaf
Hardy
BEACON ROCK STATE PARK
Hamilton
Cedar Creek
Carpenters Lake
Moffetts Hot Springs
Aldrich Butte
Lookout
Hamilton Mtn
Substation
VANCOUVER 33 MI.

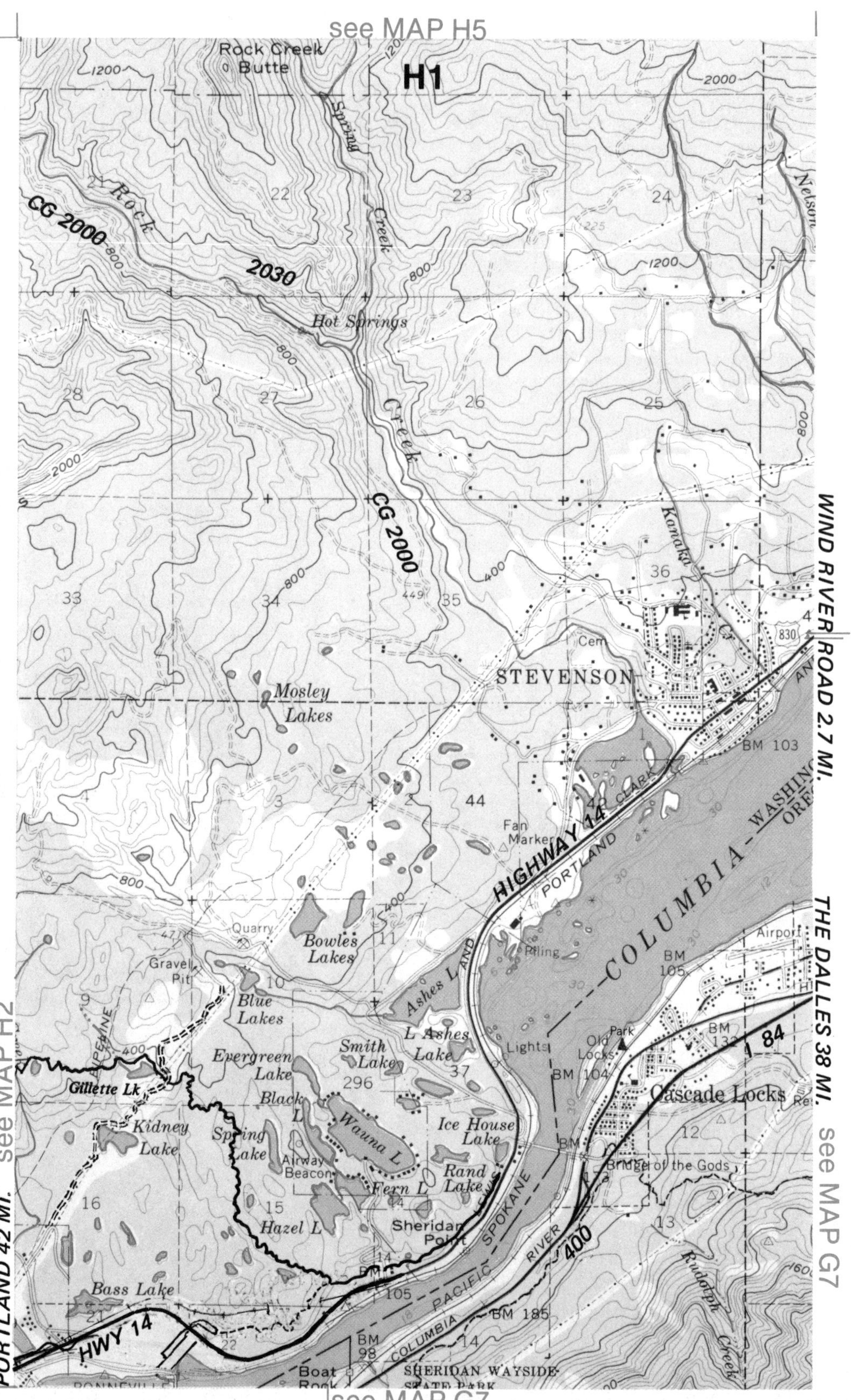

see MAP H5
H1
Rock Creek Butte
Spring Creek
Rock Creek
CG 2000
2030
Hot Springs
Nelson
Kanaka
STEVENSON
Cem
830
Mosley Lakes
Fan Marker
HIGHWAY 14
PORTLAND
CLARK
WASHINGTON
OREGON
COLUMBIA
BM 103
BM 105
Airport
Quarry
Gravel Pit
Bowles Lakes
Blue Lakes
PIPELINE
Ashes Lake
L Ashes Lake
Smith Lake
Evergreen Lake
Gillette Lk
Kidney Lake
Black L
Wauna L
Spring Lake
Airway Beacon
Fern L
Ice House Lake
Rand Lake
Hazel L
Sheridan Point
Piling
Lights
Old Locks
Park
BM 104
BM 132
84
Cascade Locks
Bridge of the Gods
SPOKANE
PACIFIC
RIVER
400
Rudolph Creek
Bass Lake
HWY 14
BM 185
BM 98
Boat Rock
COLUMBIA
SHERIDAN WAYSIDE STATE PARK
see MAP G7
see MAP H2
PORTLAND 42 MI.
WIND RIVER ROAD 2.7 MI.
THE DALLES 38 MI.
see MAP G7

The gorge's north wall is more prone to landslides than is the south wall because the volcanic rocks that compose both walls dip to the south. Naturally, then, rocks tend to slide south along this incline, and resulting landslides push the Columbia River against the south wall. Such landslides can temporarily dam the Columbia River, and such temporary dammings perhaps provided a basis for the Indian legend about Bridge of the Gods. It is known that certain Oregonian Indians witnessed the eruption of Mt. Mazama 7700 years ago, leaving Crater Lake basin in its aftermath, and it is therefore quite likely that the Multnomah Indians witnessed one or more devastating landslides in the last few millenia.

After about an hour of seemingly aimless wandering—more of it up than down—you temporarily break out of forest cover at a utility road (410–2.1), which serves three sets of Bonneville Dam powerlines. Across this major road, the PCT follows an abandoned road down toward Gillette Lake (280–0.3).

Side route (from official PCT only). You'll find a 75-yard spur trail heading east to the lake's northwest shore, which may be your first possible campsite in this section. On private land in a setting that is anything but pristine, the lake is, nevertheless, utilitarian, and swimmers will find the water relatively warm.

Now the trail re-enters forest, in a couple of minutes passes the lake's seasonal inlet creek, and then climbs for ¼ mile to a "firebreak." From it you follow an old road 70 yards west before leaving it. Eastbound trekkers could be led astray if they miss the PCT tread starting from the east side of the firebreak. On trail tread, westbound trekkers make an easy climb to a lily-pad pond before momentarily dropping to a horse bridge across Greenleaf Creek (510–0.9). This is your last totally reliable, *on-trail* water source until Rock Creek, 15.5 miles farther. Fortunately, some near-trail water sources are available.

Switchback upward from the creek and get your only views of sprawling Bonneville Dam as you make a short traverse southwest. Then angle northwest to a gully with a seasonal creeklet, ramble west to a second creeklet, and

See maps H1, H2

SECTION H

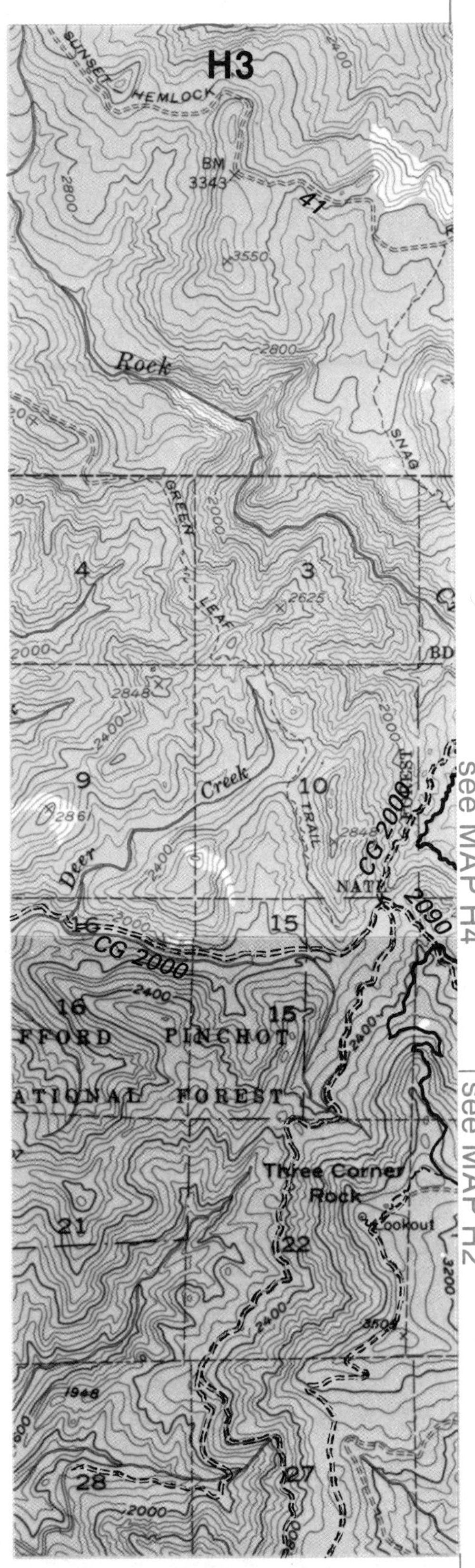

then climb north along a third before switchbacking up to a low ridgecrest (1100–1.9). Here, you turn north and parallel a little-used road up Cedar Creek canyon.

Water access (from official PCT only). Along this stretch, you can drop to the nearby road, camp along it, and wade through dense vegetation to get water from Cedar Creek.

After a crest walk northward, you cross the road (1300–0.6), and then in ⅓ mile recross it.

Water access (from official PCT only). The trail unfortunately climbs above Cedar Creek's headwaters, but at the recrossing, you can continue 0.2 mile north up the road to a campsite with water.

In about ⅓ mile, the climb north takes you to a creeklet, just beyond which you meet Table Mountain East Way, which climbs very steeply up a minor ridge. On a moderate grade, you climb northwest, then southwest, up to a larger ridge (1970–1.2) that has Table Mountain West Way along it.

Now you exchange the Cedar Creek drainage for the larger Hamilton Creek drainage. The trail drops a bit, quickly emerges from forest cover, and then drops some more to avoid steep slopes on the west side of towering Table Mountain. Enjoy the panoramic views while you can, for you still have 1500 feet of climbing ahead. On a hot, muggy summer's day, you may be too tired to enjoy anything, particularly with that heavy pack on your back. The earlier in the morning you make this protracted climb out of the Columbia Gorge, the better.

On a shady bench due west of Table Mountain, the PCT latches onto an abandoned roadbed which, fortunately, is alder-shaded along its first half mile. You'll need the shade, for the gradient averages a stiff 17%. Just before the gradient abates, you get a view (2480–1.3). Stop and listen for music to your ears—a never-failing creek.

Water access (from official PCT only). Reaching the creek is another problem. It could use a spur trail down to it, but unfortunately the creek is on private land. Drop your pack and cautiously head downslope, trying to keep slipping and sliding to a minimum. (Equestrians have a real dilemma: horses can't reach this spring-fed creek, and they may not be able to reach Cedar Creek, mentioned earlier. Horses could get heat prostration on a hot summer afternoon—you may have to walk your horse up this demanding stretch.)

Onward, in about 140 yards, the trail reenters forest cover and bends west. Soon you leave the old roadbed, pass under a buzzing powerline, traverse a short stretch of beargrass turf, and then ramble over to a nearby road (2790–0.8). You climb briefly north and then head east on a rather steep, very rocky tread across a rubbly open slope that offers fine views south down Hamilton Creek canyon. Mt. Hood also comes into view, poking over the shoulder of multilayered Table Mountain. With

See map H2

PCT bridge across Trout Creek

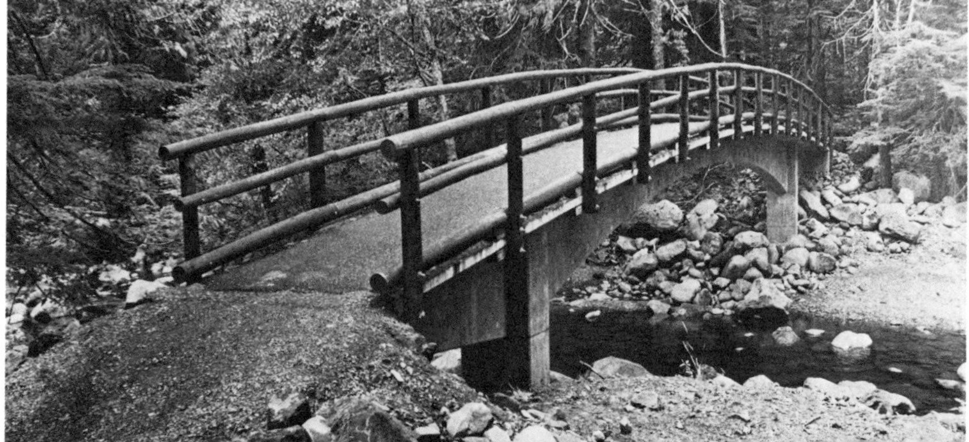

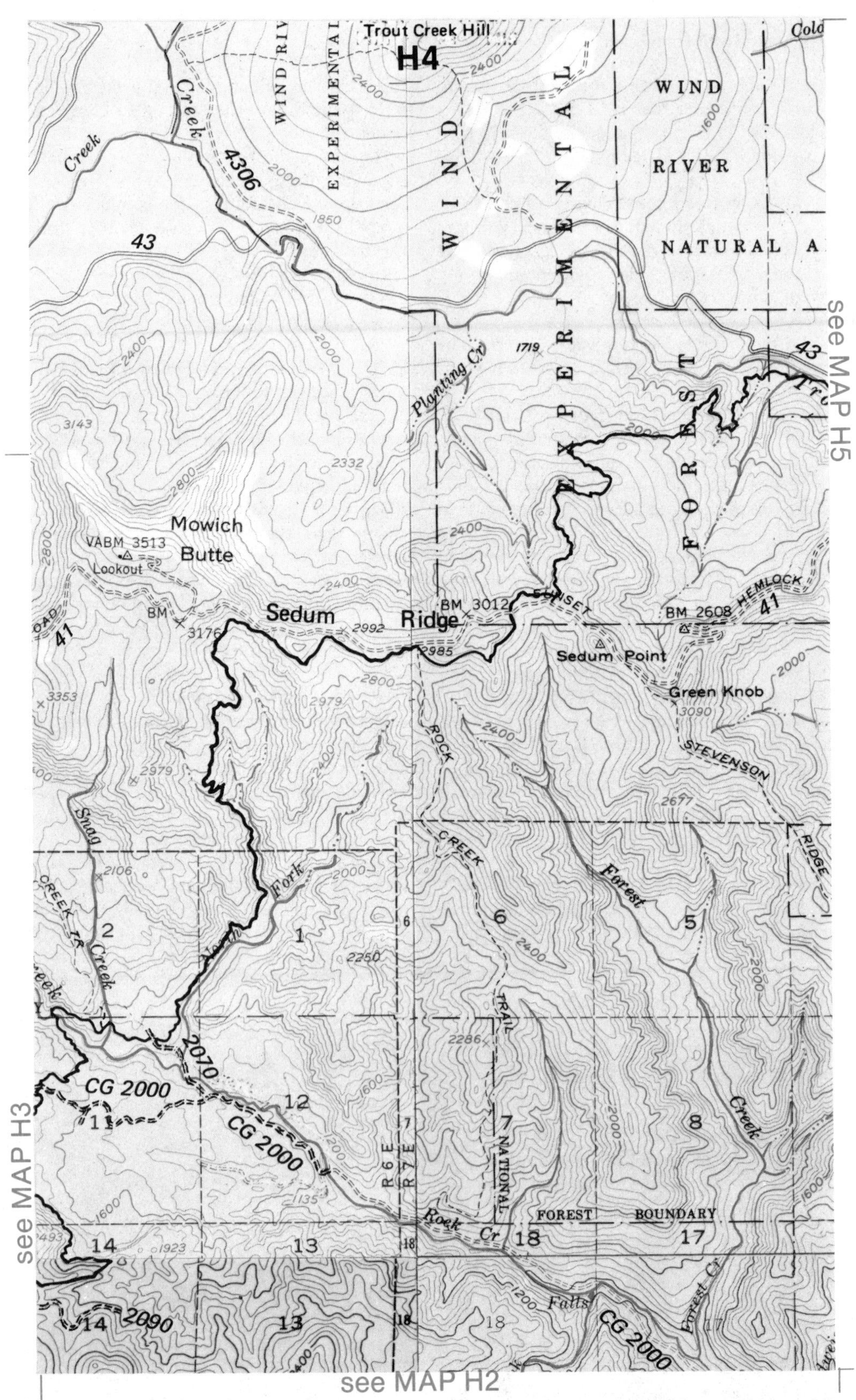

see MAP H5
see MAP H3
see MAP H2

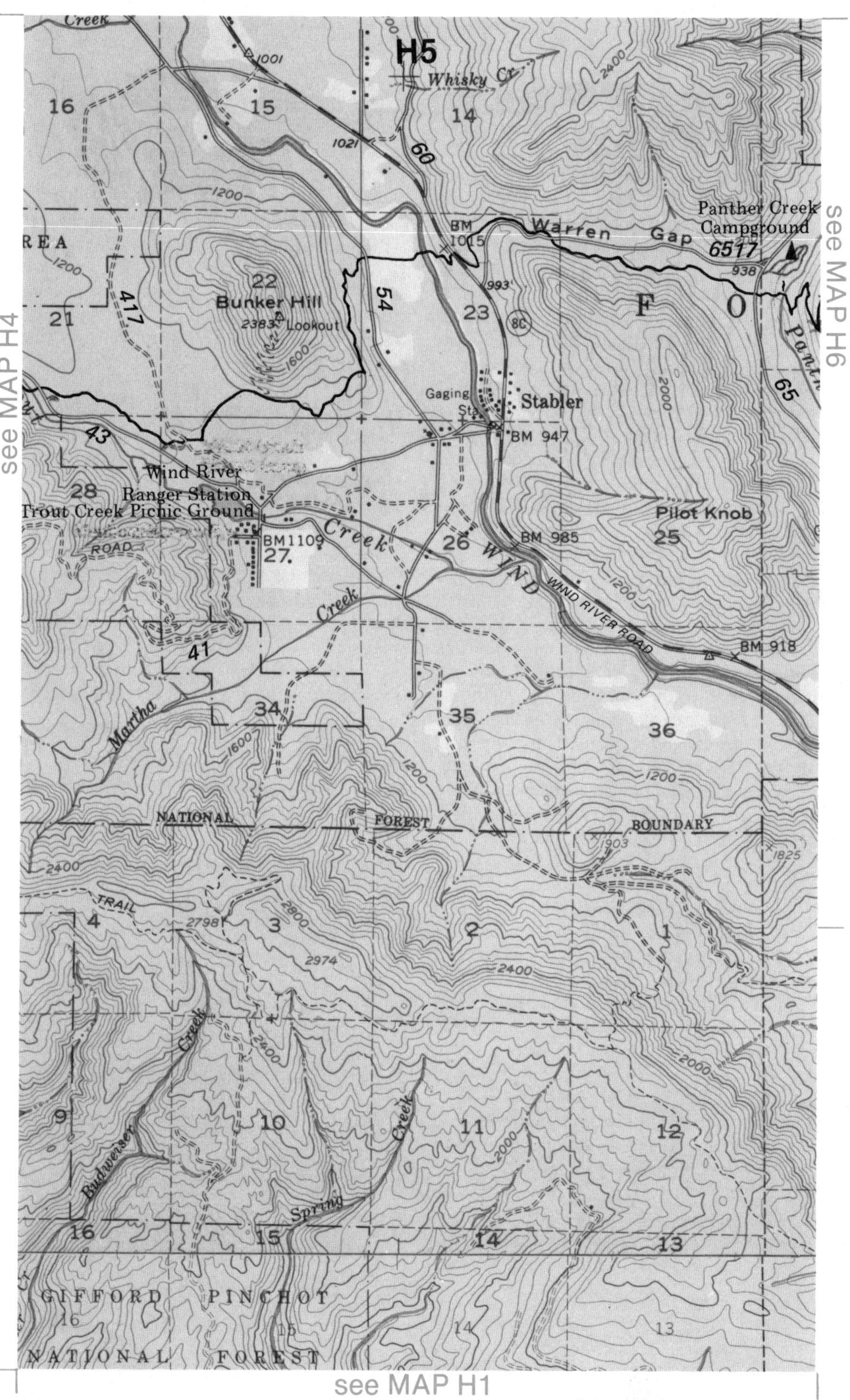

see MAP H4
see MAP H6
see MAP H1

a final burst of effort, you reach a ridge (3120–0.5) above a powerline saddle. Welcome back to a crest route; you've struggled 11 miles to reach it.

Having put most of the elevation gain behind, you can enjoy the next stretch, which has views east past Greenleaf Basin and Peak to the Columbia Gorge and south past Table Mountain to Mt. Hood. Typical of a crest route, the PCT climbs to a saddle and crosses it (3400–0.7), giving you your first view of Three Corner Rock, a conspicuous knob to the northwest. The trail climbs briefly, topping out at just over 3400 feet, and then makes a minimal descent over to flowery, bushy slopes, immediately beyond which you come to a seep (3370–0.3). It may be dry, so don't count on it.

Next, you wind around a ridge, absorbing panoramic views to the south, west, and northwest, and then submerge in a forest canopy for a descent to a saddle with a crestline road (3020–1.3). This jeep road heads over to Three Corner Rock, and the PCT parallels it in the same direction. Along this stretch, a newer road crosses the PCT and quickly meets this jeep road. Traversing along the PCT, you get sporadic views to the north and east, with Mt. Adams and clearcuts catching your attention. Views disappear about ¼ mile before the trail touches the jeep road, and ahead you climb, first viewlessly southwest and then viewfully west, up to a spur trail (3320–2.0). The next on-trail water is way down at Rock Creek, a hefty 5.0 miles away.

Water access (from official PCT only). If you really need water, you can gamble and take the narrow, bouldery spur trail ⅓ mile over to a water trough. You'll find it about 30 yards west of the trail at a point just 40 yards before the trail ends at a jeep road. The trough is bathtub-size, and when author Schaffer visited it, it looked like folks had bathed in it. You'll certainly want to treat the water! The trough, unfortunately, could have sprung a leak, leaving you thirsty and frustrated. If you've hiked as far as the water trough, you might as well scramble up the jeep road to close-by Three Corner Rock for unrestricted views, which include Mts. Hood, Adams, St. Helens, and, weather permitting, Rainier.

From the junction, you get a few views of unaesthetic clearcut slopes as the trail winds and switchbacks northward down to a viewless saddle (2360–1.9), which is crossed by Road 2090. Next, you skirt east just below a ridgecrest, soon enter a clearcut, and then gratefully leave it just before ducking through a crest gap (1980–0.5). After immediately switchbacking west below the gap, you quickly plunge into a deep forest and wander in and out of numerous, usually dry gullies before crossing Road 2000 (1720–1.8). This is found after a ½-mile hike through a former clearcut.

Side route (from official PCT only). If you need to abort your trip, take this well-maintained road 11 miles down to Stevenson.

Otherwise, follow the PCT down and across gullies to an ultimate bridging of Rock Creek (1420–0.8). ▮ *This 5.0-mile stretch from the spur trail has been a well-graded, very steady descent across a generally viewless, intricately complex terrain. Hats off to whoever surveyed this route; it must have been a formidable task, particularly with such dense vegetation.* ▮

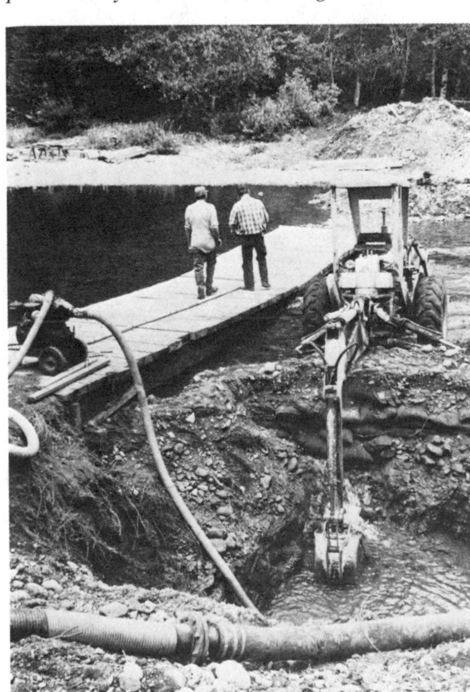

1978 PCT bridge construction at Wind River

See maps H2, H3, H4

Water availability now is less of a problem, at least until you leave Panther Creek Campground, some 15+ miles ahead. You quickly climb above Rock Creek, traverse east to a junction with the Snag Creek Trail, and then, in 120 yards, reach its namesake, Snag Creek (1470–0.4). Ahead, you soon emerge from forest cover, cross a clearcut with crowding, waist-high vegetation (very miserable on a rainy day), and then reach Road 2070 (1450–0.3). Prepare for a challenging ascent.

Side route (from official PCT only). If you're in need of a campsite, you can head about 250 yards down this rocky road and set up camp along the North Fork of Rock Creek.

At first, you have a pleasant stroll through a forest of Douglas-firs, alders, and vine maples. The North Fork stays close by for the first ¾ mile; then the trail enters and leaves a prominent gully and climbs to a north-trending North

See map H4

see MAP H7

H6

see MAP H5

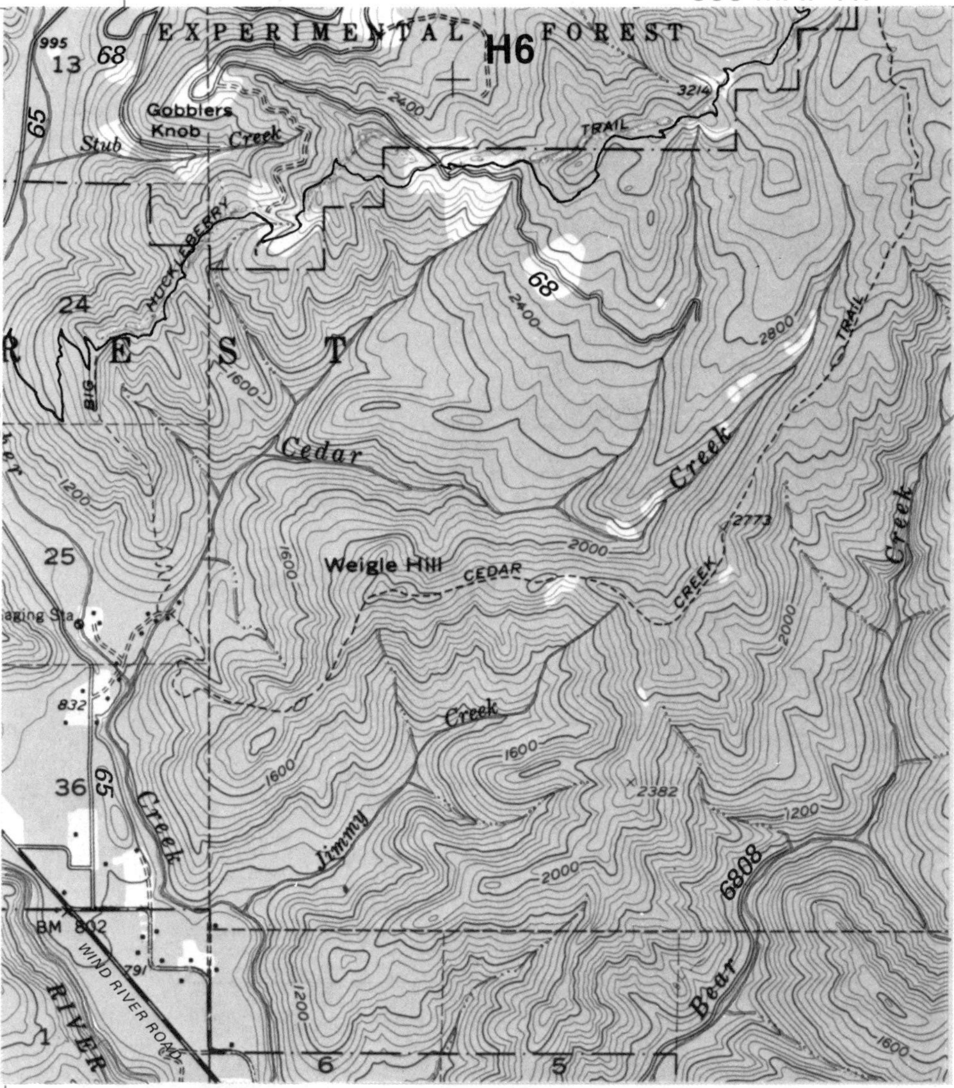

CARSON 3.9 MI.
HIGHWAY 14 4.9 MI.

Fork tributary. It is usually flowing but is a problem to reach because the PCT typically stays 200 feet above it on steep, densely vegetated slopes. Finally, the trail crosses a seasonal creeklet (2080–1.8), your last hope for any water until a Trout Creek tributary 7.0 miles away. Switchbacks carry you up to gentler slopes, across which you climb to a lushly vegetated, though dry, gully. Ahead, the trail climbs east to a ridge and then north to the base of steep slopes below crest-hugging Sunset-Hemlock Road 41. Southeast, you climb a short half mile, obtaining poor views before reaching a south-trending ridge (3080–1.8). Next, you skirt over to an adjacent crest saddle and then, just beyond it, have your first good views as the trail skirts the base of a lava cliff. At a second saddle (2985–0.7), the trail almost touches Road 41, and here you might note the abandoned Sedum Ridge Trail, descending 4 miles to Road 2000 along Rock Creek. The trail climbs once more, topping out at 3130 feet

See map H4

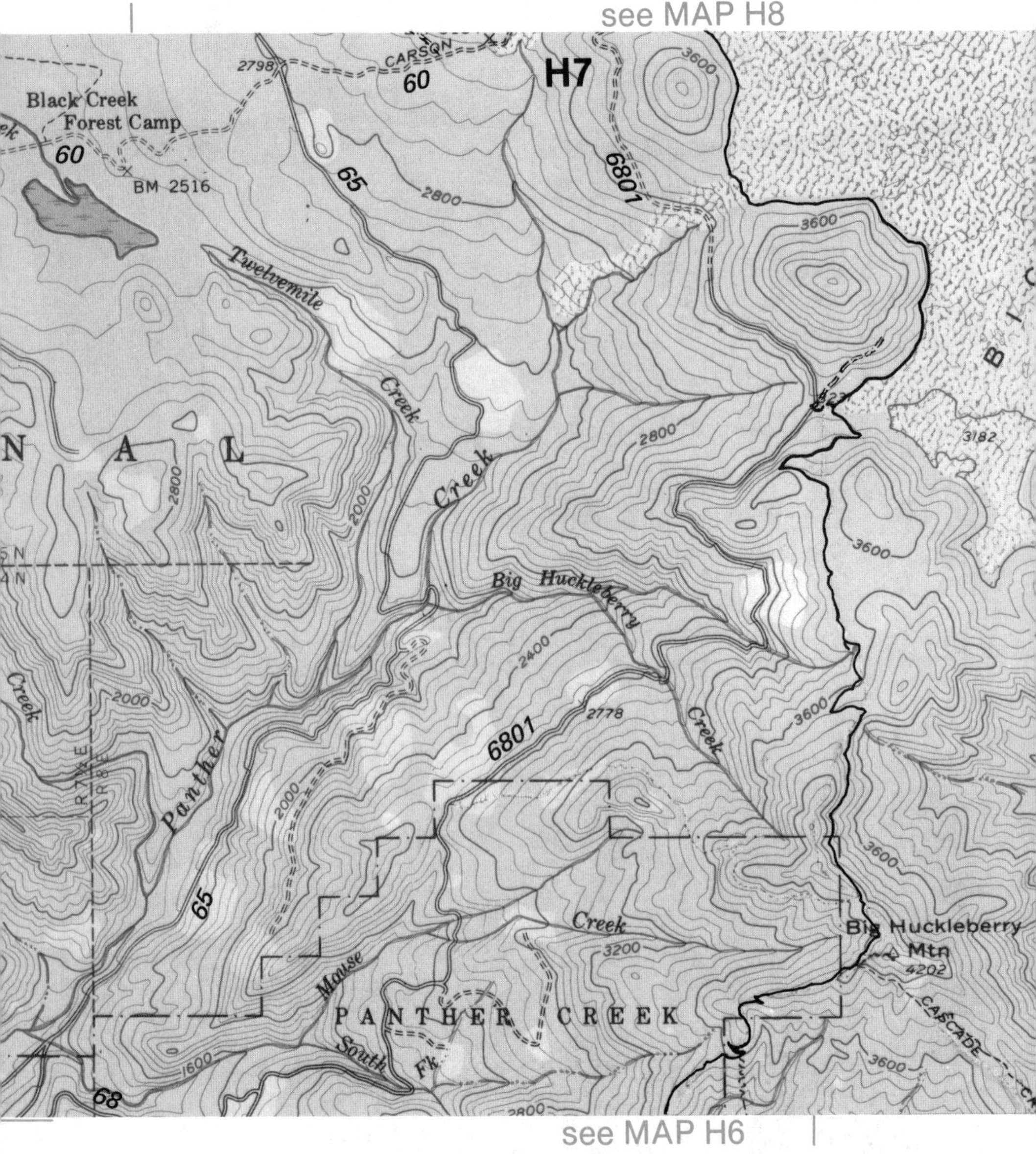

see MAP H9

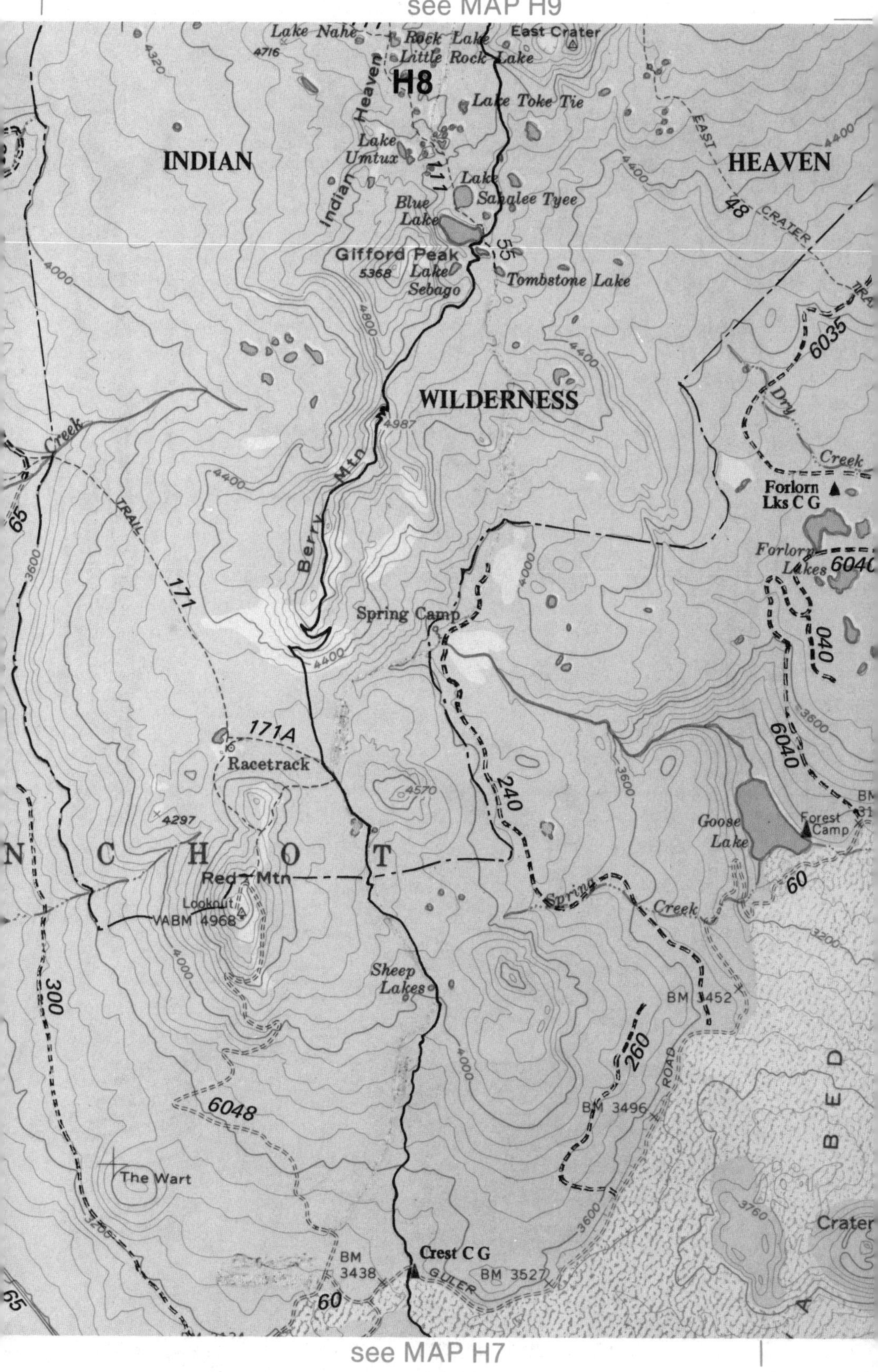

see MAP H7

see MAP H1

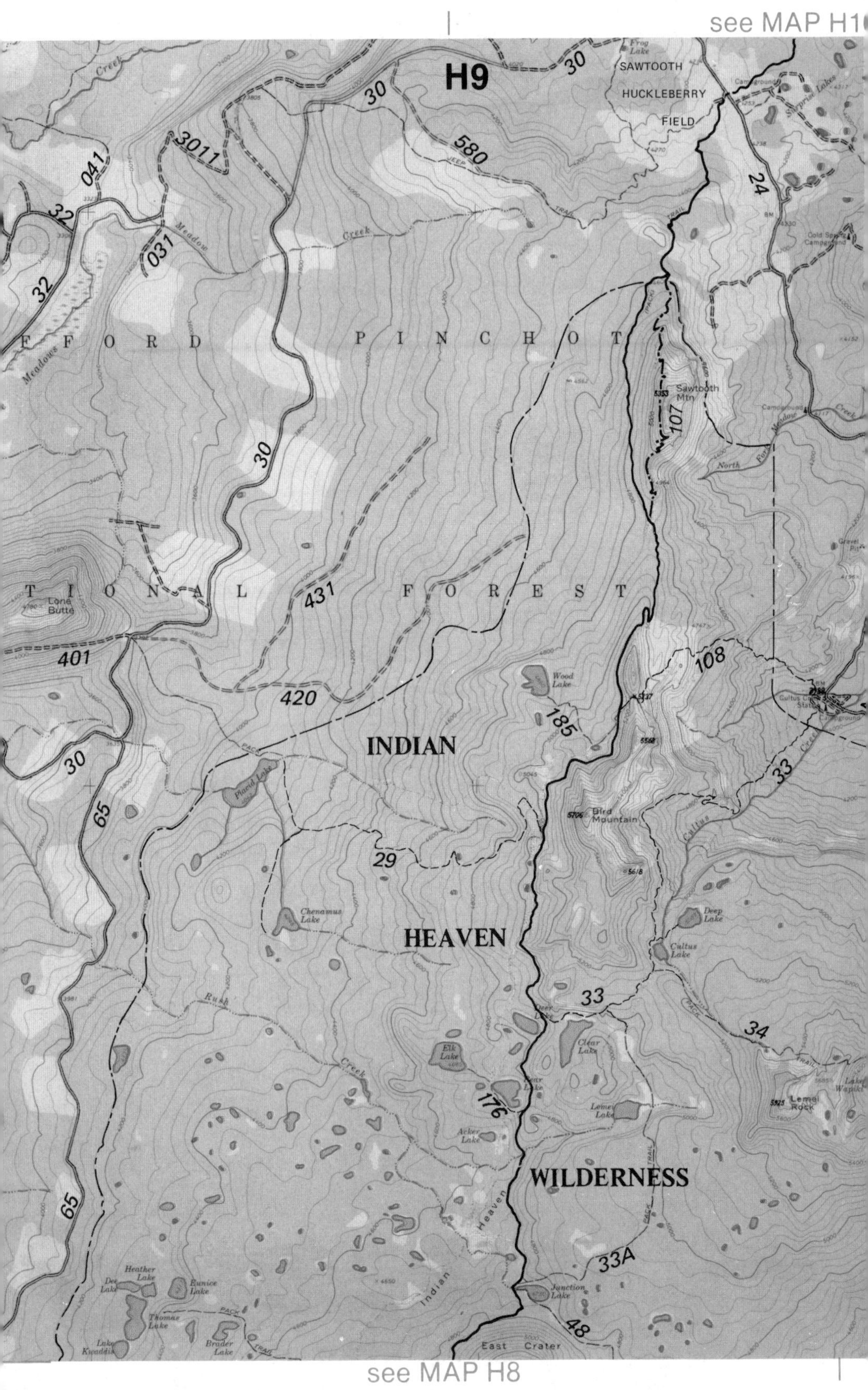

see MAP H8

near a viewful, south-trending ridge, and then descends to Sedum Ridge, where it finally crosses Road 41 (2950–0.8).

Leaving the road, you meet what's left of Greenknob Trail 144 in ¼ mile, and on this PCT descent, you are likely to see traces of this former trail. The PCT reaches a gully, descends briefly north, turns east around a knifeblade ridge, and then drops north through a lush forest to the main ridge (2550–1.0). Here you get the first good view north and see Bunker Hill to the east, standing alone in a flat-floored valley.

The view disappears, and once again you disappear into a lush forest. ▮ *If you are hiking the trail on one of those damp, misty days so common to this area, you may see a dozen or more rough-skinned newts.* ▮ The trail quickly reaches gentler slopes, angles northeast down to a viewless saddle (2150–0.7), and then continues northeast down into several gullies that often, though not always, provide water. The trail leaves these gullies and in ⅓ mile crosses a wide, splashing tributary (1210–2.0) of Trout Creek. Now on nearly level ground, the trail curves east to Trout Creek and crosses it on a concrete span built to last as long as the PCT does. This is a good spot to camp. Immediately past the bridge, the trail crosses Road 43 (1180–0.3), which gently descends 1.3 miles to the Trout Creek Picnic Ground, with a good swimming hole.

From the road, hike 280 yards over to a bend in the trail, where a faint path heads 75 yards west over to a nearby campsite at the end of a short spur road. Past the campsite, the PCT soon parallels unseen Road 43 southeast to Road 417 (1120–0.8). Walking east 30 yards on this road, you locate the PCT's tread, which follows the road's north edge 120 yards to a road junction (1120–0.1). From here, a road goes ½ mile southeast to the Wind River Ranger Station, which is near Trout Creek Picnic Ground. Road 417 heads northwest along one edge of a tree farm, while the PCT heads east along the tree farm's fenced-in south edge.

Briefly parallel the tree farm's east edge, hiking northward, and then in 100 yards angle northeast for a steepening walk up to a junction with the Bunker Hill Trail (1210–0.5), which switchbacks up to the summit. The PCT now winds, dips, and climbs eastward along the hill's viewless lower slopes, crosses a crest (1250–0.7), and then descends gradually north, down to a crossing of Little Soda Springs Road 54 (940–0.8).

See maps H4, H5

Mt. Hood and Columbia River gorge from summit of Big Huckleberry Mountain

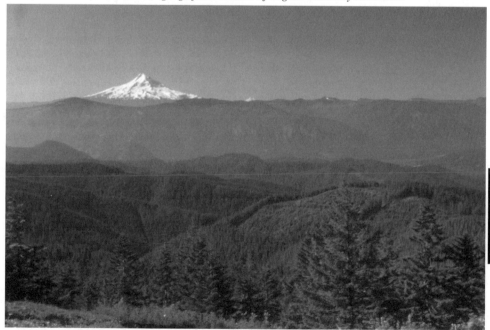

East of the road, a row of trees bisects a large meadow, and the PCT stays along the row's north side as it traverses east. It leaves this meadow just before crossing Wind River (940–0.3) on a major bridge, built in 1978, which is one of the largest bridges to be found along the entire PCT. You could camp in this vicinity, but Panther Creek Campground, less than an hour's walk ahead, is better for logistical reasons.

From this river, climb to busy Wind River Road (1020–0.2) and cross it just 0.2 mile northwest of this road's junction with Warren Gap Road 6517. The PCT starts a climb southeast, almost touches Road 6517, eventually crosses it (1180–0.8) just past Warren Gap, and then winds east down to Panther Creek Road 65 (930–1.2) to meet the alternate route, following, near Panther Creek Campground.

Alternate route. The alternate route starts north from the west end of Bridge of the Gods toll road (180–0.5, if you're counting the mileage from the end of Oregon's Section G).

This route follows obvious, well-signed roads, and is generally off the east edge of this book's maps.

Highway 14 curves past Ashes Lake and then heads northeast to the town of Stevenson (110–2.7), which has stores and cafés, plus the Stevenson Post Office, located at the corner of First and Russell, one block south of the highway. In Stevenson, you should be able to buy food, boots, packs, and other equipment.

East of Stevenson, the highway climbs rocky bluffs and provides scenic views up and down the river. Douglas-fir and maple provide plenty of shade even if you're doing this stretch on a sunny afternoon. The road eventually descends slightly to a junction with the Wind River Road (280–3.4), an "all weather" route you take northeast. It curves over to the sleepy settlement of Carson (450–1.0), which has a post office on the road's east side. This is the last one you'll find until you reach White Pass Village, a very long 119 miles away. If you're doing the whole PCT or at least the Oregon-Washington part, you'll want to mail your heavy packages here rather than carry them from the Cascade Locks or the Stevenson post office.

The Wind River Road leaves Carson, bends northwest, crosses a bridge spanning the 200-foot-deep Wind River gorge (570–2.5), and reaches a junction (802–2.3), where you turn right and follow the Old State Road briefly east to Panther Creek Road 65 (802–0.1). On this, you walk one mile north and soon begin a winding stretch of road up along Panther Creek to the PCT (930–2.7–14.7). This trail crosses the road only 230 yards south of Warren Gap Road 6517 and its adjacent Panther Creek Campground.

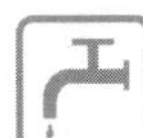

Water access (for official PCT and alternate route). The entrance to Panther Creek Campground is just 230 yards up the road, opposite the end of Road 65. You should plan to camp there, for once you leave Panther Creek, you won't have any campsite with *good* water until Blue Lake, 23 miles farther.

Official PCT route and alternate route rejoined. From the Panther Creek Road, the PCT winds east 300 yards to Panther Creek; immediately before it is a lateral trail that goes 150 yards to the southeast corner of Panther Creek Campground. After bridging Panther Creek, you switchback upward, passing two trickling springs long before reaching the westernmost end of a ridge (2100–2.3). Now you largely follow the old Big Huckleberry Trail up to Big Huckleberry Mountain. The trail starts by paralleling a slightly climbing ridgecrest northeast to a saddle (2300–1.1), from which a good dirt road starts a northeast descent and a vegetated one starts a southeast traverse. Take the vegetated road and follow it for 300 yards, curving around a brushy wash and then meeting a trail once again, just before the road curves south around a ridge. Hike east up this trail, recross the head of the wash, and wind around two minor ridges before coming to a saddle. This you cross; then, after a ½-mile climb across south slopes, the trail becomes an old road that quickly arrives at a junction with Road 68 (2810–1.3), on a saddle.

The trail continues east from the road, staying just south of the crest as it traverses a logged-out area, and then, just before a saddle, curves around the forested south slopes of the ridge, soon returning to the crest. Now you stay fairly close to the crest, which narrows to 5 feet

See maps H1, H5, H6

in one spot. and then soon descends to a broad, open saddle (3214–1.7). Next, you climb and then traverse to an important junction (3550–1.1).

Water access. From here, a steep trail makes tight switchbacks southward 0.3 mile down to Cedar Creek, and just 20 yards south of it is a small campsite.

Onward, the PCT immediately switchbacks to climb up and around a small, open lava cap, from whose top there is a fine view of Mt. Hood. Better views await at the summit of Big Huckleberry Mountain. From the lava cap, the PCT climbs ⅔ mile to a junction with southeast-traversing Grassy Knoll Trail 146, a stretch of Washington's pre-PCT Cascade Crest Trail. In several paces, you reach a junction with the steep, 300-yard-long Big Huckleberry Mountain summit trail (4010–1.1).

Side route. Don't miss this opportunity to survey the lands of southern Washington and northern Oregon from Big Huckleberry's little summit. To the south is Mt. Hood, rising prominently, and, just right of it, the summit of Mt. Jefferson. To the northeast is your next major volcano, Mt. Adams. All around are patches of clearcuts in various stages of reforestation.

The PCT now eases off and curves northward to cross a saddle 0.4 mile from the last junction; you could make an emergency dry camp on this saddle. Onward, the trail skirts across open slopes that provide excellent views of Mt. Adams, and then it soon enters viewless forest. From a second saddle crossing (3730–1.3), the trail descends to a gully

See maps H6, H7

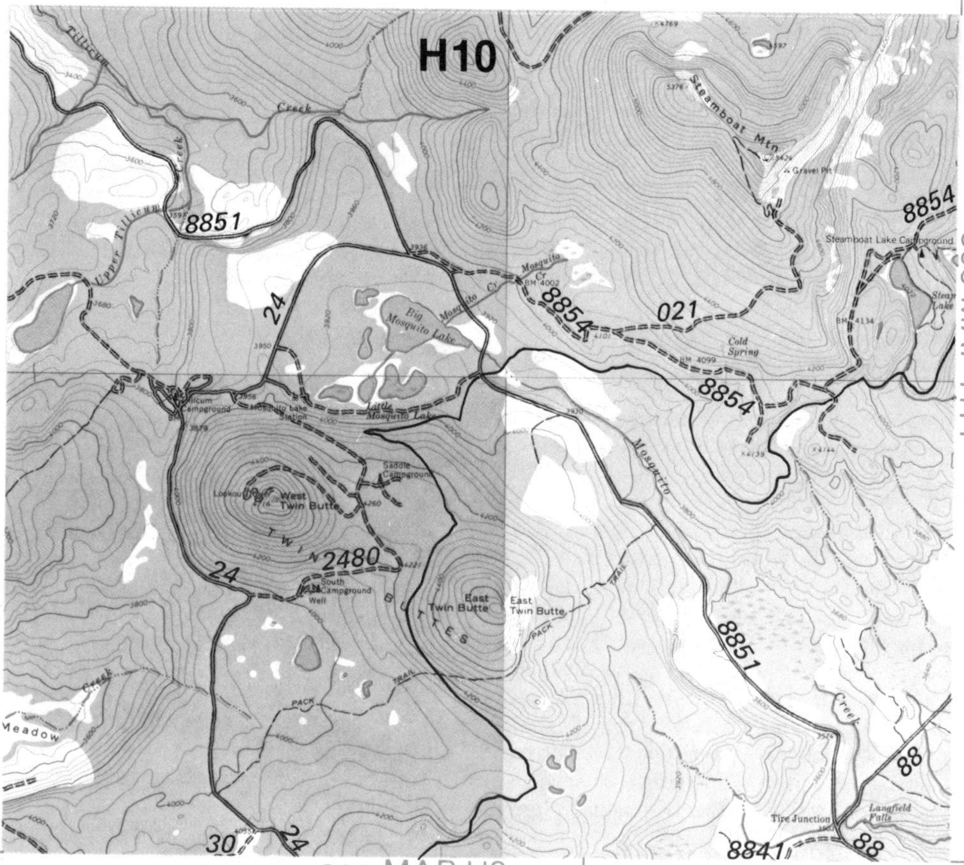

H10

see MAP H11

see MAP H9

(3550–0.5) that has a fairly reliable spring. This spring, 10.3 miles beyond Panther Creek, will be your last on-trail water until the Sheep Lakes, 7.0 miles farther. About 130 yards past it is a spur trail.

Side route. This spur trail goes 50 yards southeast to a developed campsite. It certainly beats waterless, roadside Crest Campground, which can have lumber-related traffic very early in the morning.

Onward, you contour northward through a shady forest of Douglas-fir, western hemlock, and western white pine to reach a viewless, broad saddle (3580–0.8) and then wind down to the edge of Big Lava Bed, also by a broad saddle (3220–0.8).

Alternate route. From this vicinity, a lateral trail winds 200 yards north to a northeast-climbing spur road, on which you can walk 50 yards west to Road 6801. If you've been having snow problems you might consider following this road 2-½ miles north to Road 60 and then ¼ mile east up it to the PCT and Crest Campground.

Contouring counterclockwise around Summit 4170, you may quickly encounter one or two springs, neither absolutely reliable. You follow the edge of geologically recent Big Lava Bed, cross one of its western overflow channels—which reveals the detailed intricacies of the flow—and then contour around another summit and cross another channel to the back of the Crest Campground (3490–3.5), which is on the south side of Carson-Guler Road 60.

The campground has a horse corral but no water, so pick your pack off the table, put it on your back, and trudge north up the signed PCT. ▮ *This moderate ascent up a fern-decked path is really quite nice if you aren't running short of water.* ▮ Climb to a flat and reach a duck pond (4020–1.9), which is no more than an oversized mud puddle after your arrival frightens the ducks away. Nevertheless, it boasts the name *Sheep Lake*. If necessary, you can camp by this trailside "lake" or by the adjacent western or eastern Sheep Lakes. After climbing northwest through a more open forest, you enter Indian Heaven Wilderness and reach another pond, a 35-yard-wide puddle, Green

See maps H7, H8

Lake (4250–2.2), which gets as deep as a foot in early summer and serves as a vital water supply.

If you find Green Lake too polluted to suit your standards, prepare for a dry march. Start northwest past a meadow and then reach a junction with Shortcut Trail 171A (4240–0.4), which strikes west-northwest half a mile to a large, stagnant pond and to the Racetrack, which supposedly was used by Indian equestrians. Hike north-northwest through a forest, and then climb several long switchbacks up the sunny south slope of Berry Mountain before reaching its crest. The PCT provides excellent

See map H8

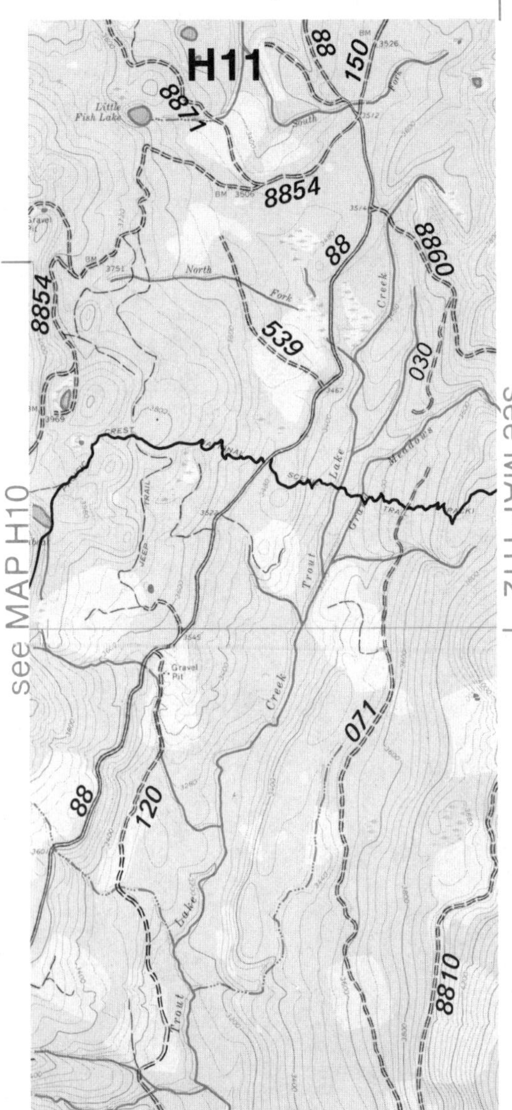

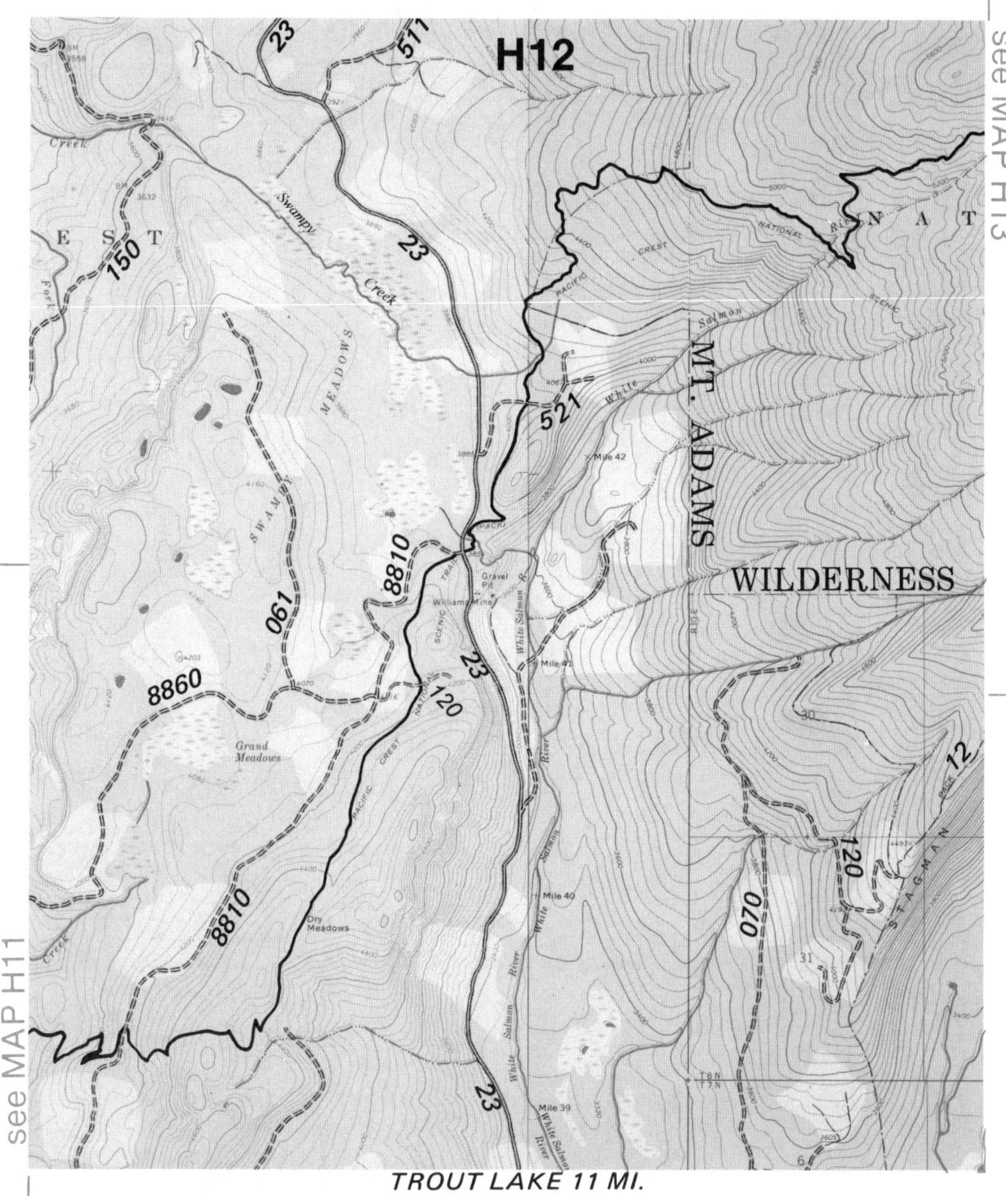

views of Mt. St. Helens (8364) to the northwest, Mt. Adams (12,276) to the northeast, and Mt. Hood (11,235) to the south. Upon reaching the north end of linear Berry Mountain, you descend short switchbacks to a saddle (4730–2.9), follow a rambling path down past the seasonal outlet creek of Lake Sebago (4640–0.9), and come to an overlook of a 100-yard-wide stagnant pond beyond which you finally reach the welcome, clear waters of Blue Lake (4630–0.2), nestled at the foot of Gifford Peak (5368). Here you'll find the first good campsites since Panther Creek Campground, 23 miles back.

Side route. Starting along the lake's east shore, Thomas Lake Trail 111 heads ¼ mile northwest over to an additional good campsite at shallow, circular Lake Sahalee Tyee. Camp at it if the Blue Lake campsites are full.

The PCT, which barely touches Blue Lake, starts northeast from the lake's southeast corner and then winds north up to a west arm of East Crater. The trail curves northeast around this youthful feature and then angles north for a short drop to a junction with East Crater

See maps H8, H9

see MAP H14

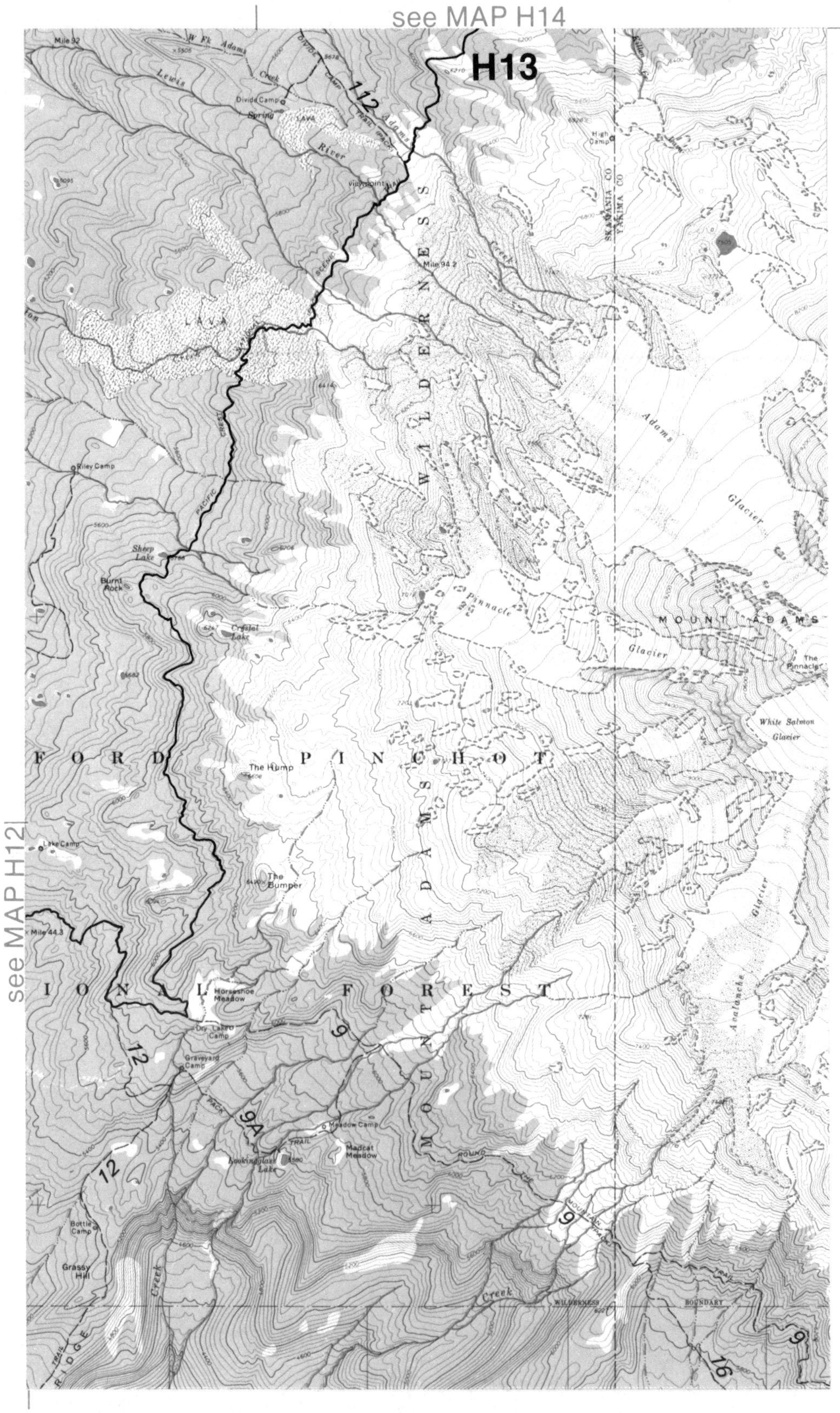

see MAP H12

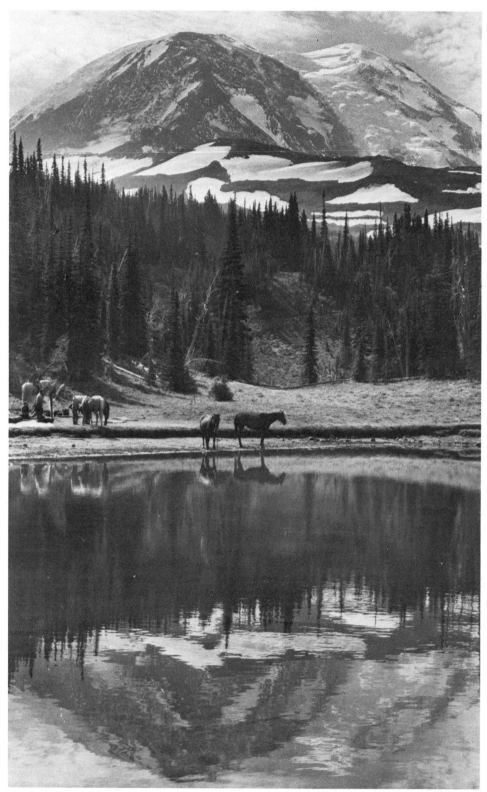

Mt. Adams and Adams Glacier

see MAP H15

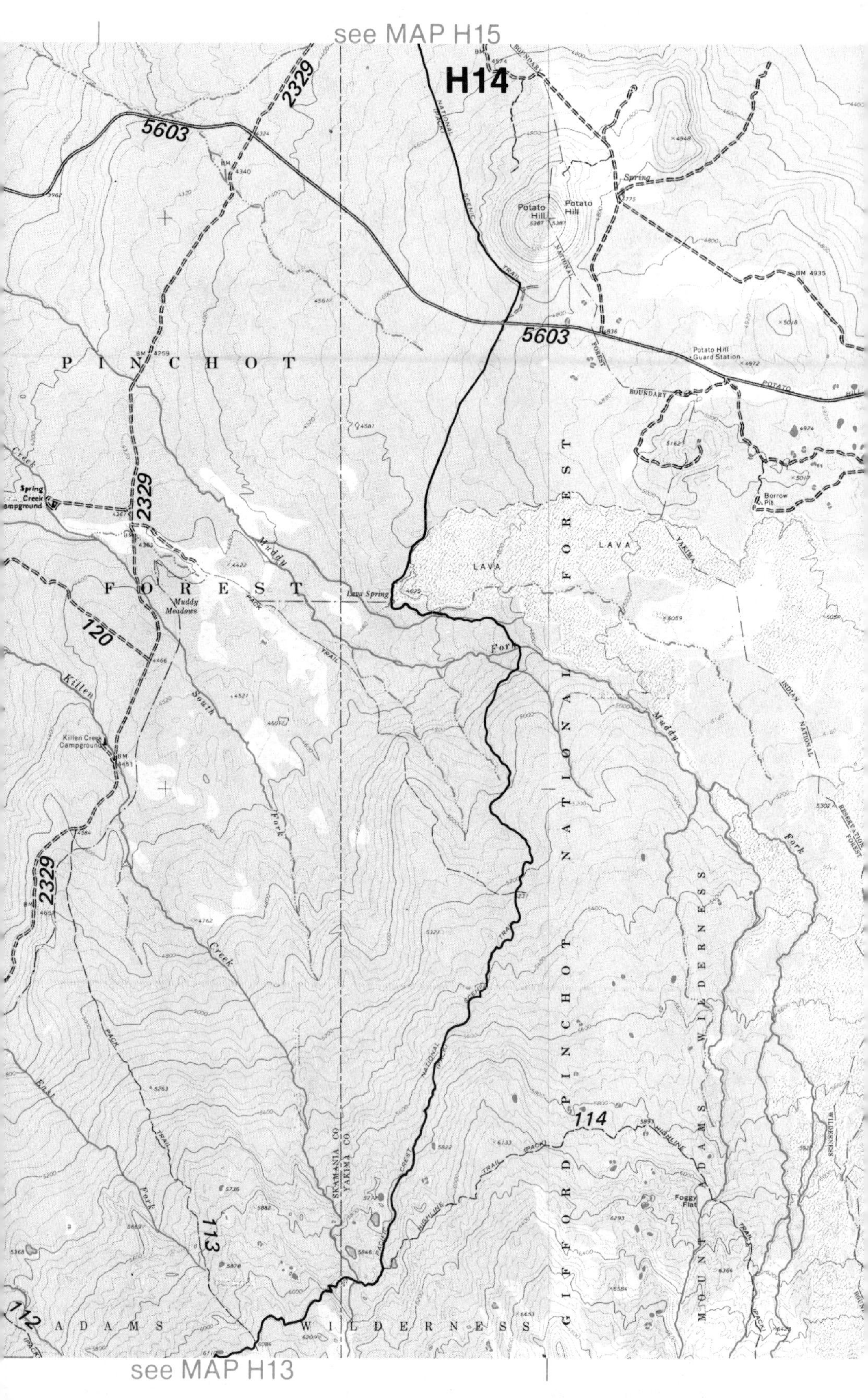

see MAP H13

Trail 48 (4730–1.9), which starts east along a skinny west finger of pleasant Junction Lake. You'll find a good campsite near its southwest shore and a poorer one near its northwest shore.

At the tip of the finger, you cross the lake's outlet and meet Lemei Lake Trail 33A (4730–0.1), which climbs east before swinging north past Lemei Lake to Indian Heaven Trail. Whereas the old Cascade Crest Trail skirted Indian Heaven's mosquito-populated ponds and lakes, the newer PCT stays on lower slopes just east of and above them.

By adhering to the lower slopes, the PCT avoids the bogs that were found along the old Cascade Crest Trail, but in early season, snow patches may be quite a problem. One-quarter mile past the crossing of usually dry Lemei Lake creek, you meet a junction with Elk Lake Trail 176 (4790–1.0) above the southeast corner of Bear Lake.

Side route. From above the southeast corner of Bear Lake, this trail first skirts the southwest shore, offering you access to a campsite or two. Both Acker and Elk lakes, which are nearby, are less desirable.

Onward, you traverse above Bear Lake and then over to a slope (4830–0.4) above the east end of Deer Lake, whose shoreline camps are fewer and poorer than those at Bear Lake. Rounding slopes above the lake, you meet Indian Heaven Trail 33 (4880–0.1).

Side route. This 3.8-mile-long trail takes the long way out to fairly large and often popular Cultus Creek Campground, which usually has a summertime host present, should you need help. By going just ⅓ mile on this trail, you can reach an adequate campsite by the northeast corner of Clear Lake. A couple of more-remote lake campsites can be reached with some cross-country effort.

With no more trailside lakes before Road 24, you continue north, pass two seasonal ponds, and then soon reach Placid Lake Trail 29 (4980–1.1), offering neither nearby camps nor water. Still northbound, the trail crosses a saddle, and then traverses northeast to another one (5110–0.5).

Side route. From this saddle, you can head 150 yards down to a campsite by a pleasant, unnamed lakelet.

Staying high, the PCT contours around the lakelet and soon meets Trail 185 descending to Wood Lake, which is not worth a visit. Also by Trail 185 is the west end of Cultus Creek Trail 108 (5150–0.4).

Side route. Cultus Creek Trail 108 climbs briefly northeast to a wooded saddle and then drops 1.5 miles at a hefty 15% gradient to the aforementioned Cultus Creek Campground, along Road 24.

The trail now stays close to a well-defined crest, which it eventually crosses and thereby gives you views of massive Mt. Adams and the terrain being logged around it. Just past the crest crossing, the trail heads briefly south, only to switchback north and descend to a crest saddle. ▮ *At the switchback, you'll see a prominent huckleberry field just below, with berries in season from about mid-August until mid-September. You might sample these if you haven't already made a side trip to huckleberry fields back near Indian Heaven.* ▮ There is a junction here; you can stay on the official PCT route, following, or take a viewful alternate route, below.

If you keep to the official PCT route, the PCT stays low as it traverses north gently down the west slopes of Sawtooth Mountain to a reunion with that summit's footpath (4570–1.4) and the alternate route.

Alternate route. From the crest saddle (4850–1.2), a 1.7-mile-long footpath switchbacks almost up to the knife-edge crest of Sawtooth Mountain before switchbacking down to the PCT. From the serrated crest, which can be reached by a short scramble, you get an exhilarating view down its east cliff as well as an unobstructed view of Mt. Adams. On a clear day, you also see three other snowy peaks: distant Mt. Hood in the south, bleak Mt. St. Helens in the west-northwest, and distant Mt. Rainier in the north.

See map H9

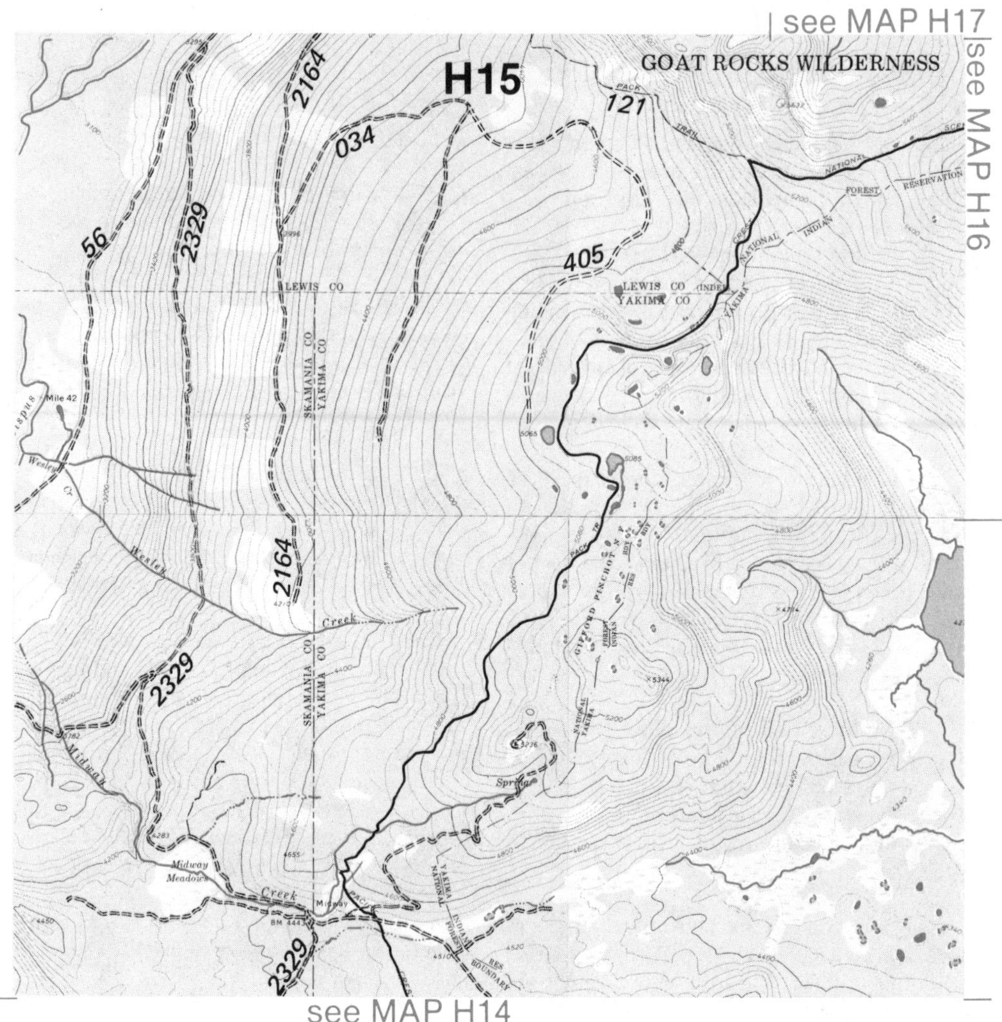

see MAP H17
see MAP H16
see MAP H14

Official PCT route and alternate route rejoined. The PCT then leaves Indian Heaven Wilderness as it descends into the Sawtooth Huckleberry Field, reaches a spur road, and parallels it 60 yards northeast to a signed PCT crossing of Road 24 (4260–1.2). ▮ *The large berry field at this flat was being harvested by Indians when George B. McClellan's exploration party came through in 1854. Needless to say, it had probably been harvested for countless generations. Roads were built up to it around the turn of the century, and today the Indians have exclusive rights only to the berries* east *of the road.* ▮

The trail now descends gently east-northeast, enters forest, and passes above the little-developed Surprise Lakes Campground, which, like Cold Spring and Meadow Creek campgrounds south of it, is for *Indians* only. Continuing northeast on the 1972 Surprise-Steamboat lakes section of the PCT, you descend to a saddle (4070–1.4), climb northwest up this well-graded trail, and then round the west slopes of East Twin Butte (4690). You reach a platform between the two Twin Buttes, which are obvious cinder cones, descend northwest below unseen, dumpy Saddle Campground, switchback northeast, and descend to a crossing of a trickling creek immediately before reaching Road 8851 (3915–2.5) at a junction 35 yards southeast of the west-trending Little Mosquito Lake road. The PCT bears northeast from Road 8851 and quickly reaches the wide, refreshing outlet creek from Big Mosquito Lake (3892). Just northeast beyond this creek is a campsite.

See maps H9, H10

see MAP H17

see MAP H15

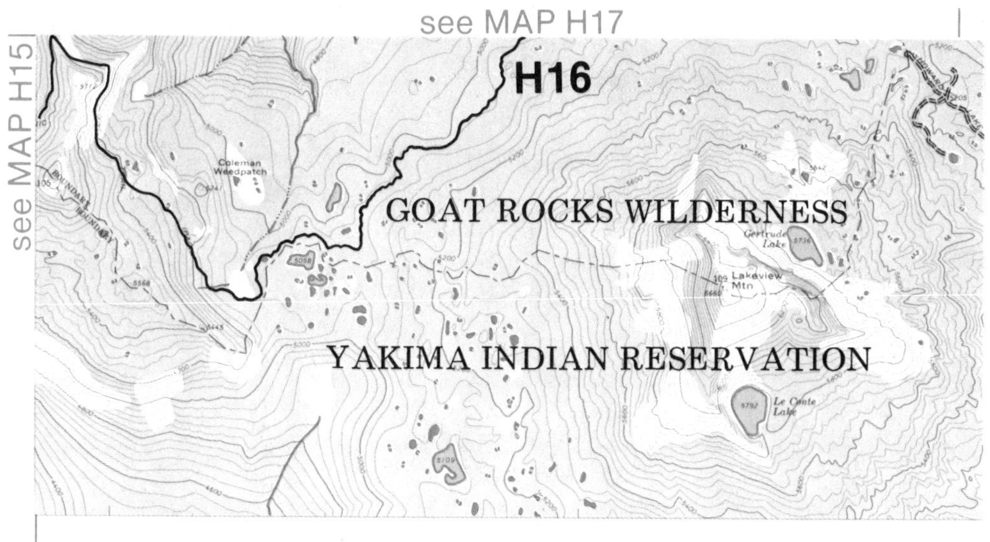

Side route. When conditions are boggy, you might prefer to follow Road 8851 north briefly down to where it bridges the creek. Just beyond it, on the left, is a parking area, which could serve as an early-season campsite.

The PCT leaves the creek and climbs gently east along the upper margin of a sheep-inhabited clearing, rounds a spur, and shortly crosses a dirt road (4090–2.5) that snakes northwest 130 yards up to Road 8854. Continue northeast and descend to a small gully with a seasonal creek (3980–0.4) to meet a spur trail to Steamboat Lake. You can stay on the official PCT, following, or take an alternate route via Steamboat Lake, below.

Official PCT route. From the Steamboat Lake spur-trail junction, the PCT curves counterclockwise from the gully, makes a gentle descent to an outlet creek 70 yards downstream from an unseen, unnamed lake, and then climbs briefly northward to a saddle, where it meets the end of the alternate route (3970–0.8), which climbs west to Steamboat Lake Campground.

Alternate route. This spur trail to Steamboat Lake climbs north moderately 0.2 mile up to Steamboat Lake (4022), and from it you can climb to waterless Steamboat Lake Campground, ¾ mile from the

See map H10

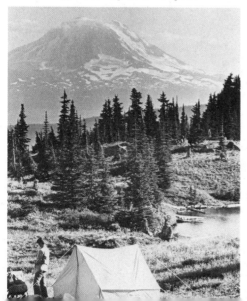
Mt. Adams, from Sheep Lake campsite

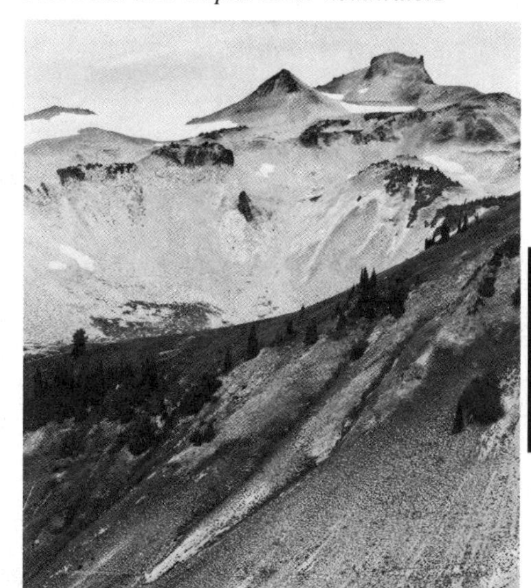
Ives Peak and Cispus River headwaters

see MAP H18

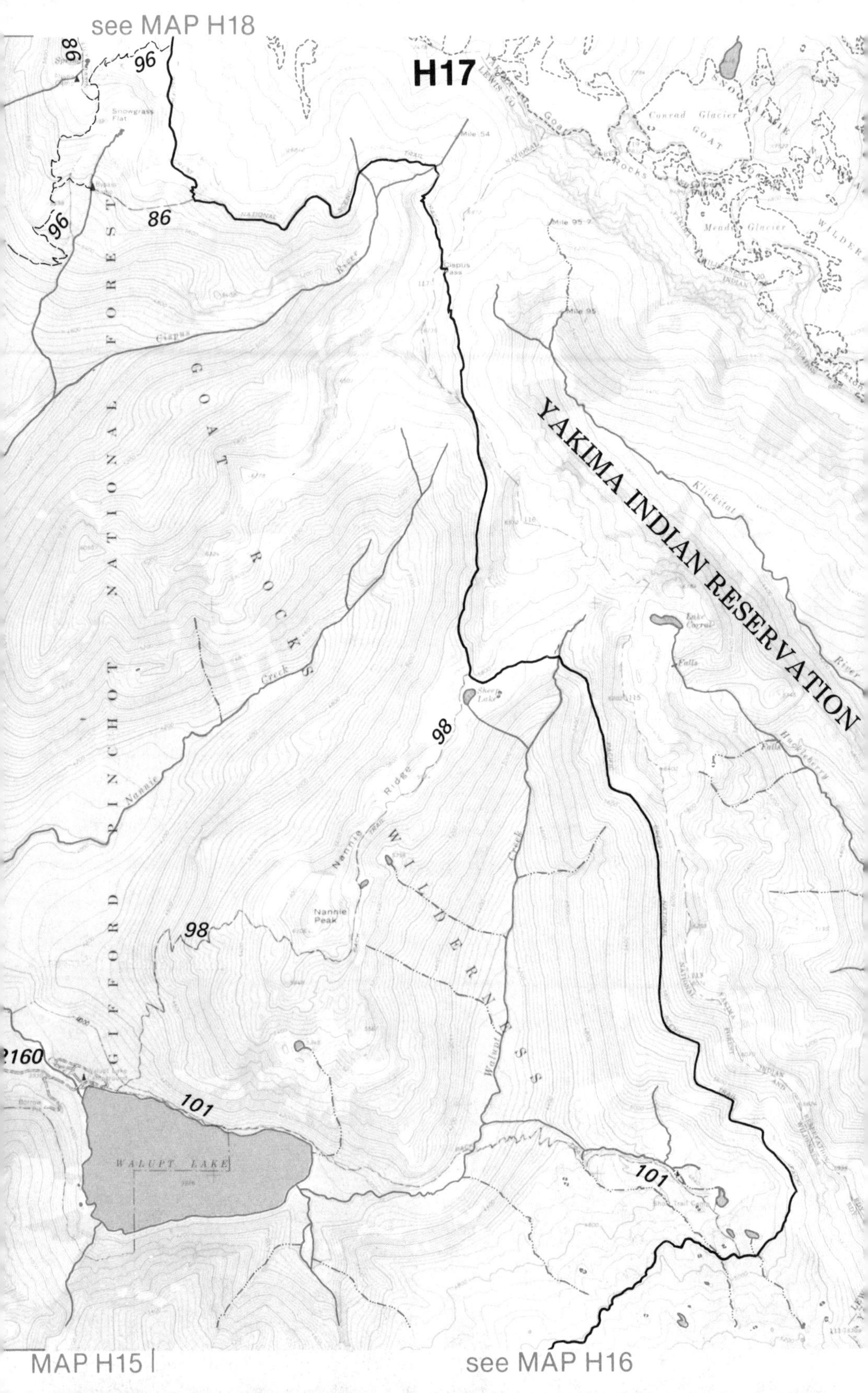

MAP H15

see MAP H16

PCT. At the northeast edge of the camp, a ½-mile-long trail descends to a shallow, unnamed lake and then rejoins the PCT at a bend.

Official PCT route and alternate route rejoined. Here, the PCT descends first northeast, then east, weaving through a quiet forest down to a junction with Road 88 (3470–1.2). The swath this road cuts through this forest is so oriented that it affords an open view directly at Mt. Adams.

The PCT recommences 50 yards northeast up this road, and on it you top a minor ridge before descending to 3-yard-wide Trout Lake Creek (3310–0.4). North of the trail at a point 25 yards east of this creek, you see a very good campsite, and, 100 yards later, cross the smaller Grand Meadows Creek. The trail now ascends eastward, crossing Road 071 one-third of the way up to a ridge. Soon it momentarily descends to a tributary before making a final, stiff climb up to Road 8810 (4140–2.1). Continuing east up the slope, you reach the crest (4570–0.6) and then begin a generally descending route north-northeast along the ridge down to a trailhead at Road 8810 (3854–2.7), reaching it ⅔ mile after crossing minor, east-heading Road 120. Walk east 50 yards to this road's junction with north-trending Road 23 and a trailhead for Mt. Adams Wilderness.

From Road 23, the PCT heads 140 yards over to a creek, and 90 yards later, you reach an old roadbed on which you could camp. The trail then climbs north before traversing the slopes of a low summit and then briefly

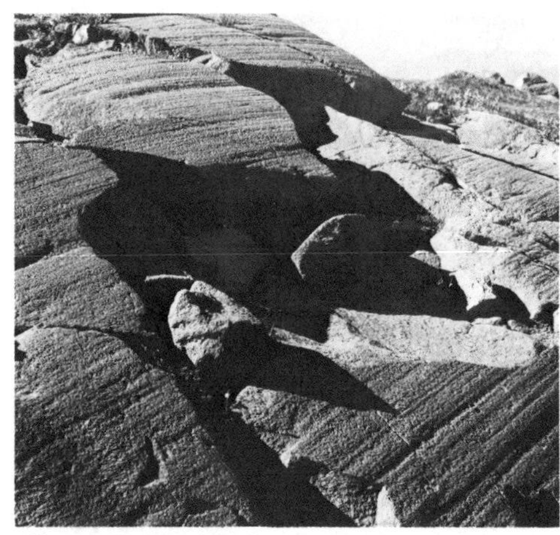

Glacier-striated rocks

descending to a crossing of east-trending Road 521 (4020–0.9). After hiking ¼ mile north, you reach a small, good campsite near a bridge over a permanent creek. In the next ¾ mile, you cross two usually flowing creeks.

Now you continue up an increasingly steep trail to the Mt. Adams Wilderness boundary, switchback northeast, traverse east, and finally drop gently to a barely recognizable, often dry creek known as the White Salmon River. About 100 yards past it (4900–2.7), you'll see a spring gushing from thick vegetation 50 yards below the trail. This is your last reliable water until Sheep Lake, 6.5 miles later.

The trail then switchbacks, crosses the "river" in a shady bowl, switchbacks again, and then makes a long, snaking ascent to a junction with Stagman Ridge Trail 12 (5790–2.5),

See maps H11, H12, H13

Forty-foot-high "Split Rock" along PCT

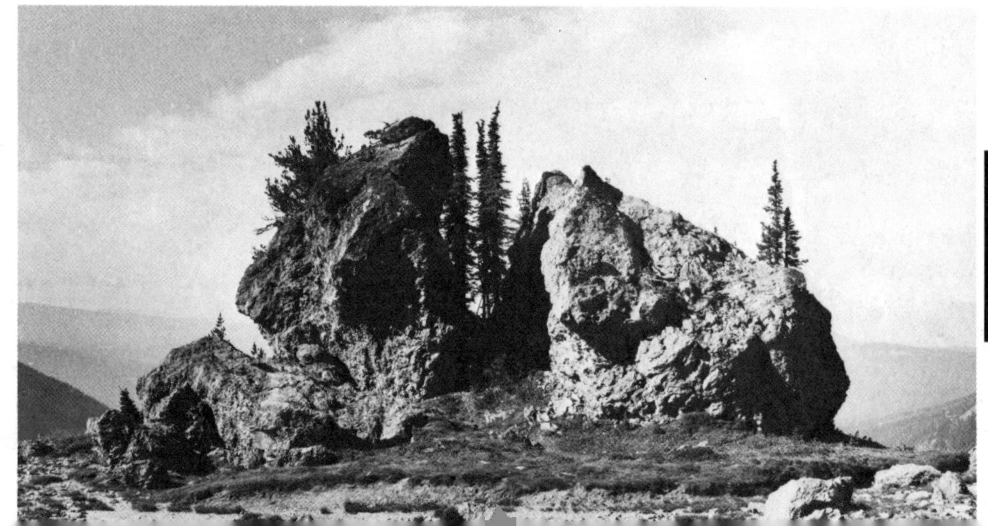

see MAP H19

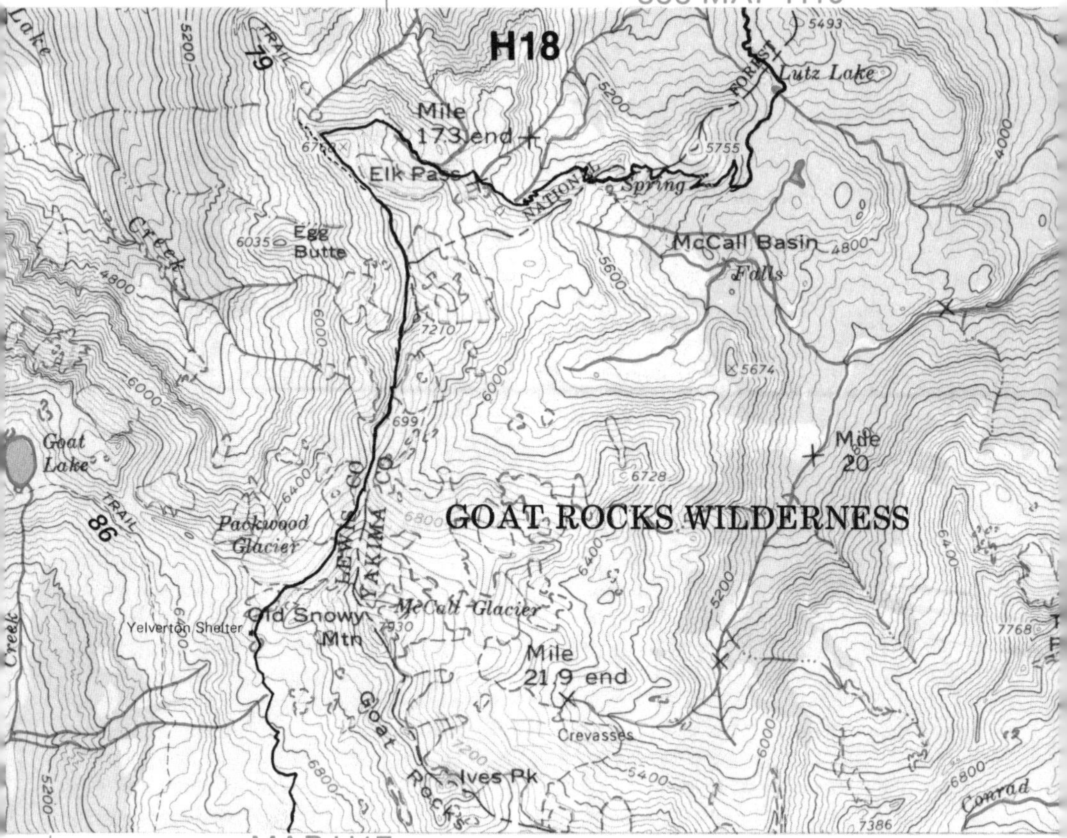

H18
Lake
TRAIL
79
5200
5493
Lutz Lake
FOREST
Mile
17.3 end
6750
5755
Elk Pass
NATIONAL
Spring
Creek
6035
Egg
Butte
McCall Basin
4800
Falls
5600
4800
7210
6000
5674
6000
6991
Goat
Lake
TRAIL
86
Mile
20
6400
6728
LEWIS CO
YAKIMA CO
6800
GOAT ROCKS WILDERNESS
Packwood
Glacier
6400
5200
6400
McCall Glacier
Old Snowy
Mtn
7930
Yelverton Shelter
Creek
7768
Mile
21.9 end
Crevasses
Goat
Rocks
6000
7200
Ives Pk
5400
6800
6800
Conrad
5200
7386

see MAP H17

Goat Lake and Mt. Rainier

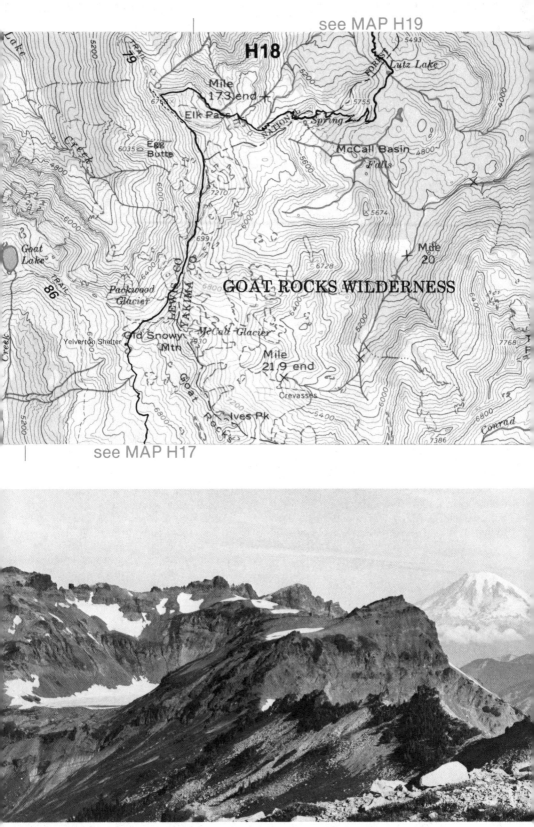

which starts a descent south. Pressing onward, you climb east up to a junction with Round the Mountain Trail 9 (5900–0.5).

Side route. This traverses ¼ mile east to Dry Lake Camp and then continues 6¼ miles to Timberline Camp, above the end of Road 8040. The easiest and most popular route to the summit of Mt. Adams (12,276) starts there and climbs up the south ridge. You should have no trouble attaining the summit in good weather, for this is the route that mule trains used in the 1930s. ▮ *Back then, a sulfur claim had been staked out on the summit, but it didn't pay off. This massive andesitic stratovolcano, like the others you've seen, should still be considered active. Its last eruption may have been 1000 to 2000 years ago, and in May 1921 its near-surface magma generated enough heat to initiate a large snow-slide that eradicated the forest on the slope below it.* ▮

On the high slopes east of this junction with Trail 9, you can see the White Salmon Glacier. ▮ *Some PCT mountaineers prefer to climb Mt. Adams via that icy route, which starts from this junction and crosses Horseshoe Meadow.* ▮

The PCT climbs northwest around a ridge that separates this glacier from the Pinnacle Glacier immediately north of it. This northward, round-the-mountain route is quite a contrast with that on Mt. Hood; it stays at a relatively constant elevation, and where it climbs or descends, it usually does so on a gentle gradient. To the north and the northwest, you can often see Goat Rocks and Mt. Rainier. After traversing to a saddle (5950–3.2) just east of Burnt Rock, the trail descends toward 70-yard-wide, 5-foot-deep Sheep Lake (5768–0.3), which is 40 yards northwest of the trail, and then reaches milky, jump-across Riley Creek (5770–0.2).

Next on the menu, you approach Mutton Creek (5900–1.3) and follow it up beside a geologically recent, rather barren lava flow over which you eventually diagonal quite a distance up. The route then bounds from one wash to the next, crosses milky Lewis River (6060–1.3), and in 200 yards reaches a spur trail. ▮ *This spur goes 110 yards north to a viewpoint. From it, you'll see distant, snowy Mt. Rainier standing above a nearer, clearcut-patched landscape.* ▮ The PCT quickly crosses some silty tributaries of West Fork Adams Creek before it curves north-northwest to a junction with Divide Camp Trail 112 (6020–0.3), which descends northwest toward Road 2329. ▮ *Directly upslope from you is the overpowering, steeply descending Adams Glacier, which appears to be a gigantic, frozen waterfall. Along this journey north, glances back toward this massive peak will always single out this prominent feature.* ▮

The trail heads northeast across a 330-yard swath of bouldery glacier outwash sediments and then jumps across silty Middle Fork Adams Creek. After climbing its bank, the route contours northeast past a 70-yard-wide pond (6110) and in a few minutes arrives at a junction with Killen Creek Trail 113 (6084–1.4), which starts beside a seasonal creek as it descends northwest toward Road 2329. Contour onward, descend to a large flat through which flows clear Killen Creek, and cross this creek as it reaches a brink (5920–0.8) and cascades merrily down 30 feet to a small meadow and a beautiful campsite nestled under a cluster of subalpine firs.

▮ *As you are about to head north away from the mountain, reflect upon another characteristic of this crescentic trail which distinguishes it from its counterpart on Mt. Hood: this trail stays on the mountain's lower slopes, and you never feel like you've set foot on the mountain itself—the upper slopes don't begin until a "distant" 2000 feet above you. In this respect, the trail resembles those around Mt. Jefferson and the Three Sisters.* ▮ A short distance from the campsite, the trail meets Highline Trail 114 (5900–0.2), upon which you may find *footprints* leading east toward the Yakima Indian Reservation.

Side route. About 100 yards along this trail, you'll find a shallow lakelet near which you can camp.

Side route. Just north beyond this junction, you spy a 70-yard pond a hundred yards northwest. It is better to descend 80 feet down the slope to this pond than to continue onward to a second, readily accessible one that receives too much impact from packers.

See maps H13, H14

The PCT passes the second pond (5772–0.4) and becomes a rambling, evenly graded pathway that descends north-northeast into a subalpine fir/lodgepole-pine forest whose monotony is broken by an intersection with a trail (5231–2.0) that starts north-northeast toward a junction two miles later with the Highline Trail.

Meeting no traffic other than perhaps chickadees or juncos, you continue northward and eventually reach a sturdy bridge across the 5-yard-wide Muddy Fork (4740–1.6), by which you find a small campsite. Curving northwest, the path soon reaches and then parallels an alder-and-willow-lined, silty creek westward to a very good campsite (4590–0.5) nestled between two of this creek's branches. A short distance farther, you round the nose of a recent lava flow and head north to the vibrant, crystal-clear waters gushing from trailside Lava Spring (4520–0.3) at the foot of the flow. Since its water is among the best you'll find along the *entire* PCT, you might as well rest and enjoy it.

Leaving it, you follow the 40-foot-high edge of the flow a short way, leave Mt. Adams Wilderness, and then climb gently through a predominantly lodgepole forest to a small trailhead parking lot a few yards north of paved Road 5603 (4750–1.6). From the lot, you walk northeast 50 yards along an old jeep road and then veer north-northeast along a trail that ascends gently toward Potato Hill (5387). Although motorized vehicles are specifically barred from the PCT, they or their tracks are likely to be encountered along this rather unscenic stretch through second-growth forest. The trail quickly reaches the jeep road again, follows its northwest-curving path around Potato Hill, and then takes this dusty road north-northwest past huckleberries and mountain ash to a junction with Road 115 (4490–2.0). Walk 50 yards up a road and then branch left for a grassy diagonal up a trail to closed Road 655 (4520–0.1), which descends west-southwest 0.1 mile to Road 115. You'll walk across no more roads until Highway 12 near White Pass, 40½ miles distant.

The trail starts west-northwest up toward Midway Creek (4690–0.4), with an adjacent excellent, spacious campsite, and then climbs up through alternating forested and cleared land toward the crest. As the gradient eases off, you enter forest for good and follow a winding

See maps H14, H15

Old Snowy Mountain and McCall Glacier

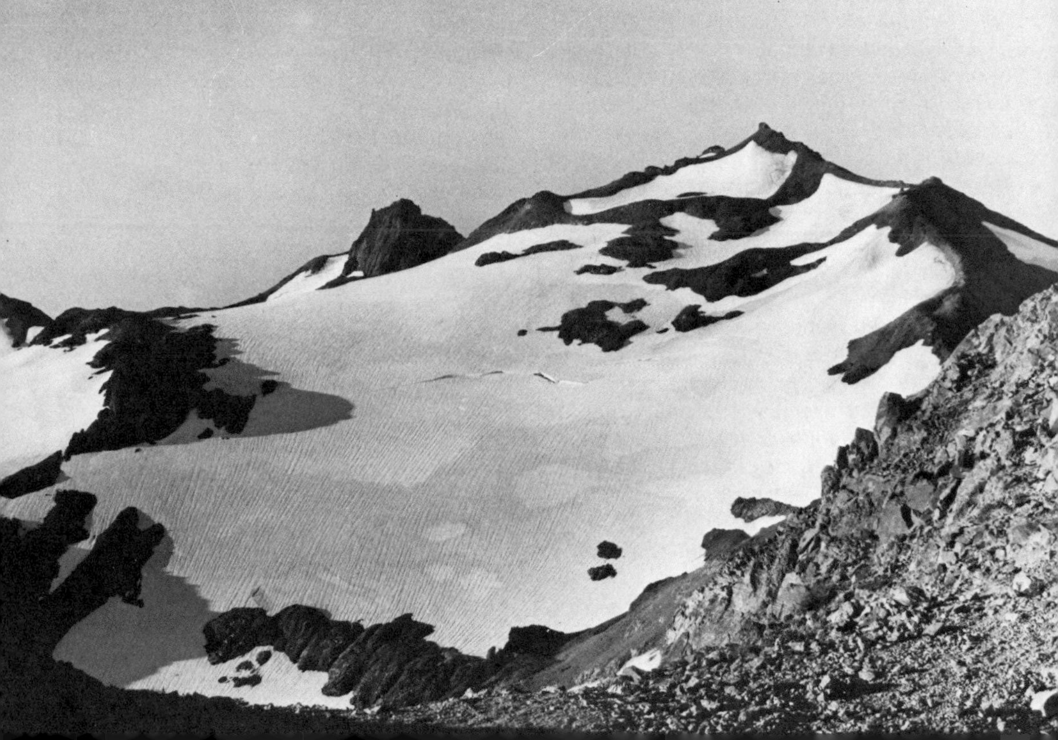

see MAP I1

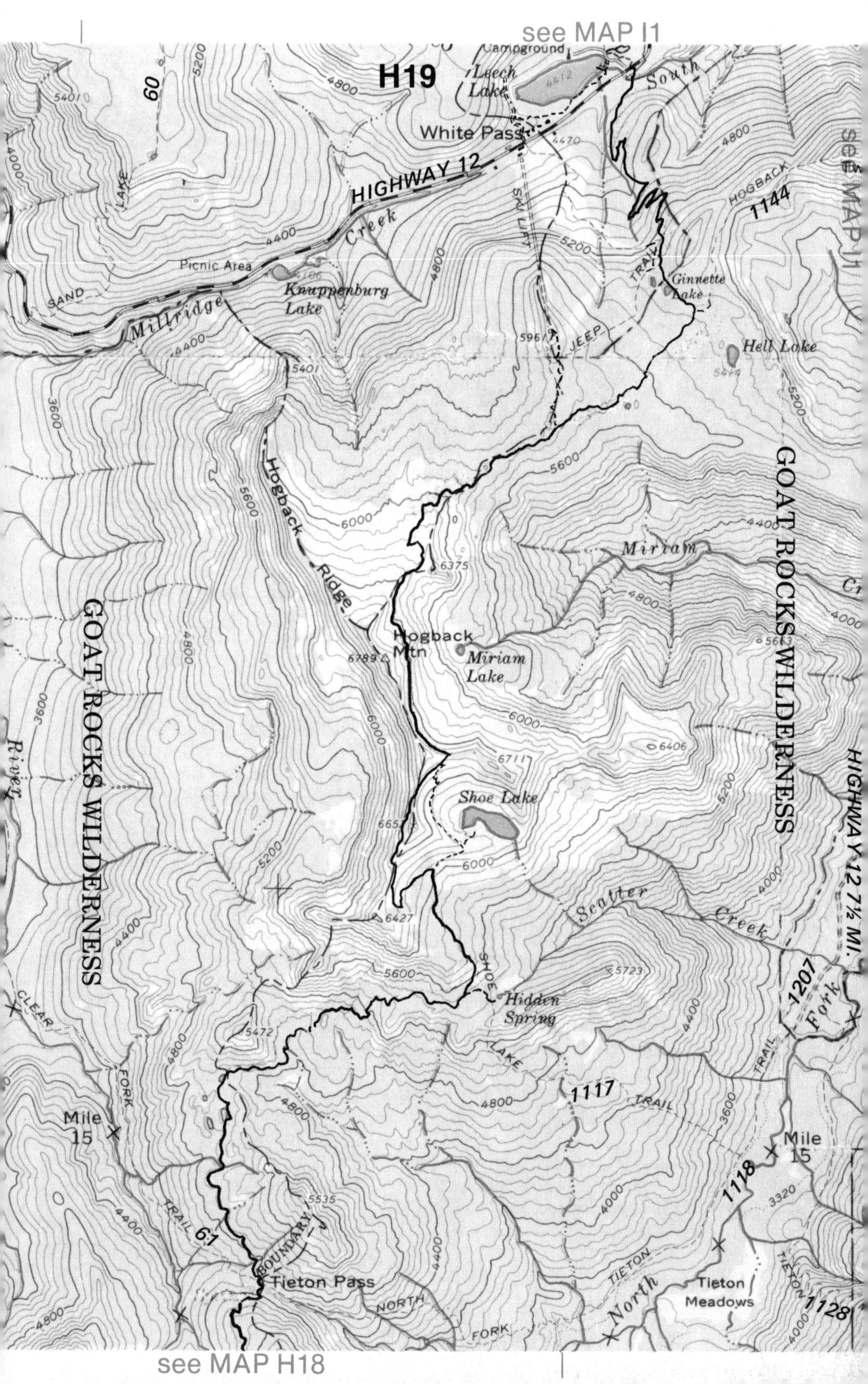

see MAP H18

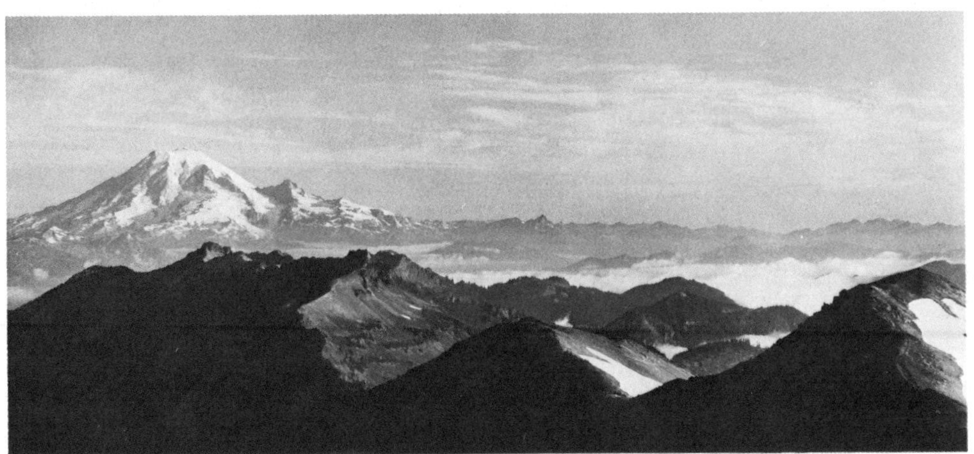

Mt. Rainier above the Chimney Rock-Elk Pass crest

path that takes you past eight stagnant ponds. You could have an adequate campsite at any of them. After leaving the last pond (5070–2.8) on the left (west), you hike around the west slope of a knoll, descend gently to the west side of a broad saddle, and then climb moderately to a switchback (5220–1.6), from which Trail 121 descends to Walupt Lake Horse Camp. Now within Goat Rocks Wilderness, the trail climbs east to a saddle (5450–0.7) and passes two small ponds on the left. Then it climbs north to a prominent ridgecrest (5600–0.8) that stands directly south of Walupt Lake (3926). North, you see the glistening summit of Old Snowy Mountain (7930) in the heart of the Goat Rocks country, over whose slopes you must soon climb.

The route now winds southeastward down auxiliary ridges and enters a forest of mountain hemlock, western white and lodgepole pines, and Alaska yellow cedar. You pass near two undesirable ponds before crossing a trickling creek (5140–1.4) that you shouldn't overlook, for it contains the best water you'll taste for miles. After descending gently eastward, you curve counterclockwise around boggy Coleman Weedpatch to a 50-yard pond (5050–0.5).

Side route. An old trail east from the pond goes to a nearby, shallow lake (5058) on a forested, flat saddle immediately within the Yakima Indian Reservation.

On the PCT, you arc eastward, north of the unseen lake, and then follow the easy path northeast, through a dense mountain-hemlock forest across the lower slopes of Lakeview Mountain (6660). As the trail veers east, the forest transforms into an open stand of lodgepoles, and the path finally curves southeast to a junction with Walupt Lake Trail 101 (4960–3.4).

Side route. This goes 4.4 miles to its trailhead at Walupt Lake Campground. You will find several fair-to-good campsites ⅓ to ½ mile down this trail.

Beyond the junction, the countryside is quite open, and the topography stretches out below as you hike the trail up the west slope of a long, north-trending ridge. Fireweed, yarrow, lupine, and pearly everlasting proliferate along the trailside before you reach the shady confines of a coniferous forest. Now you contour for several miles before reaching the diminutive headwaters of Walupt Creek (5480–3.9). If there were enough level ground here, a primitive campsite by the stream would be nice. Instead, it is better to continue west up toward a saddle where you'll see shallow, clear, 130-yard-long Sheep Lake (5710), which has good campsites. Just north of it, you meet a junction with Nannie Ridge Trail 98 (5760–0.6).

Side route. This trail descends 4.5 miles to its trailhead at mile-long Walupt Lake.

See maps H15, H16, H17

▮ *Your route through the Goat Rocks country will take you on ridges high above glaciated canyons. Walupt Creek canyon was the first major one you've seen in this wilderness, and the ones north of it are even more spectacular.* ▮ From this junction, you descend ⅓ mile before diagonaling up a mid-1970s stretch of PCT to a crest saddle (6100–1.4). Now in Yakima Indian territory, you traverse north across barren slopes that have snow patches through most of the summer. The trail steepens as it approaches often-snowbound Cispus Pass (6460–0.9), where you leave the Indian reservation.

The timberline trail drops north and passes by dwarfed specimens of mountain hemlock and subalpine fir as it descends toward the headwaters of the Cispus River. The basin is much smaller than it first appears, and you quickly reach an open campsite beside the easternmost tributary (6130–0.6). ▮ *The scale of the canyon is put in true perspective when backpackers hike past miniature conifers that are now seen as only 30 feet high instead of as 80, as you might suppose.* ▮ After descending west, jump across the base of a splashing, 20-foot-high waterfall and then make a winding contour to a junction with Trail 86 (5930–1.6).

Side route. This trail goes 0.6 mile west down to wind-shielded Bypass Camp on the east side of Snowgrass Creek. Westward, the trail continues 0.2 mile to Trail 96, which offers the shortest route into the Goat Rocks area. Northward, Trail 96 connects with the PCT north of your Trail-86 junction. Southwestward, Trail 96 goes about 3 miles to a fork from which the south branch goes over to a nearby hikers' trailhead on spur road 405, and the north branch goes about ⅓ mile farther to an equestrians' trailhead near the end of Road 2150.

Leaving the Trail-86 junction, the PCT switchbacks up to a saddle, traverses slopes above Snowgrass Flat, and arrives at a junction with Trail 96 (6420–1.0). After a fairly steep climb north for 0.2 mile, you pass the old junction with the abandoned route of the old Trail 96, which is about 40 yards from a 40-foot-high "Split Rock." ▮ *This broke apart eons ago, for full-sized conifers now grow in the gap between the two halves.* ▮ The route next climbs north-northeast up past the rock and then switchbacks west over to a nearby ridge. From about this point north to Elk Pass and then east to the saddle above McCall Basin, you can expect to find quite a number of snowfields through most of the summer. About ¾ mile past the newer Trail-96 junction, you tread across rocks with deep striations, convincing "fingerprints" of past glaciers. Climbing up to the low west ridge of Old Snowy Mountain, you find the Dana May Yelverton Shelter (7040–1.1), 12 feet square, which provides plenty of protection from the frequent summer storms (no fires allowed). Sometimes the shelter needs periodic repair, and without it the shelter might provide no shelter at all. The 6-inch-high junipers here attest to the severity of this environment. Above lies the realm of rock and ice, the habitat of the alpine mountaineer.

As you climb briefly north from the shelter, you may see one or two low windbreaks, neither giving you much protection if you are caught in a storm. Crossing a snowfield takes you to the brink of the severely glaciated, 3000-foot-deep Upper Lake Creek canyon. ▮ *This canyon will become even more impressive as this northbound trail provides even better views down and across it. To the northwest you see usually frozen Goat Lake (6450) nestled in a classic glacial cirque at the southeast end of the Johnson Peak ridge.* ▮ At this brink, ¼ mile beyond the shelter, the official PCT route traverses northeast along the gentle, upper slopes of the Packwood Glacier. Typically, this leg is mostly snowbound and potentially dangerous; the older PCT route, given as an alternate below, is sometimes passable for stock. When you start across these slopes, you leave the second highest PCT point in Washington—7080 feet. ▮ *Before 1978, hikers left the official PCT route at this brink to traverse cross-country northeast across these slopes rather than climb 550 feet higher on the official PCT to the north shoulder (7630) of Old Snowy Mountain (7930). In 1978 the Forest Service blasted this newer route that more or less follows the old cross-country one.* ▮

Official PCT route. The newer PCT route cuts rather precariously across the upper part of Packwood Glacier before curving north down to a crest saddle (6850–1.0), where it rejoins the alternate route, below.

See maps H17, H18

Alternate route. In a way, it is unfortunate that the old trail up Old Snowy is not taken by everyone, for from it you have an almost full-circle panorama of the Goat Rocks country. From this brink, the old Cascade Crest route makes short switchbacks eastward for 0.8 mile to the north shoulder of Old Snowy Mountain. Up there, at 7630 feet, you are almost as high as on the alternate hikers' route along Crater Lake's rim (Section C). From that point, you then have a steep descent 0.6 mile north to a saddle where you meet the newer PCT route. ▮ *Looking above the canyons to the northwest, you see the monarch of the Cascade Range, mighty Mt. Rainier (14,410), ruling above all the other stratovolcanoes. To the south is Mt. Adams (12,276), the crown prince and third highest peak in the range (California's Mt. Shasta, at 14,162 feet, rivals Mt. Rainier in size). Off to Adams' west lies the youthful, one-time princess, Mt. St. Helens (8364); before Mt. St. Helens (8364) blew its top off in 1980, it was a symmetrical peak 9677 feet in elevation. The Multnomah Indians had a legend about Mts. Adams and St. Helens and about Mt. Hood (11,235), the Cascades' fourth highest peak. They said a feud developed between Klickitat (Adams) and Wyeast (Hood) over the beautiful Squaw Mountain (pre-1980 St. Helens), who had just moved into the neighborhood. (In geological terms, Mt. St. Helens is the youngest of these stratovolcanoes.) She loved Wyeast, but Klickitat triumphed in a fight, so she had to reside in Klickitat's domain. She refused to bed down with him, however, and after a while, as would be expected, his flames of love for her died, and both volcanoes became dormant. A modern-day account would say she couldn't stand Klickitat any longer, so finally, on May 18, 1980, she blew her top. Literally. You'll find traces of Mt. St. Helens' ashes along the PCT in much of this section.* ▮

This Egg Butte section of the PCT, constructed with heroic efforts in 1953–54, now continues along the jagged ridge, contours around its "teeth," and provides alpine views across McCall Glacier toward Tieton Peak (7768), due east of Old Snowy. You reach a small saddle from which the trail makes a precarious descent across a steep slope as it bypasses summit 7210. You can expect this narrow footpath to be snowbound and hazardous through most of July. Crampons may be required, particularly in early summer, and stock animals may be forced back. Reaching the ridge again, you follow it down to Elk Pass, where you meet the upper end of Coyote Trail 79 (6680–1.3). ▮ *Here, the windswept whitebark pines stand chest-high at most, and the junipers creep but inches above the frost-wedged rocks.* ▮

Pushing toward supplies at White Pass, you first drop northwest, paralleling Coyote Trail 79, below you, and then in ⅓ mile angle east across the sometimes-snowy north slopes of Peak 6768. You trade breathtaking views down Upper Lake Creek canyon to the northwest for views north down larger Clear Fork Cowlitz River canyon. Just below the peak's northeast ridge, the trail reaches bleak, undesirable alpine campsites (6320–0.3). If you're hiking south, these are the last campsites you'll see until the west flank of Old Snowy.

The trail descends east-southeast to the foot of the Elk Pass snowfield, down which hikers sometimes ski. Cross its runoff creek and several others, pass by glacially striated bedrock, and then slip and slide down short, steep switchbacks etched on a narrow ridge. The grade abates and ends near a small pond at the foot of another snowfield. By late afternoon, the snowfields in this basin are melting at a good rate, as evidenced by the roar of the cascade to the west. From the pond, you switchback steeply but briefly up to a saddle (5820–1.3). The Cascade Crest Trail formerly dropped east-southeast from here to wet, meadowy, overused McCall Basin, but the PCT switchbacks east. It almost touches a crest saddle (5580–0.6), on which you could set up an emergency camp, and then it switchbacks down into forest cover to a junction with the old Cascade Crest Trail (5200–0.5).

Side route. Following the Cascade Crest Trail about ¼ mile southwest would take you down to McCall Basin.

On the PCT, you traverse over to a saddle that holds knee-deep Lutz Lake and several small campsites (5100–0.6). Beyond this viewless spot, the trail descends north around the west slope of Peak 5493 to Tieton Pass (4570–1.0) and a junction by a dry campsite.

See maps H18, H19

Water access. From this junction, North Fork Tieton Trail 1118, which at 4.6 miles is the shortest trail approach to this pass, descends east before curving northeast down to North Fork Tieton Road 1207. You can usually find creek water by descending about ¼ mile along this trail.

Side route. Also from this junction, Clear Fork Trail 61, starting a moderate descent west-northwest from Tieton Pass, takes a long way out toward U.S. Highway 12.

The PCT starts a gentle descent northwest, gradually makes a winding route north past two stagnant ponds, crosses east over the divide (4930–1.5), and rounds Peak 5472. Now you continue on this viewless path east until it climbs the southeast spur of Peak 6427 and reaches a junction with Trail 1117 (5520–1.8).

Side route. This first goes about 280 yards east to the abandoned northern segment of the Shoe Lake Trail. On that trail, you can head southeast about a similar distance to an area with several small campsites. One or more short spur trails in this vicinity head east to Hidden Spring, which lies just above a beautiful meadow. Note that this is your last real opportunity for camping and for good water this side of U.S. Highway 12, about 8.5 trail miles from the spring.

On the PCT, climb north and then northwest, and where an old segment of the PCT bends northeast, branch west (6040–0.9) on a newer segment. This first curves southwest as it climbs toward Peak 6427 and then curves north, leaving forest cover as it approaches a ridge. Cross this and then traverse steep slopes on the west side of Peak 6652. These at first are bouldery and open, offering views west into steep Clear Fork Cowlitz River canyon, whose floor lies a half mile below the trail. Boulders give way to firs and hemlocks and, through midsummer, some snow problems. Soon you recross the ridge and have views southeast of Shoe Lake as you contour over to the old Shoe Lake segment of the PCT. ▮ *Overuse at the lake led to the creation of the newer, less desirable route.* ▮ You meet the old segment, which still switchbacks down to the lake (no camping allowed!), and then in 90 yards top a narrow ridge (6620–1.2). From it, you see Mt. Rainier poking its head above Hogback Ridge, while Mt. Adams just manages to lift its crown above Goat Rocks.

▮ *The volcanic flows around here superficially resemble sedimentary rocks, for they have broken along close, evenly spaced horizontal joints to give the illusion of alternating, stepped beds of sandstone and shale.* ▮ You make one switchback, descend a well-graded trail past a thumb above you and Miriam Lake below you, and then reach the stepped slope of Hogback Mountain (6789). Descending its northeast ridge, you obtain more views of Mt. Rainier. Then you enter forest once again, cross a vaguely defined saddle, and climb gently to a nearby junction with Trail 1112 (5830–2.5).

From the junction, the PCT makes a viewless, winding descent northeastward to a junction with little-used Hogback Trail 1144 (5400–1.2), which starts on a gentle descent east before curving north. The trail curves northwest, passes a small, stagnant pond, and reaches green, 100-yard-long Ginnette Lake (5400–0.2). You now leave Goat Rocks Wilderness, get a glimpse of the chairlift jeep road northwest of the trail, and then switchback down to a trailhead parking lot 50 yards south of U.S. Highway 12 (old State Highway 14) (4405–2.2). (From the highway, the short road to the trailhead begins just 30 yards east of, and on the other side of the highway from, the Leech Lake spur road to White Pass Campground.)

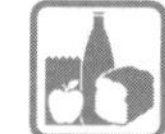

Resupply access. About 200 yards up the Leech Lake spur road, where it bends from west to north, an old, closed road starts south and then quickly bends southwest for a rambling traverse over to White Pass Village, reaching a north-south road that starts from the west side of the village. This usually soggy, mosquito-ridden route is supposedly for campers, hikers, and equestrians, but author Schaffer much prefers walking southwest along the broad highway shoulder to reach the Kracker Barrel Grocery and White Pass Village.

See map H19

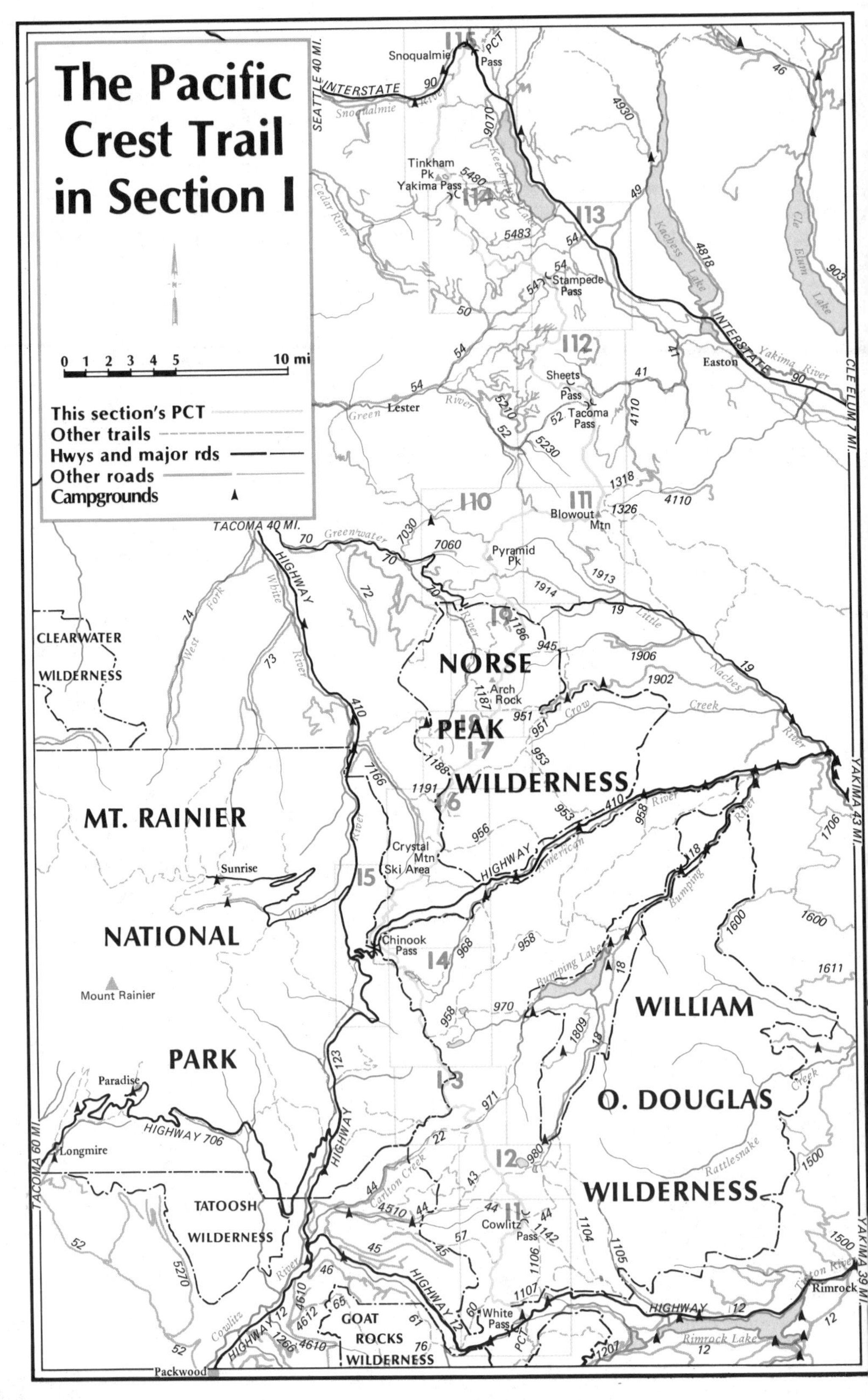

The Pacific Crest Trail in Section I
0 1 2 3 4 5 10 mi
This section's PCT
Other trails
Hwys and major rds
Other roads
Campgrounds
Snoqualmie Pass
PCT
SEATTLE 40 MI.
INTERSTATE 90
Tinkham Pk
Yakima Pass
Stampede Pass
Sheets Pass
Tacoma Pass
Lester
Easton
Kachess Lake
Cle Elum Lake
Yakima River
CLE ELUM 7 MI.
Blowout Mtn
Pyramid Pk
TACOMA 40 MI.
CLEARWATER WILDERNESS
NORSE PEAK WILDERNESS
Arch Rock
MT. RAINIER NATIONAL PARK
Sunrise
Mount Rainier
Crystal Mtn Ski Area
Chinook Pass
Bumping Lake
WILLIAM O. DOUGLAS WILDERNESS
YAKIMA 43 MI.
Paradise
Longmire
HIGHWAY 706
TACOMA 60 MI.
TATOOSH WILDERNESS
GOAT ROCKS WILDERNESS
Cowlitz Pass
White Pass
Rimrock
Rimrock Lake
YAKIMA 39 MI.
Packwood

Section I:
Highway 12 near White Pass to Interstate 90 at Snoqualmie Pass

Introduction: Graphic contrasts in land use separate this section into two very different segments. The southern half is largely a subalpine parkland glistening with lakes cupped in forests and meadows. Most of this backcountry lies protected within the boundaries of two wilderness areas and Mt. Rainier National Park. The northern half, on the other hand, being lower, is totally within the montane forest belt so favored by the lumber industry, and it blisters with a lot of barren earth, some of the most extensively clearcut land in the West.

Moderate topography characterizes both halves of this section, and fit border-bound hikers can make good time. From White Pass, the trail sloshes through soggy muskeg country, crossing a plateau pocked with pools and lakes. As the Cascade divide rises into a knobby backbone, the trail follows it faithfully, swinging from saddle to subalpine saddle, passing within 12 miles of massive Mt. Rainier. Not quite one-third of the way through this section, at Chinook Pass, the broadest of these flower-rich saddles, State Highway 410 crosses the crest.

Halfway through this section, the craggy divide slopes below the subalpine zone, and though fir and hemlock forests dominate here, meadows and crest-top vistas keep the hiking varied and interesting. Still 40 miles from Snoqualmie Pass, the trail enters land shared in a checkerboard pattern by the Forest Service, Weyerhauser, and Plum Creek, the land-holdings subsidiary of Burlington Northern railroad. The railroad received title to every other square mile during the railroad subsidies of the 1880s in return for laying tracks across Stampede Pass. Neither owner being fully responsible for the territory, the forests have been mined, and nearly one half of this last stretch goes through clearcuts laced with logging roads and bulldozer tracks. By 1984, most of the timber-company sections that the PCT passes through had been logged and the trail permanently rerouted through them. By 2000, the Forest Service began acquiring private land, and hopefully in a few years all of Section I's PCT will be on public land.

Declination: 19½°E

Points on Route	S➛N	Mi. Btwn. Pts.	N➛S
Highway 12 near White Pass	0.0		99.0
Buesch Lake	5.9	5.9	93.1
Bumping River ford by Bumping Lake Trail	14.6	8.7	84.4
Dewey Lake	26.3	11.7	72.7
Highway 410 at Chinook Pass	29.5	3.2	69.5
Sheep Lake	31.7	2.2	67.3
Big Crow Basin Spring near Norse Peak Trail	40.2	8.5	58.8
Arch Rock shelter spur trail	47.3	7.1	51.7
Camp Urich at Government Meadow 5	2.3	5.0	46.7

Unnamed spring 2.1 miles NE of Windy Gap	57.1	4.8	41.9
Granite Creek Trail on Blowout Mountain	63.1	6.0	35.9
Sheets Pass	71.1	8.0	27.9
Stampede Pass	80.4	9.3	18.6
Stirrup Creek	85.5	5.1	13.5
Mirror Lake	89.9	4.4	9.1
Lodge Lake	96.8	6.9	2.2
Interstate 90 at Snoqualmie Pass	99.0	2.2	0.0

Supplies: For White Pass, see "Supplies" in the previous chapter. For Snoqualmie Pass, see "Supplies" in the next chapter.

Wilderness Permits: No wilderness permits are required along this section, unless you venture some distance west of the PCT into Mt. Rainier National Park.

Problems: Mosquitoes can be especially bad in the marshy terrain north of White Pass. On the crest-top route between Government Meadow and Stampede Pass, though, water is scarce, partly because logging has obliterated some springs. By mid-July, only one reliable water source can be found for the last 23 miles of this stretch, and even it is somewhat inconvenient. In early season, snow clinging to north and east slopes between Bumping River and Blowout Mountain can make carrying an ice ax worthwhile.

In some of the logged areas, blowdowns and generally battered soil make following the trail less than easy, although few hikers get off-route. The trail crosses many logging roads and follows a few for very short distances. *Most* of these crossings and followings are clearly posted with PCT emblems or diamonds, but a few might require a brief search.

Maps:

White Pass, WA
Cougar Lake, WA
Chinook Pass, WA
White River Park, WA (PCT barely enters map)
Norse Peak, WA
Noble Knob, WA
Raven Roost, WA
Lester, WA
Blowout Mountain, WA
Stampede Pass, WA
Lost Lake, WA
Snoqualmie Pass, WA

THE ROUTE

Hikers driving to White Pass will want to turn north off Highway 12 just 0.5 mile northeast of White Pass and park, after 0.2 mile, at the trailhead parking lot near Leech Lake. The PCT crosses Highway 12 only 30 yards east of the Leech Lake PCT trailhead turnoff and passes an old shelter on its way to this parking lot.

Pulverized duff and "trail apples" evince this trail section's popularity with equestrians as you start from the lot (4415–0.2) in a gentle, switchbacking climb before entering William O. Douglas Wilderness. ▮ *A staunch conservationist, the late U.S. Supreme Court Justice Douglas grew up near Yakima, and he hiked throughout his life in the lands now named after him, loving the area enough, despite his world travels, to establish his home in Goose Prairie, on the Bumping River.* ▮ After leveling out in the fir-and-spruce forest, you pass a junction with Dark Meadows Trail 1107 (4780–1.1), which descends east to Dog Lake. Resuming a gradual climb, you skirt a meadow, rise beside and then cross Deer Lake's out-

See maps I1,

see MAP I2

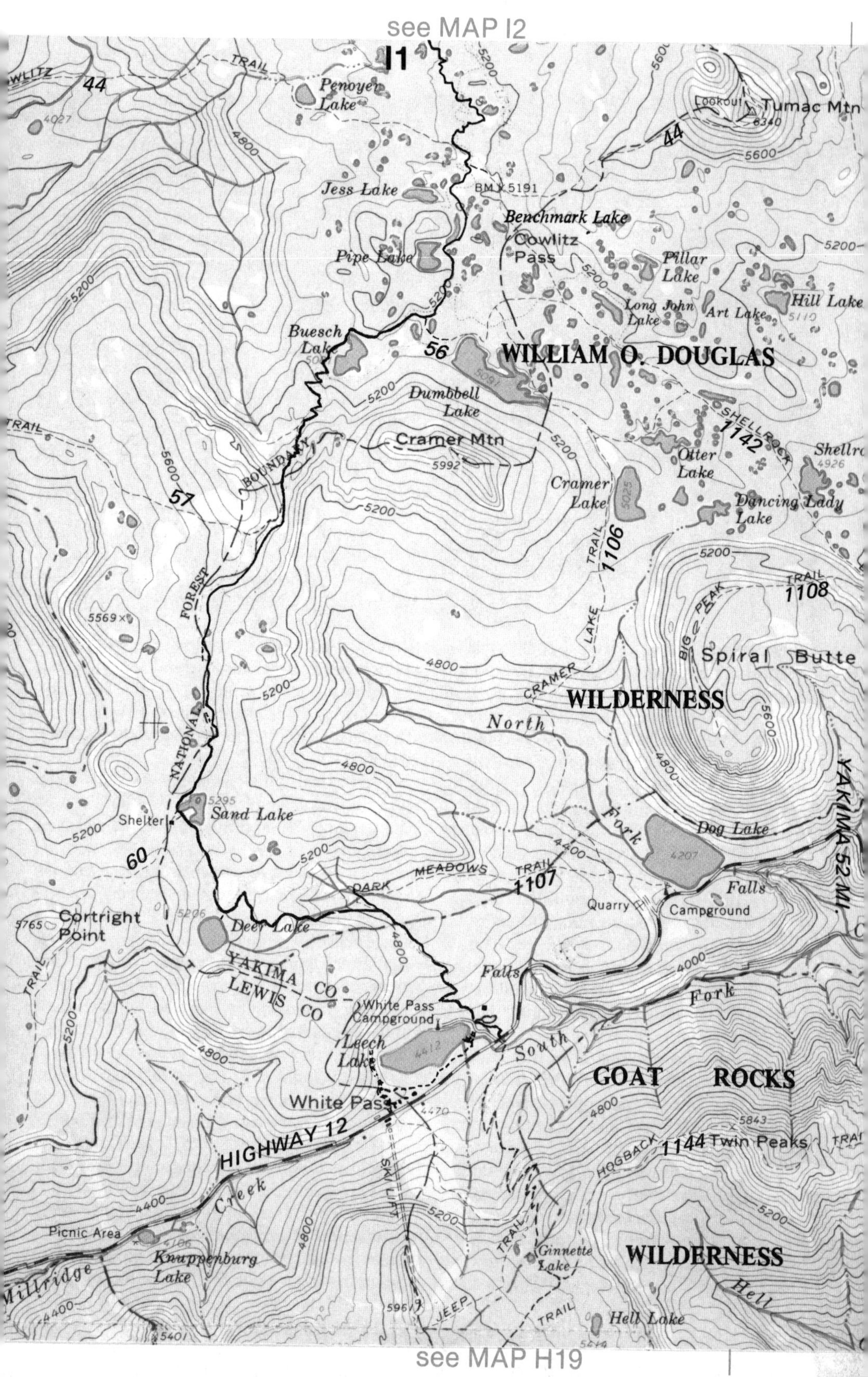

see MAP H19

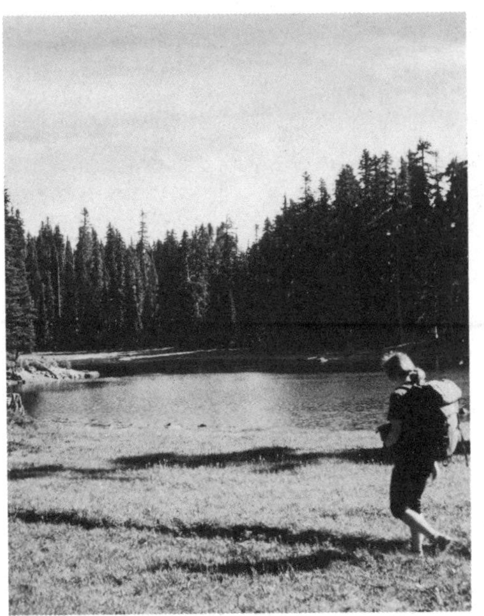

Sand Lake

let creek, and switchback up to a much larger meadow just before reaching Deer Lake (5206–1.0). Here, there is an extensive and beaten-down camping area.

Ahead, a barely ascending walk north through forest and lupine-rich glades brings you to Sand Lake (5295–0.5) where, from the base of the lake's peninsula, a spur leads south to a shelter that's barely large enough to sleep three. Just beyond this spur, a sign points west to Highway 12, along obscure Sand Lake Trail 60. The PCT, however, continues north on an essentially level track, past the curious spikes of beargrass, to meet Cortright Creek Trail 57 (5520–2.0) coming from the southwest. Under subalpine firs, the trail contours around a rocky knob to a gap, where it starts winding down a few steep switchbacks.

The brief descent ends at Buesch Lake (5081–1.1), entry point onto the heart of the plateau that caps this part of the gentle divide between the Cowlitz and Yakima rivers. ▮ *Andesite lavas erupted in the Pliocene and Pleistocene epochs to form this plateau, and during the cooler Pleistocene, a small ice cap formed over it and helped smooth it out.* ▮ For half a dozen miles now, the trail runs across hummocky flatlands riddled with ponds, puddles, mudholes, and muskeg. Patchily forested with droopy hemlocks and pointy subalpine firs, and carpeted with heather, huckleberry, and azalea, this area supports only acid-tolerant plants.

Turn east along the north shore of Buesch Lake and soon come to Dumbbell Lake Trail 56, which forks south between two pools. From here, you curve north to pass within close view of Pipe Lake and then pass a long, slender lake with a good picnic spot (5180–1.1). A few minutes north from here, the trail arcs northeast around a couple of grassy ponds and arrives at ill-defined Cowlitz Pass (5160–0.5). In this open area, snags from an old fire stand over spiraea and azalea and allow a view of Mt. Rainier. Trail 44 heads east from here for Shellrock Lake; this trail briefly joins the PCT northward.

The PCT soon turns northwest, leaves the westbound stretch of Cowlitz Trail 44 (5140–0.2) behind, and starts a twisting, winding course, first northeast and then trending northwest. Although the topo map shows almost no contours through here, dozens of hillocks and gullies dimple this land, and the trail takes great pains to avoid every hint of meadow or soggy ground. On the way, you pass just north of one unnamed lake and wind into dark forest and then down to Snow Lake (4935–2.1).

You cross a bridge over Snow Lake's outlet and weave a north-trending course, barely descending. Peeking in and out of fir groves, you come to Twin Sisters Trail 980, tracking east, and then intersect Pothole Trail 45 (4900–0.8), which to the south meets Trail 44 and to the north parallels the PCT some distance east of you. Still avoiding meadows while trending north-northwest, you hike just west of a creek that is gradually gathering water and momentum. The track channels into a steady, gentle descent as you pass the forested slopes of Fryingpan Mountain and a junction with southbound Jug Lake Trail 43. With more easy walking, you come to a bridge over the creek, at a packer campsite (4620–2.9).

From this bridge, the PCT skirts east of a large meadow and decidedly drops off the Cowlitz-Yakima plateau. The steady descent ends at the outlet of Fish Lake (4100–1.1), headwaters of the Bumping River. Across this creek is a large campsite and a junction with Bumping Lake Trail 971, where the PCT cuts

See maps I1, I2, I3

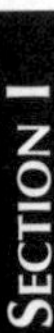

west to touch the north shore of long, shallow Fish Lake. The PCT promptly leaves the lakeside path and starts working up long switchbacks that take you above Buck Lake, across Crag Lake's outlet, and then back to a spur that drops to Crag Lake itself, where there are some comfortable campsites. As the PCT contours just beyond this spur, it passes a reliable, drinkable rill (5170–2.7).

A couple more long, lazy switchbacks have you rising across meadowy slopes verdant with aster, spiraea, blueberry, and corn lily. Marveling at Mts. Rainier, Adams, and St. Helens, you then turn north around the Cascade divide and pass Laughingwater Trail 22 (5690–1.6), which drops southwest. ▮ *Here, at the start of a long tour high along the Cascade backbone, you can, in good weather, look forward to miles of glorious, expansive views; in bad weather, you'll find yourself shrouded in clouds, exposed to the brunt of wet, westerly storms.* ▮

Contouring now, you soon recross the divide to traverse above One Lake and eventually meet Trail 380 (5660–1.6), which descends 0.3 mile to Two Lakes. Next, the trail makes a quick climb back to the west side, where Mt. Rainier's overwhelming presence hardly lets you notice the many wildflowers underfoot, of which partridge foot is the most common flower. Along here there's a junction with Cougar Lakes Trail 958A, which heads back over the crest. You start another long traverse, contouring through forest and meadow across a couple of spur ridges before dropping via abrupt switchbacks to a saddle and a junction with American Ridge Trail 958 (5320–2.6), which departs eastward. Just past this junction, there's a campsite, although finding water here requires a bit of a walk downhill. ▮ *Here, you look down the long, forested (and previously glaciated) valley of the American River.* ▮

Now the PCT makes a brief climb north to cross a crest saddle and then contours through subalpine-fir groves before winding down to visit Anderson Lake (5340–1.4), just within Mt. Rainier National Park. It has a nice campsite, and you don't need a permit to camp at it. Continuing north, the trail barely climbs as it crosses a seasonal trickle, traverses scree, and rounds a spur ridge. It then arcs down toward Dewey Lake, first meeting Dewey Way Trail 968A, which splits northeast to connect with Trail 968. Just beyond the junction, Dewey Lake's expansive waters and numerous campsites along the shore-hugging PCT invite a pause (5112–1.8); be aware, however, that no campfires are allowed within ¼ mile of the lake.

After rounding Dewey Lake's shore and bridging its inlet, the route passes Dewey Lake

See maps I3, I4

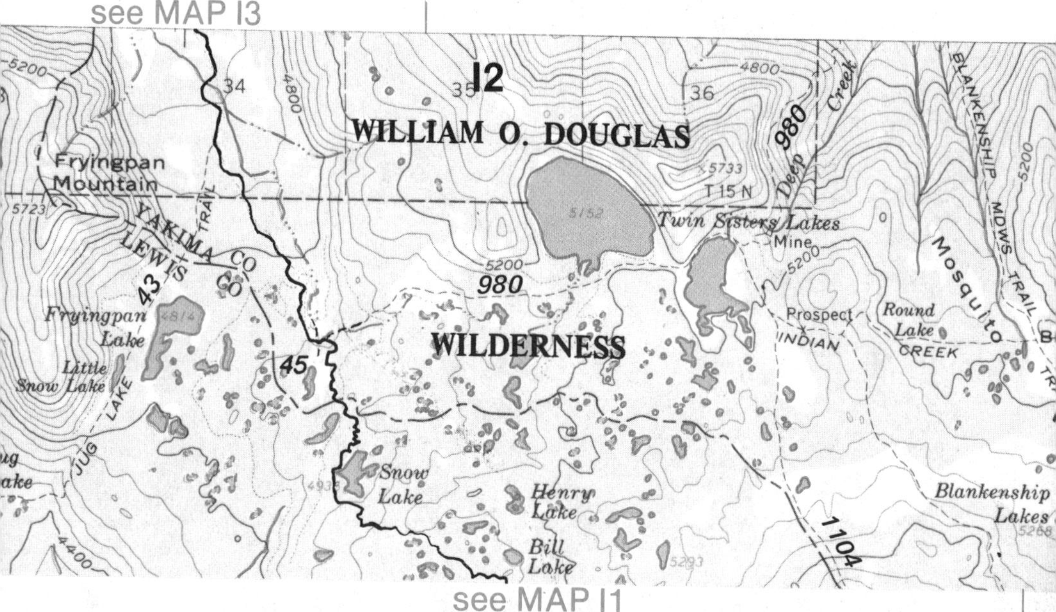

Trail 968 (5130–0.5), which branches east to the American River valley. Then the PCT climbs out of the soggy lake basin, working west through dark forest before emerging onto meadowland. After this, the trail switchbacks and immediately meets the Tipsoo Lake Trail, a dayhiker's path that reaches Highway 410 only ⅓ mile south of Chinook Pass. ▮ *Here is an introduction to some amazingly colorful flora. Paintbrushes, pasqueflowers, lupines, avalanche lilies, and a galaxy of other blossoms spill over the PCT.* ▮ The trail tops the rise and then descends, first abruptly and then in a long traverse past a tarn, to Highway 410's fairly steady traffic at Chinook Pass (5432–2.7). In this vicinity, there are junctions with a spur trail to the highway's rest area and a trail to Tipsoo Lake. ▮ *From Chinook Pass, it's 68 miles east to Yakima, 41 miles northwest to Enumclaw, and 34 miles southwest to Paradise, the starting point for the challenging "standard" route to the top of Mt. Rainier.* ▮

Water access. For water, take the trail which leaves the pass` for a ⅓-mile descent to a picnic area beside Tipsoo Lake.

Beyond the footbridge over the highway, the PCT turns north onto an old roadbed, crosses a bench, and then, once more a trail, approaches traffic as it makes a rising traverse. ▮ *This steep slope supports a scrubbier flora than that at Chinook Pass proper. Fireweed, huckleberry, manzanita, pearly everlasting, and bedraggled Alaska cedars, hardy plants all, testify to tougher conditions.* ▮ The gradual ascent turns up a ravine and then steepens into a couple of switchbacks before reaching Sheep Lake (5750–2.2), a popular spot for dayhikers and overnighters. After following the lakeshore for a bit, the PCT starts upslope, weaving and switchbacking generally northeast across meadowy bowls and up into ptarmigan and pika country. It then traverses under small

See maps 14, 15, 16

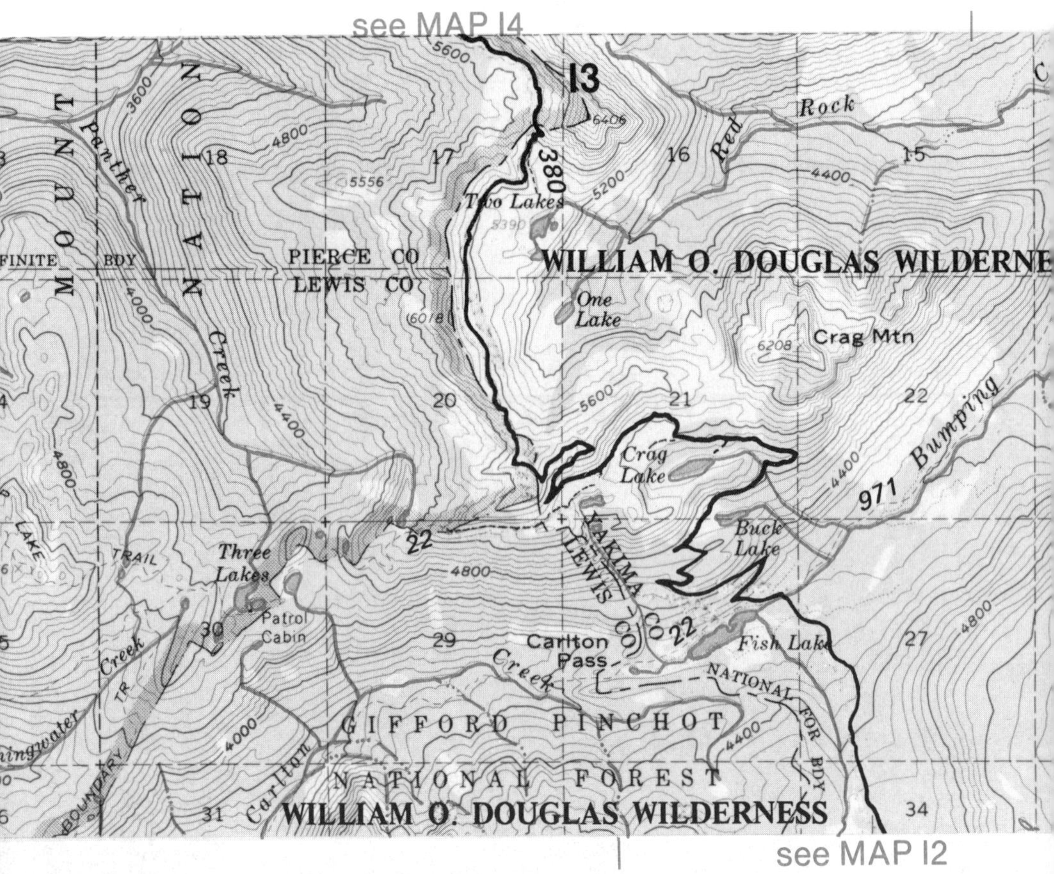

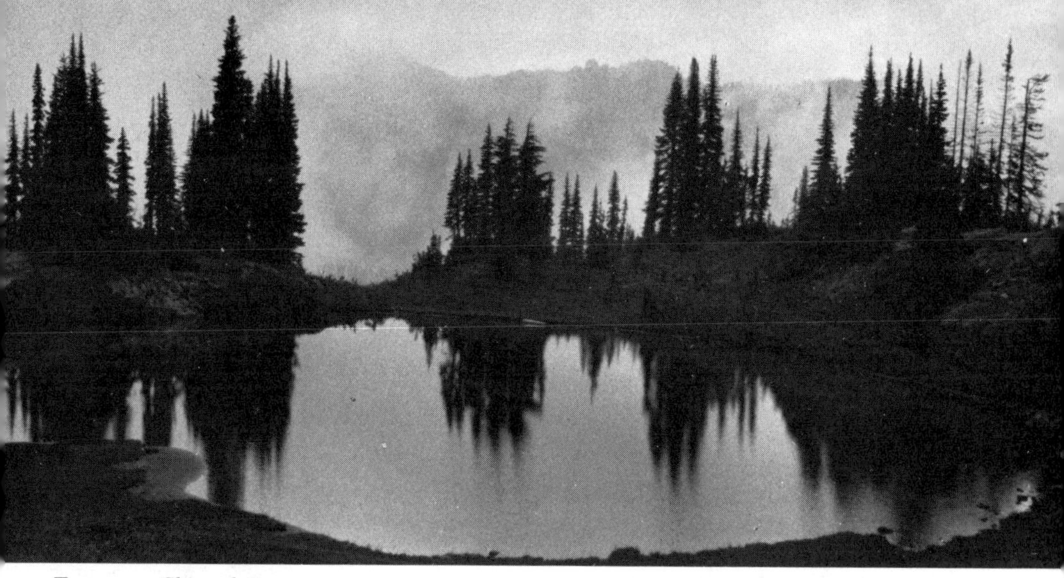

Tarn near Chinook Pass

crags to Sourdough Gap (6440–1.2). ▮ *The names of this saddle and of other features to the north recall the gold and silver prospectors who worked this region.* ▮ Just after the gap, you may find a trail climbing northwest.

Admiring Mts. Adams and St. Helens, you can savor here the start of another long stretch of high traverse, which is wonderfully scenic if the weather is good. Skidding down scree off the gap, you come to an unsigned spur at the first switchback, and, after another hairpin, settle into a long, gently descending traverse near treeline. Placer Lake comes into view 600 feet below as you approach Bear Gap, where you find a major trail plexus (5882–2.1). ▮ *From here, Silver Creek Trail 1192 drops northwest to civilization at Crystal Mountain Ski Area, Hen Skin Lake Trail 1193 starts a traverse*

See map I6

Sourdough Gap

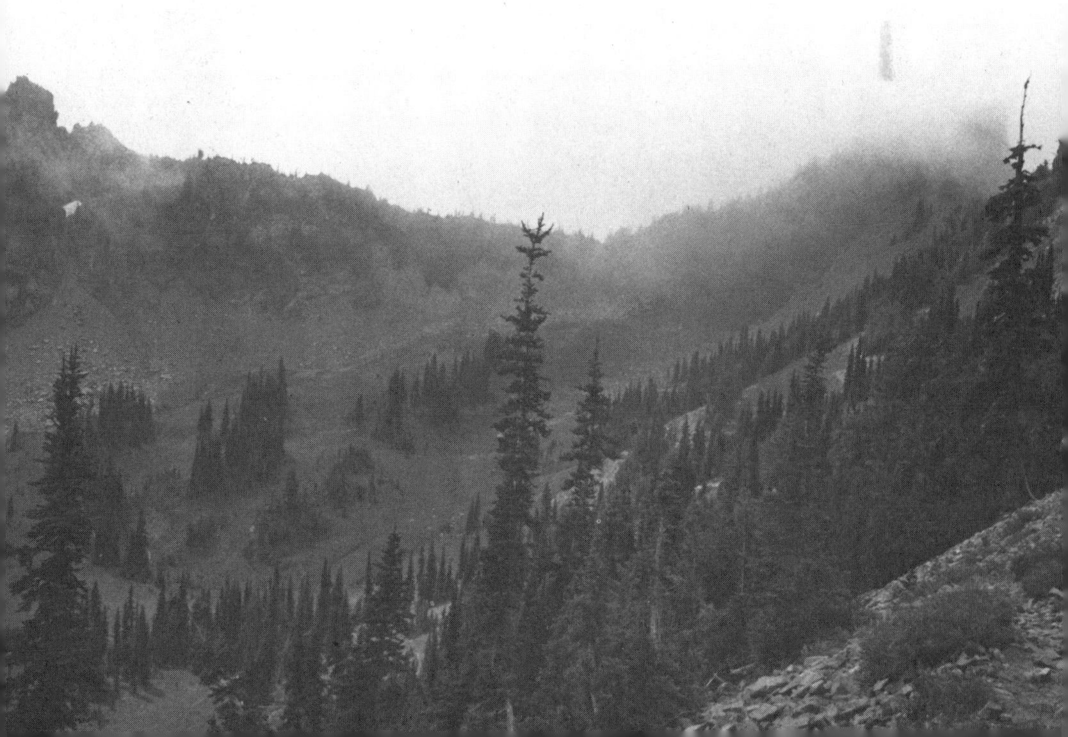

southwest, and Bear Gap Trail 967 comes up from Morse Creek and Highway 410 to the east. ▮ You, however, take the PCT in a slant across the gap and then contour north, viewing ski lifts and condominiums well below, until the PCT turns southeast on its way around the steep flanks of Pickhandle Point.

Next, the trail angles back across the crest at Pickhandle Gap and promptly meets a trail (6040–1.1) dropping east and bound for Fog City and Gold Hill. Then the PCT rises along the open south slopes of Crown Point and, at the breathtaking crest between Crown Point and Gold Hill, reaches the southern boundary of Norse Peak Wilderness. Here, there's a junction with two other trails (6200–0.3), one following the ridgecrest east to Gold Hill and the other, Union Creek Trail 956, dropping north off the crest 50 yards west of where you gain it. Follow the PCT on a steady climb west and then north around Crown Point, before long coming onto the narrow watershed divide at Blue Bell Pass (6390–0.4).

From this saddle, the trail contours north, and, as it approaches the spur dividing Pickhandle and Bullion basins, it intersects an unsigned path. The lower track drops steeply into Bullion Basin, while the upper one climbs to the top of summit 6479. Contour around this summit, which takes you to narrow Bullion Pass. Balancing astride this narrow saddle, you first meet a steep, unsigned trail crossing the ridge and then meet Bullion Basin Trail 1156 (6150–0.9) descending to the west. As the crest rises to a summit again, you ascend along its west flank in a long, meadow traverse to Scout Pass (6530–1.5). ▮ *Here, you have a view across Lake Basin's gentle parkland, bossed over by one of the area's larger crags.* ▮

A gentle descent leads you across the head of Lake Basin, and you first pass a trail that beelines down into the basin and then a designated trail (6390–0.6).

Side route. This trail descends to excellent camping at Basin Lake, ½ mile below.

You round the northeast spur of Norse Peak and descend into Big Crow Basin. As you near the bottomland at the head of this basin, you pass 30 feet above a welcome and reliable spring (6290–0.4). Some 40 yards beyond this, you meet the junction with Norse Peak Trail

See map 16

Lake Basin and Basin Lake

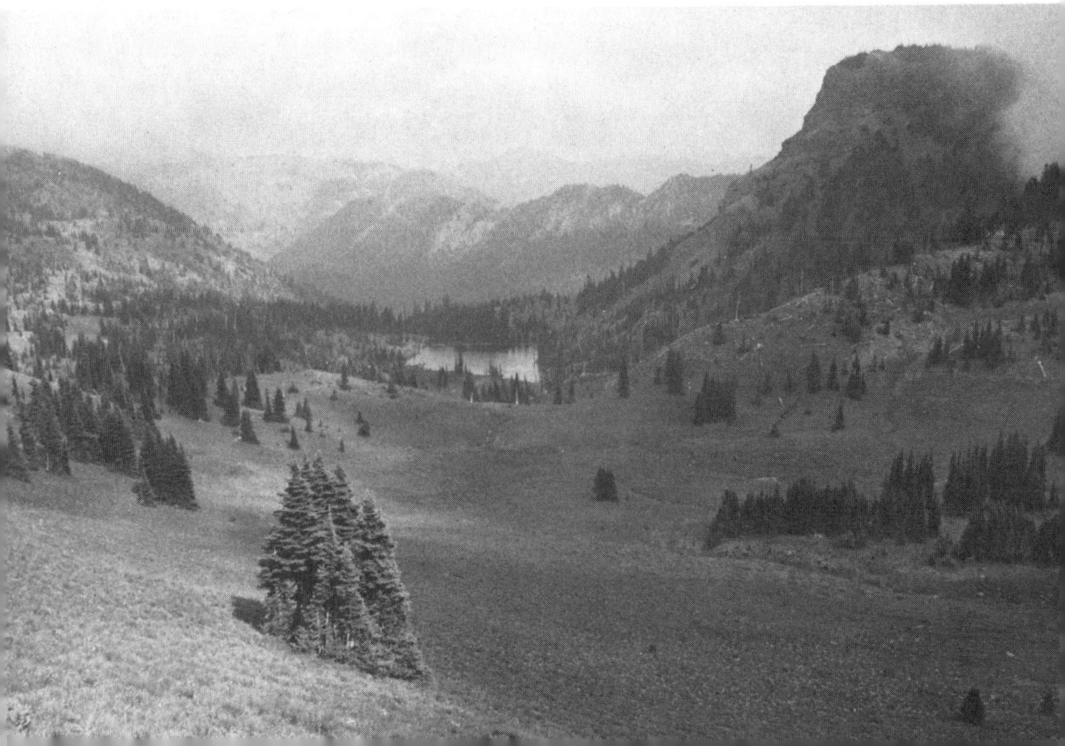

see MAP I6

see MAP I5

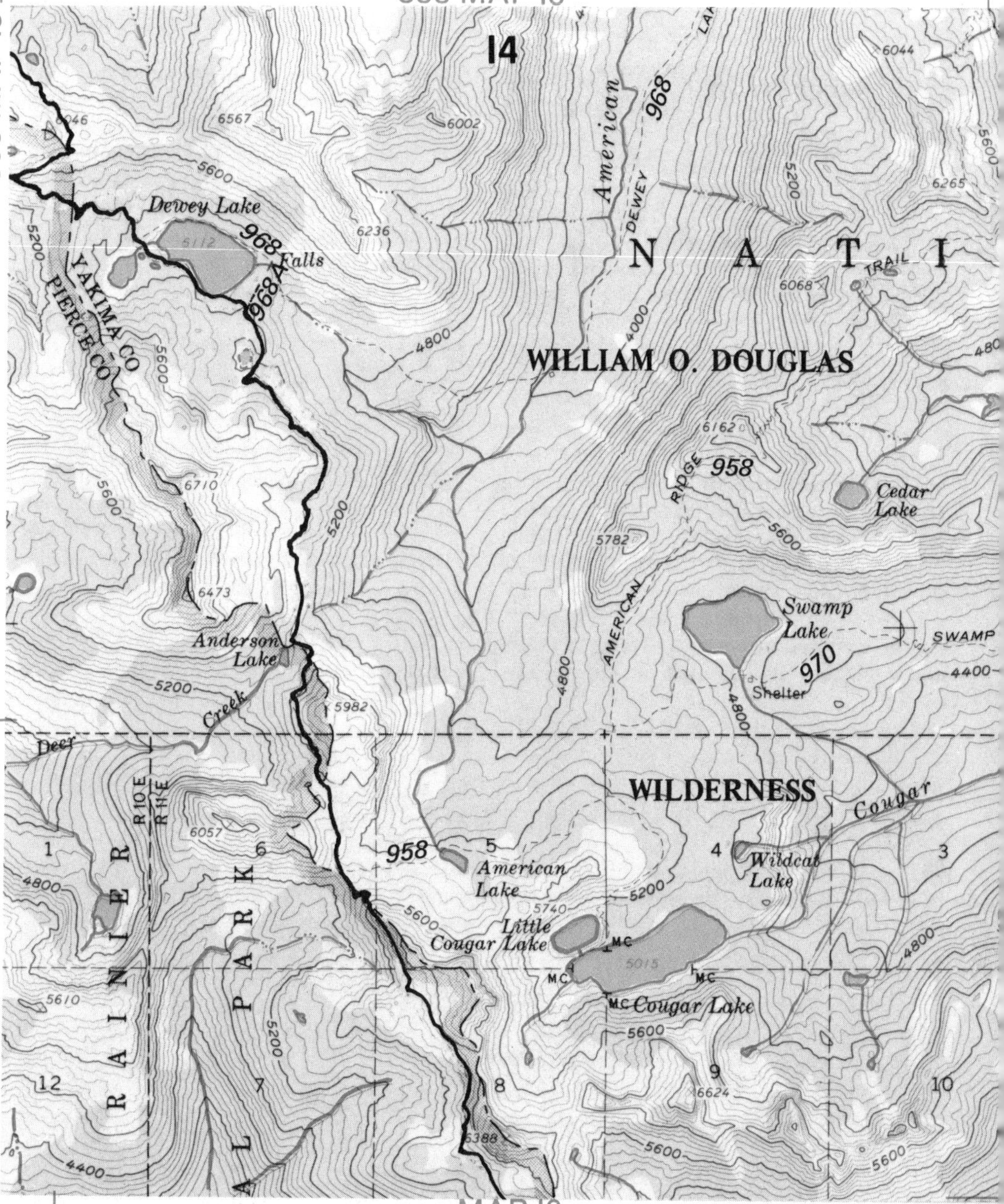

see MAP I3

1191, which climbs west, and Crow Lake Way 953, which passes an old shelter ½ mile away on its eastward descent. Next, the PCT passes a campsite as it rounds Big Crow Basin, and then it rises along a bench and back to the crest at forested Barnard Saddle (6150–0.8). After weaving through a couple of small, crestline ravines, passing an unsigned track that drops west in the first ravine, the PCT returns to the east side of the divide at Hayden Pass (6150–0.3), and you get a view over Little Crow Basin.

The PCT makes a steep slant down into this basin and then gradually descends across its upper glades and fir forest to a sign, LITTLE CROW BASIN (5930–0.4).

See maps I6, I7

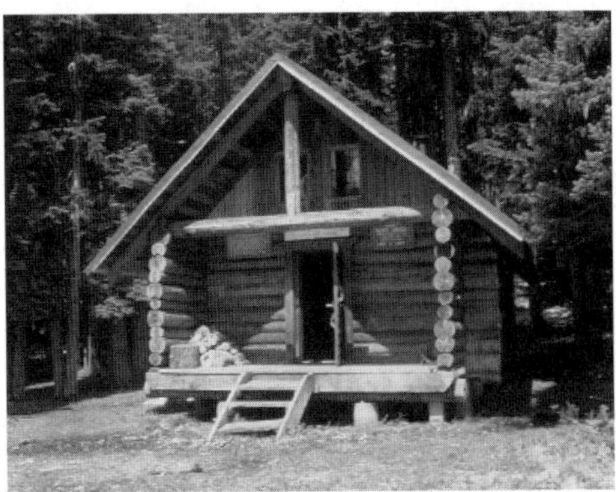

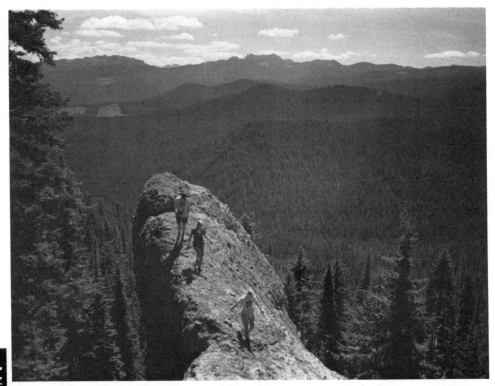

Camp Urich

Water access. Twenty yards before this sign, you can drop off the trail 75 yards to an established campsite. In a draw another 100 yards below and south of this site, water trickles much of the summer.

The PCT soon crosses an avalanche gully and continues slanting down and out of Little Crow Basin. Then it traverses northeast for some time before making a brief climb up to Martinson Gap (5720–1.4). Beyond this gap, the track turns northwest to angle up the slopes of Peak 6373, passing an old burn. Next, the trail pivots and arcs around the south and east slopes of 6373, recrosses the crest, and gradually settles onto the broadening Cascade divide, still presenting Mt. Rainier's massive white dome through the scattered and stunted subalpine firs. Along this stretch, the PCT intersects Arch Rock Way 1187 (5930–2.1).

Water access. Arch Rock Way, on its way to Echo Lake, descends past nearby Saddle Springs. Although these springs are convenient to the PCT hiker, in many years they trickle only into midsummer, so see Morgan Springs, below.

Half a mile beyond that junction, the PCT intersects yet another trail (5700–0.5).

See maps 17, 18

Hikers on an andesite rock outcrop west of Green Pass

See maps 11,

Water access. This trail drops east ¼ mile to a packer camp known as Morgan Springs, and these springs are a more enduring water source than Saddle Springs, above.

Beyond this junction, easy walking for ¼ mile takes you to the Cougar Valley Trail (5780–0.3), which heads east along a spur ridge. More strolling along the crest brings you to an unsigned trail junction (5920–0.5) at the base of an open rise. Avoid the fork that climbs directly up this broad summit and take the one contouring to the east—the PCT—passing through more blends of forest and meadow on the way to the spur trail (5760–0.8) to Arch Rock shelter.

Water access. At the end of this 200-yard-long spur, you find a perennial spring trickling from a pipe, as well as an old, four-sided shelter. Camp spots can be found in the forest below.

Beyond the junction, the PCT descends past the northern access to the shelter, and then it crosses a seasonal branch of South Fork Little Naches River. Well-sheltered now under silver fir and western hemlock, the route loses elevation along the broad crest to Louisiana Saddle (5220–1.5), from which obscure Middle Fork Trail 945 traverses east. The PCT continues descending through deep forest to Rods Gap (4820–1.1), from which it abruptly gains back 400 feet. After leveling out for a bit, your forested trail gently descends northwest and meets Maggie Way Trail 1186 (4850–1.6) heading west for a deep drop to the Greenwater River. Not much farther northwest, the PCT's descent takes you out of Norse Peak Wilderness and ends at perennial Meadow Creek in Government Meadow. After bridging this creek, you go 100 yards to Camp Urich (4750-0.8), a large camping area with a conspicuous shelter plus fire ring and outhouse. ▮ *This camp is named for Mike Urich, a trail worker in this area during the 1940s and '50s. On the shelter you may see a sign warning that the wrath of Mike's ghost will fall on anyone who harms the area's trees.* ▮

From the back side of the shelter, you continue 200 yards north to a sign that recalls the first wagon trail to cross the Cascades east of Puget Sound. ▮ *In 1853 the party, headed by David Longmire, rested here, by Government Meadow, before starting a rough descent into the Greenwater River canyon. By 1855, a military road was completed through this area, crossing gentle Naches Pass, ½ mile to the east.* ▮ From the sign, your path continues 40 yards to a parking area, and then you continue 80 yards on an east-southeast bearing to cross a jeep road (4780–0.2) that provides access to a parking area. Paralleling the north edge of the jeep road is Naches Trail 942.

Now you climb briefly to a minor gap and then make a winding traverse of ½ mile over to Road 787, up which you trek ¼ mile northwest to a junction (4840-1.1) from which a crest road starts northeast. Take this road just 20 yards to a resumption of trail tread, branching left; the winding crest road goes about ⅓ mile before giving rise to a short spur road. The PCT, more or less paralleling the crest road, also takes about ⅓ mile to reach the spur road. Just a few paces up this road, look for the resumption of trail tread, take it, and in 70 yards reach a junction with the Pyramid Peak Trail (5000–0.4). ▮ *You could take this trail steeply up to the top and then steeply down to the PCT. However, the energy expended isn't worth the effort. You'd see plenty of clearcuts, and most folks will see more of them than they want to long before they reach Snoqualmie Pass.* ▮ The PCT, traversing northwest through forest, offers glimpses of Mt. Rainier, and then, after ½ mile, it traverses northeast to offer a

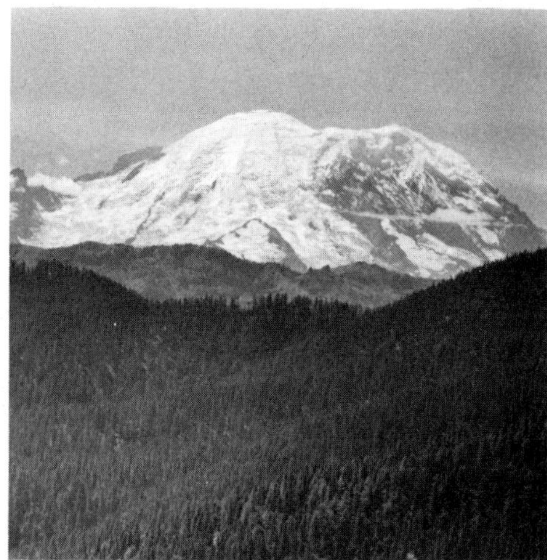

Mt. Rainier, from above outcrop

See maps I8, I9, I10

TACOMA 63 MI.

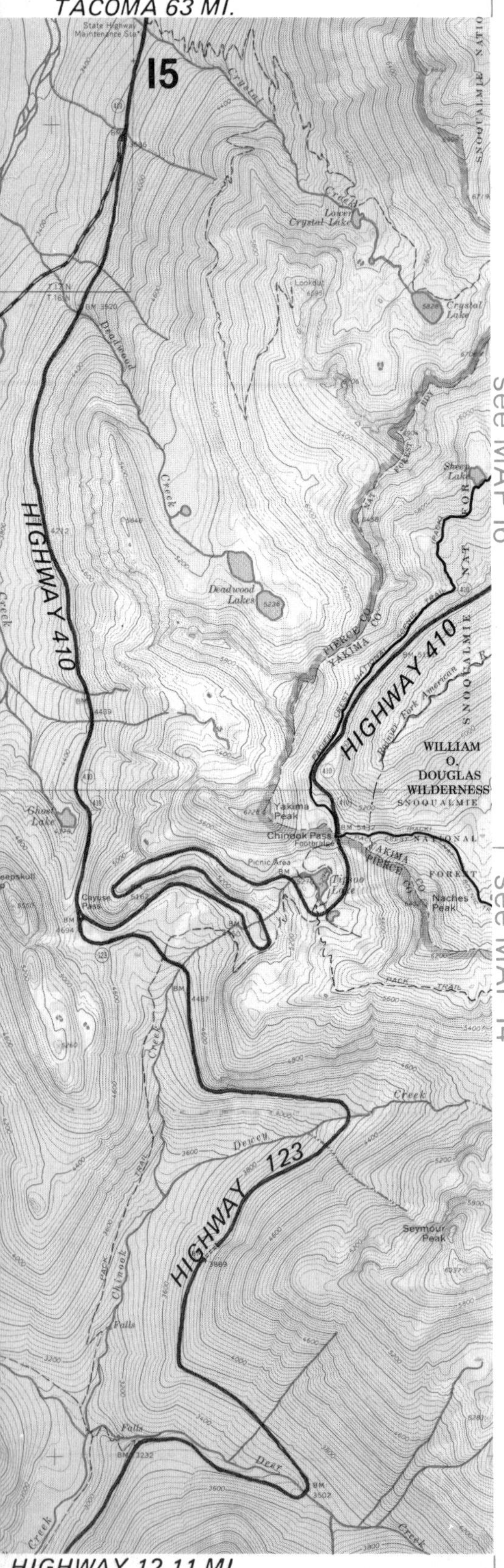

HIGHWAY 12 11 MI.

see MAP I6

see MAP I4

view or two of clearcuts. On this tack, there is one short stretch that, when snowbound, could expose you to a fatal fall if you slip and go over the brink.

Leave the slopes of Pyramid Peak behind at Windy Gap (5200–1.0) and now begin a fairly long stretch across east- and south-facing slopes. You start with a one-mile traverse northeast and then ½ mile east to a point where you cross a spur ridge. ▮ *This stretch fell victim to the 1988 Falls Creek Burn, which covered over 3000 acres. At the start of the new millennium, this stretch had hundreds of blowdown snags, and over the years, more snags will fall.* ▮ From the spur ridge, hike about ¼ mile northwest through untouched forest, but where the PCT curves north, you encounter a clearcut and traverse partly through its upper part. Within forest again, you head northeast and soon hear a noisy spring immediately below the tread. In 240 yards, you diagonal across a major road (5020–2.4). Ahead, the PCT makes an east-northeast, usually viewless, descending traverse to another road (4640–1.0), which climbs 250 yards west to an old crest road. Onward, you contour ⅓ mile to a gully and then gently ascend to a road-laced crest saddle (4900–1.4). Between two of these roads, the PCT starts a moderate-to-steep ascent southeast, levels off near the crest, follows it about ½ mile southeast, and then curves east-northeast to descend to a crossing of major Road 784 (4920–1.3). ▮ *Down, Road 784 and then Road 1913 together descend an even 6 miles to Forest Route 19, a paved, relatively heavily-used road. Up, Road 784 goes 140 yards to often windswept Green Pass. From there, a ridgecrest spur road heads 250 yards east before dying out.* ▮

From the Road 784 crossing, the PCT climbs 150 yards northeast to the end of that spur road, and now you face the first significant climb in many miles: up the west ridge of Blowout Mountain. You follow a couple of switchbacks and then, viewing Goat Rocks and much of the broad Naches River drainage to the south, you slant up to the ridgecrest, from which the obscure but signed West Fork Bear Creek Trail (5340–1.0) drops off to the south. The PCT continues climbing, switchbacking once, and enters a small stand of subalpine firs where you meet a sign pointing out obscure Granite Creek Trail 1326 (5480–1.0), bound

See maps I10, I11

see MAP I7

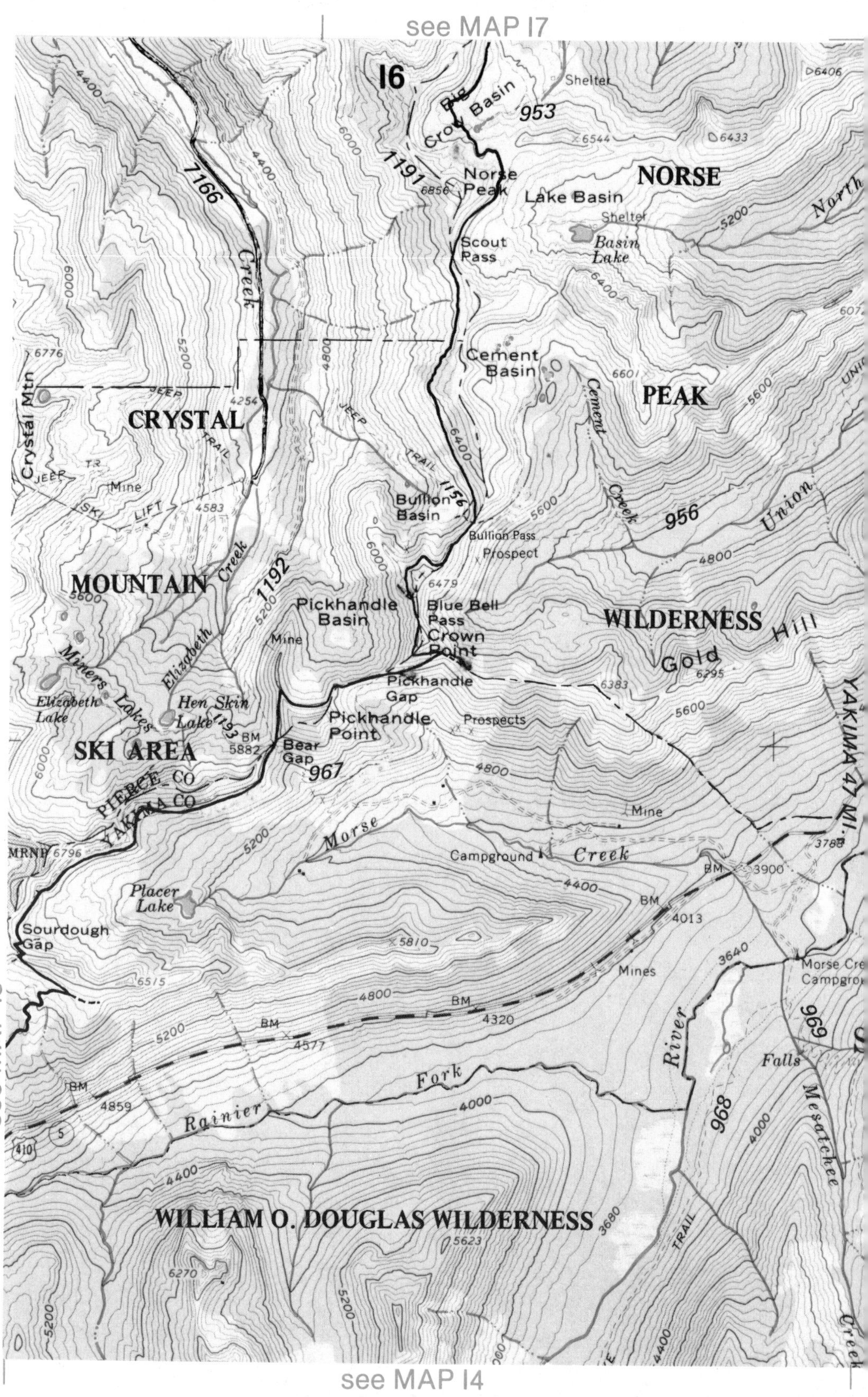

see MAP I5

see MAP I4

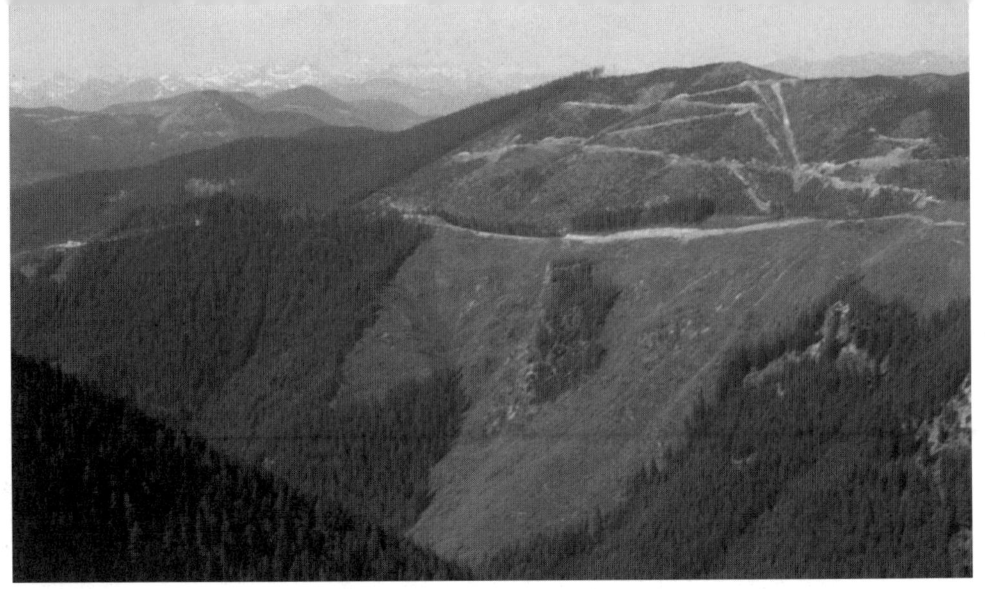

Green Pass vista

see MAP I9

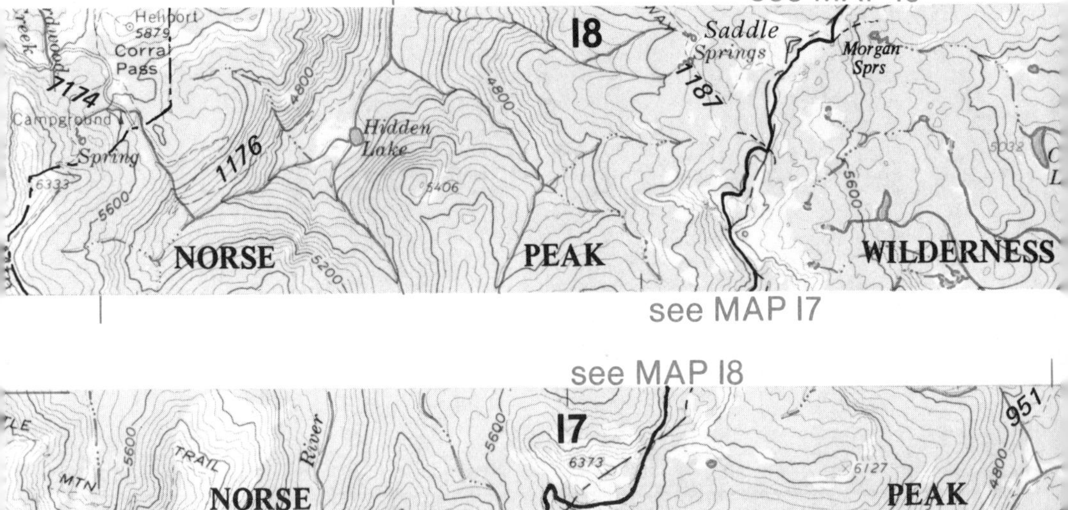

I8
Heliport
5879
Corral
Pass
7174
Campground
Spring
6333
5600
1176
4800
Hidden
Lake
5406
Saddle
Springs
1187
Morgan
Sprs
5600
5032
NORSE
PEAK
WILDERNESS
5200

see MAP I7

see MAP I8

I7
MTN
TRAIL
5600
River
NORSE
Greenwater
5200
Castle
Mountain
6658
6546
1188
6703
6000
6373
Martinson Gap
PIERCE CO
YAKIMA CO
Little
Crow Basin
Hayden
Pass
6290
Reese
Lake
Goat
Lake
Barnard
Saddle
953
5200
WILDERNESS
Crow
4800
5600
953
6127
PEAK
951
4800
Creek
6220

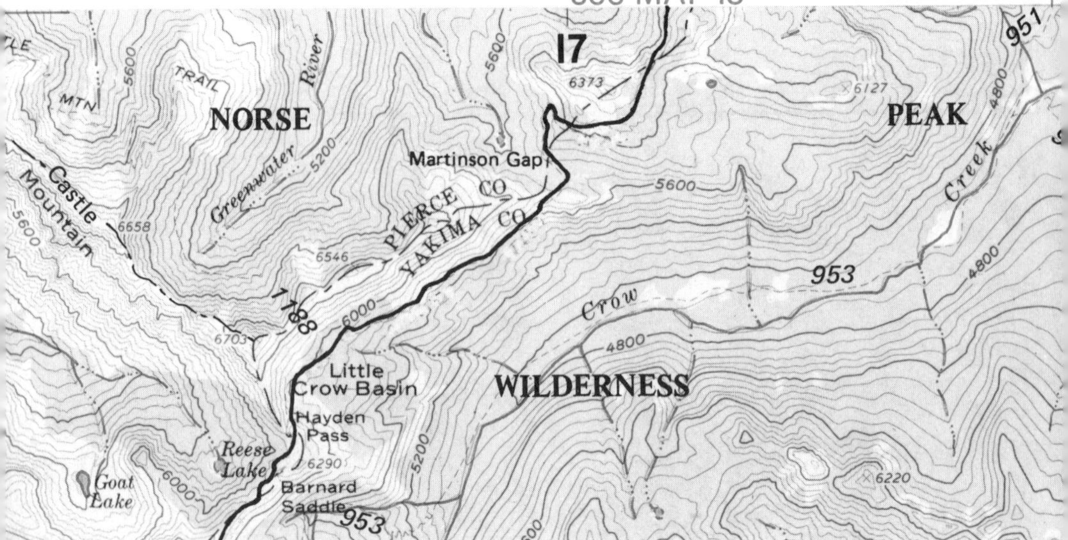

see MAP I10 | see MAP I11

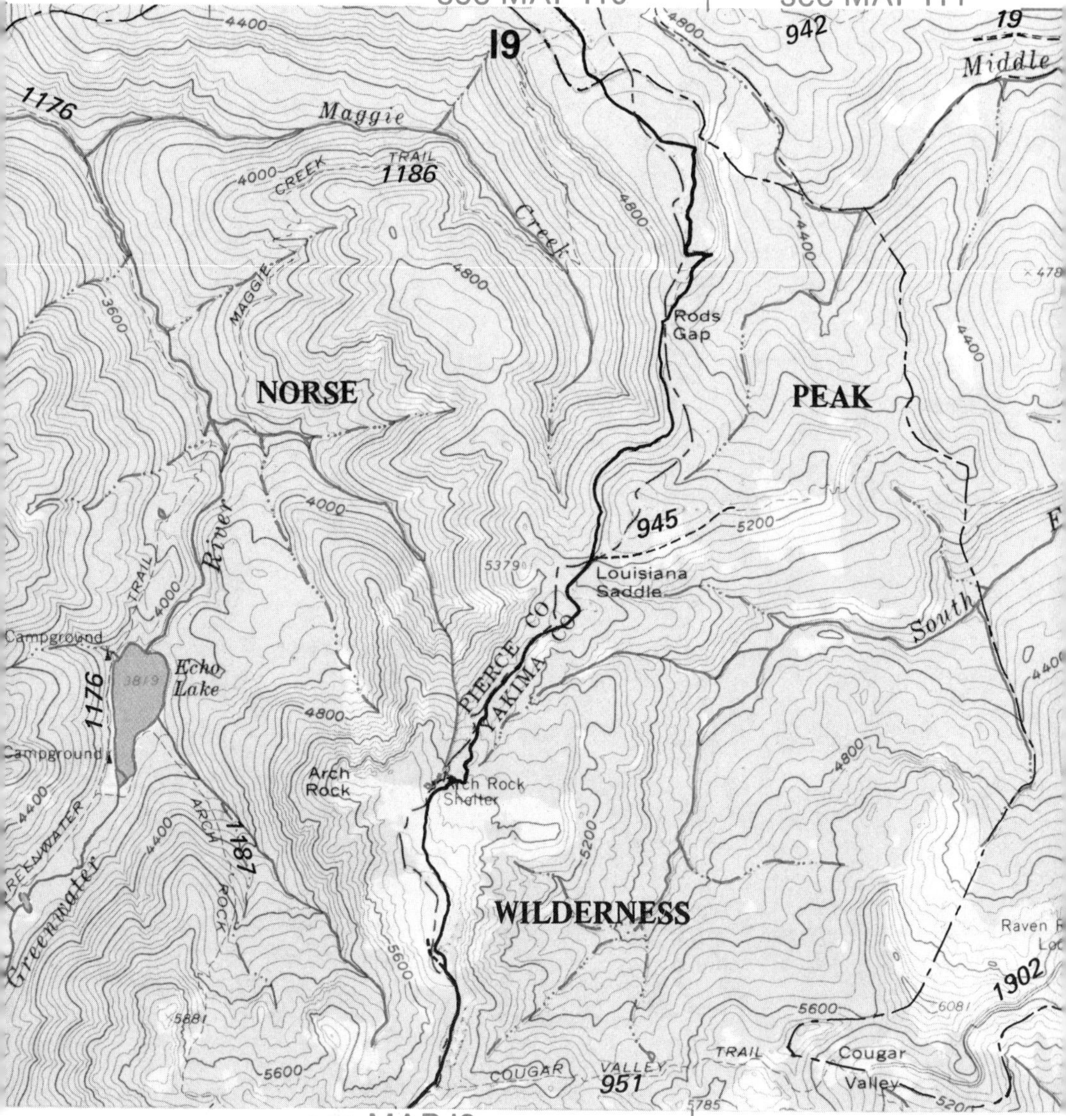

see MAP I8

for Mt. Clifty and Quartz Mountain. You can continue on the official PCT, following, or divert on an alternate route using Trail 1326 to an "oasis," below.

Staying on the official PCT from the Granite Creek Trail 1326 turnoff, you climb a bit more to the crest of Blowout Mountain, where you get the most expansive views in some time, once again seeing Mt. Rainier dominating the central Washington hinterlands. Now you follow the trail along a narrow summit ridge and look east down to the aforementioned pond, which could be the last water source for a *long* way. The PCT then rounds the north summit of Blowout Mountain and switchbacks down through a dense fir forest to Blowout Mountain Trail 1318 (5260–1.1), the northern access to the oasis described in the "Alternate route," following.

Alternate route. Granite Creek Trail 1326 is the southern end of a 1.2-mile alternate route to what, by mid-July, may be the only water at all convenient to the PCT for 6 miles to the south and over 17 miles to the north. This oasis is on a bench on the northeast side of Blowout Mountain, a bench that cups a marshy pond and

See map I11

I12

I10

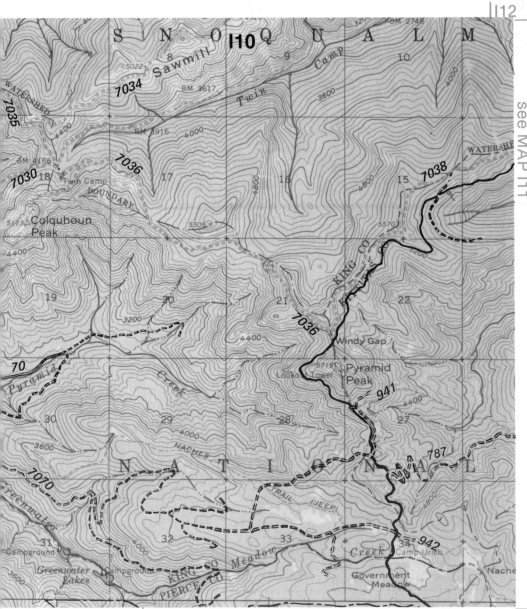

see MAP I11

see MAP I9

contains a spring. To reach this oasis from the south, turn onto hard-to-follow Trail 1326, traverse east, and descend, first steeply and then more reasonably, to a saddle on the east ridge of Blowout Mountain. Here, 0.4 mile from the PCT, you meet Manastash Ridge Trail 1388. Take this trail north 0.3 mile to the pond and its adjacent campsites. To rejoin the PCT, climb north on eroding Trail 1388 to crest the east-west ridge north of the pond's bench. Turn west here on Blowout Mountain Trail 1318 and join the PCT in 100 yards. PCT hikers coming from the north, or northbound hikers not wanting to hassle with route-finding along obscure Trail 1326, can branch off at Trail 1318 and follow the description in reverse to the pond.

Official PCT route and alternate route rejoined. North from the junction, a steep ridgeline descent ends your hiking through extensive, unmarred terrain as you emerge onto a vast, clearcut landscape. ▮ *Your first*

See map I11

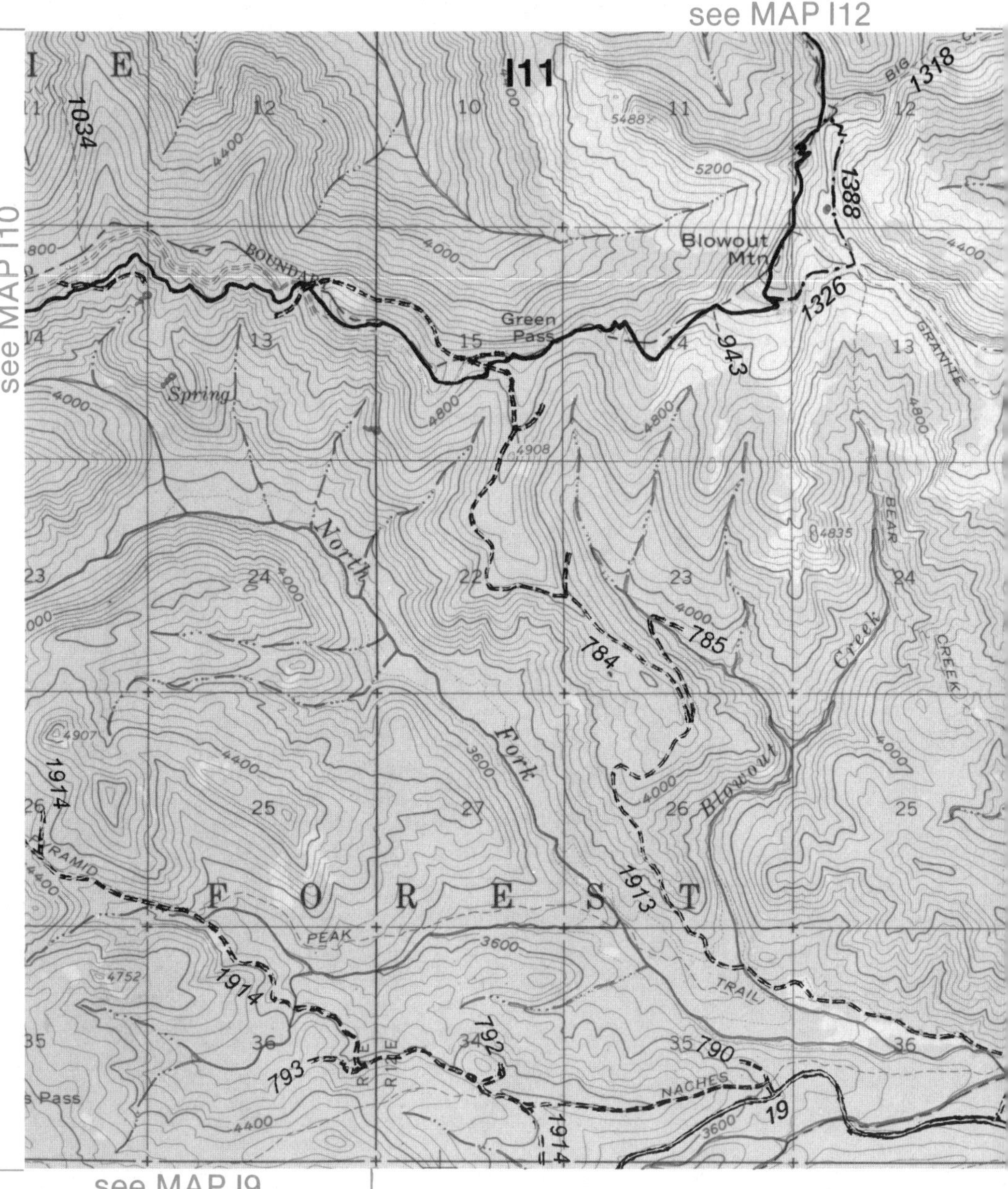

reaction might be revulsion at ridge after ridge riddled with roads and shaved down to soil, but PCT hikers might consider that hiking the PCT is more than just a pleasant walk through beautiful scenery. ▮

For quite some time, the trail keeps on or near the ridge dividing the Yakima and Green rivers. At first, it is barely east of deforested private land, but then it follows the flat but narrow ridge across a section line back into fully forested government land. The track eventually emerges from the woods just east of the crest, where you can see the PCT rising around barren Point 4922, ahead, at the end of a logging road. The route barely touches this road and then contours before climbing 50 yards onto the adjacent crest. From this, it then switchbacks down, crossing two roads on its way to a major saddle (4400–2.8).

From this saddle, the PCT traverses around the east side of Point 4922 and then re-enters forest to make a long, lazily switchbacking

See map I11, I12

see MAP I13

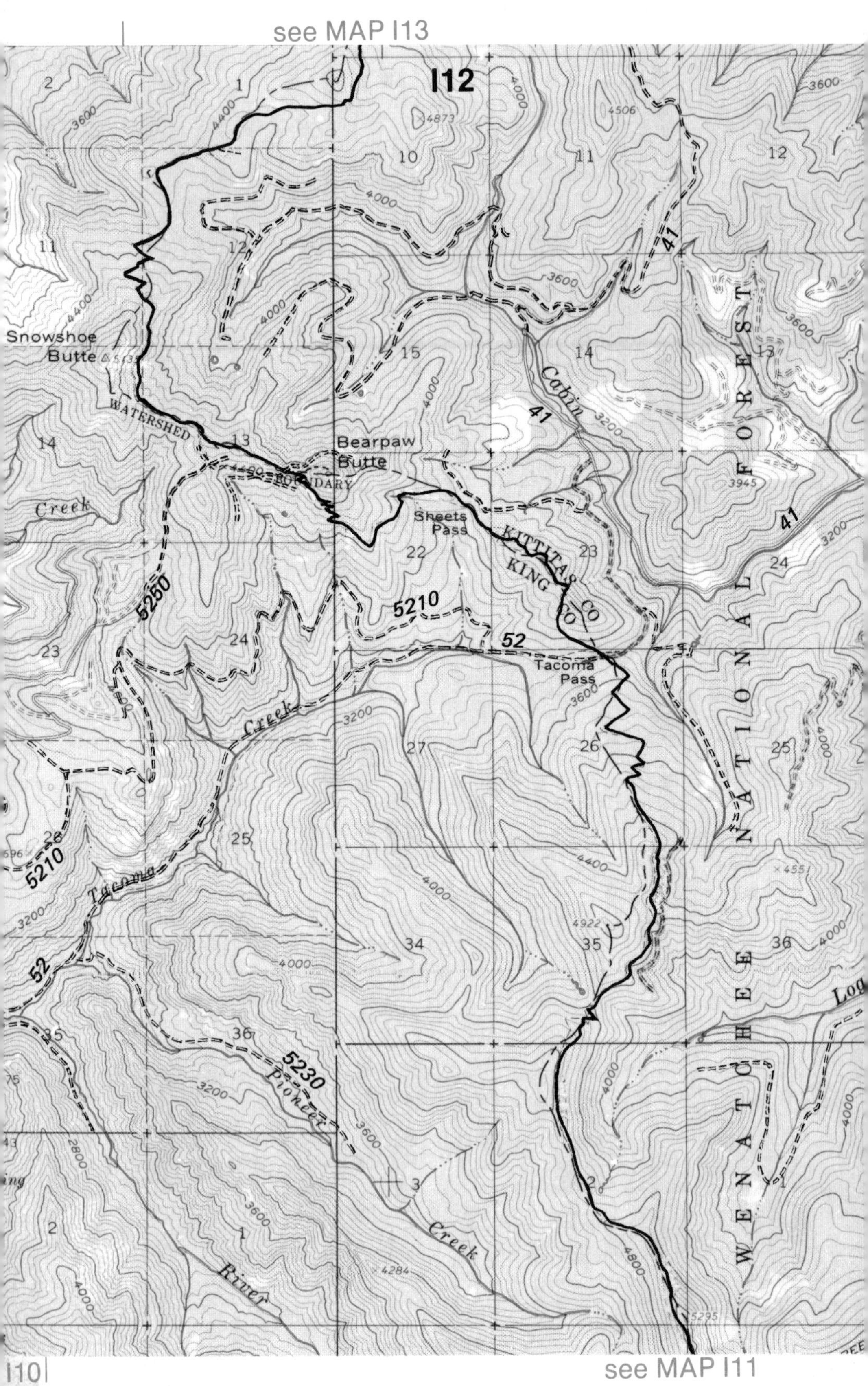

see MAP I11

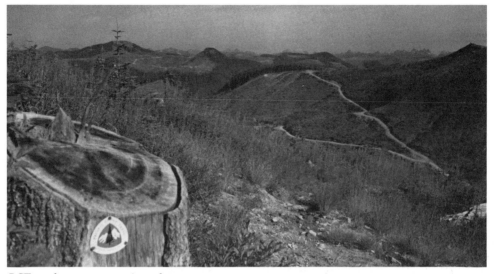

PCT marker on a stump in a clearcut

descent to Tacoma Pass (3460–2.7). Road 52 crosses this pass, and you jaywalk this logger's thoroughfare to ascend northwest into clearcut land again. With Mt. Rainier in full view, you now stride northwest along the divide as the PCT crosses one old logging road and then follows another one downhill for 30 yards before crossing it.

Now in forest, you cruise across Sheets Pass (3720–1.4) and then climb and contour through pleasant woods to a campsite and a seasonal creek (3860–0.4). This rill might carry water into mid-August of a *wet* year. From here, the route turns south and climbs around the south ridge of Bearpaw Butte. Climbing in and out of the next clearcut, you find the trail a bit grassy and overgrown, but you follow short hairpins trending northwest. As the PCT leaves the hairpins and traverses northwest, you spot a stagnant pond about 300 feet below the trail, a pond that the truly desperate might find refreshing.

The climb takes you to the crest, which the PCT follows northwest across an old log landing, across an old road, and then across another landing. Shortly, the trail drops a few yards south to avoid a ridgetop road and, as it traverses toward Snowshoe Butte, it makes the short climb back to cross the ridgetop road where the road curves. Next, the trail turns north along the east slope of Snowshoe Butte and passes through a corner of forested public land into more-razed earth on the butte's north ridge. A switchbacking descent takes you in and out of this clearcut, across one road, and then lands you on a second road. Follow this second road 250 yards northeast downhill, leave it on the same side as that on which you entered it, and walk back into the forest onto a broad saddle (4200–3.8).

As you then follow the low crest from here, the trail branches left, north-northeast, at a trail junction, back into a clearcut and, at the crest of a small knob, turns east onto a track. Follow this for 200 yards past an old slash pile and continue east, more or less directly up the adjacent ravine, passing a glade of corn lilies before reaching the edge of the clearcut near the crest of a knob, where the trail turns north. The track traverses just east of the knob's summit and then descends just east of the rounded divide to a pass where fast-growing grasses and shrubs, especially huckleberries, partly obscure the trail. ▮ *Huckleberry and blueberry bushes favor cleared and burned land, and so they cover a great deal of this country. By mid-August, most PCT hikers here develop a purple tongue from sampling the abundant fruit.* ▮ At the low point of the pass (4290–2.3), you cross a road, not far west of a flight-navigation complex.

From here, make a short climb up the next knob north before starting a descent toward the Stampede Pass weather station, visible ahead.

See maps I12, I13

see MAP I15

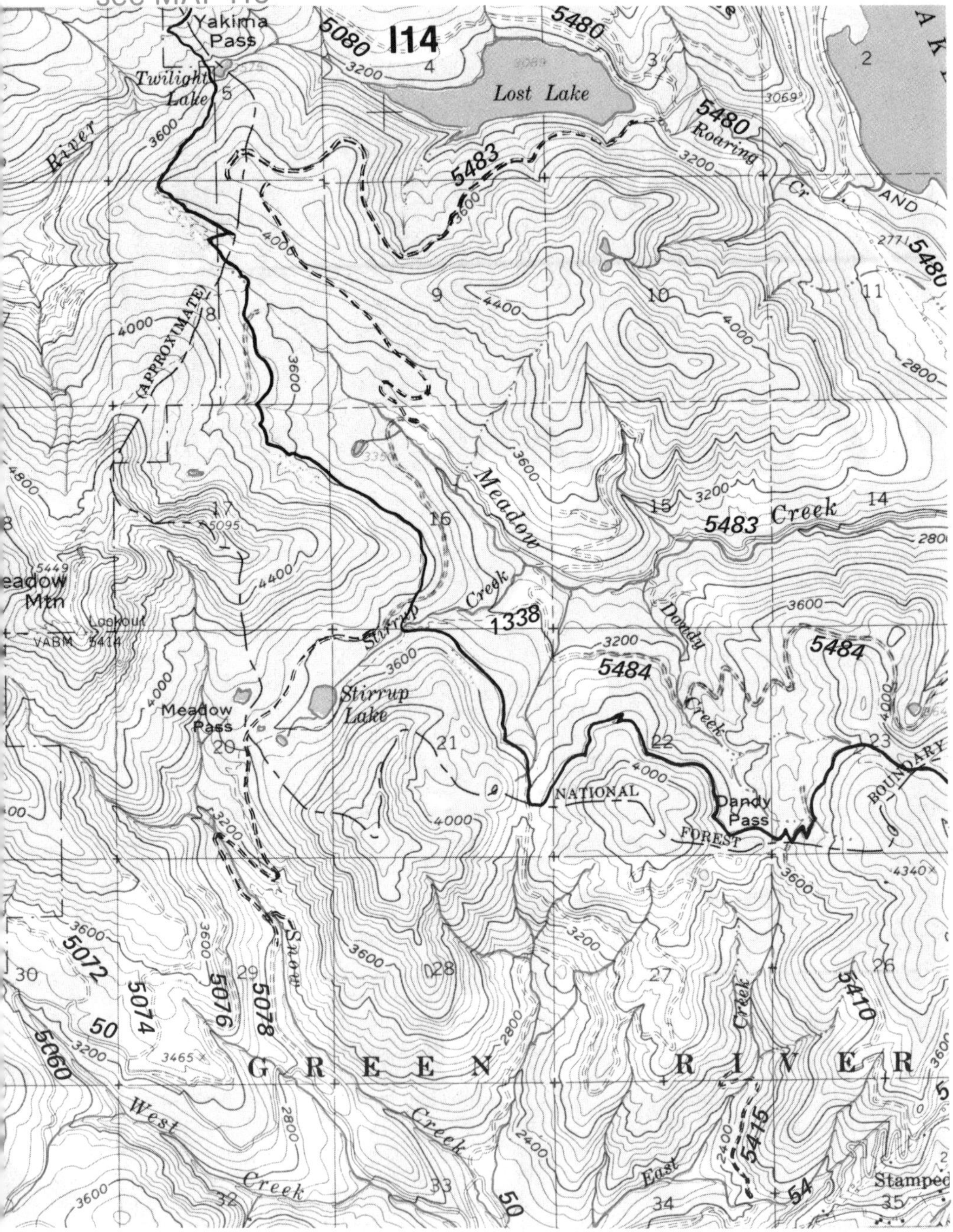

I14

Yakima Pass
Twilight Lake
Lost Lake
Roaring Cr
River
(APPROXIMATE)
Meadow Creek
Stirrup Creek
Stirrup Lake
Meadow Mtn
Lookout
VABM 5414
Meadow Pass
Dandy Creek
Dandy Pass
NATIONAL FOREST BOUNDARY
Snow
G R E E N R I V E R
West Creek
Creek
East Creek
Stampede
1338
5080
5480
5483
5484
5072
5074
5076
5078
5060
5410
5415
50
54

see MAP I13

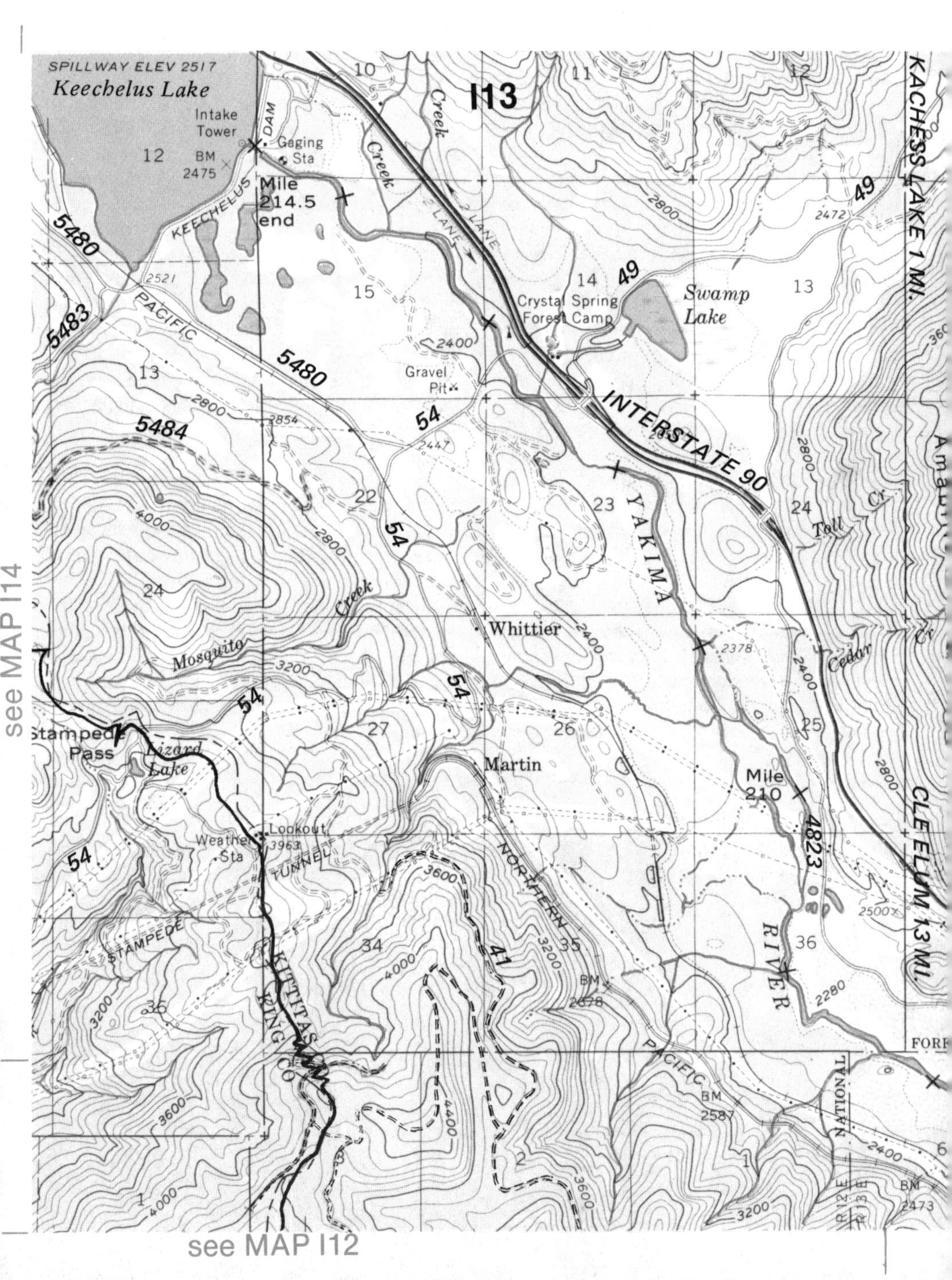
I13
SPILLWAY ELEV 2517
Keechelus Lake
Intake Tower
Gaging Sta
DAM
KEECHELUS
Mile 214.5 end
2 LANE
Creek
Crystal Spring Forest Camp
Swamp Lake
Gravel Pit
INTERSTATE 90
KACHESS LAKE 1 MI.
PACIFIC
YAKIMA
Whittier
Mosquito Creek
Toll Cr
Cedar Cr
Stampede Pass
Lizard Lake
Lookout 3963
Weather Sta
TUNNEL
Martin
NORTHERN
STAMPEDE
KITTITAS CO
KING CO
Mile 210
RIVER
CLE ELUM 13 MI.
NATIONAL
FORE
see MAP I14
see MAP I12

Steep switchbacks take you across a track and then across a more substantial road. The last switchback takes you into dense forest where an overgrown 4WD track might lead some hikers astray. Trail blazes help you head nearly straight down the divide to a dry campsite at a notch from which you ascend to traverse the east side of the next knob. You emerge from forest at a powerline cut and then soon reach another powerline cut with old log poles. ▮ *Deep beneath this latter cut runs the Northern Pacific railway tunnel.* ▮

A short distance farther on, you cruise behind the weather station and cross its access road (3950–1.8). The station is about 200 yards up this access road, and it has well water, which is much better than the water at upcoming Lizard Lake. However, there is no good camping here or along the stretch down to that lake. Now you follow the low Cascade divide as it turns west, crossing another road and then another powerline cut on your way through a regrowing forest of silver fir, Douglas-fir, lodgepole pine, white pine, and western hemlock. The trail makes a gradual descent to Stampede Pass Road 54 (3680–1.0) at a point a couple of hundred yards south of the pass proper.

Water access. About 0.2 miles south down this road lies Lizard Lake, a swampy, fetid pond next to crackling powerlines, with a fouled campsite on its south shore. Unpleasant though it may be, any campsite with water is rare along this stretch of PCT, and author Selters camped here and drank the water, after having properly treated it, with no ill effects.

From Road 54, the PCT next strikes steeply uphill, switchbacking through the second-growth forest. Soon after cresting the rise, the trail turns north, parallel to a logging road, and enters a former clearcut. After a slight climb, the PCT cuts west across the divide and cruises through huckleberry prairies and across two logging roads on its way to the forested headwater ravine of Dandy Creek, which might carry water through July. The trail barely descends into the ravine before contouring south out of it, and then it slants southwest down through thick fireweed and other pioneers of clearcuts. It crosses a logging road and then empties onto and follows the same road to a hairpin (3840–2.1) where a rill might trickle through July. Dropping from the road here, the PCT descends gradually, switchbacking across another logging road before reaching Dandy Pass (3680–0.3).

Here you enter forested public land and circle halfway around a hill under the shade of a magnificent forest of giant, old-growth hemlocks. This mile-long arc is a now-rare glimpse at the quality of tree for which the Pacific Northwest is famous. Eventually, you cross the section line and enter brushy country again, just shy of a saddle. You turn north here and skirt the saddle to cross and then parallel a logging road, and, in a few minutes, you come to a creek (3600–1.9) that probably cascades

See maps I13, I14

Lizard Lake and Mt. Rainier

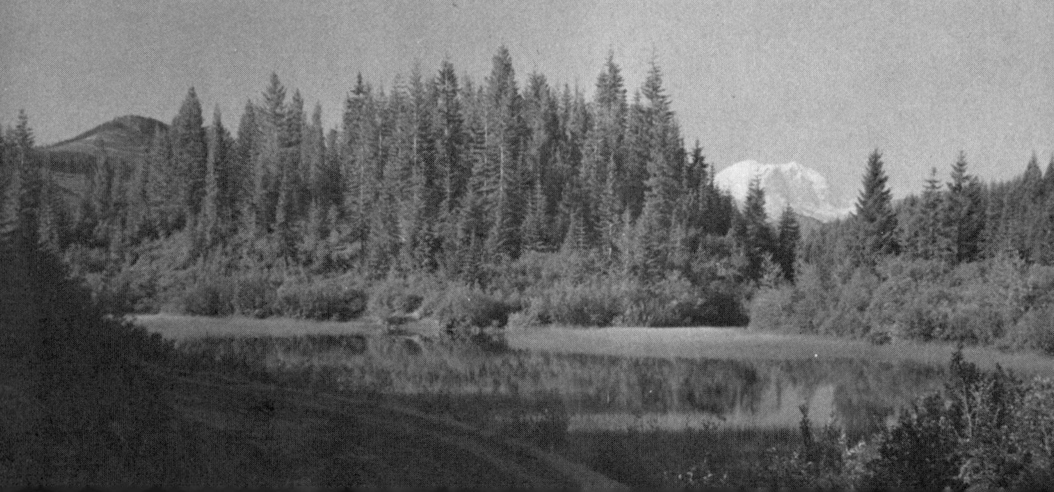

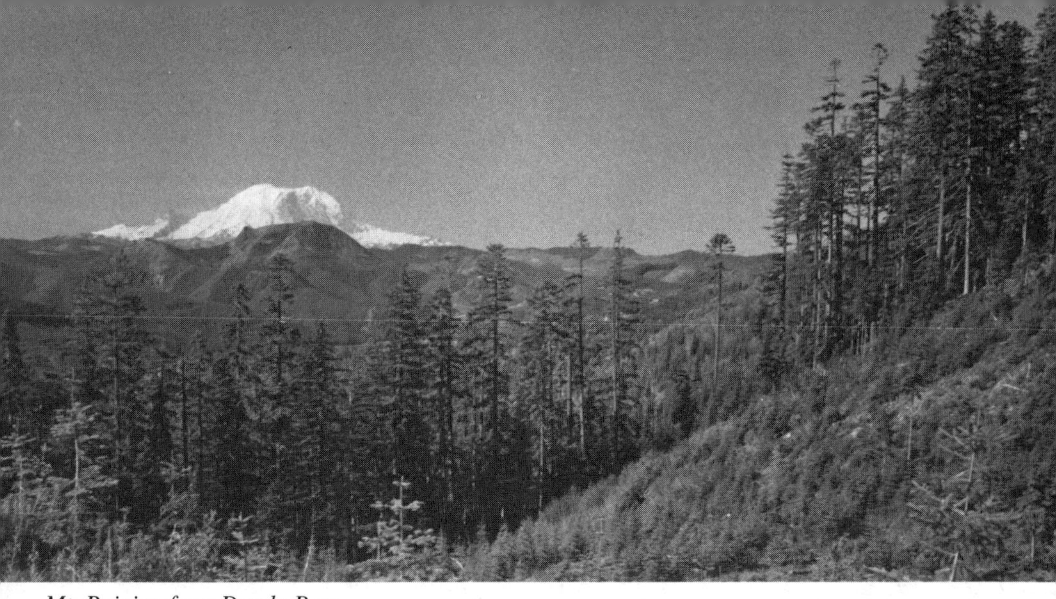

Mt. Rainier, from Dandy Pass

year-round. A rough, rocky traverse north from here, paralleling and then dropping across a road, brings you to an even more-certain stream, Stirrup Creek (3480–0.8).

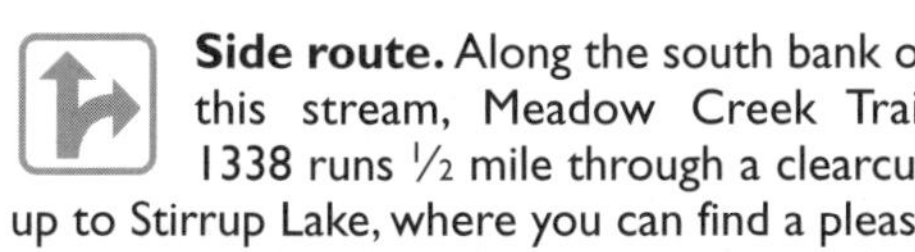

Side route. Along the south bank of this stream, Meadow Creek Trail 1338 runs ½ mile through a clearcut up to Stirrup Lake, where you can find a pleasant campsite barely in the trees.

Climbing gradually from here among tall cedars, the trail crosses a well-graded logging road and rounds a ridge before striking northwest on a level traverse through a 1989-vintage clearcut. ▮ *Note what kind and how much growth has occurred since then.* ▮ Eventually, the trail re-enters forest at the Forest Service boundary and traverses to the dribbling headwaters of Meadow Creek (3660–2.1). From here, work up a couple of hairpins, gaining 350 feet to a ridgeline that overlooks the mostly clearcut headwaters of North Fork Cedar River, a major feeder into Seattle's water supply. At the valley's head, you see Yakima Pass cupping Twilight Lake which, at the bottom of a massacred amphitheater, looks like a forlorn island of natural beauty trying to hide behind a relict forest curtain. The trail then slants down to the pass, crossing a logging road en route, and skirts Twilight Lake along its west shore (3575–1.4). Campsites can be found in the scant trees on the east shore.

From the pass—part of an old Indian route—the PCT strikes northwest directly uphill, crosses a road, and then cuts northeast to ford the creek that issues from Mirror Lake. Just beyond this first ford, the PCT turns across the end of a logging road and then climbs steeply to cross and recross the outlet creek on the way to Mirror Lake (4195–0.9). Suddenly, you've entered a refuge of undisturbed mountain landscape: craggy Tinkham Peak looks over the sapphire waters that periodically ripple with feeding trout, and the rimming fir forest invites secluded access to a scenic swim—in warm weather, anyway.

After passing a number of campsites on the way around the east shore of this lake, you exit the lake basin and meet Mirror Lake Trail 1302 (4220–0.4) coming up from the Lost Lake trailhead only a mile to the southeast. Here, the PCT merges with Twin Lakes Trail 1303, continues north for a bit, and then climbs some steep hairpins to a spur of Tinkham Peak. At a junction (4500–0.5), Twin Lakes Trail 1303, here signed as Cold Creek Trail, drops away north from the PCT, which turns west on a hillside below andesite bluffs. ▮ *In early 2000, the Forest Service obtained this section of land in an exchange, and so the trees of Tinkham Peak should remain part of an unlogged segment, connecting those of Silver Peak and Mirror Lake. This was one of the first actions in Washington conservationists' hopes to protect and rehabilitate this Central Cascade crest as*

See maps I14, I15

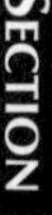

see MAP J1

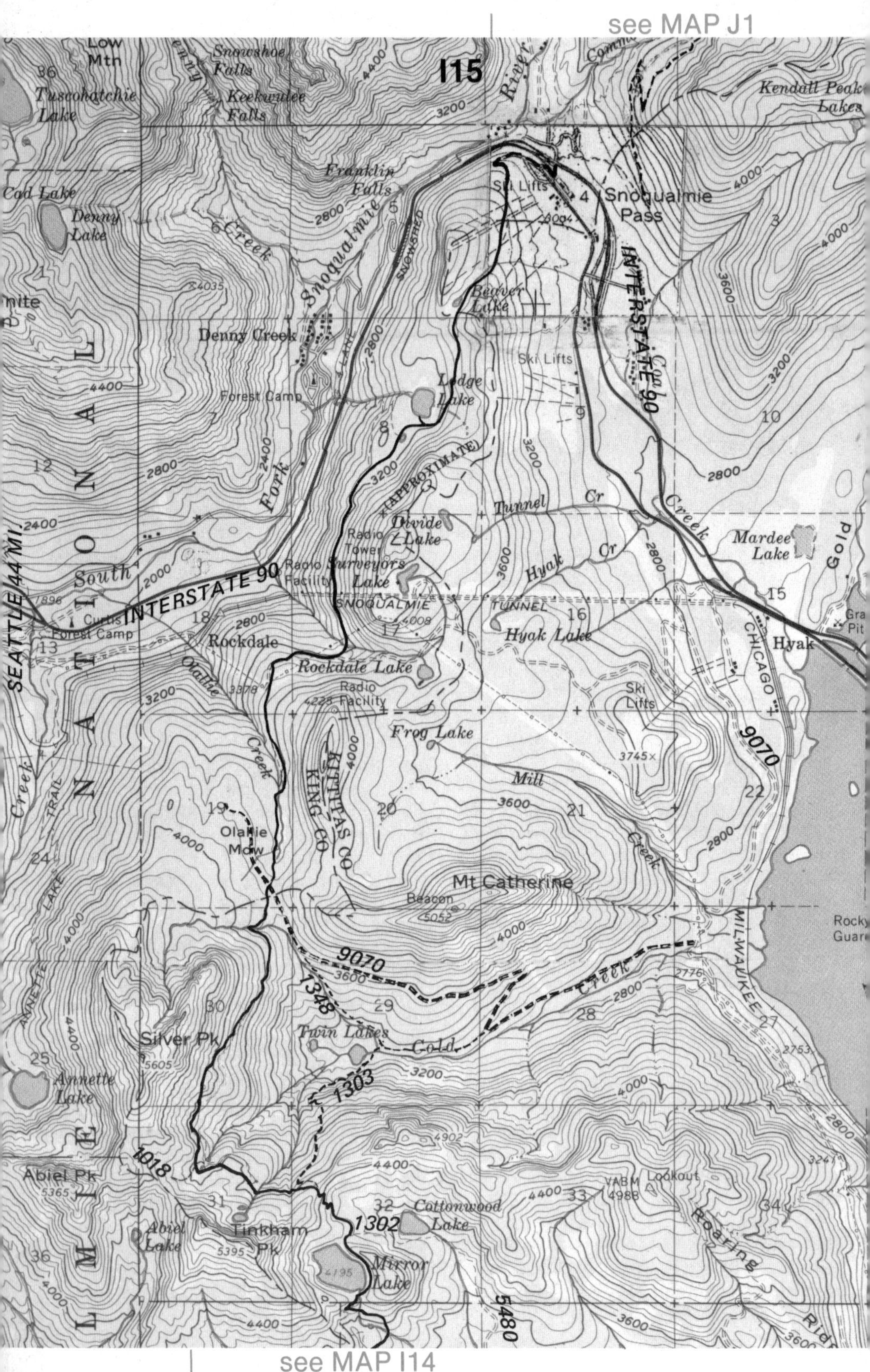

see MAP I14

a continuous forest habitat. ▮ Soon you cross a small creek on the way down to a soggy bowl with a couple of tiny ponds and a rug of marsh marigolds. Next, the PCT turns north and passes unmaintained Garren Ridge Trail 1018, which climbs west. The PCT then begins a very steep, rocky climb of its own as it traverses the slopes of Silver Peak. This climb takes you to a tiny side valley behind a knob, from which you make a steep and then a moderate, traversing descent among silver firs to a perennial creek (3900–2.5).

After crossing this creek, the PCT continues north, soon entering a clearcut that allows a view of Chair Peak and its satellites across the gash of the Snoqualmie River valley. Then the trail descends to and follows Olallie Creek. You cross a road and then a feeder of Olallie Creek and finally cross to the east bank of Olallie Creek itself (3620–0.8). Along the creek, you pass through a patch of forest and then break back into logged land where you hear the roar of Interstate 90 some 1400 feet below. Soon you follow a logging road a few yards north before descending from it, traversing under powerlines, and dropping onto the powerline access road (3350–0.7). The PCT follows this road west and downhill for 0.4 mile, past a spur road climbing east, and then drops beside Rockdale Creek, which tumbles under a canopy of maples and firs. Cross the creek, turn north under powerlines, proceed across talus slopes dotted with vine maple, and then enter deep fir-and-cedar forest for a long, flat traverse.

Eventually, the steep slope you traverse levels into a bench, and the path skirts a small pond where an unsigned track branches northwest. Quickly, the PCT then comes to a sign pointing out a 100-yard spur to Lodge Lake (3180–2.0).

Side route. Down this spur, you'll find the lake's campsites, some close to the PCT, although a number of them, popular with overnighters, are set around the shallow, muskeg-rich lake.

The PCT rises as it rounds Lodge Lake's bowl and then traverses slopes up past a creek ford to cross a forested saddle and enter a swale holding Beaver Lake (3480–0.8). Here the trail passes under ski lifts of the Snoqualmie Pass ski area before starting a long, descending arc down the groomed ski slopes. The trail slowly curves far to the west, presenting views of Interstate 90 and the complex of cute buildings at Snoqualmie Pass below the craggy peaks across the valley. The latter promise a more ruggedly scenic and pristine section of PCT to the north. A final switchback quickly takes you down to a trailhead (3030–1.0) at the end of a broad road with ample room for parking. The next set of directions may seem confusing as you read them, but the route is plain when you're actually there. On this road, you make a curving descent 250 yards east to a very broad snow-parking area that branches southeast, then continue 150 yards straight ahead to a point where you branch northeast for a 40-yard descent down a road to a longer road. This goes 140 yards southeast to the main road, which curves north 130 yards to pass under Interstate 90 (3000–0.4). Here, Section I's PCT ends by the freeway's West Summit exit. If you're a long-distance hiker, you may first want to head southeast along the main, freeway frontage road, which is Highway 906. Along it, you'll find a choice of eating establishments, groceries, and lodgings. About 0.4 mile along this road, on the left, is the Time Wise Grocery, where you'll also find the Snoqualmie Pass Post Office.

See map I15

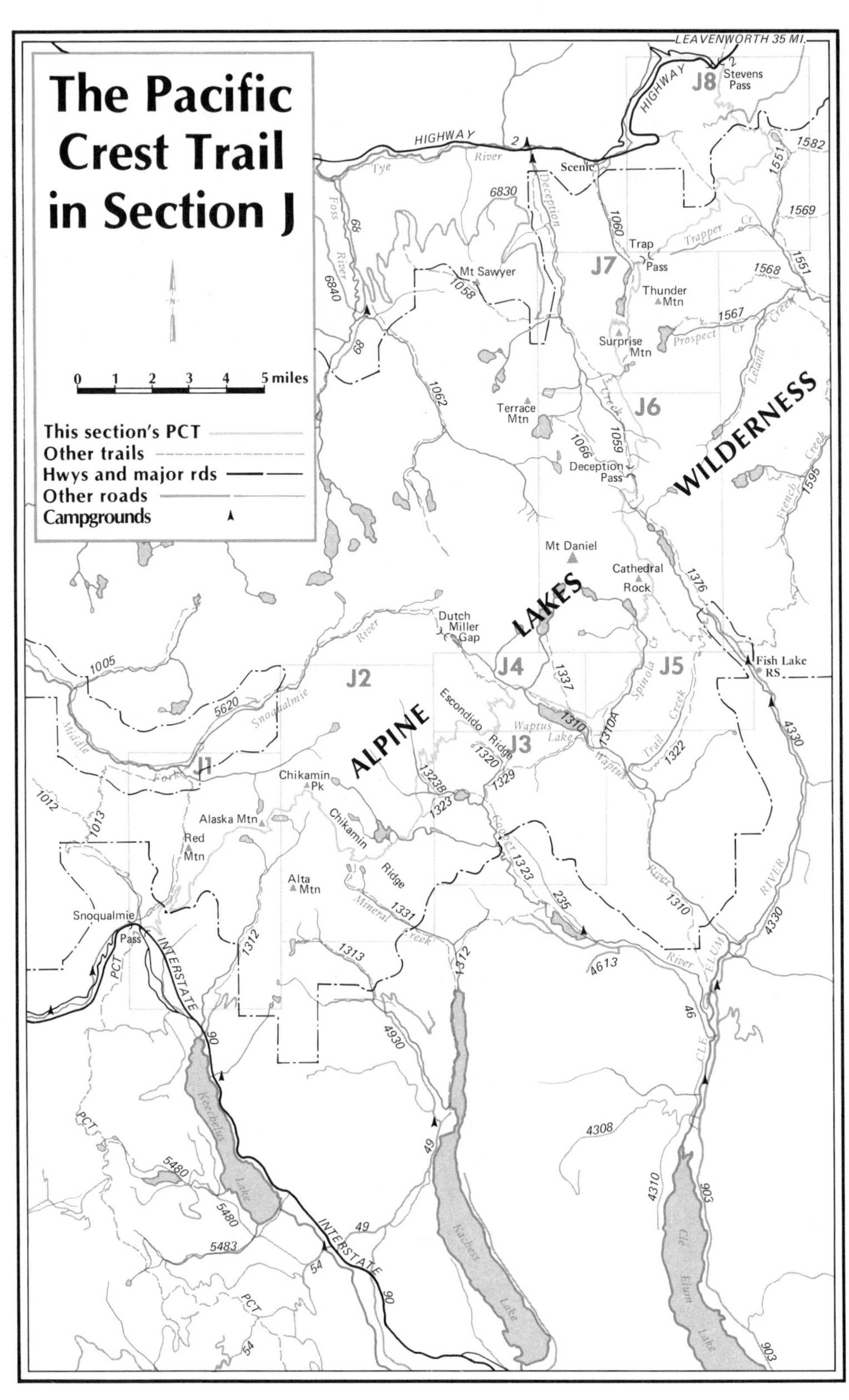

The Pacific Crest Trail in Section J
0 1 2 3 4 5 miles
This section's PCT
Other trails
Hwys and major rds
Other roads
Campgrounds
LEAVENWORTH 35 MI.
HIGHWAY
Stevens Pass
J8
HIGHWAY 2
Scenic
Tye River
Foss River
Deception
6830
1060
Trap Pass
Trapper Cr
1582
1551
1569
J7
Mt Sawyer
1058
6840
Thunder Mtn
1568
1567
Surprise Mtn
Prospect Cr
Leland Creek
68
1062
Terrace Mtn
J6
1066
1059
Deception Pass
WILDERNESS
French Creek
1595
Mt Daniel
Cathedral Rock
1376
LAKES
Dutch Miller Gap
River
1005
J2
J4
1337
J5
Fish Lake RS
Spinola Cr
5620
Snoqualmie
Middle Fork
Escondido Ridge
Waptus Lake
1310
1310A
Trail Creek
1322
4330
ALPINE
J3
1320
1329
J1
Chikamin Pk
1323B
1323
1012
1013
Alaska Mtn
Chikamin Ridge
Red Mtn
Cooper
Alta Mtn
River
Snoqualmie Pass
PCT
INTERSTATE
1312
Mineral Creek
1331
235
4613
River
CLE ELUM
1313
4930
90
46
Keechelus Lake
PCT
49
4308
5480
4310
903
5483
49
INTERSTATE
54
Kachess Lake
Cle Elum Lake
PCT
90
54
903

Section J:
Interstate 90 at Snoqualmie Pass to Highway 2 at Stevens Pass

Introduction: From high traverses along craggy crests, to meadowland tours past swimable lakes, to forest walks near churning rivers, this section bisects a spectacular variety of Cascades backcountry, making for a classic, week-long backpack. This is the land of Alpine Lakes Wilderness, an area that was so designated after one of the 1970s' most bitter wilderness battles.

From Snoqualmie Pass, the PCT climbs directly to the crest-top crags and boldly traverses right among them. Confronted by Chikamin Peak and brutal Lemah Mountain, it relinquishes the divide, swerving east to where summer storms generally dissipate into clear skies. On this stretch, the route dips into and climbs out of two major watersheds, Lemah Creek and the Waptus River. It then works back to and weaves along the descending divide, visiting a number of memorably scenic lake basins on its way to Stevens Pass. In all, this section will challenge your legs, lift your spirits, and probably confirm your reasons for backpacking.

Declination: 19½°E

Mileages:	S→N	Mi. Btwn. Pts.	N→S
Interstate 90 at Snoqualmie Pass	0.0		74.7
Ridge Lake and Gravel Lake	7.2	7.2	67.5
Park Lakes campsites	15.4	8.2	59.3
Lemah Creek	21.9	6.5	52.8
Waptus Burn Trail	31.7	9.8	43.0
Waptus River	36.5	4.8	38.2
Deep Lake	44.2	7.7	30.5
Cathedral Pass	47.4	3.2	27.3
Deception Pass	52.7	5.3	22.0
Deception Lakes outlet creek	56.1	3.4	18.6
Glacier Lake campsite	60.1	4.0	14.6
Hope Lake	66.6	6.5	8.1
Lake Susan Jane	70.4	3.8	4.3
Highway 2 at Stevens Pass	74.7	4.3	0.0

Supplies: A host of services are available at the settlement of Snoqualmie Pass. From the West Summit exit off Interstate 90, a frontage road heads southeast through the settlement, and you'll first encounter The Summit at Snoqualmie, with a restaurant. Just beyond it is a Chevron station, which, besides dispensing fuel, is the local Greyhound bus stop. Adjacent to it is another restaurant, followed by the Summit Inn. You'll find more services, but the most important one may be the Time Wise Grocery, just ahead, which has the Snoqualmie Pass Post Office (98068). Onward, you'll soon see Yellowstone Trail Road branching left to head under Interstate 90. About ½ mile along this road, you'll find the Ward Home West Bed & Breakfast. They have a trekker rate and laundry service. Since they are about a mile out of the way, you might phone them first at (425) 434-6540, for two reasons. The first is that they may be full; the second is that if they have the time, they'll pick you up.

At this section's end, Stevens Pass, there are no facilities. The closest town to this pass is at Skykomish (post office: 98288), about 14 miles west, with a choice of eating and lodging establishments.

Wilderness Permits: None are required along this section, but the Forest Service asks that all hikers self-register at the post just beyond the Snoqualmie Pass trailhead.

Problems: Snow typically lingers through mid-August on some of the steep traverses during the first 15 miles, making for some treacherous gully crossings.

Maps:

Snoqualmie Pass, WA
Chikamin Peak, WA
Polallie Ridge, WA
Mount Daniel, WA
The Cradle, WA (alternate route)
Scenic, WA
Stevens Pass, WA

THE ROUTE

To reach the trailhead, eastbound drivers take the West Summit exit off Interstate 90 and turn left to immediately cross under Interstate 90. Westbound drivers take the East Summit exit, take the frontage road (Highway 905) briefly through the settlement of Snoqualmie Pass, and then, by the West Summit exit offramp, cross under Interstate 90.

See map J1

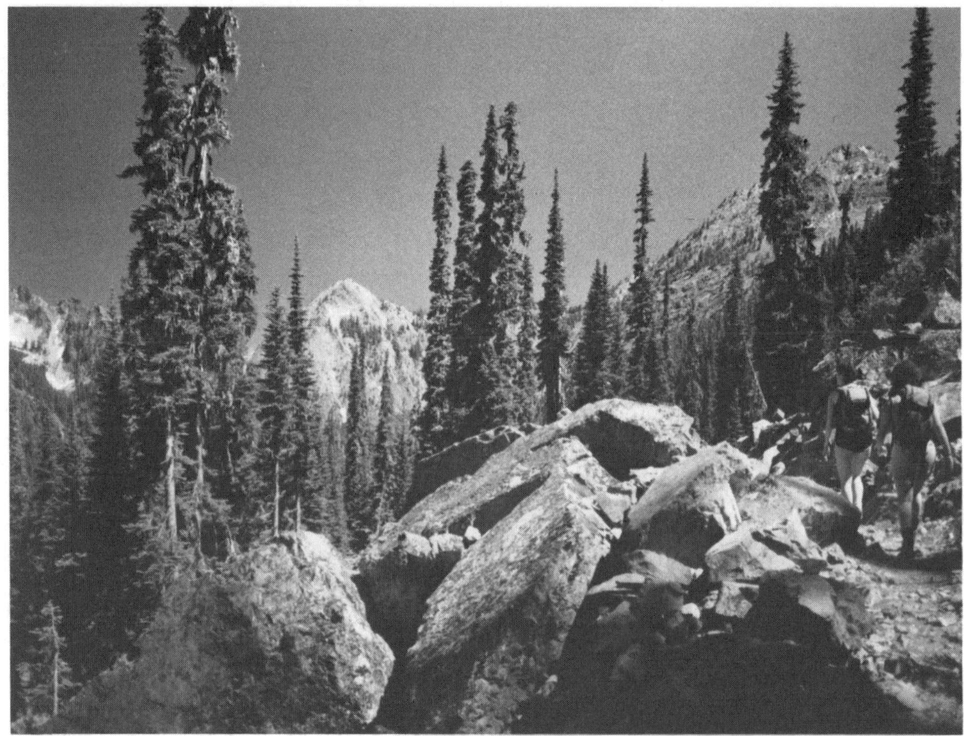

Red Mountain, from PCT in Commonwealth Basin

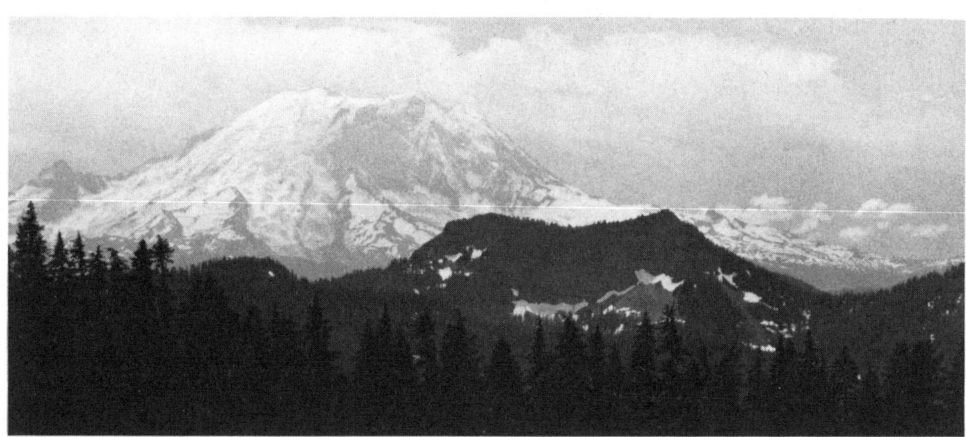

Mt. Rainier, from above Commonwealth Basin

On the road north from it, you'll quickly reach a spur road that branches right, climbing to the nearby main trailhead parking lot and its adjacent equestrian parking lot.

This book begins PCT mileage from I-90. On the road north from it, you walk just a few yards to a footpath starting up the road's cut. If you're on foot, take this path, which winds up to the far end of the trailhead parking lot (3080–0.2). Here, those on horseback or starting from the lot join you. With fir and hemlock above you, and bunchberry, spring beauty,

See map J1

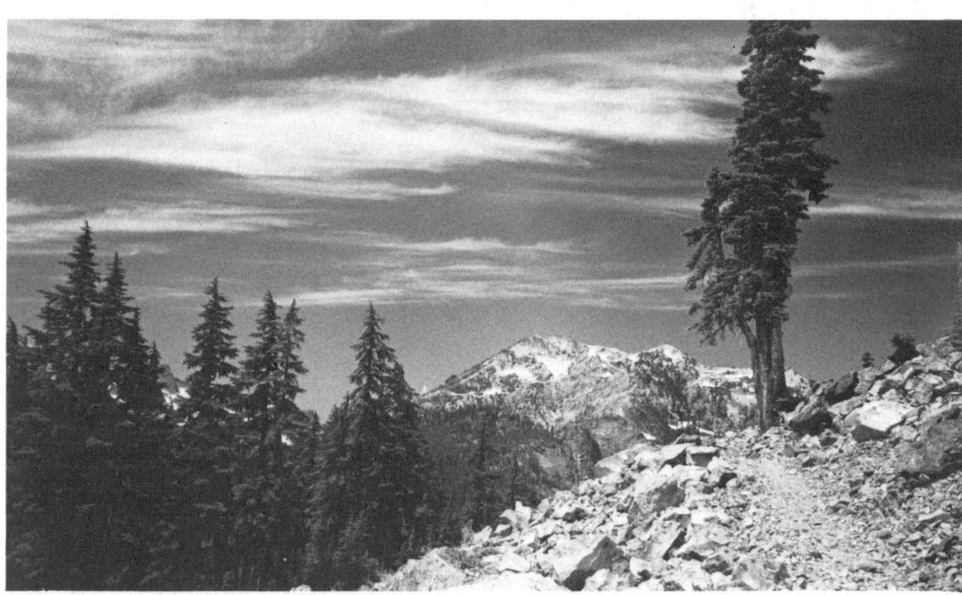

PCT, outlying fir and Snoqualmie Mountain

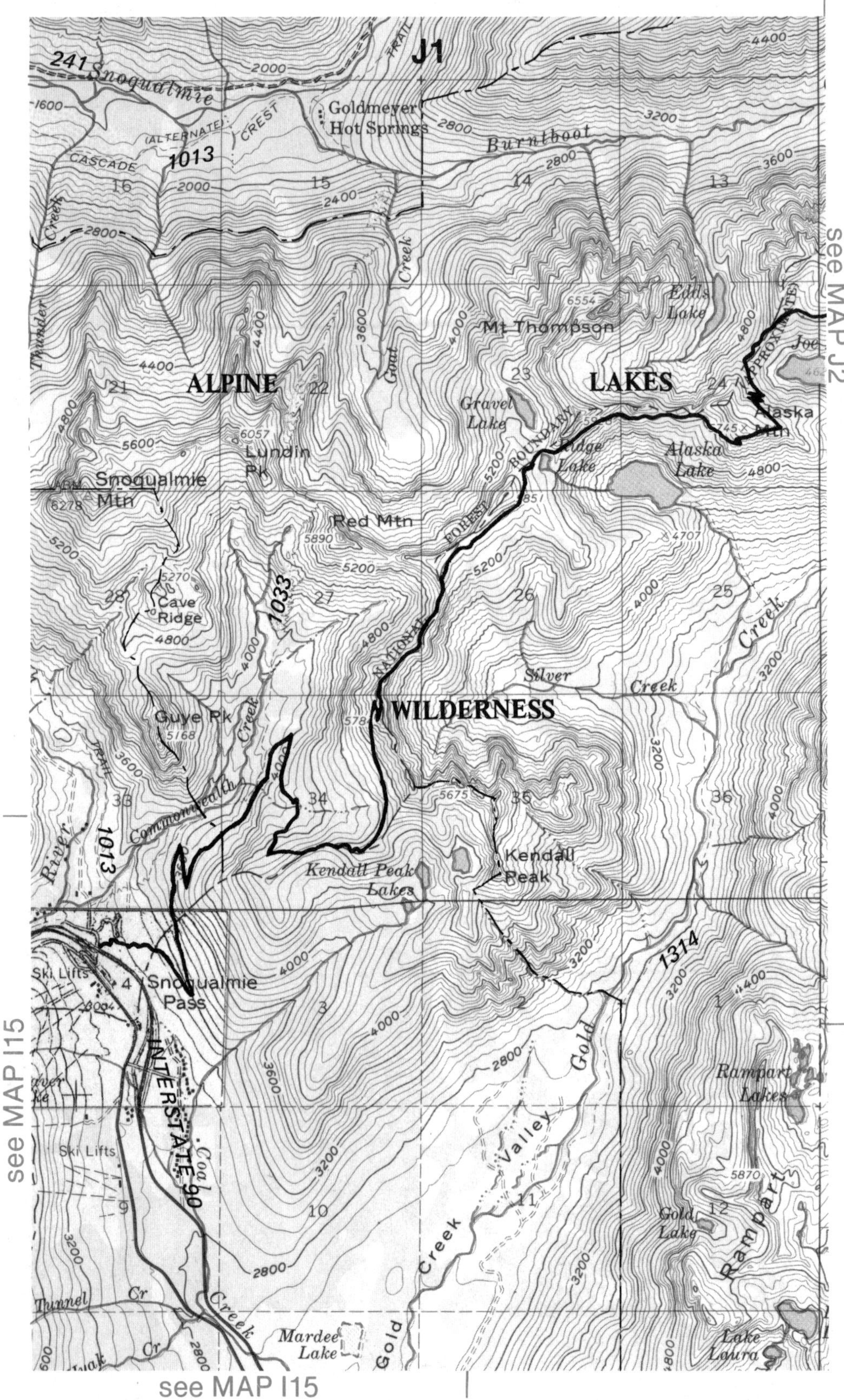

see MAP J2
see MAP I15
see MAP I15

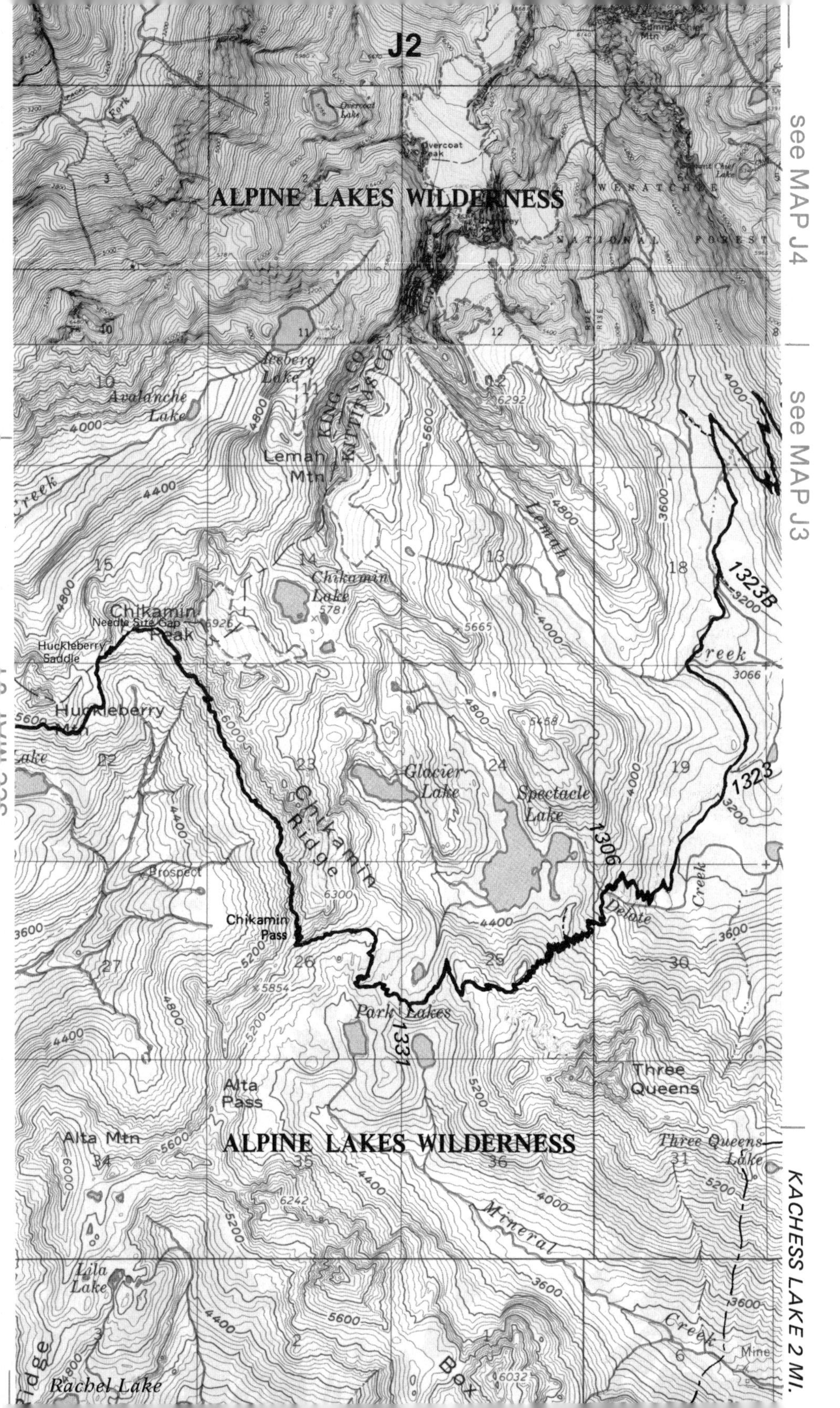

J2
ALPINE LAKES WILDERNESS
Overcoat Lake
Overcoat Peak
WENATCHEE NATIONAL FOREST
Iceberg Lake
Avalanche Lake
KING CO.
KITTITAS CO.
Lemah Mtn
Lemah
Creek
Chikamin Lake
Chikamin Peak
Needle Site Gap
Huckleberry Saddle
Huckleberry Mtn
1323B
1323
Creek
Glacier Lake
Spectacle Lake
Chikamin Ridge
1306
Prospect
Chikamin Pass
Delate
Creek
Park Lakes
1331
Alta Pass
Alta Mtn
Three Queens
ALPINE LAKES WILDERNESS
Three Queens Lake
Mineral
Lila Lake
Creek
Mine
Box
Ridge
Rachel Lake

see MAP J4
see MAP J3
KACHESS LAKE 2 MI.

huckleberry, and devil's club at your feet, cross an abandoned road and before long start climbing three long, well-graded switchbacks. They lift you around a ridge, away from the freeway noise and into the valley of Commonwealth Creek. As the trail traverses above this valley's floor, the route crosses a tributary right below a spraying waterfall and then comes to a junction with Red Mountain Trail 1033 (3820–2.5).

Side route. Heading up Commonwealth Creek, this trail takes you to a number of creekside campsites in a few minutes' walk. These are the only suitable ones between Snoqualmie Pass and Gravel Lake.

From the junction, the trail resumes climbing on newer tread, heading for high country that was seldom visited before the completion of this PCT segment in 1978.

To the west and north, Chair Peak, Snoqualmie Mountain, Red Mountain, and other summits already hint at the alpine terrain awaiting as the trail next switchbacks south. Returning into deeper forest, you continue climbing steadily on another switchback leg, up to the divide between the Snoqualmie and Yakima rivers. Along here, you glimpse Kachess Lake to the southeast and then immediately angle back onto the west flank of the steepening divide to continue the ascent.

Before long, the route emerges onto talus, and the high country opens up all around you. Besides the craggy, multicolored peaks to the west, Mt. Rainier rises like a huge apparition to the south. ▌ *Even if bad weather obscures this view, you can still find your spirits lifted by brilliant pockets of paintbrush, columbine, spiraea, valerian, tiger lily, and other flowers.* ▌ The PCT continues rising gradually, with dwarfed mountain hemlocks clinging to trailside craglets, while more peaks come into view to the north, including Mt. Thompson and distant Mt. Stuart. Cross to the east side of the crest (5440–3.2), from which level hiking shows you Chikamin Ridge at the head of Gold Creek Valley, and Alta Mountain and some amazing cliffs of Rampart Ridge draw your eye across the valley.

Water might seep from late snow patches on this trail, but otherwise, this airy section, often just a ledge blasted from the rocky crest, is fairly dry. Soon the trail rounds a narrow spur ridge well above glistening Alaska Lake, and then it cuts down to the crest saddle (5270–1.1) between Ridge and Gravel lakes. Campsites away from the west shore of Gravel Lake, the northwestern of the two lakes, are the last sites until Park Lakes, 8.2 miles distant. Camping is not allowed at well-worn Ridge Lake.

From the north side of Ridge Lake, the PCT takes off on a talus traverse around the rim of the cirque holding Alaska Lake and then climbs some as it rounds the sharp east ridge of Alaska Mountain. Next, steep switchbacks that hold snow into August take you down the north slope of this peak, and then a traverse leads you to a narrow, forested saddle (5030–2.2), between Joe and Edds lakes. These lakes lie, respectively, 400 feet below to the east and 800 feet below to the west.

The trail slants off the saddle into a meadowy ravine and then rises across the open, rocky south flank of Huckleberry Mountain. As you turn north around the east side of this peak, which is a summer pasture for wary mountain goats, you enter a beautiful hanging vale. Here, with a full view of Mt. Rainier, the trail meets a stream that cascades among rock slabs and heather gardens. At the head of this ravine, you pass a couple of small pools before coming to the crest at Huckleberry Saddle (5560–1.5), which is a broad pass with a fragile carpet of bilberries. This scenic gap has remained nearly pristine largely because the Forest Service prohibits camping at it.

Short switchbacks among dwarfed hemlocks take you above the saddle, allowing views of Mt. Index and the Olympic Mountains in the distant northwest. This climb then leads to a traverse below the tip of a crag to Needle Sight Gap (5930–0.6). After a glimpse through this notch beyond the Burntboot drainage to distant Glacier Peak, the PCT turns southeast for a long alpine traverse along the meadow and rocky southwest face of Chikamin Ridge. ▌ *Whole platoons of marmots may whistle loudly and then scurry from approaching hikers as the latter make their way across this headwall of Gold Creek, from which they can admire the placid sheen of Joe Lake, the twin thumbs of Huckleberry Mountain and Mt. Thompson, and the miragelike*

See maps J1,

dome of Mt. Rainier. ▮ On the way, the trail crosses a few steep chutes that usually shelter slippery tongues of snow well into midseason.

After climbing gently on the last third of this traverse, the PCT reaches Chikamin Pass (5780–2.5), where you can look across Park Lakes' basin to Three Queens, Box Ridge, and, in the distant northeast, the granite pyramid of Mt. Stuart. Now brake down a couple of switchbacks into the lake basin, where mosquitoes swarm in the subalpine meadows much more thickly than at the breezy crests just left behind. Once on gentler ground, the route passes campsites, then a junction with southbound Mineral Creek Trail 1331, and finally an access spur (4960–1.4) that leads to more campsites. Weaving through this hummocky plateau, which actually straddles the divide between Mineral Creek and Delate Creek, you follow the PCT generally east and then northeast around the bowl of the northernmost Park Lake. With the lake behind you, climb a pair of switchbacks to pass some ponds and gain a northwest spur of Three Queens (5350–0.8). Here you can look north over turquoise Spectacle Lake to the spiny, metamorphic fangs, hanging glaciers, and alpine waterfalls of Lemah Mountain. The rolling Wenatchee Mountains rise in the more distant east.

Now start a bone-jarring, 2000-foot descent, twisting and pounding down literally scores of tight switchbacks—hairpins that continue from a chute on the east side of a knob down to the runout of Three Queens' avalanche slopes. As the trail drops into thicker forest, you pass Spectacle Lake Trail 1306 (4440–1.6), which forks north, and below this junction, you walk on a sturdy bridge across roaring Delate Creek (3920–1.2); this spot has a one-tent campsite. Just beyond, you find the old, steeper Spectacle Lake Trail branching up the drainage and then find a small campsite (3800–0.3). The last series of switchbacks finally drops you onto a bottomland forest with fern glades, and later you cruise past eastbound Pete Lake Trail 1323 (3210–1.8).

Northbound, the PCT rounds a small knob and then gently descends northwest to the trunk stream of Lemah Creek (3200–0.8), where there are many sandy-gravelly campsites. From

See map J2

View across Joe Lake toward Alta Mountain and the Three Queens

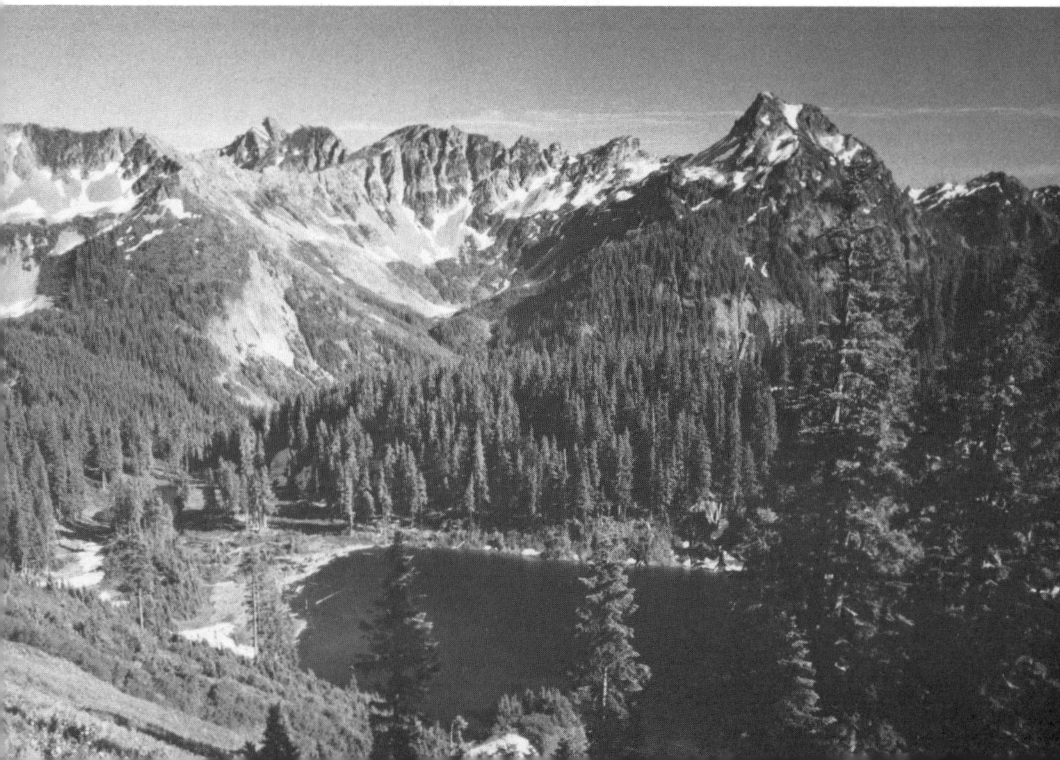

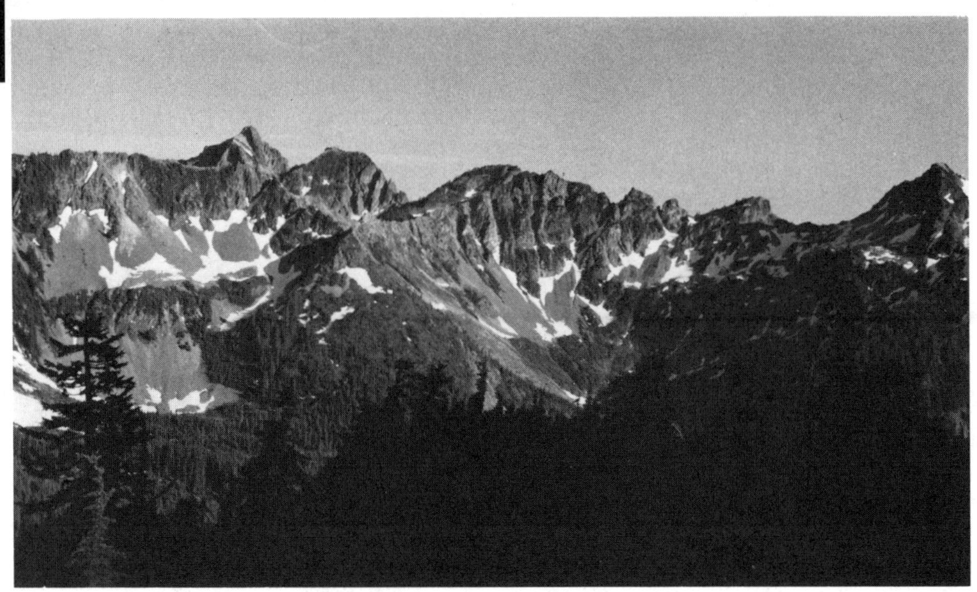

Three Queens and Alta Mountain

here, the trail continues north, rising over a small moraine and then dropping to cross a bridge over North Fork Lemah Creek. Immediately after climbing out of this stream's ravine, the PCT meets Lemah Meadow Trail 1323B (3210–0.7), which climbs northwest from Pete Lake. The PCT continues north past a couple of campsites (3240–0.7), gradually leaving behind Lemah Creek, and then passes through forest and meadow and across a freshet. The trail then comes to a spot (3370–0.7) from which an access spur descends ¼ mile to more campsites back at Lemah Creek's north fork. Here the PCT embarks on a 2200-foot climb to the top of Escondido Ridge, a climb best started early in the morning if it's to be a warm day.

Not far into this climb, you cross a couple of seasonal streams, but beyond those you must count on vistas through the cedar, hemlock, and vine-maple forest to inspire you on. Brief though these are, these impressive alpine views of Lemah Mountain, Chikamin Ridge, and Three Queens broaden with every switchback. Eventually, the montane forest wanes, and smaller mountain hemlocks and subalpine firs spread around you as the trail turns up a ravine into a secluded cirque with a chilly tarn (5520–5.3). Camping is prohibited here, but after you switchback once more and contour southeast 0.3 mile through subalpine parkland, you come to some designated campsites.

Continuing around point 5984, you reach another cirque, where camping is also prohibited, and cross the inlet (5300–1.3) of the lowest of a chain of crystalline tarns before starting a gradually rising traverse across the next ridge. From the top of this ridge, the PCT arcs around a sheltered vale, jumping its creek and passing a campsite a few hundred yards farther southeast. Next, you exit this meadowy glen and emerge onto the edge of Escondido Ridge, where you have a view over Waptus Lake and beyond to ever-closer Mt. Stuart. Not far along the ridge, you find Waptus Burn Trail 1329C (5180–1.7), which continues down the ridge while the PCT switchbacks down and begins a 2200-foot descent to the Waptus River.

▮ *A grand alpine panorama oversees these well-graded switchbacks. Across the valley, long waterfalls drain the lofty Mt. Daniel-Mt. Hinman massif, and, at the valley's head, the impressive sedimentary slabs of Bear's Breast Mountain thrust skyward.* ▮ As you stomp down the first switchbacks, pointy subalpine firs give way to open brush (a scar from the 1929 Waptus Burn fire); then you traverse north to the main bank of switchbacks, the last three touching a cascading stream.

See maps J2, J3, J4

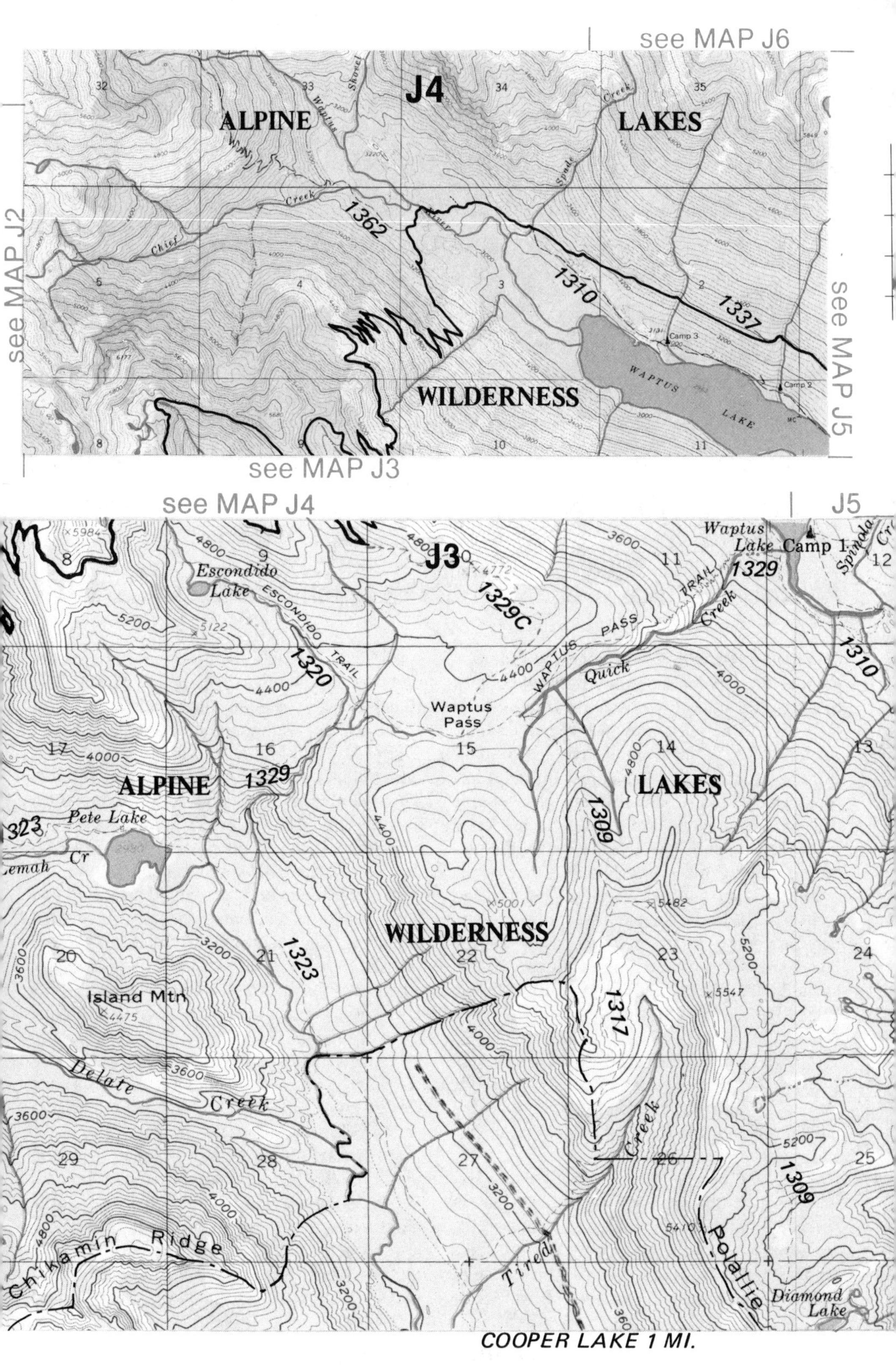

see MAP J6
J4
ALPINE
LAKES
WILDERNESS
Chief
Creek
Waptus
Spade
1362
1310
1337
Camp 3
Camp 2
WAPTUS
LAKE
see MAP J2
see MAP J5
see MAP J3
see MAP J4
J5
J3
Escondido
Lake
ESCONDIDO
TRAIL
1320
1329C
Waptus
Lake
Camp 1
1329
Spinola
WAPTUS
PASS
TRAIL
Quick
Creek
1310
Waptus
Pass
ALPINE
1329
LAKES
1309
Pete Lake
Cr
WILDERNESS
1323
Island Mtn
1317
Delate
Creek
Chikamin
Ridge
Tired
Creek
1309
Polallie
Diamond
Lake
COOPER LAKE 1 MI.

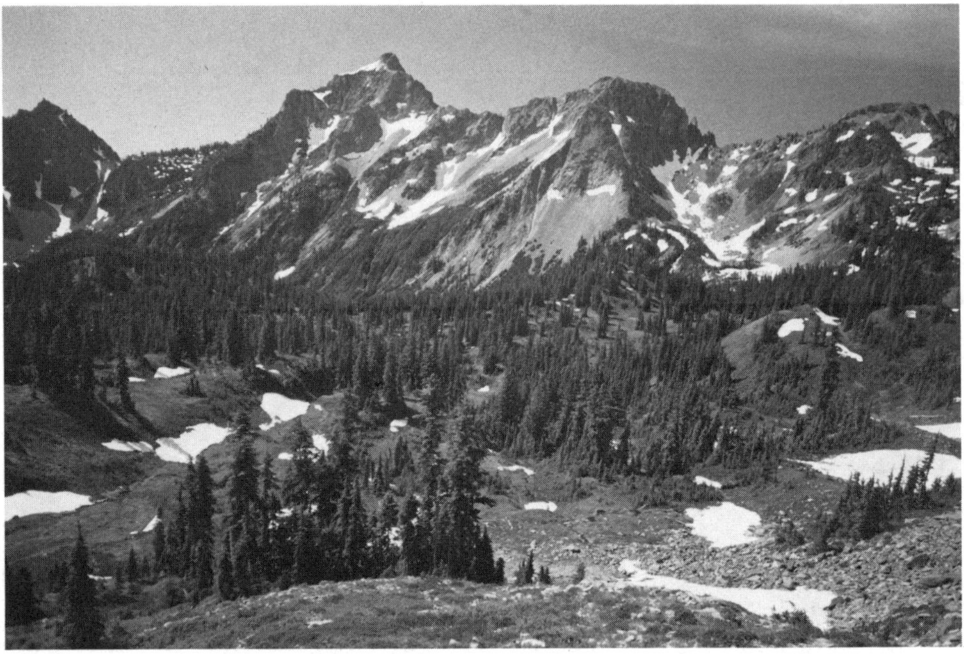

Box Ridge, from the Park Lakes basin

Western redcedar droops over the trail as it empties onto the broad valley floor and comes to a campsite at northwest-bound Dutch Miller Gap Trail 1362, but you won't find water until 0.1 mile later, at the Waptus River (3020–4.8). A girdered bridge gets you across this cold torrent, and you turn downstream alongside a *roche moutonnée*, a "dome" of rock that stood fast even though it was overridden by the glaciers that filled this valley. The PCT then winds northeast past a connection to the Dutch Miller Gap Trail and continues under Douglas-firs that rise above a carpet of ferns and vanilla leaf. As you start rising off the valley floor, you cross Spade Creek and meet Waptus River Trail 1310 (3070–0.8).

Side route. This trail comes up from campsites ¾ mile away at Waptus Lake and ultimately from the Cle Elum River, about 12 miles away.

The PCT proceeds on a gently rising traverse above the valley, well-shaded under spruce, fir, and cedar boughs, but you get the occasional blue glints of large Waptus Lake below. On the way, the path crosses a couple of fairly reliable streams. Between them, Spade Lake Trail 1337 climbs north, and at the second stream, there is a campsite (3400–1.5). Eventually, your trail turns north into the Spinola Creek valley and meets Spinola Creek Trail 1310A (3440–1.1), which climbs about one mile from the outlet of Waptus Lake. Through alternating patches of forest, meadow, and talus, the trail steepens somewhat and even switchbacks in several places as it works up this valley, keeping some distance above the creek. A second series of switchbacks gets you around a knob and onto a bench from which Cathedral Rock marks your direction. ▮ *From about this vicinity onward, a mid-1990s fire ravaged much of central Alpine Lakes Wilderness, and you see evidence of this burn for miles ahead.* ▮

Now in a meadowy subalpine realm, you continue north and, not long after crossing a feeder creek, meet Lake Vicente Trail 1365 (4440–3.8), which ascends west. The PCT immediately turns through a small gap and then follows the bank of now-quiet Spinola Creek, soon crossing another tributary at a campsite. A bit farther north, the PCT approaches Deep Lake's indigo surface, only to fork from the lake's campsite-access trail (4400–0.5) and turn east to wade its ankle-deep

See maps J4, J5, J6

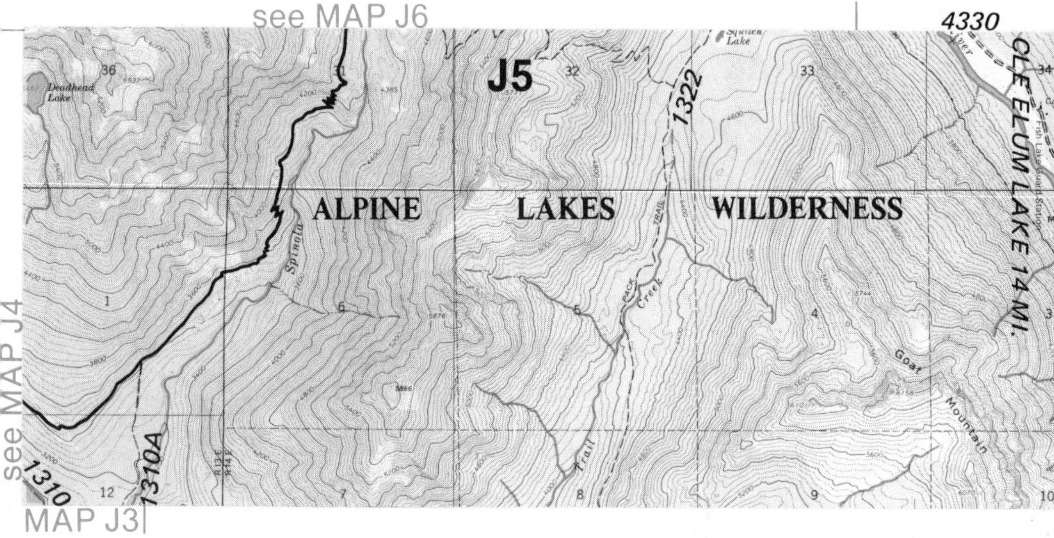

outlet. Now you head for the east side of Deep Lake's basin to the start of a 1200-foot climb to Cathedral Pass.

Well-graded switchbacks take you far above the lake to the scraggly outliers of the subalpine-fir forest, where you get a new perspective of the alpine bluffs of Mt. Daniel. From the last hairpin, Trail 1375 (5560–3.0) forks northwest to Peggys Pond. Under the towering and resistant andesite of Cathedral Rock, the trail tops a crest at Cathedral Pass (5610–0.2) for a view across the upper Cle Elum River valley to the gray, alpine uplands of Granite Mountain.

From the pass, the Rainier View spur trail heads south down the ridge, while the PCT descends briefly east onto a parkland bench

See map J6

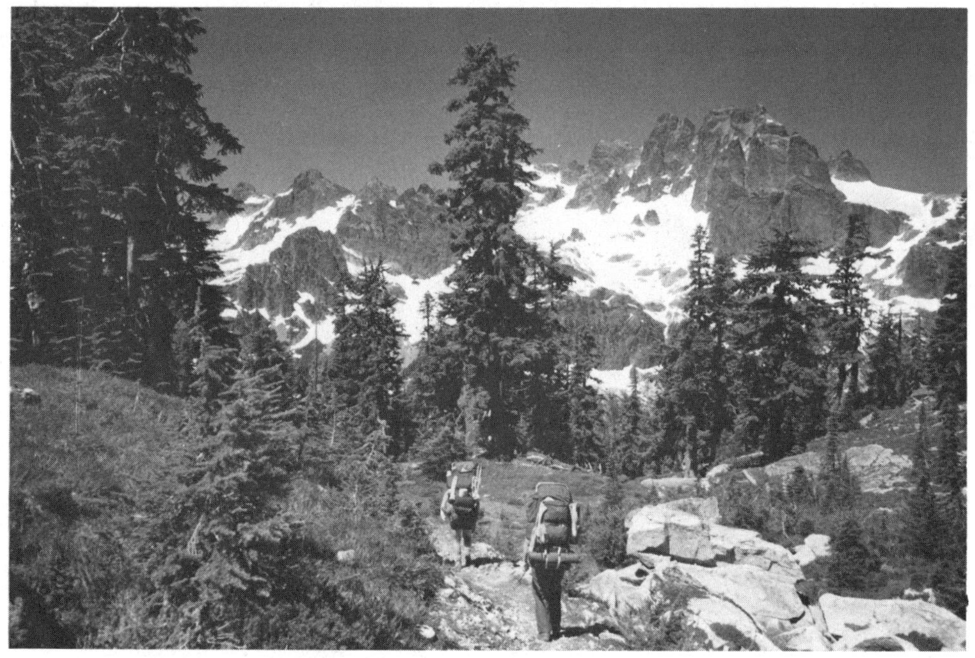

Lemah Mountain, from Escondido Ridge

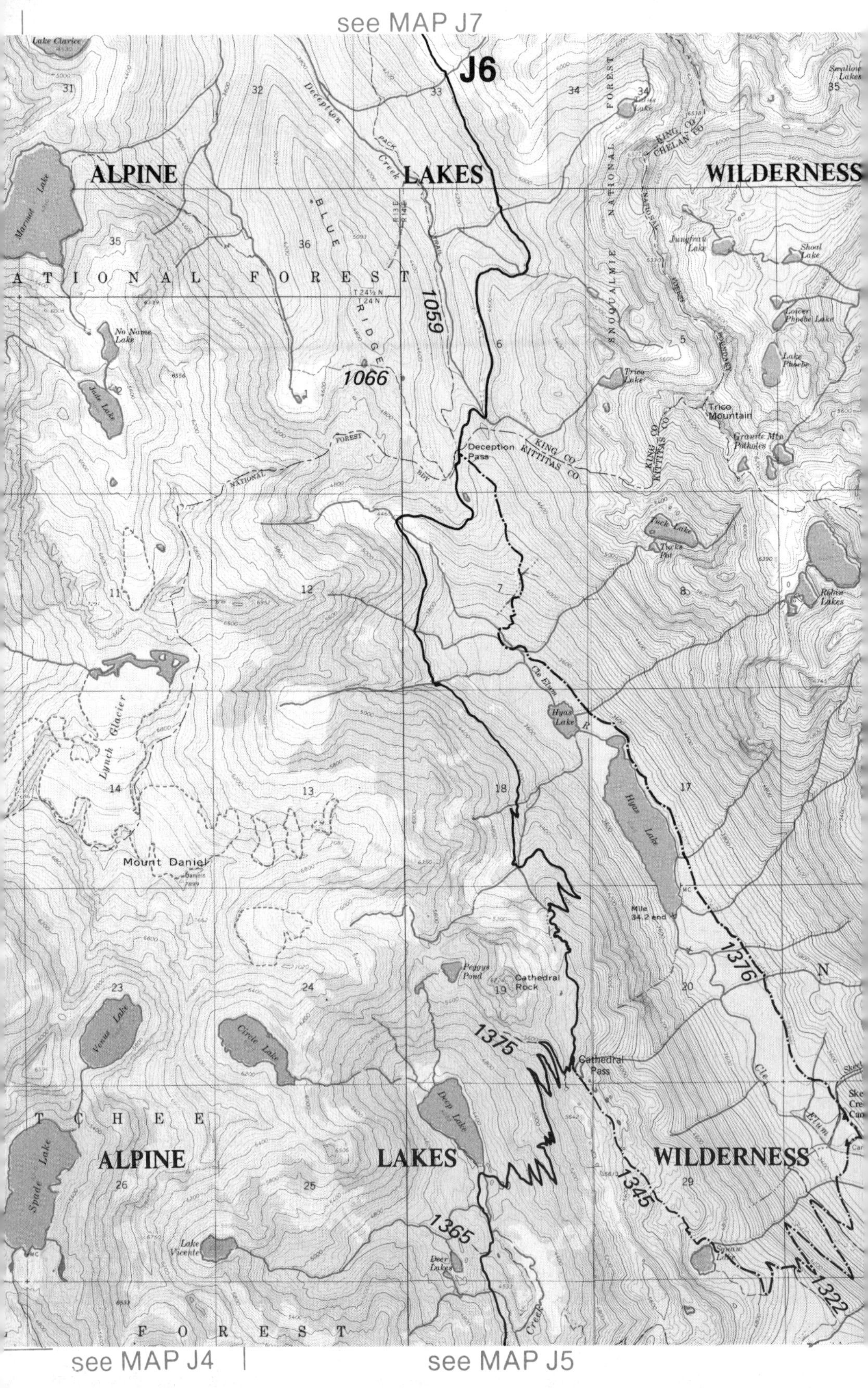
see MAP J7
J6
ALPINE LAKES WILDERNESS
NATIONAL FOREST
Lake Clarice
Marmot Lake
Deception Creek
PACK TRAIL
BLUE RIDGE
1059
1066
No Name Lake
Jade Lake
Deception Pass
KING CO
KITTITAS CO
CHELAN CO
SNOQUALMIE NATIONAL FOREST
Swallow Lakes
Jungfrau Lake
Shoal Lake
Lower Phoebe Lake
Lake Phoebe
Trico Lake
Trico Mountain
Granite Mtn Potholes
Tuck Lake
Tucks Pot
Robin Lakes
Cle Elum R
Hyas Lake
Lynch Glacier
Mount Daniel
Mile 34.2 end
1376
Peggys Pond
Cathedral Rock
1375
Cathedral Pass
Venus Lake
Circle Lake
Deep Lake
Spade Lake
ALPINE LAKES WILDERNESS
1345
1365
Lake Vicente
Deer Lakes
Squaw Lake
1322
FOREST
see MAP J4
see MAP J5

with a few campsites and a few small tarns (5460–0.1). From here, Cathedral Rock Trail 1345, the old PCT, drops south 2000 feet to the Cle Elum River. You can take the official PCT, where there is a potentially treacherous stream crossing, or the old PCT as a long alternate route. In author Selters's opinion, the stream crossing in question is rarely dangerous enough for the average backpacker to warrant the 9½-mile detour on the old PCT route. Still, we've drawn it on Map J6 for those who may want to take it.

The official PCT route, wandering around hillocks as it continues north, proceeds in the shadow of Cathedral Rock along the edge of the scenic bench. It then starts twisting down a ridgeline, steepening as it goes, until it traverses into montane forest, where it makes a couple of longer switchbacks. These end at a bench that has shady campsites at a junction of two streams (4600–2.0). North from this bench, the trail continues descending steadily across slopes forested in complex patches of mountain hemlock and subalpine fir, then red-cedar, Douglas-fir, and alder. The route crosses one creek and then comes to a second, which is

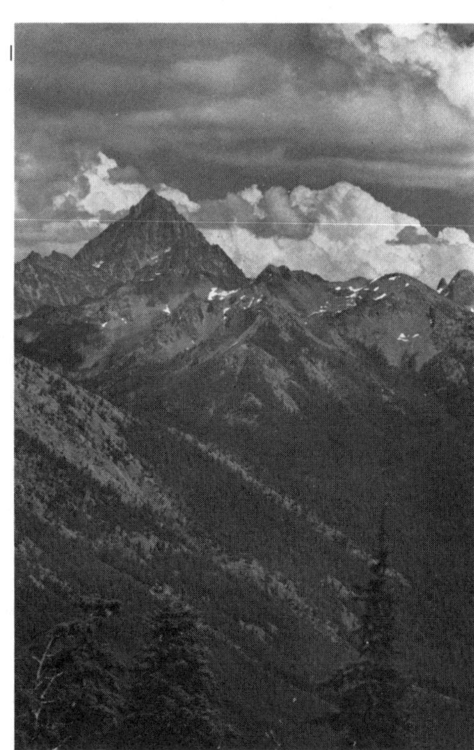

Mt. Stuart, from Cathedral Pass

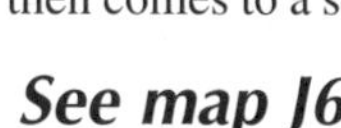

See map J6

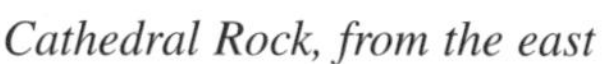

Cathedral Rock, from the east

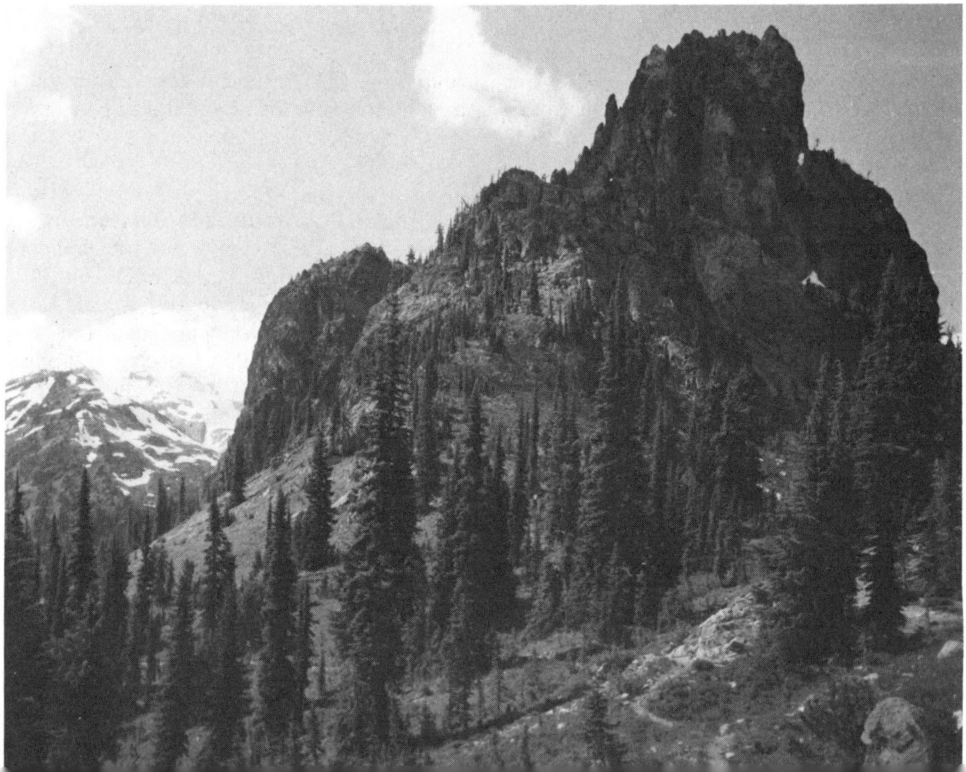

HIGHWAY 2 3½ MI. HIGHWAY 2 and SCENIC 3½ MI. see MAP J8

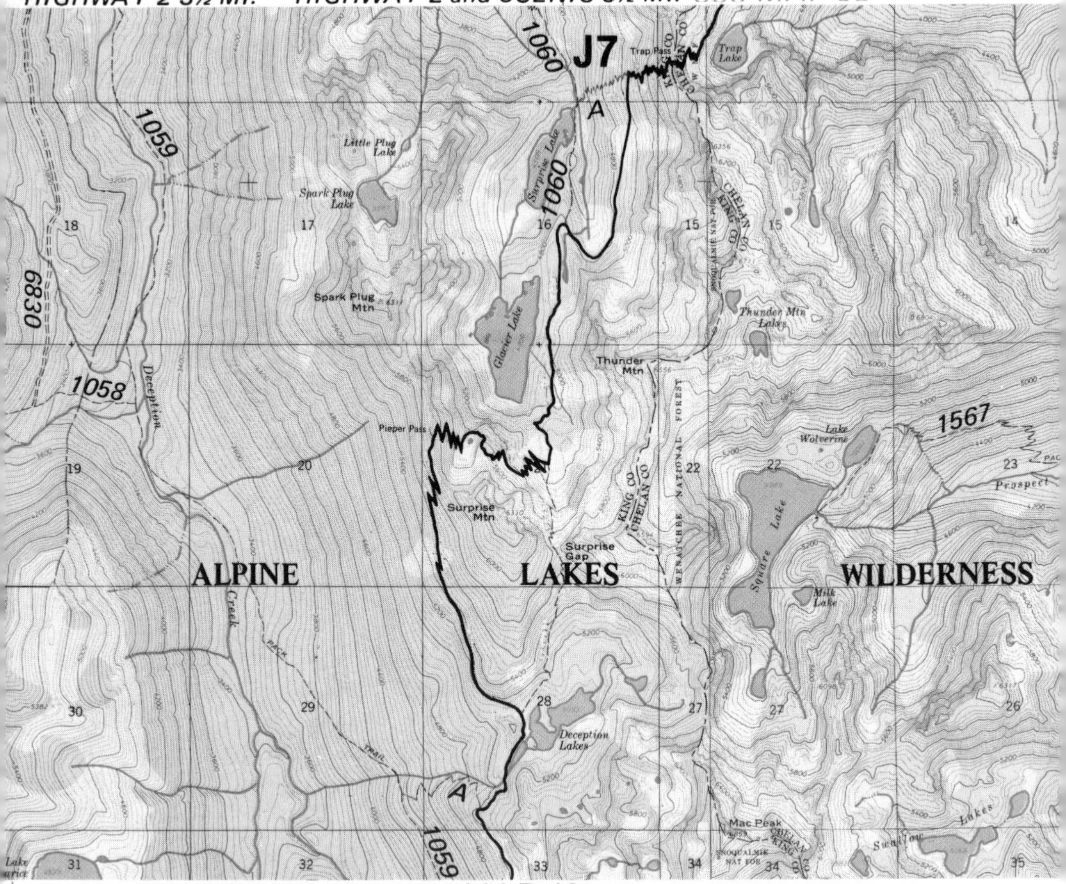

see MAP J6

potentially treacherous (3770–1.4). This stream, which drains Mt. Daniel's northeast slopes, is swift and cold, and you'll want to wear shoes or boots to cross its stony bed. However, the current is not capable of carrying a person away. Before the sun gets high, or on a cloudy day, the ford won't be more than a shin-deep swash for a few short strides.

From this ford, the trail ascends steadily across avalanche swaths and two or three more streams. The last, where the trail turns east at the head of the Cle Elum drainage, will likely require another, less vigorous footbath (4180–1.0). The gradual climb turns north again in a forest of unusually large subalpine firs and tops out at Deception Pass (4470–0.8) to meet the end of the alternate route, following.

Alternate route. To avoid the potentially treacherous stream crossing, some hikers might take the old route, Trail 1345, from this junction and climb back up to rejoin the newer trail at Deception Pass. This route is 4¼ miles longer than the official PCT.

Official PCT route and alternate route rejoined. Here at Deception Pass, a number of trail options confront the hiker. The old PCT (now Trail 1376) comes up from the Cle Elum River and Hyas Lake to rejoin the official PCT. Marmot Lake Trail 1066 branches west, and Trail 1059 forks north for Deception Creek, meeting Highway 2 about 6 miles east of Skykomish. Beyond these junctions, the PCT heads north-northeast.

Now the PCT contours around a knob to drop to nearby Deception Creek, a small stream in a deep and eroding drainage. ▮ *This gully is cutting along the Straight Creek fault, a major crustal weakness traceable from near Yakima well into British Columbia. In the past,*

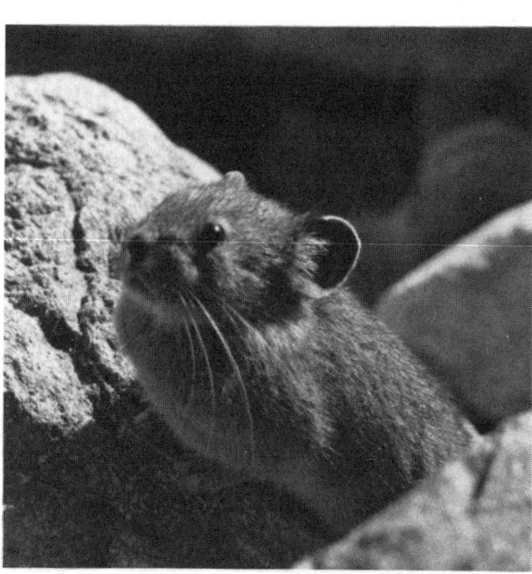

Pika

land to its west was shifted north, displaced 100–200 miles over the millennia. ▮ Continue out of the gully on a level track, getting a glimpse back to the glimmering heights of Mt. Daniel and its massive Lynch Glacier. Next, you round a ridge, jump one stream, and then, near a campsite (4400–1.9), jump another stream as you continue through cedar-and-fir forest. The PCT starts a long, gradually rising traverse above the valley of Deception Creek, passing through the skeletons of an old forest fire and eventually rounding a ridge to meet Deception Creek Trail 1059A, which drops west. About 0.1 mile east of this junction, you cross the outlet (5040–1.5) of Deception Lakes and then follow the west shoreline of the narrow lower lake. Although these lakes offer fine swimming and a pleasant rest, their accessibility has lured hordes who have beaten their campsites and much of their shorelines to dust.

Just as it nears the large upper lake, the PCT climbs northwest and enters a draw at the end of which an unsigned and unmaintained trail drops off to the west. You, on the other hand, angle northwest uphill and around a ridge to resume the ascending traverse high above Deception Creek. Now, however, you can see northwest beyond a checkerboard of clearcuts to the jagged teeth of Mt. Index, Mt. Baring, and Three Fingers, as well as across the valley, where Lake Clarice nestles against Terrace Mountain. Turn up a steep slope and, with a few switchbacks, surmount it at Pieper Pass (5920–2.0). From here, the abandoned Cascade Crest Trail follows the ridgecrest north, but the PCT turns east toward inviting Glacier Lake and then drops off the pass for a braking descent.

Steep switchbacks take you down to a small bench with a tarn and a view of distant Glacier Peak, and then you wind among the granite

See maps J6, J7

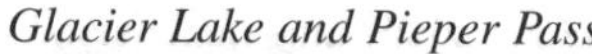

Glacier Lake and Pieper Pass

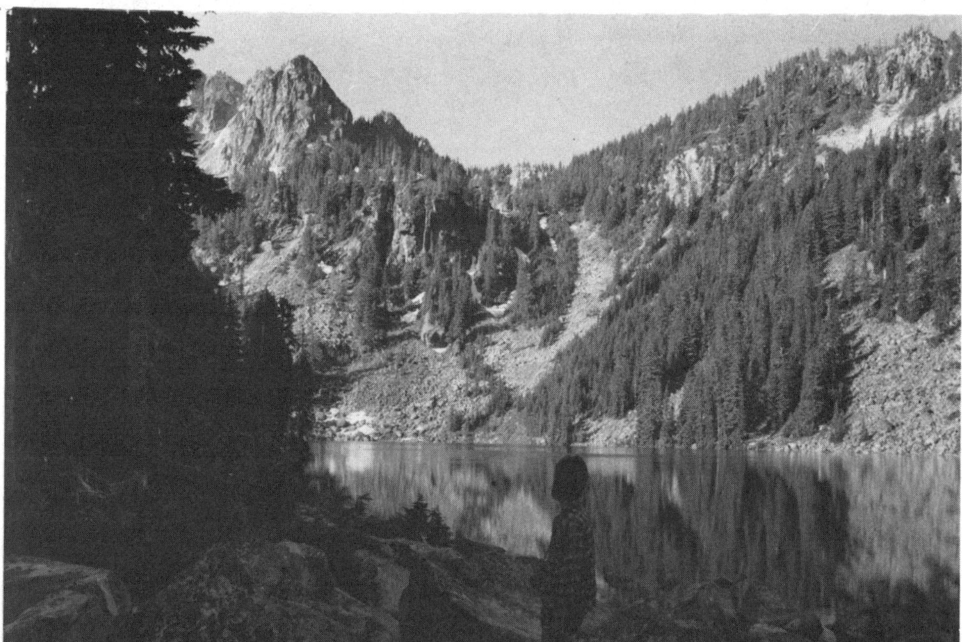

see MAP K1

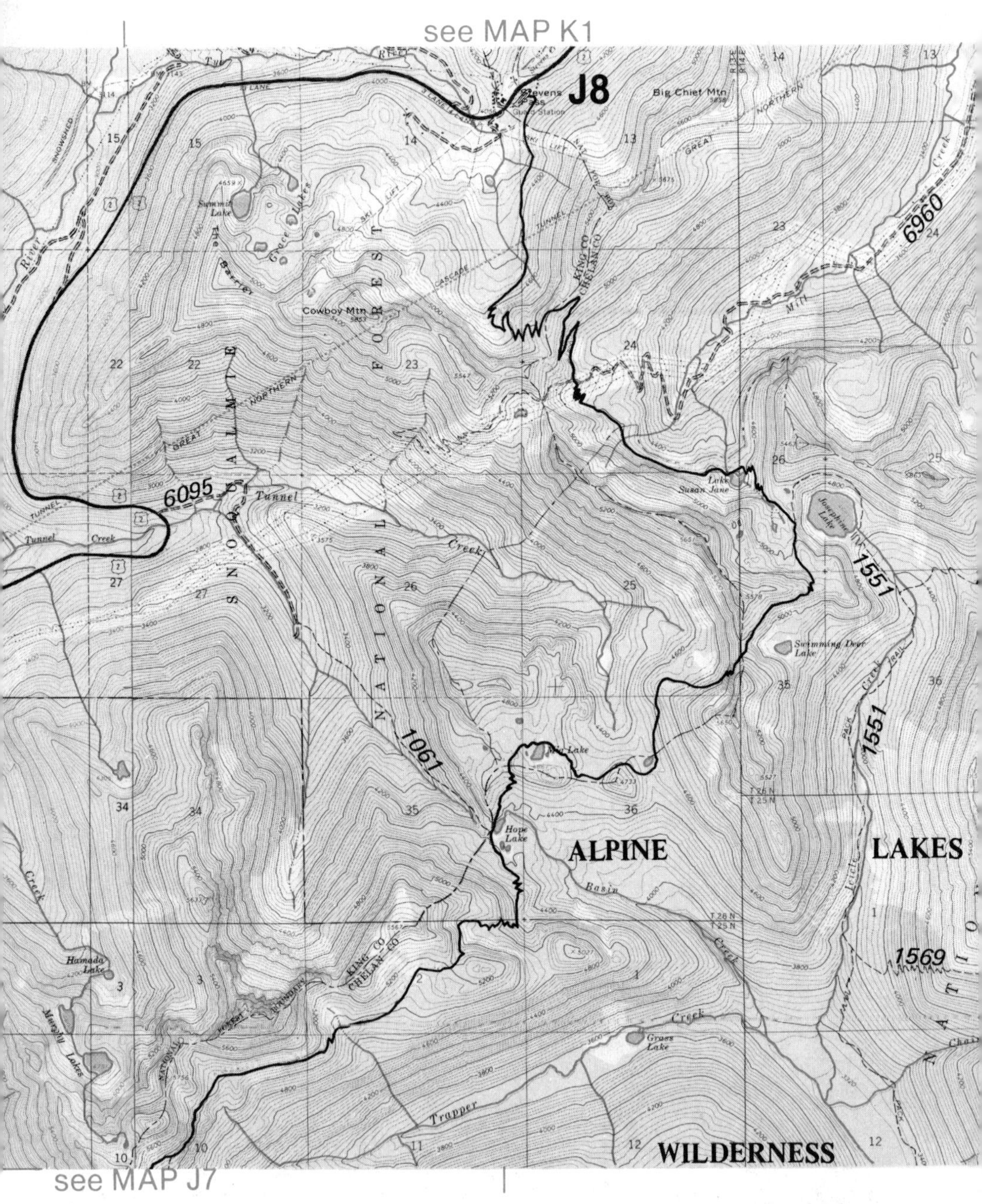

see MAP J7

boulders of a lower bench before descending a talus slope to the cirque floor. From here, you descend into the forest past a campsite (5000–2.0) that is above the southeast shore of Glacier Lake. Beyond this, you cross a creek and hike around the bottom of a talus slope as you parallel Glacier Lake's glistening east shore 50–100 feet above it. Then continue away from the lake past a narrow pond with another campsite and shortly meet Surprise Lake Trail 1060 (4840–0.8), which heads north for about four miles to meet Highway 2 about

See map J7

8 miles east of Skykomish. At the junction, the PCT pivots southeast to arc around the head of a ravine and start a rising traverse north.

This traverse takes you through forests and rocky fields, ever higher above Surprise Lake, ever closer to gnarly crags atop the crest. It ends where the PCT joins Trap Pass Trail 1060A (5080–1.0) in the middle of a bank of steep switchbacks and then grinds up the rest of the switchbacks to the Cascade divide at Trap Pass (5800–0.9). With the blue disc of Trap Lake seemingly a straight drop below, you switchback and traverse down and across its steep cirque wall to a sharply descending access trail (5350–0.8) to the lake. After leaving the lake's bowl, the PCT keeps to flowery avalanche slopes and shady forested slopes high above Trapper Creek. At a small bench, it passes a campsite beside a seasonal creek (4970–1.2) and then climbs briefly to a notch (5210–0.7). From here, you slant and switchback down through steep forest and across another bench, dropping before long to a gentle terrain at overused Hope Lake (4400–1.1). From here, at a curiously low spot in the Cascade crest, Tunnel Creek Trail 1061 drops 1.4 miles northwest to Road 6095, which descends 1.2 miles to Highway 2.

North from the turbid waters of Hope Lake, you climb through fir-and-hemlock forest onto a somewhat-swampy parkland plateau on which you turn east to the north end of Mig Lake (4670–0.7). By midsummer, this shallow lake warms to a pleasant swimming temperature. East from it, the PCT drops to a crest saddle, rounds a knob, and curves around a swampy pond. Onward, climb around a forested ridge and confront steeper climbing beneath cliffbands, topping out at an unnamed crest saddle (5190–1.8). Here a slice of Swimming Deer Lake tempts you to drop 300 feet through very steep forest, but more accessible water is just down the trail, which contours east to a spur ridge, beyond which it drops along a rill in a grassy swale to the rim of Josephine Lake's cirque (4980–0.8). From here, Icicle Trail 1551 descends around the cirque to the turquoise lake's outlet.

From the Icicle Trail junction, the PCT proceeds northwest down a ravine and then down

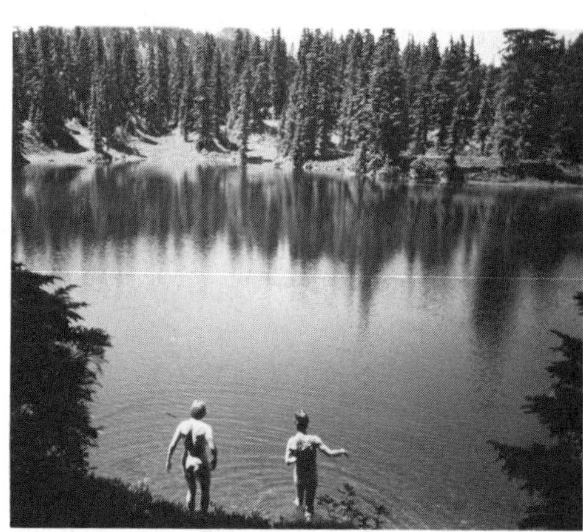

Swimmers at Mig Lake

a talus slope to the north shore of Lake Susan Jane (4600–0.5). With powerlines and the crest of Stevens Pass Ski Area in sight, and probably with a number of overnighters at this pretty and accessible lake, a wilderness-accustomed PCT hiker strongly senses re-entry into civilization. Next, the trail traverses west under steep but well-flowered bluffs where snow lingers across the track until August. Soon after crossing a tumbling stream, the trail passes a campsite near the edge of the swath cut for the immense powerlines overhead. ▮ *These buzzing cables carry hydroelectricity from the rural Columbia basin east of the Cascades to the cities of the coast.* ▮ A couple of rough roads run through the logged swath, and you depend on trail signs to follow the climbing, switchbacking path across the former roadbeds.

North of the powerlines, the trail continues climbing, taking long, meadowy switchbacks up to the Cascade crest at a saddle (5160–2.2) near the top of a chairlift. Steeper, tighter switchbacks then take you down beneath this and other chairlifts to lower-angled slopes from which you make a long, descending traverse north, crossing a creek on the way to four-lane Highway 2. The trail ends at a parking area, and you head southwest through it as it quickly narrows to a road and is joined by another short road coming in from the left. On this road, you momentarily reach Highway 2 (4060–2.1). This spot is 100 yards north-northeast of signed Stevens Pass (4061) and its obvious ski area.

See maps J7, J8

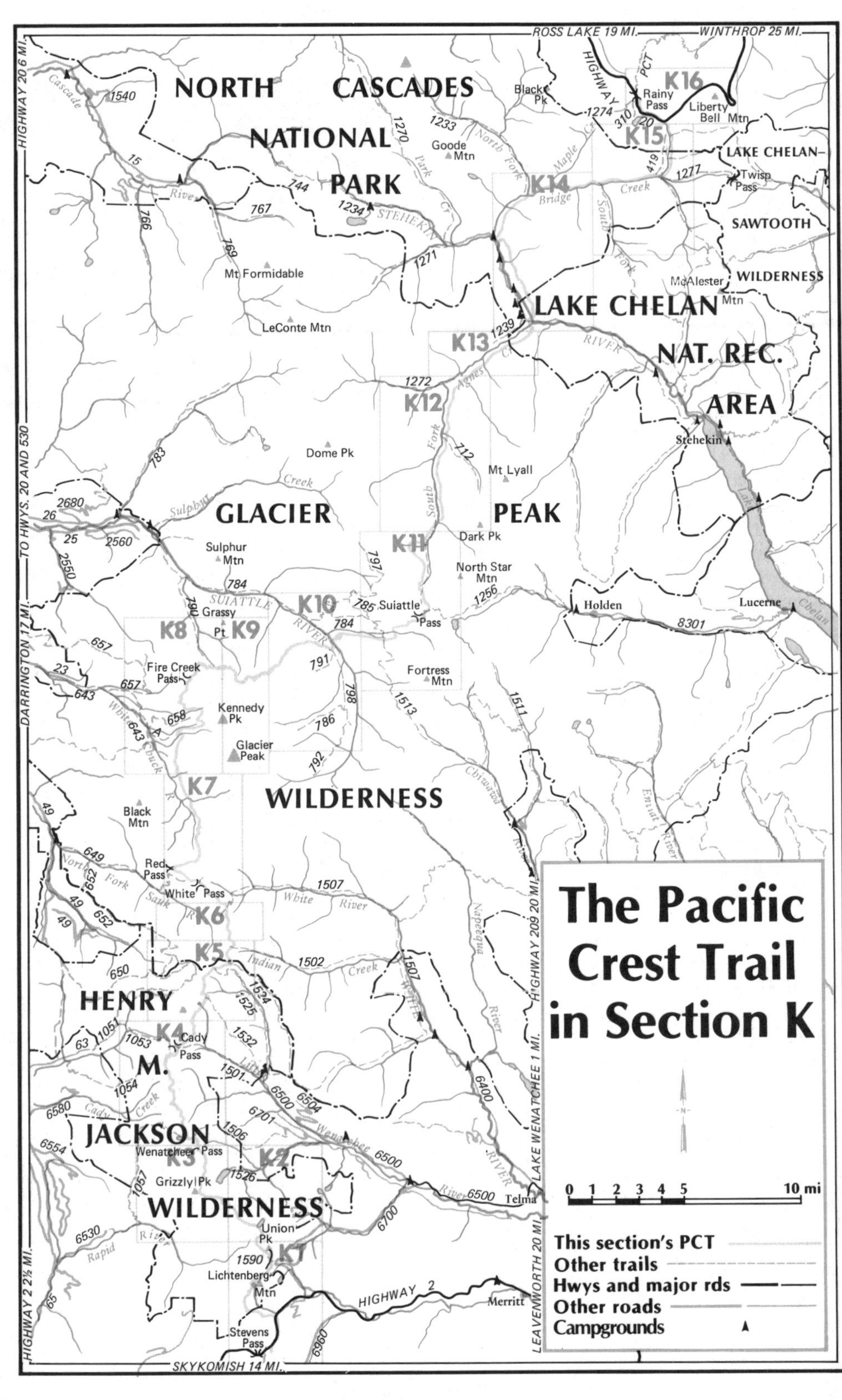
The Pacific Crest Trail in Section K
NORTH CASCADES NATIONAL PARK
LAKE CHELAN NAT. REC. AREA
SAWTOOTH WILDERNESS
GLACIER PEAK WILDERNESS
HENRY M. JACKSON WILDERNESS
ROSS LAKE 19 MI.
WINTHROP 25 MI.
HIGHWAY 20 6 MI.
TO HWYS. 20 AND 530
DARRINGTON 17 MI.
HIGHWAY 2 2½ MI.
SKYKOMISH 14 MI.
LEAVENWORTH 20 MI.
LAKE WENATCHEE 1 MI.
HIGHWAY 209 20 MI.
LAKE CHELAN—
Rainy Pass
Liberty Bell Mtn
Twisp Pass
McAlester Mtn
Black Pk
Goode Mtn
Mt Formidable
LeConte Mtn
Dome Pk
Mt Lyall
Dark Pk
North Star Mtn
Sulphur Mtn
Grassy Pt
Suiattle Pass
Fortress Mtn
Fire Creek Pass
Kennedy Pk
Glacier Peak
Black Mtn
Red Pass
White Pass
Cady Pass
Wenatchee Pass
Grizzly Pk
Union Pk
Lichtenberg Mtn
Stevens Pass
Stehekin
Holden
Lucerne
Telma
Merritt
HIGHWAY 2
K1 K2 K3 K4 K5 K6 K7 K8 K9 K10 K11 K12 K13 K14 K15 K16
0 1 2 3 4 5 10 mi
This section's PCT
Other trails
Hwys and major rds
Other roads
Campgrounds

Section K: Highway 2 at Stevens Pass to Highway 20 at Rainy Pass

Introduction: In this section, you will traverse along a very rugged section of the North Cascades. This hike ranks second only to Volume 1's John Muir Trail section in difficulty. Traversing around Glacier Peak, the hiker brakes down to and then labors up from, a number of deep-floored canyons that radiate from that peak. Unfortunately, a nice, contouring trail, such as the one around Mt. Adams, is impossible to route around Glacier Peak proper, for such a trail would be too snowbound and too avalanche-prone.

Not only does this section have rugged topography, but it sometimes has dangerous fords, cold, threatening weather, and persistent insects. Why then do thousands of backpackers flock to Glacier Peak Wilderness? Well, perhaps because it is a *real* wilderness and not, like so many others, a wilderness in name only. It provides a definite challenge to modern-day people, who are so protected from the elements. This area's intimidating, snowy terrain, which is contrasted with lovely, fragile wildflower gardens, will draw you back time and time again.

Declination: 19¾°E

Mileages:	S➛N	Mi. Btwn. Pts.	N➛S
Highway 2 at Stevens Pass	0.0		117.5
Lake Valhalla	5.5	5.5	112.0
Lake Janus	9.5	4.0	108.0
Wenatchee Pass	16.6	7.1	100.9
Trail 1057 to Pear Lake	17.9	1.3	99.6
Lake Sally Ann	27.9	10.0	89.6
Indian Pass	32.6	4.7	84.9
White Pass	36.5	3.9	81.0
Red Pass	38.4	1.9	79.1
White Chuck Trail	45.7	7.3	71.8
Kennedy Ridge Trail	47.3	1.6	70.2
Fire Creek Pass	54.5	7.2	63.0
Milk Creek Trail	58.5	4.0	59.0
Dolly Vista campsite	63.8	5.3	53.7
Suiattle River access trail	71.3	7.5	46.2
Miners Creek	76.2	4.9	41.3
Railroad Creek Trail to Holden	79.2	3.0	38.3
Hemlock Camp	85.7	6.5	31.8
Five Mile Camp	92.7	7.0	24.8
Agnes Creek trailhd. on Stehekin River Rd.	97.7	5.0	19.8
Bridge Creek trailhd. on Stehekin River Rd.	103.0	5.3	14.5
Six Mile Camp	109.2	6.2	8.3
Highway 20 at Rainy Pass	117.5	8.3	0.0

Supplies: See "Supplies" in the previous section for the facilities at Stevens Pass, this section's starting point. There are no other on-route supply points. However, upon reaching the Stehekin River near the end of the section, you can take a Park Service shuttle-bus, $5.00 each way in 2000, over to Stehekin, which has a resort, post office (98852), hiker-oriented store, and information center. If you need boots, clothes, or other special items, you can take a ferry from Stehekin to Chelan and then return.

Wilderness Permits: These are required for all backcountry stays in North Cascades National Park. The PCT enters the park about a mile north of the High Bridge Ranger Station and leaves the park about 3 miles south of Highway 20's Rainy Pass. If you're heading north on the PCT and don't already have a wilderness permit, you can get one in Stehekin at the Golden West Visitor Center or the Stehekin Ranger Station (in early or late season, when the visitor center is closed). If you're heading south on the PCT from Rainy Pass, then get a permit from the Marblemount Ranger Station, Wilderness Information Center (if coming from the west) or from the Methow Valley Visitor Center in Winthrop (if coming from the east). While in the park, you are required to camp in designated trailside camps only. If you don't have a permit, you may find that you also won't have a campsite!

Problems: In this section of heavy rain and snow avalanches, bridges periodically are washed away. Generally, the bridges are replaced within a year or two, but this is no consolation to you if you encounter a bridgeless stream. In particular, if either the bridge across the White Chuck River or the one across the Suiattle River is gone, the ford may be dangerous.

Additionally, this section is located in the central part of Washington's North Cascades, a part of the greater Cascade Range, extending roughly from Snoqualmie Pass north to the Canadian border, and composed largely of granitic and metamorphic rocks. These rocks aren't the problem, but the snowfall they collect is: the North Cascades accumulate more snow than anywhere else in the United States. In the 1998–99 weather season, the Mt. Baker Ski Area, lying west of the PCT, received a world record 1140 inches of measured snowfall. What this means for you, the trekker, is that even in a normal year, you may encounter a lot of snow-covered trail, which slows you down and sometimes causes you to get off route. Don't try hiking across snow in a whiteout; you may get lost.

A final problem is bears, which are quite common from Stehekin north up the Stehekin River and up Bridge Creek. You can bearbag your food, which usually works, although rodents such as mice and even flying squirrels have gotten into suspended food bags. The Park Service recommends you use a bearproof canister. Hopefully in the future, there will be bearproof food-storage boxes at all the Park's PCT campsites, much as in Yosemite National Park, but until money becomes available, the area remains "boxless".

Maps:

Stevens Pass, WA
Labyrinth Mountain, WA
Captain Point, WA
Bench Mark Mountain, WA
Poe Mountain, WA
Glacier Peak East, WA
Glacier Peak West, WA
Lime Mountain, WA
Gamma Peak, WA
Suiattle Pass, WA
Agnes Mountain, WA
Mt. Lyall, WA
McGregor Mountain, WA
McAlester Mountain, WA
Washington Pass, WA

THE ROUTE

Look for the trailhead about 250 yards north-northeast from Stevens Pass (4061) on Highway 2, by the east side of a power substation. The PCT route begins on a maintenance road that contours north across granitic terrain. On this open, bushy stretch, you pass an assortment of aster, bleeding heart, bluebells, columbine, fireweed, lupine, monkeyflower, paintbrush, parsnip, and Sitka valerian before curving west into a forested environment. You reach a 3-yard-wide tributary (3850–2.5) of Nason Creek, beside which you could camp, but you elect to continue up to a meadow (4220–1.0) through which Nason Creek flows. Here among the cinquefoil, shooting stars, red heather, and grass are good campsites. ▮ *Mosquitoes and several species of biting flies, common in northern Washington through midsummer, will not bother you if the day is cold or misty.* ▮

Now within Henry M. Jackson Wilderness, the trail climbs up to a second meadow where you could camp, and then it switchbacks up to a saddle (5030–1.7) from which you can look down at beautiful Lake Valhalla and across it at the challenging west face of dark-gray Lichtenberg Mountain (5844). Descending north from the saddle, the trail reaches meadow campsites and a spur trail (4900–0.3) that descends southeast 200 yards to the northwest shore of deep, cool, sparkling Lake Valhalla (4830).

The PCT now climbs east to a saddle, snowbound through late July, and then steadily descends northeast to Union Gap and a junction with Smithbrook Trail 1590 (4700–1.8), which descends eastward 0.7 mile to Road 6700. From the gap, the trail descends northwest along a lower slope of Union Peak (5696) before turning north and ascending to a delightful, singing cascade (4200–1.8). Tree frogs and evening grosbeaks may join in a dusk-time chorus as you approach a large campsite (4150-0.4) beside shallow Lake Janus (4146), which is somewhat disappointing after Lake Valhalla. The warmer temperatures of this semiclear lake, however, do allow you a comfortable dip. Just northwest is the clear outlet creek.

Beyond this creek, the PCT switchbacks west up to a gully, on your left, in which you

See maps K1, K2

Glacier Peak, from atop Grizzly Peak

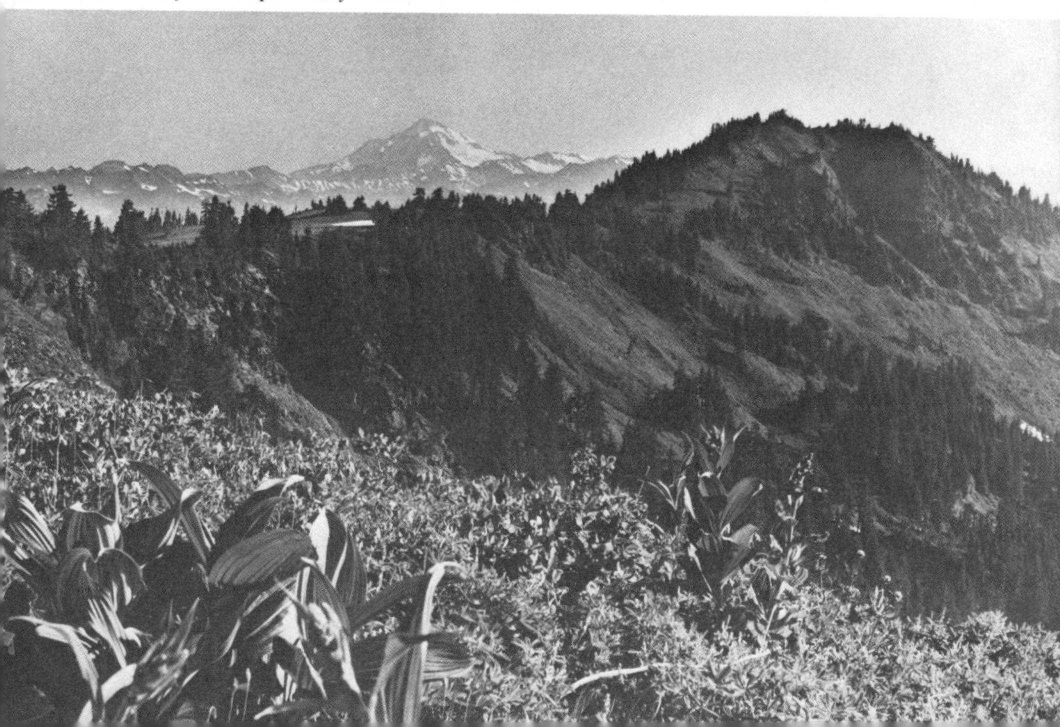

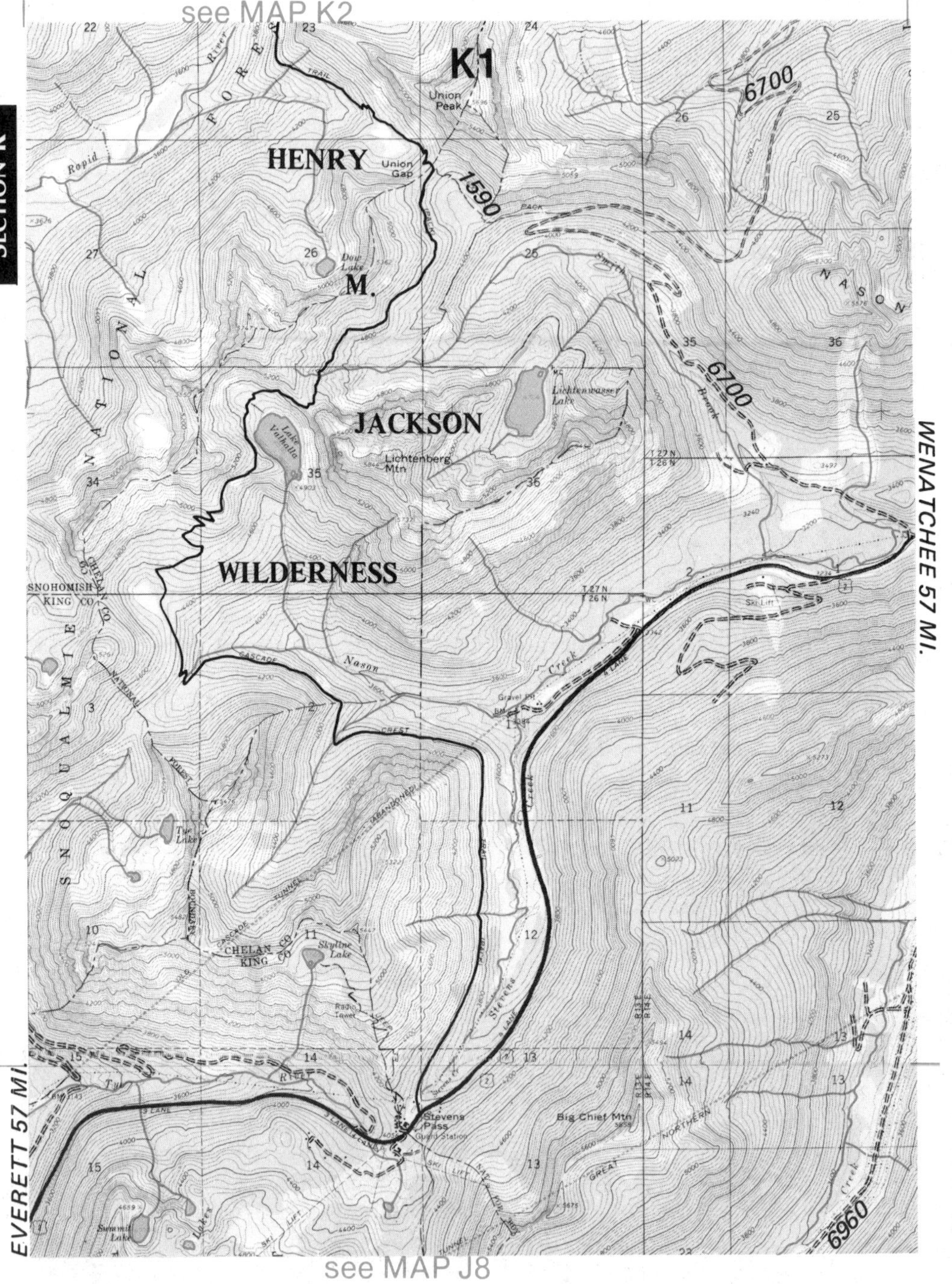

could camp. In ¼ mile, the trail reaches the crest (5180–1.6), traverses a short, northeast slope with a view due north of distant, regal Glacier Peak (10,541), and then reaches a saddle. A moderate descent northwest leads to a meadow (5070–0.8) from which a faint trail leads 40 yards northeast and then descends a moderately steep gully toward Glasses Lake (4626). At the west end of the meadow, the trail passes a good, designated campsite and then

See maps K2, K3

follows a winding crest route up past outcrops of mica schist before it reaches the upper west shoulder (5580–2.1) of Grizzly Peak (5597).

From it you hike north along the ridge, round another summit, and then come upon a designated but poor campsite on a saddle. Leaving it behind, the trail descends moderately across a west slope, passes well above shallow Grizzly Lake (4920), crosses the crest (5120–1.4), and reaches a good but shadeless campsite (5030–0.2) on a grassy flat. Descending north on a moderate-to-steep, sometimes-soggy trail, you reach the crest again and then switchback down it to broad, forested Wenatchee Pass (4230–1.0), where there is another good campsite. Climbing north to a flat, you reach a junction with Top Lake Trail 1506 (4570–0.6), which curves east one-half mile to that lake (4590). You can camp 50 yards southwest of this junction, but with Pear Lake next on the itinerary, you'd be foolish to stop here if you can still make it to that lake by dusk.

The PCT heads west to a gully whose west side is composed of large boulders. Gushing from them is the outlet of Pear Lake, which is dammed behind them. Climb several short switchbacks, pass through a saddle with a view of Glacier Peak, and then climb a few more hairpins to a ridgeline, the edge of Pear Lake's cirque (4880–0.7).

Side route. From here, Trail 1057 (formerly the PCT) heads west down to excellent campsites at the nearby, cliff-backed lake.

The late 1980s PCT climbs northwest just below the crest of the ridge—a moraine—allowing glimpses down to the aquamarine lake, and then it weaves between mossy boulders atop the moraine. Next, a switchback drops you to a notch where you leave the cirque and start a traverse around Peak 5548. Scattered hemlocks stand over the trail until it rounds 5548 and becomes a path blasted through huge granitic talus blocks. With pikas sounding off at your passage, continue traversing to a tier of tight, steep hairpins that work past a cliff and up to the crest (5350–1.6).

On the west side of the crest, climb a bit more and then settle into a contouring ramble. As you round the meadowy bench of a point

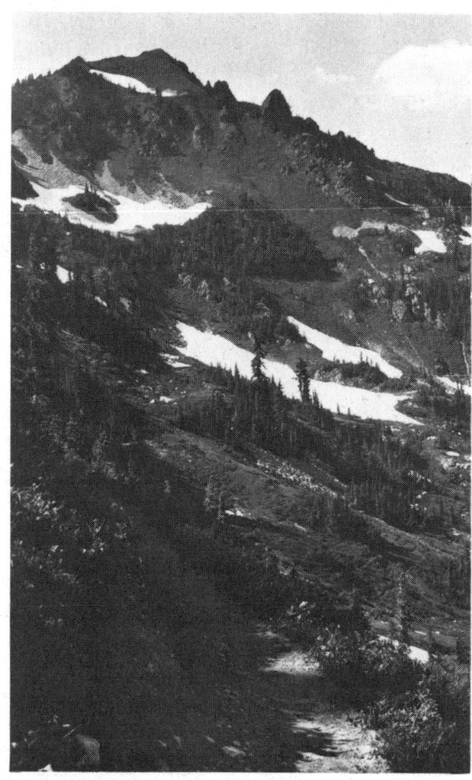

PCT below Skykomish Peak

(5504), you can see the country ahead through Saddle Gap to Skykomish Peak and Glacier Peak and to the west to the Monte Cristo peaks. For a stretch, the trail passes right below the scattered trees and glades of the crestline, and then it angles downslope into denser forest, passing one more talus slope before weaving down some switchbacks. From these, it resumes a contouring course and reaches a pair of adjacent, fairly reliable creeks (4800–2.4). Beyond these, the PCT climbs northwest gradually across steep slopes to a campsite, where a sign claims water is available not far downslope. Just up the trail from here, you reach Saddle Gap (5060–0.7).

Beyond the gap, you follow the northward-curving path down to a junction with West Cady Ridge Trail 1054 (4930–0.3), which climbs north-northwest. After descending north toward a prominent knob of metamorphic rock, the trail makes two long switchbacks down to a fair campsite west of 3-yard-wide Pass Creek. Immediately after crossing it

See maps K3, K4

on stepping-stones, you meet Pass Creek Trail 1053 (4200–1.0), which descends north alongside the creek. The PCT climbs northeast and shortly arrives at Cady Pass from which Cady Creek Trail 1501 (4310–0.4) departs northeast before dropping to that creek. At this forested pass, there's a dumpy, dry campsite that we would recommend for emergency bivouac only.

A long ascent—a taste of what's to come—now begins as the PCT switchbacks north up to a metamorphic ridge and reaches an exposed campsite at its crest (5470–1.9). This strenuous ascent does reward you near its top with scenic views to the south and east. After descending slightly to a granitic saddle, the trail rounds the east slope of a knob (5642) and then reaches another saddle. Beyond it, trailside snow patches can last into August.

Now contour across the east slope of rugged Skykomish Peak (6368), where minor PCT reroutings leave unsigned, paralleling tracks. This twisting, contouring course takes you around granitic knobs and into ravines—a couple with creeks—and eventually brings you to Lake Sally Ann (5479–1.7). ▮ *This beautiful lake has attracted many over the years, and the Forest Service has lined off much of the beaten-down spots, built a privy, and laid revegetation netting. Camping here is a privilege that, if abused, could be revoked by the Forest Service.* ▮

Beyond the lake, the PCT curves down past creeklets to a junction with Cady Ridge Trail 1532 (5380–0.4).

See maps K4, K5

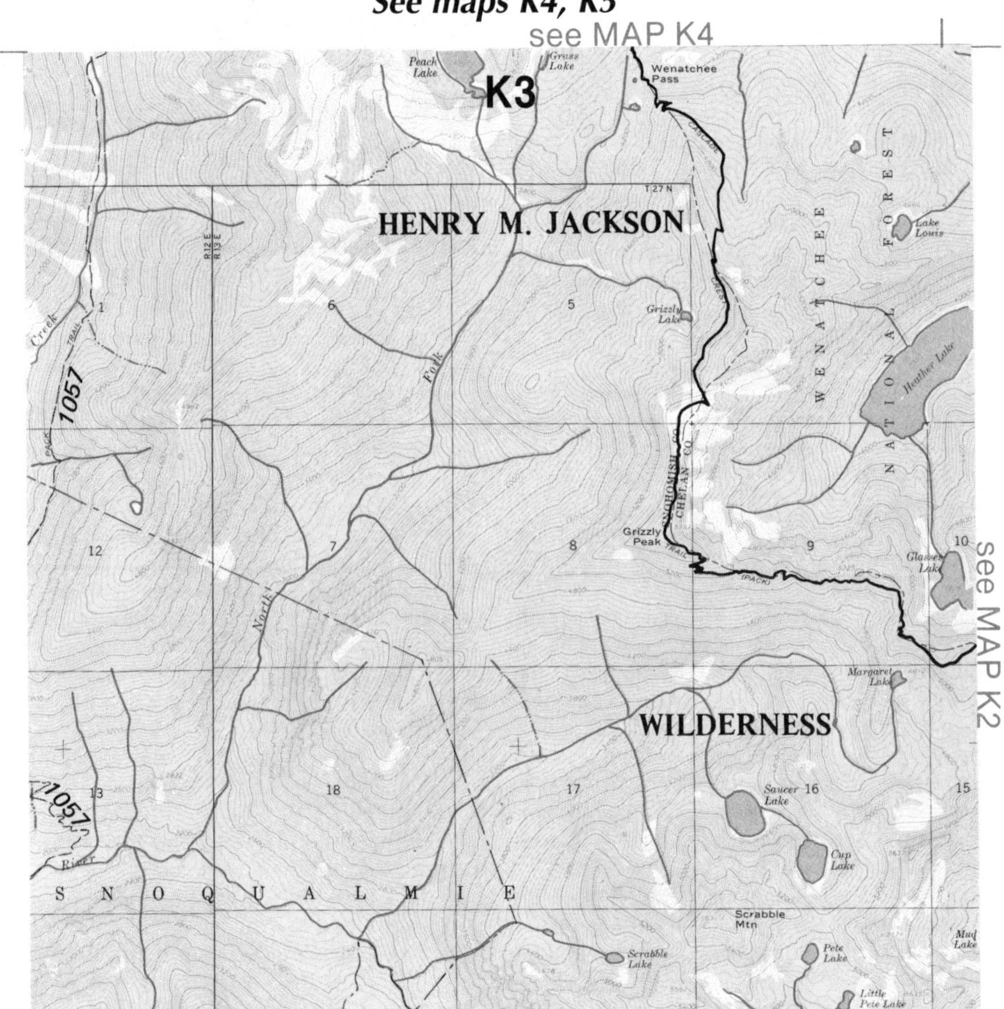

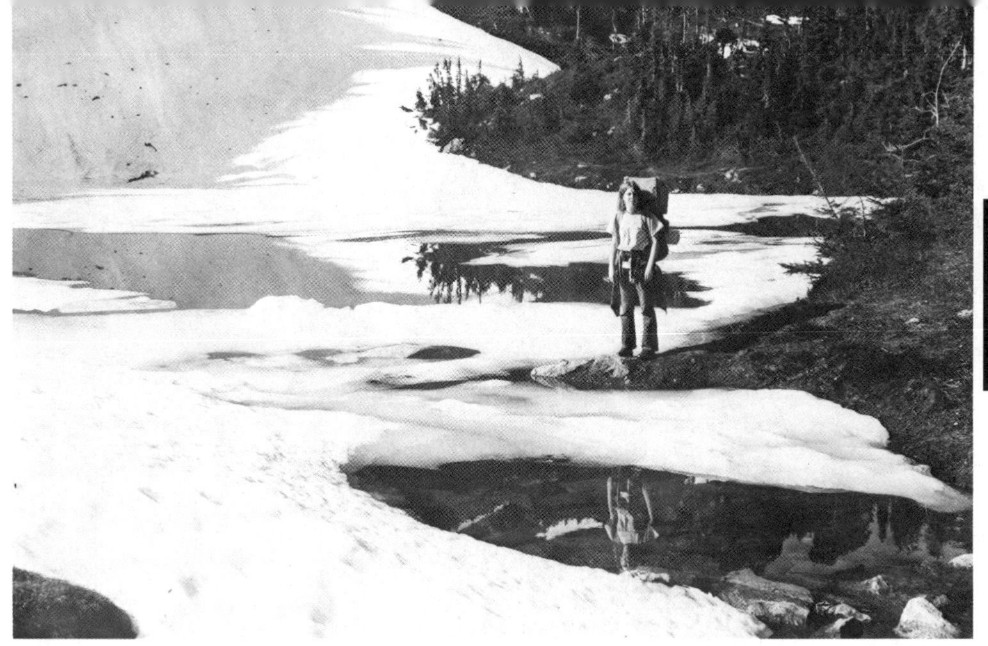

Lake Sally Ann

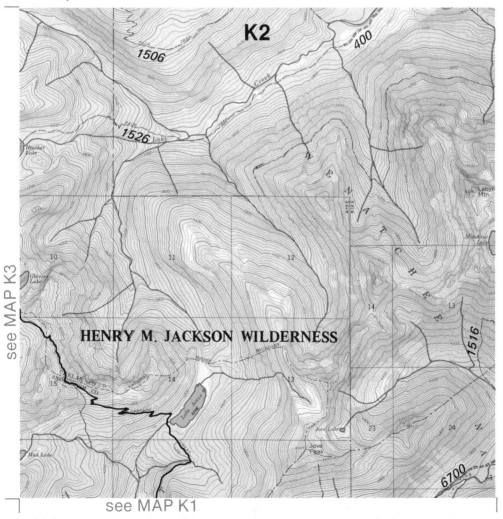

K2

1506

400

1526 Lake

Creek

Heather Lake

Glasses Lake

WENATCHEE

Labyrinth Mtn

Minotaur Lake

1516

HENRY M. JACKSON WILDERNESS

Lake Janus

Jove Lake

Jove Peak

Mud Lake

6700

see MAP K3

see MAP K1

see MAP K5

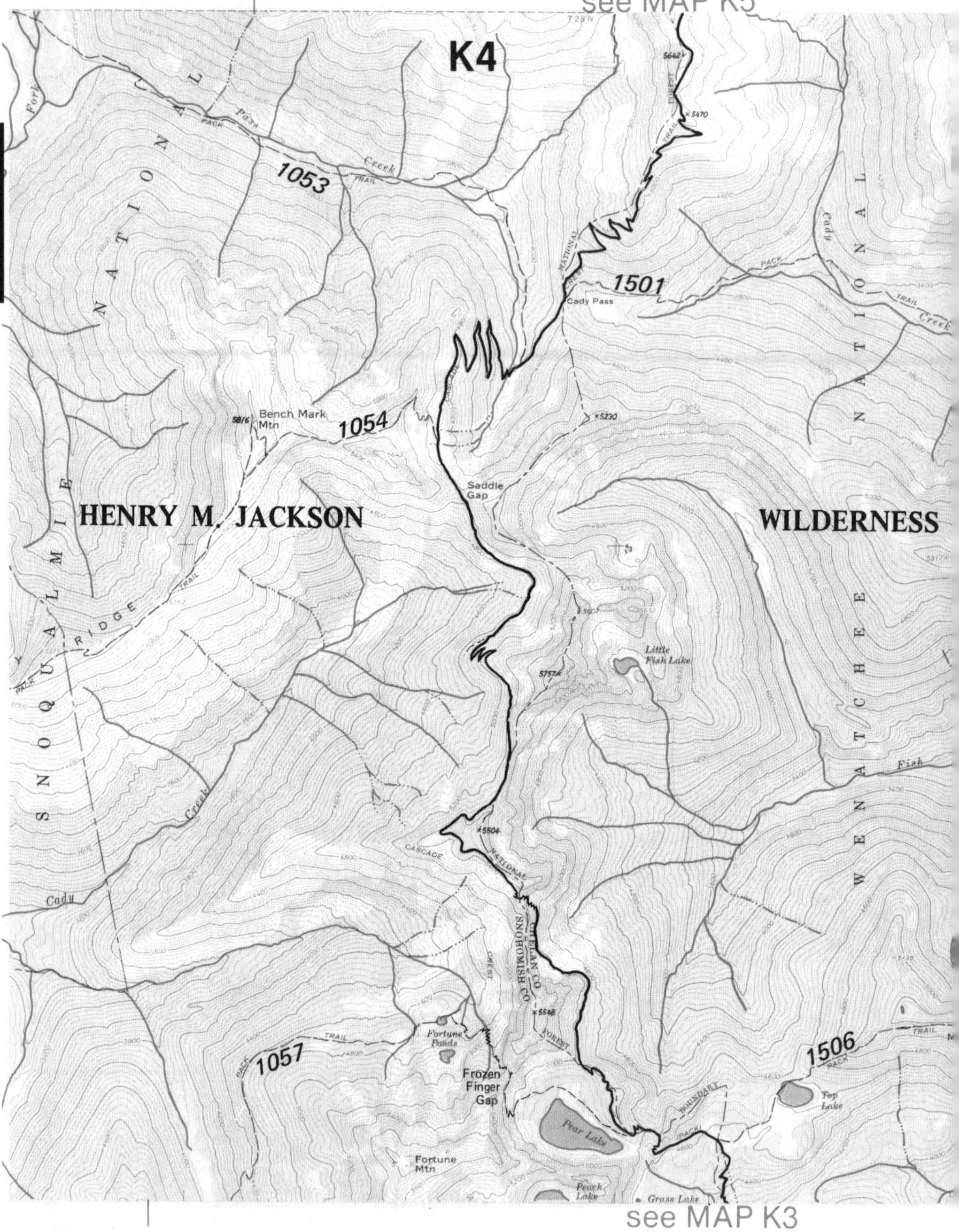

K4

HENRY M. JACKSON WILDERNESS

Saddle Gap

Cady Pass

Bench Mark Mtn

Little Fish Lake

Fortune Ponds

Frozen Finger Gap

Pear Lake

Top Lake

Fortune Mtn

see MAP K3

Side route. You can descend this trail 200 yards to a suitable campsite on an open saddle.

Beyond this junction, the sometimes-snowbound trail climbs northwest across a slope of greenish mica schist, glistening white-vein quartz, and speckled adamellite before it switchbacks up to Wards Pass (5710–0.7). Turning north, you then hike along a crest route that takes you down the soggy, volcanic soils of Dishpan Gap, where North Fork Skykomish Trail 1051 descends west and, just beyond, Bald Eagle Trail 650 (5600–0.6) veers north-northwest. The PCT veers right and crosses the southeast slope of Peak 5892 to a ridgecrest

See map K5

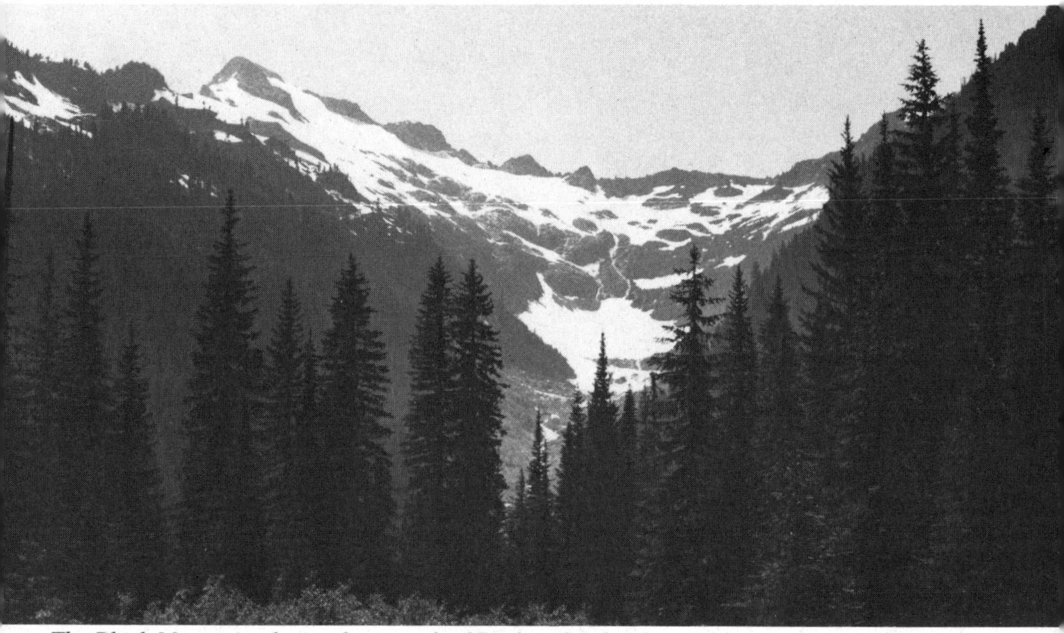

The Black Mountain glacier, from north of Baekos Creek

see MAP K6

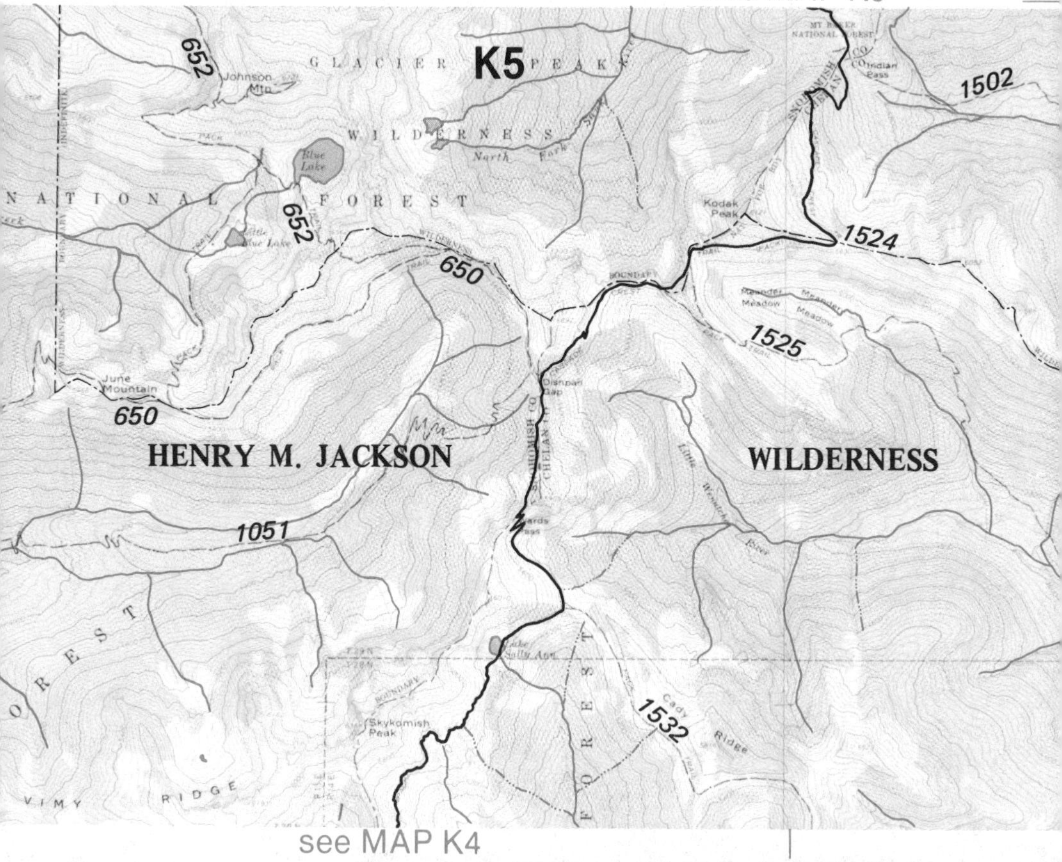

K5

HENRY M. JACKSON WILDERNESS

see MAP K4

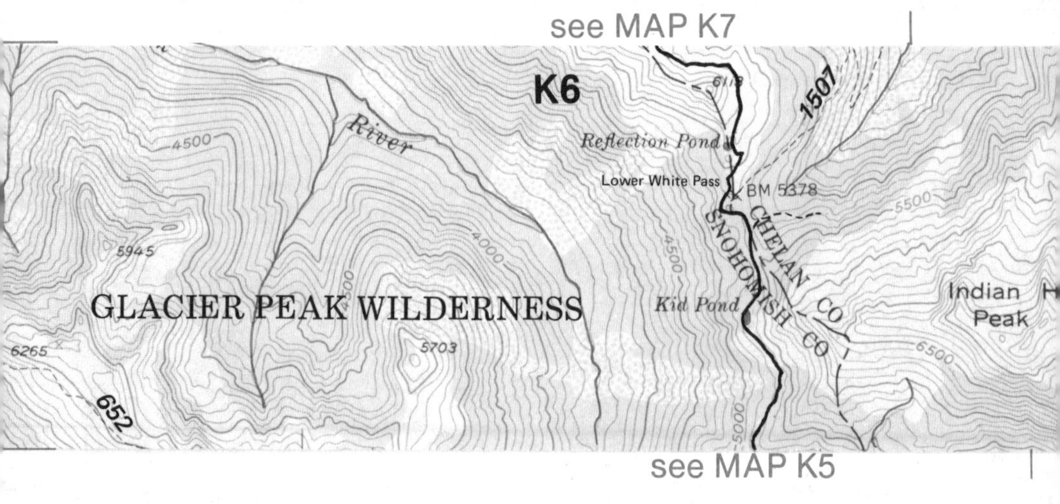

campsite (5450–0.5) on an open slope of grass, cinquefoil, and fawn lilies. *Should you camp here, don't be surprised to see deer come around and graze beside your tent.*

Following the crest east across this glaciated country, you quickly arrive at a junction with Little Wenatchee River Trail 1525 (5440–0.3), which contours southeast. You diagonal up the northwest slope of a triangular summit and then reach a saddle from which a spur trail (5500–0.2) contours south to Trail 1525. The PCT heads north toward Kodak Peak (6121) and then climbs east across its flowery, picturesque south slope of metamorphic rocks, where the distant view includes Mt. Rainier, Chimney Peak, Mt. Daniel, and the Stuart Range. Upon your arrival at Kodak Peak's east ridge (5660–0.7), Glacier Peak comes into view to the north. Little Wenatchee Ridge Trail 1524 strikes east-southeast along this ridge, the southern boundary of Glacier Peak Wilderness and the northern boundary of Henry M. Jackson Wilderness.

The trail turns northwest and descends across open slopes, July snowfields, and a couple of rivulets before it curves north and switchbacks past stalwart hemlocks down to Indian Pass (5020–1.3).

See map K5

PCT traversing southeast from slopes of Peak 6203

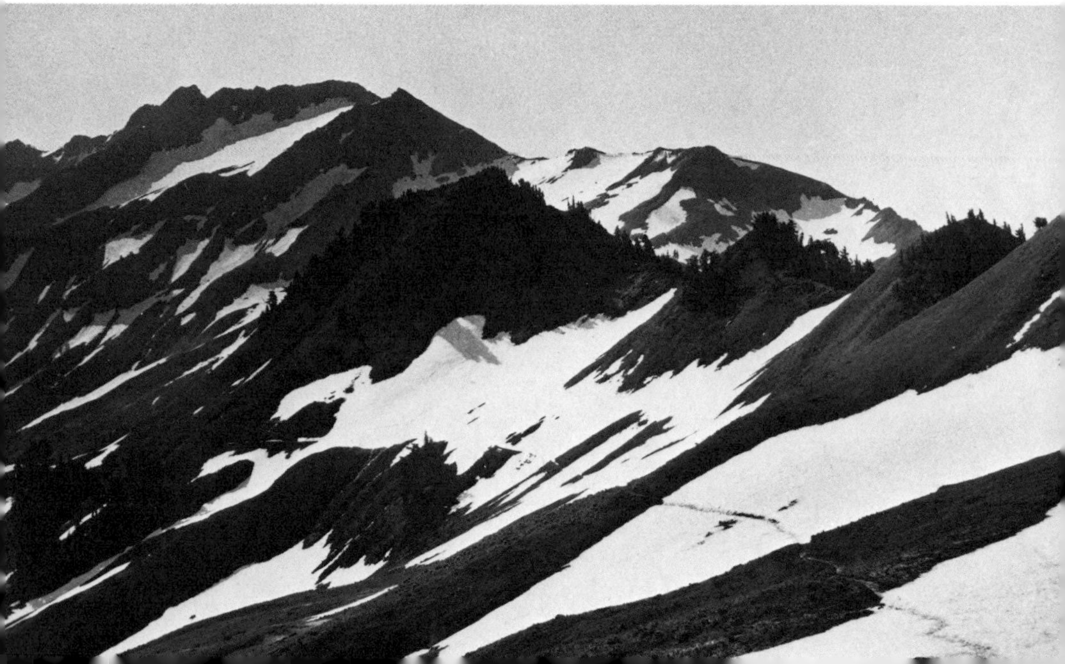

Side route. From here, you can follow a spur trail 0.1 mile west to a good campsite and then another 0.1 mile to a boggy spring.

Ascending to the PCT from the southeast is faint Indian Creek Trail 1502. From its junction, you arc northwest up to a southwest spur of Indian Head Peak (7442) and then climb

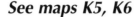

See maps K5, K6

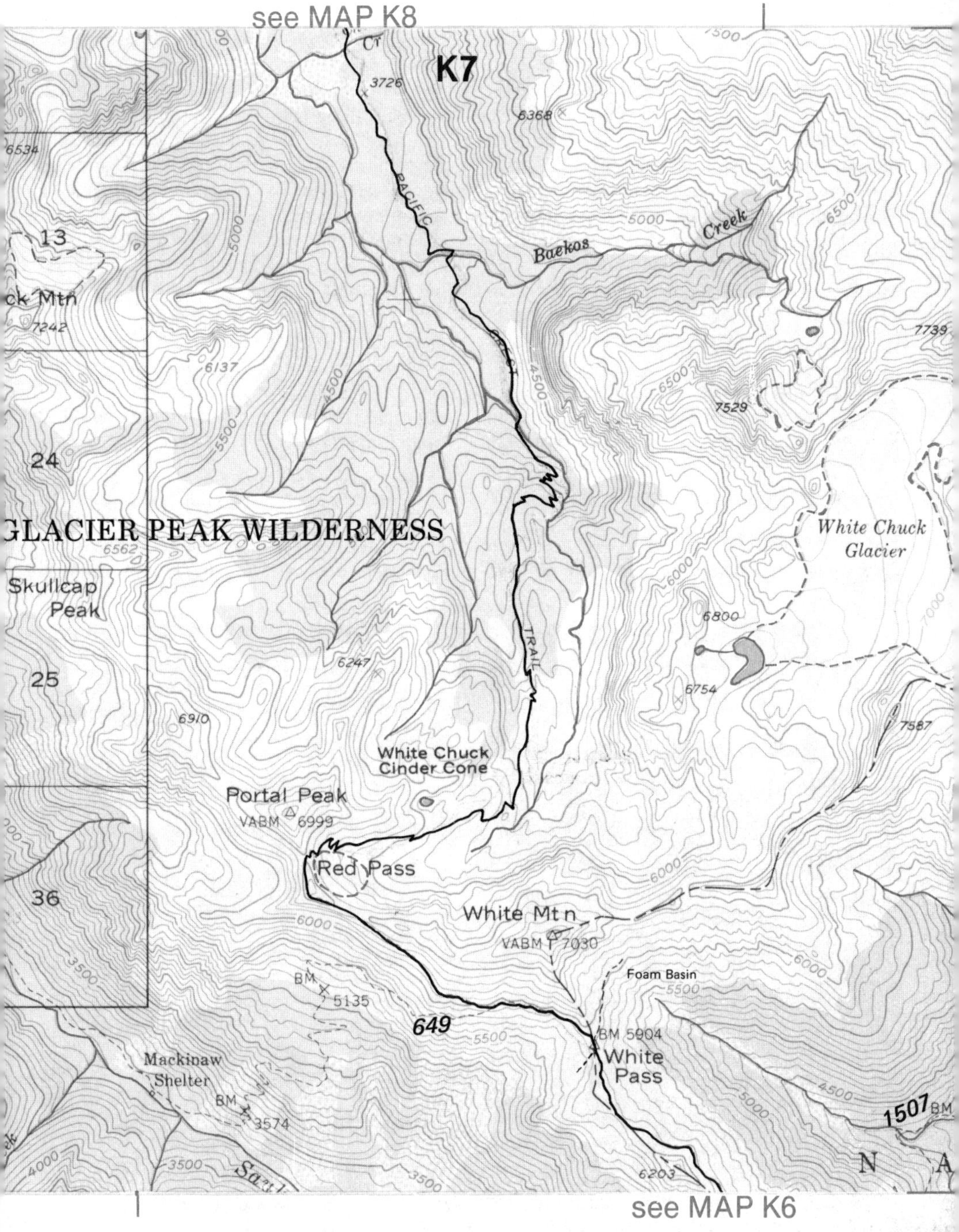

see MAP K8

K7

Cr
3726
6368
6534
PACIFIC
5000
Baekos
Creek
6500
13
ck Mtn
7242
7739
6137
CREST
4500
6500
7529
5500
24
GLACIER PEAK WILDERNESS
White Chuck
Glacier
6562
Skullcap
Peak
6000
6800
7000
TRAIL
6247
25
6754
7587
6910
White Chuck
Cinder Cone
Portal Peak
VABM 6999
Red Pass
36
6000
White Mt n
VABM 7030
6000
BM 5135
Foam Basin
5500
649
5500
BM 5904
White
Pass
Mackinaw
Shelter
BM 3574
4500
5000
1507
BM
4000
3500
3500
6203
N A

see MAP K6

northward to an adequate campsite at the north end of shallow, murky Kid Pond (5320–1.0). ▮ *The location of this pond and the nature of its surrounding rocks of garnet-graphite-mica schist both indicate that it fills a slight depression behind avalanche deposits.* ▮

The PCT proceeds north to a ridge and to a junction with an older trail that traverses the north slopes of Indian Head Peak. Staying on the PCT, you descend to Lower White Pass (5378–0.7), from which the old Cascade Crest Trail once descended northeast; nowadays, the trail is called White River Trail 1507; an adequate campsite lies 30 yards east of this junction.

The trail climbs a ridge north to good campsites on the west and southwest shores of semi-clear Reflection Pond (5560–0.3) and then traverses the snowbound northeast slopes up to a junction at White Pass (5904–1.9). No camping is allowed along the crest at White Pass.

Side routes Here, a trail begins a curving traverse northeast to Foam Basin, with an adequate campsite, about ¼ mile away. Another spur trail leads west down to good camping 200 yards from the ridgecrest, where snowmelt is reliable.

Continuing along the PCT, you follow its contouring path west-northwest to a fork from which North Fork Sauk Trail 649 (5950–0.6) descends steeply westward. ▮ *The meadow here has such an abundance of flowers and insects, it's no wonder that birds fly north to feast on them.* ▮ Flycatchers hover and snatch insects from midair as you start a steady climb west-northwest. The trail becomes dusty as it approaches a small summit (6650) affording an excellent panorama of the Monte Cristo massif and of prominent Sloan Peak. The path then turns north and shortly reaches the gray, garnet-biotite gneiss rocks of marmot-inhabited Red Pass (6500–1.3).

▮ *The view from here is nothing short of spectacular. Above you and 5 miles to the northeast is a towering volcano, Glacier Peak (10,541), which last erupted about 12,500 years ago. Below is the perennially snowclad upper canyon of the White Chuck River. To the*

See maps K5, K6, K7

Glacier Peak, from slopes above Pumice Creek; Glacier ridge is in the mid-ground, Kennedy Peak on the left skyline; Kennedy Glacier (left) and Scimitar Glacier (right) descend the flanks of Glacier Peak

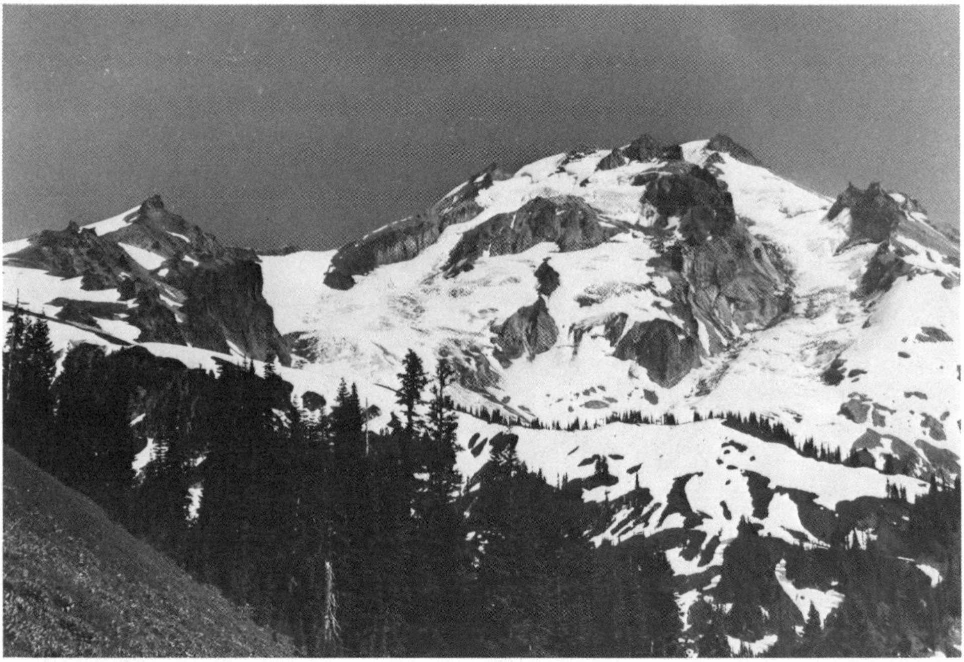

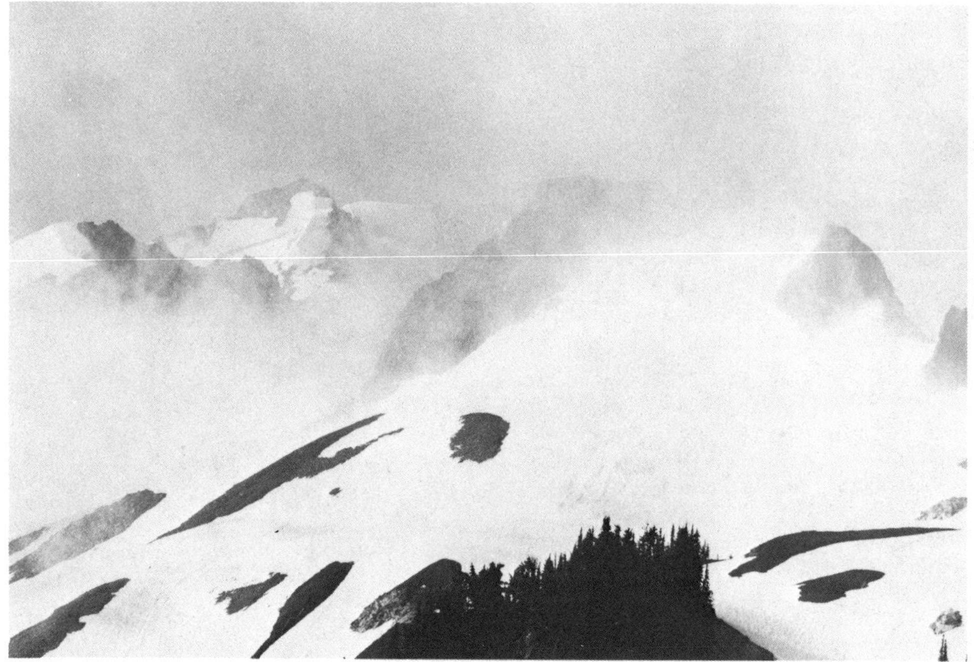

Too often, clouds roll in and obscure views; Glacier Peak, to the south, is the pointed peak left of center

distant south is lofty, glistening Mt. Rainier (14,410), cloaked in snow, giving it the appearance of a giant stationary cloud that reigns eternally over the distant forest. If you're heading south, you'll definitely remember your climb up to this pass. ▮

The PCT first switchbacks and then descends along the base of the east ridge of Portal Peak. ▮ *When this section of trail is snowbound, most hikers slide directly down the steep but safe upper snowfield and then head east down-canyon until they reach the visible trail.* ▮ Keeping north of the headwaters, the PCT descends toward a lone, three-foot-high cairn (5700–1.4) on a low knoll, turns northward, and then descends to campsites at a saddle (5500–0.3) between a 20-foot-high hill to the east and a high slope to the west. Better sites are on the hill. Just 250 yards north, you pass another campsite; then, farther down, you can see numerous campsites along the banks of the rumbling White Chuck River below and to the east.

You may spot a blue grouse and its chicks as you descend alongside a swelling creek that the PCT crosses three times via bridges. Hikers have camped beside each crossing. Leaving the last crossing (4700–1.5), the trail switchbacks down toward the White Chuck River, parallels it above its west bank, and then crosses it (4000–1.0) eastward via a wide, planked horse bridge. Leave the river's side, follow an undulating route north, and then descend to a good campsite just before a log crossing of cold, roaring Baekos Creek (3990–1.0), whose north bank contains much green mica schist. Follow the base of its high north bank downstream a short way, switchback over it, and then descend to level ground and a number of log crossings over small creeks. ▮ *Mountaineers intent on climbing Glacier Peak (10,541) usually leave the PCT between Baekos and Kennedy creeks. Should you try, bring rope, crampons, and an ice ax.* ▮

Nearing a campsite beside the north bank of Chetwot Creek (3730–1.3), the vegetation opens enough to afford views southwest to broad Black Mountain glacier, which spreads across the upper rim of a deeply glaciated side canyon. Continuing northward, you reach Sitkum Creek, make a log crossing of it, and then find yourself at an excellent campsite (3852–0.8). From this point, you can continue on the official PCT or take a 3¼-mile alternate

See maps K7, K8

ROAD 26 4 MI.

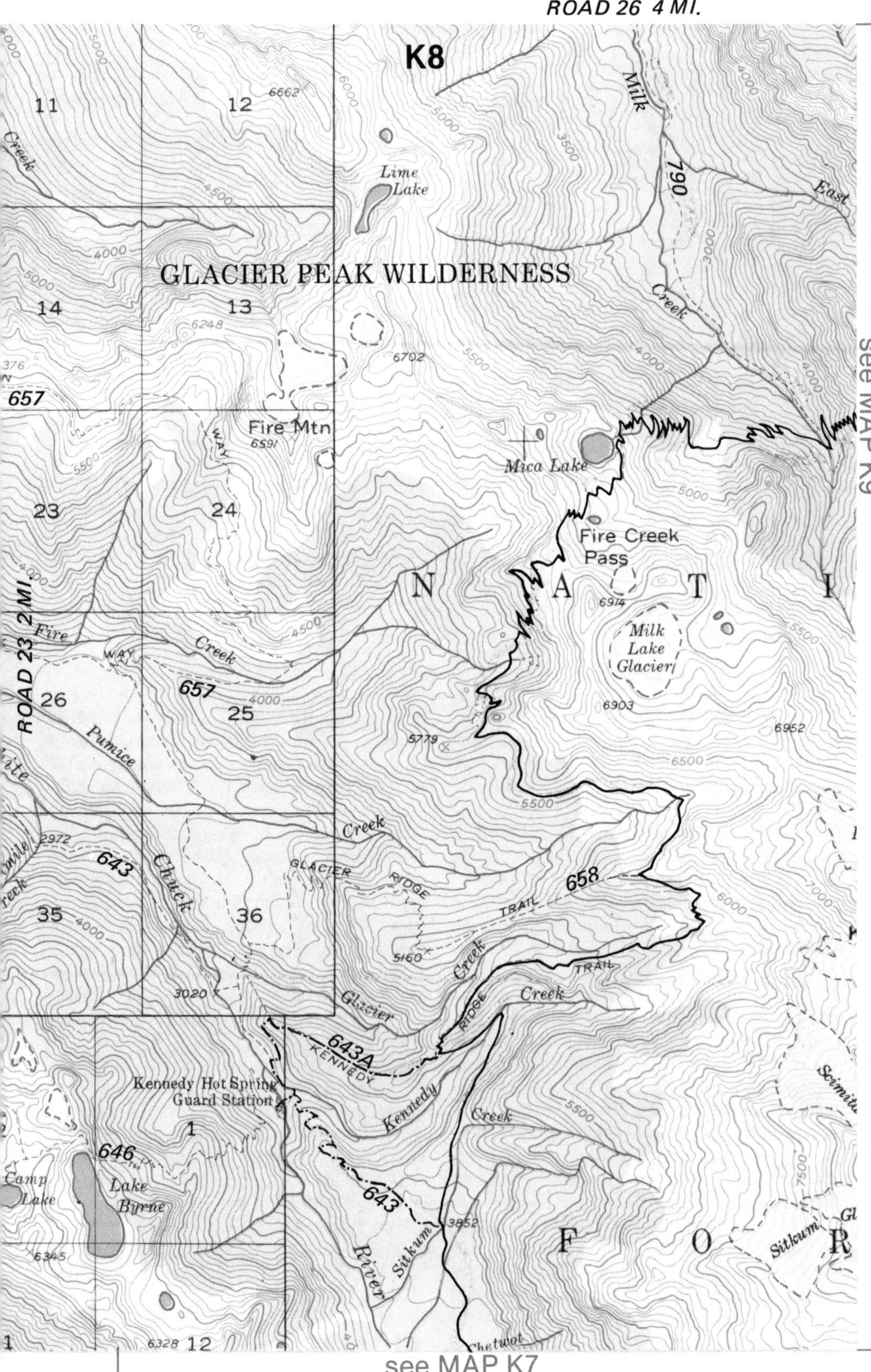

ROAD 23 2 MI.

see MAP K9

see MAP K7

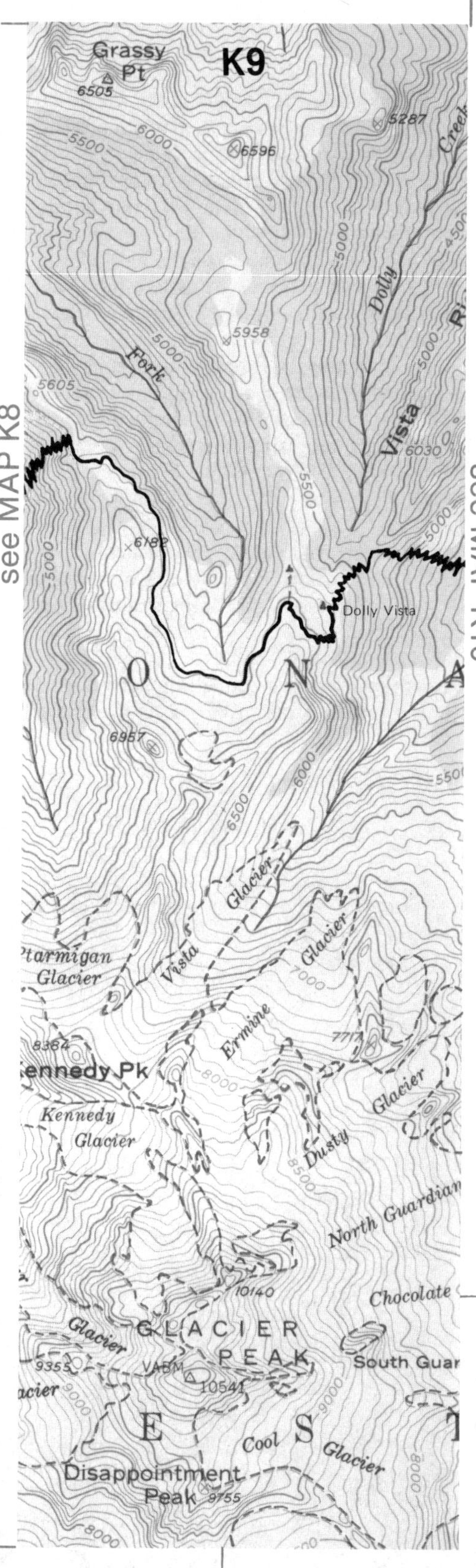

route on White Chuck Trail 643, which passes off-limits Kennedy Hot Spring.

The official PCT route. From Sitkum Creek, a long climb lies ahead. After an initial 250-yard climb north, you reach an adequate campsite. One-quarter mile later, the trail reaches a better one beside Sitkum Creek, and then it crosses an unmapped creek just before reaching a morainal ridge. Enjoying a short-lasting descent northeast, you pass by small outcrops above that are quartz-and-biotite rich, Miocene-age granitic intrusions. ▮ *The slopes above them are composed of andesitic lava flows from Glacier Peak.* ▮ You reach chilly, glacier-fed Kennedy Creek (4050–1.2), a 10-yard-wide torrent that sometimes has to be forded, since bridges built across it have a tendency to be wiped out by avalanches. Without a bridge, the ford can be treacherous. ▮ *Around July 11, 1975, one such avalanche tore down this creek and nearly overwhelmed the Kennedy Hot Spring area, 1½ miles downstream.* ▮

After crossing the creek, climb southwest up a path cut through unstable morainal material that in turn is being undercut by the creek. Soon you reach a junction with Kennedy Ridge Trail 643A (4300–0.4), where the alternate route rejoins the PCT.

Side route. You can head west down this trail for a look at off-limits Kennedy Hot Spring. ▮ *Its warm water indicates that molten magma is relatively close to the surface.* ▮

Alternate route. From a junction by this creekside campsite, follow White Chuck Trail 643 as it first traverses northwest and then switchbacks down a crest to a junction beside Kennedy Creek. Here, on a spur trail, you curve southwest immediately over to the White Chuck River and, near a ranger station, bridge the river. For a peek at the off-limits hot spring, hike 80 yards upstream to Kennedy Hot Spring (3275), a cubical, neck-deep hole in the ground. ▮ *Many hikers used to skinny-dip at this 94°F soda spring, but its increasing popularity in the 1960s led to a ban of this fun in the early 1970s.* ▮ From the bridge, you can follow the river's west bank a short way down to campsites on a gentle slope. When you are ready to leave—

See map K8

if ever, considering what's ahead—retrace your steps to the Kennedy Creek junction, cross the creek, follow Trail 643 ¼ mile downstream, and then climb 1¼ miles up Kennedy Ridge Trail 643A to the PCT.

With the official PCT route and the alternate route rejoined, the real climb begins as you ascend six short, steep switchbacks past huge andesite blocks to the lower crest of Kennedy Ridge. You struggle upward, stopping several times to catch your breath and to admire the scenery. In spots, this crest is no wider than the trail. The gradient eases off, and you eventually reach an excellent campsite by Glacier Creek (5640–1.9), which occasionally has an avalanche roar down its canyon, destroying all the trees in its path. Nevertheless, mountaineers and hikers alike camp in its track.

Side route. For mountaineers, the shortest climb to Glacier Peak's summit begins here.

Leaving the creek, you switchback north and then climb northwest past adamellite boulders to a junction with Glacier Ridge Trail 658 (6050–0.7), which is a narrow footpath that descends that ridge westward. After a short, steep descent northeast, the trail contours in that direction to jump-across Pumice Creek (5900–0.5), whose bed contains metamorphic, granitic, and volcanic rocks. ▮ *You might try to identify all three types and decipher their stories.* ▮ A fair campsite is beside the north bank. The trail descends west and then contours over to a ridge (5770–1.6). North of it, the PCT descends even more and then crosses a branch of Fire Creek (5370–0.8) just below its fork upstream.

Side route. On an open meadow atop a bluff 20 yards north of it, you'll find the last good campsite this side of Fire Creek Pass.

Now you make one final effort, and *voilà!* a magnificent panorama of the North Cascades

See map K8

The Ermine Glacier spreads out across Glacier Peak's lower flanks; viewed from switchbacks just below Vista Ridge

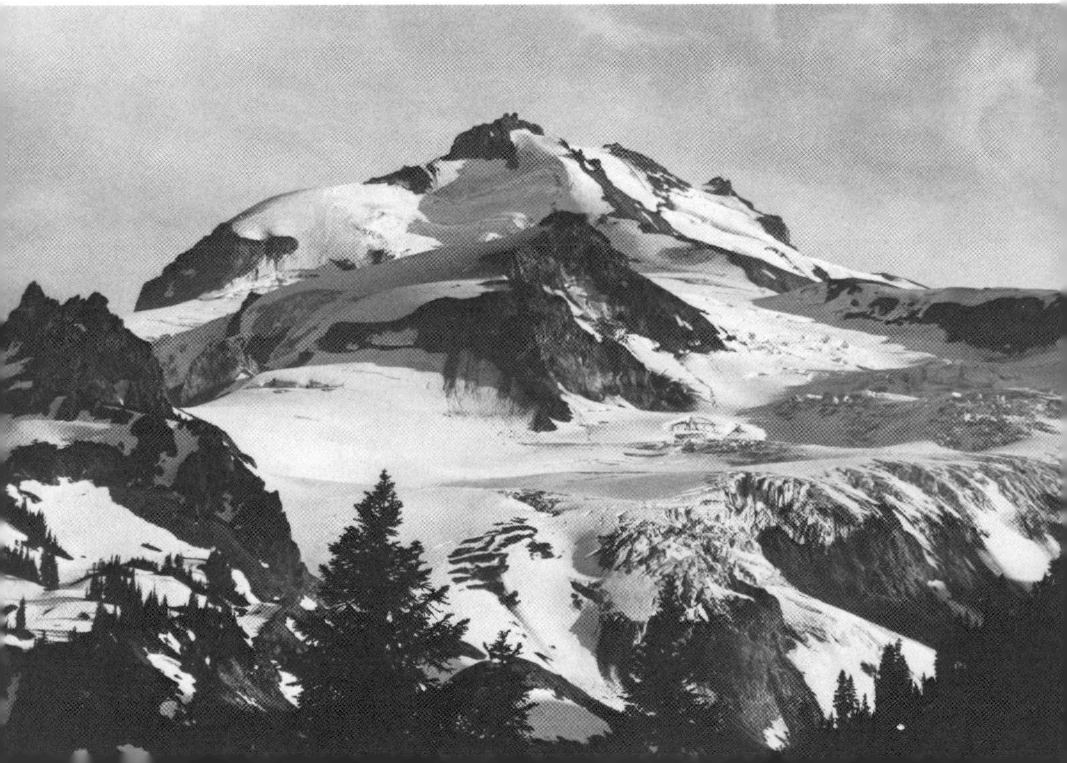

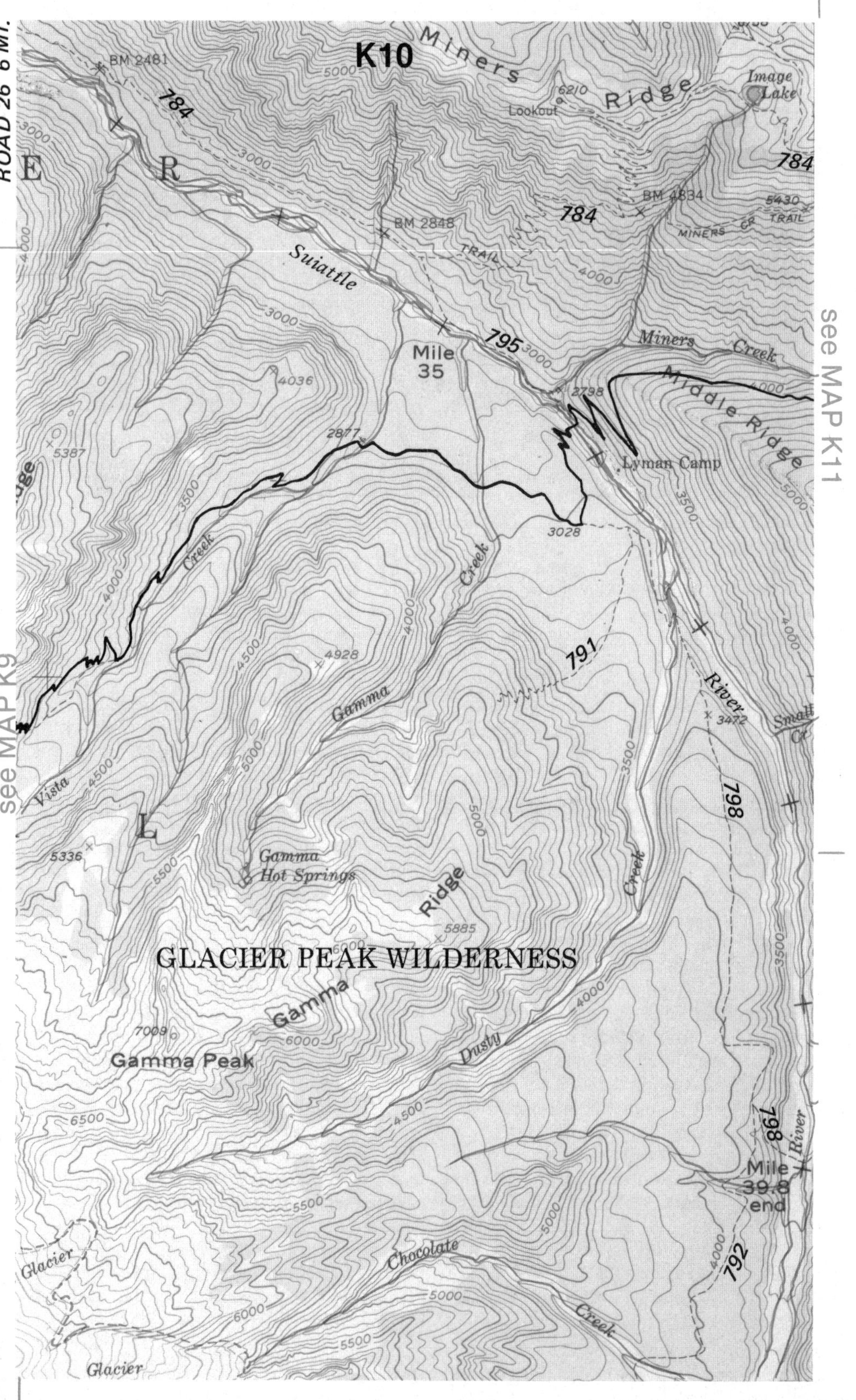
K10
ROAD 26 6 MI.
Miners Ridge
BM 2481
784
Lookout
6210
Image Lake
E
R
BM 4834
5430
TRAIL
MINERS CR
BM 2848
TRAIL
Suiattle
3000
4000
5000
Mile 35
795
Miners Creek
Middle Ridge
4036
2798
5387
2877
Lyman Camp
3500
3028
Creek
4928
791
Gamma
River
3472
Small Cr
798
see MAP K9
see MAP K11
Vista
4500
L
5336
5500
Gamma Hot Springs
Ridge
5885
GLACIER PEAK WILDERNESS
Gamma
7009
6000
Gamma Peak
Dusty
6500
River
Mile 39.8 end
792
Chocolate
Creek
Glacier
Glacier

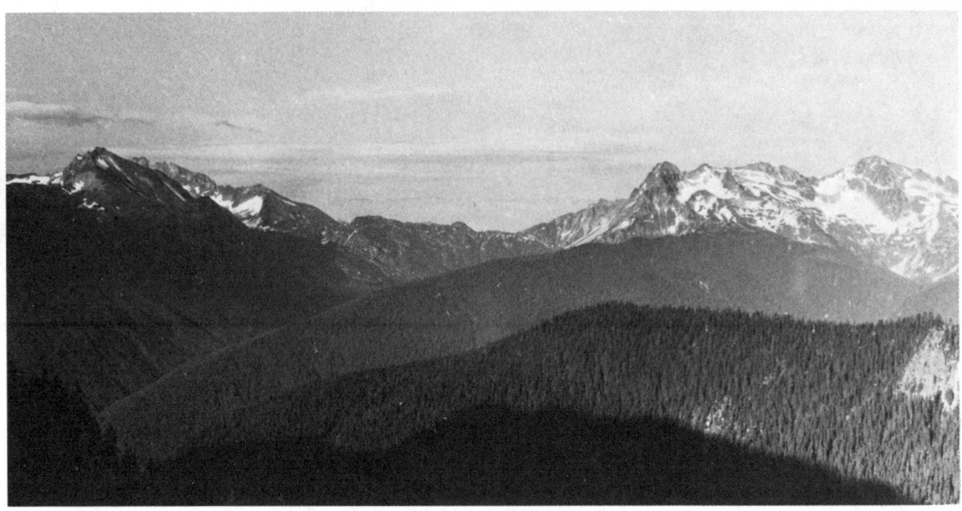

View northeast from upper Vista Creek canyon: Plummer Mountain and Fortress Mountain stand above smooth, dropping Middle Ridge

unfolds around you as you gain access to Fire Creek Pass (6350–1.7).

▮ *The North Cascades of Washington contain 756 glaciers, which account for about half of all the glacier area existing within the conterminous United States. The range's great number of fairly high summits coupled with its year-round barrage from storms accounts for its vast accumulation of ice and snow. Chances are that you'll encounter at least one storm, lasting only a few days if you're lucky, before you reach the Canadian border.* ▮

At Fire Creek Pass, the trail goes between two large cairns 30 yards northwest of an emergency campsite. The usually snowbound route switchbacks down a ridge north-northeast to a ford of the outlet of usually frozen Mica Lake (5430–1.1), whose cirque wall of dark metamorphic schist is intruded by light pegmatite dikes. From its shore, you can see dozens of unappealing switchbacks you'll have to climb to surmount the next ridge. As you descend farther, you must boulder-hop wide, shallow Mica Creek, just east of which is a good but open campsite (5110–0.5) on a small bench. Continue to switchback eastward and reach a basin, another creek, and a good, obvious campsite (4400–1.1). From it, the unrelenting descent takes you down to deep, 5-yard-wide Milk Creek. Here you'll find a fair, small campsite. ▮ *A log crossing existed in 1973 but was replaced with a $40,000 "permanent" bridge in 1974. This, however, was wiped out by an early-summer avalanche in 1975. Another bridge was built, but there's no guarantee that a bridge will be there when you reach the creek.* ▮

Immediately beyond this crossing, the PCT meets Milk Creek Trail 790 (3800–1.3), descending north, which the old Cascade Crest route used to follow before the train of switchbacks to the east of you was constructed. ▮ *Snowfields and avalanche hazards probably prevented the construction of a trail that would contour around Glacier Peak at the 6000-foot level.* ▮

When you leave the creek and an adjacent campsite, take your time switchbacking up the east wall of this canyon. ▮ *If the day is drizzly, the "fog drip" on the flowers of this heavily vegetated slope will saturate you from the thighs down. Ahead grow miles of this vegetation that you must hike through. Rationalizing this fate, you can observe that in this weather, there are no flies or mosquitoes around to bother you.* ▮ When you finally finish this creekless ascent and reach the ridgecrest (5750–2.5), a marmot may greet you; if not, you can at least expect a rest at an open campsite.

After a short, negligible climb, the trail contours the east slope of this ridge and leaves behind its outcrops of densely clustered, light-colored Miocene dikes, sills, and irregular masses. As you enter the deeply glaciated East

See maps K8, K9

see MAP K12

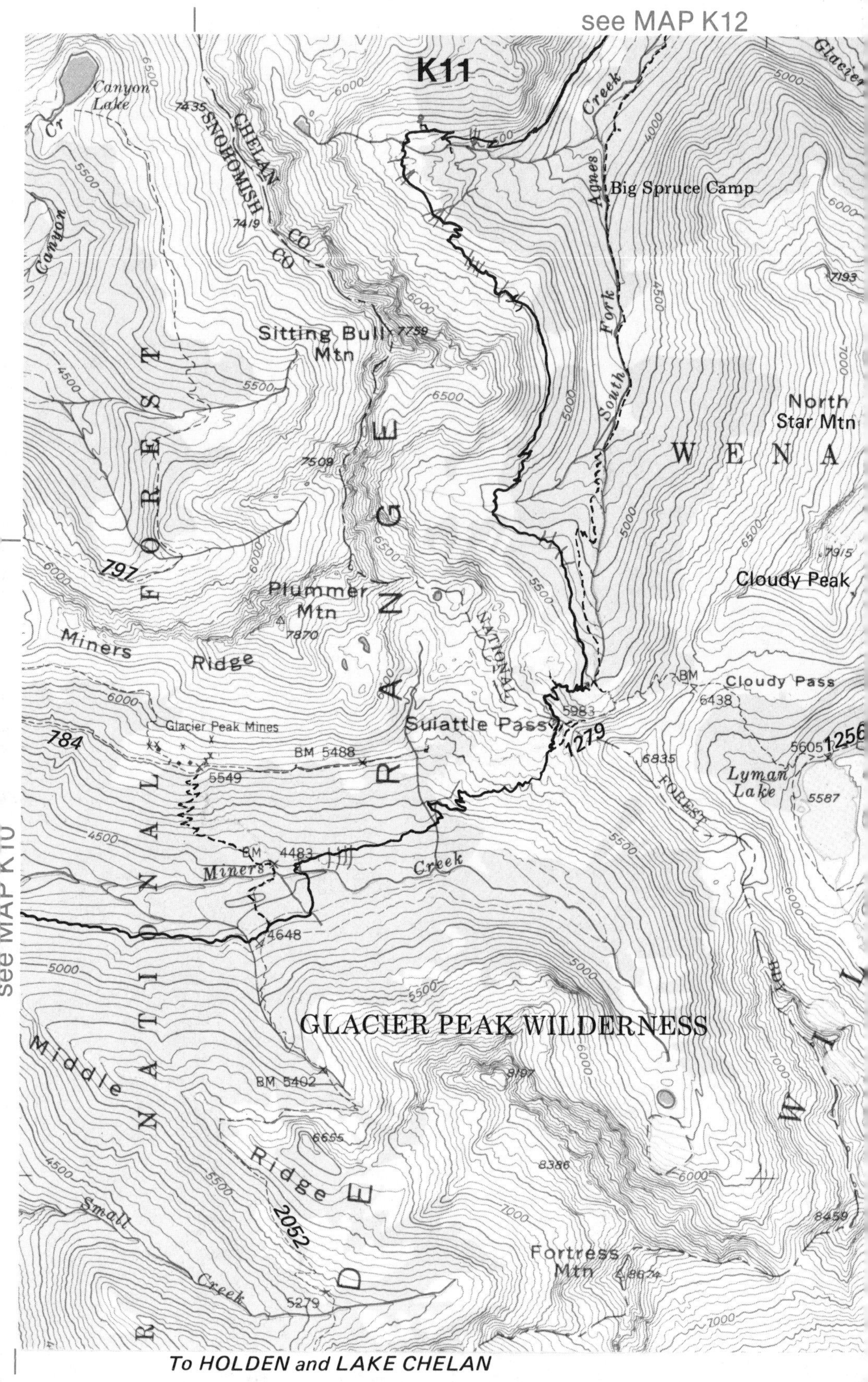

see MAP K10

To HOLDEN and LAKE CHELAN

see MAP K13

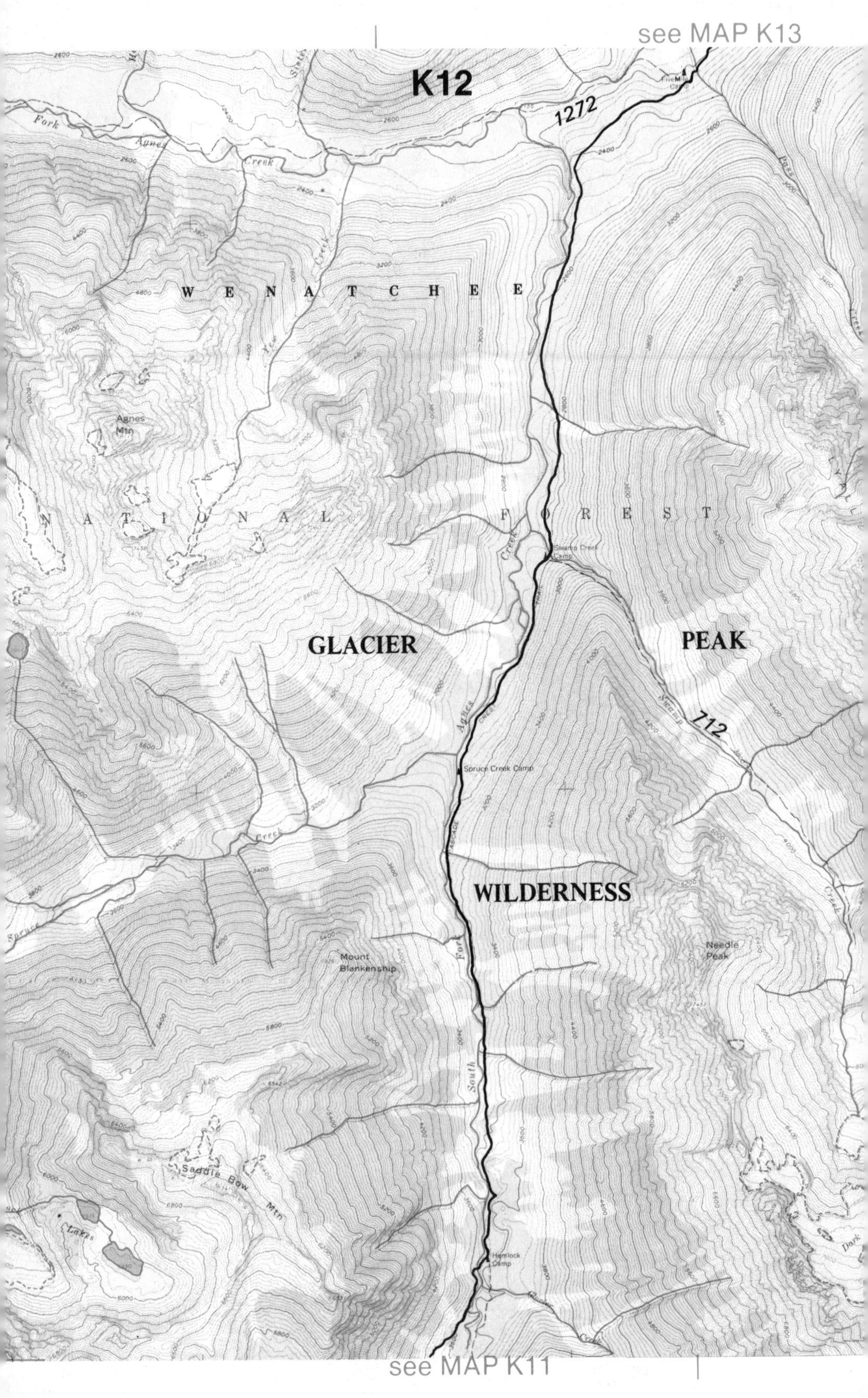
K12
1272
WENATCHEE
NATIONAL
FOREST
GLACIER
PEAK
WILDERNESS
712
Agnes Mtn
Swamp Creek Camp
Spruce Creek Camp
Mount Blankenship
Needle Peak
Saddle Bow Mtn
Hemlock Camp
Agnes Creek
South Fork
Lakes

see MAP K11

Fork Milk Creek basin, these outcrops give way to ancient, metamorphic rocks. Along the south wall of this basin, the PCT passes just below a small knoll (5860–1.5); 100 yards below this knoll is an adequate campsite. Beyond this point, the trail shortly crosses a hundred-yard-wide boulder field that is laced with creeklets. The route now climbs gently northeast to another ridge (6010–0.6) from which a short trail descends to the base of a ridge knoll about 100 yards north. The PCT switchbacks slightly up the ridge, contours southeast across it, and then starts the first of 59 switchbacks down to Vista Creek. After a few of these, you reach the Dolly Vista campsite (5830–0.7) beneath a few, protective mountain hemlocks. A pit toilet is immediately north; water is found by traversing about 100 yards southeast.

From the campsite, the PCT switchbacks northeast down through open forest to a saddle (5380–0.5) on Vista Ridge, where there is a dry, open campsite. ▮ *Northeast of you, this resistant ridge is composed of Miocene intrusive rocks that are capped with remnant Quaternary andesite flows from Glacier Peak.* ▮ Starting down into deep, glaciated Vista Creek canyon, you're grateful to be descending the last 38 switchbacks rather than ascending them. By the last switchback, 50 yards from the creek, the trail has left behind most of the "rain forest," and it continues 100 yards northeast to a large, signed campsite (3650–2.6) beside Vista Creek. From it, the PCT descends into a Douglas-fir forest that has an understory of huckleberry, ferns, and Oregon grape.

The trail curves east and the gradient eases as you approach a bridge across wide, silty Vista Creek (2877–2.1). On its southeast bank is a good campsite with a fire ring and pit toilet. Now you contour east across a gentle slope to a crossing of Gamma Creek (2910–0.8). ▮ *Part of its flow is derived from the 140°F, sodium-chloride-bicarbonate-rich waters of Gamma Hot Springs (5000), about three miles upstream.* ▮ The trail gradually curves southeast and arrives at a junction with Suiattle River Trail 798 (3028–0.7), which first bears southeast before climbing south upriver. The PCT descends north, switchbacks down to a 50-yard-long horse bridge across the silty-gray Suiattle River and then immediately reaches a junction with the Suiattle River access trail (2860–0.8).

Side route. If you follow this trail downstream, you'll pass by some good campsites and then, after 300 yards, reach a good shelter and a separate toilet, both above the south bank of Miners Creek.

The next trail segment, straight ahead, makes long, easy switchbacks up to the lower edge of Middle Ridge and then climbs east up its north slope to a junction with the Buck

See maps K9, K10, K11

Glacier Peak, viewed from near Suiattle Pass

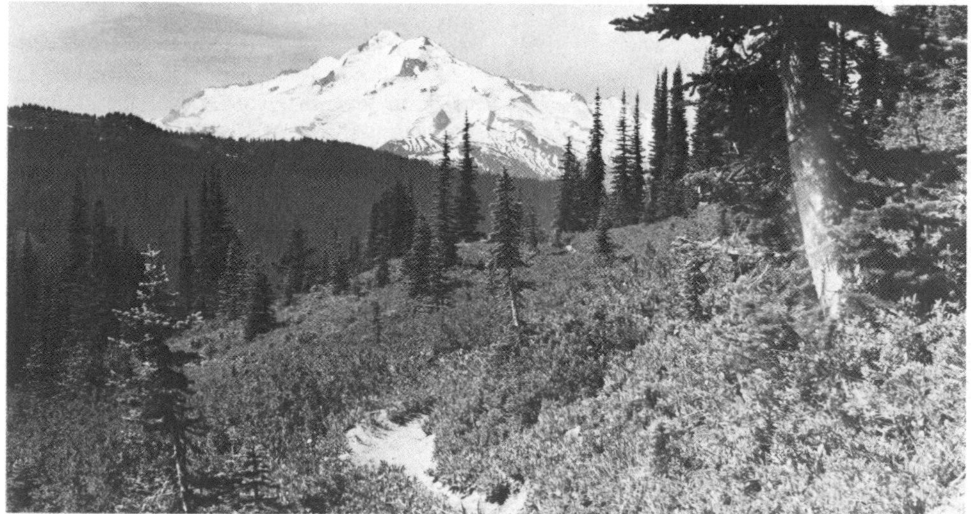

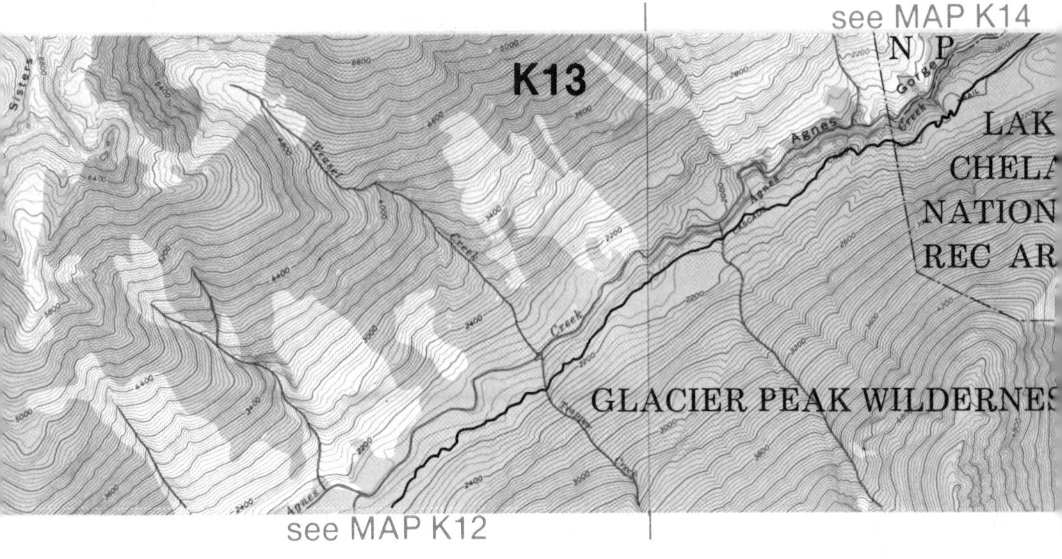

Creek Pass trail (4580–4.4), which climbs 5 miles south to the pass.

Side route. From this junction, you can follow the old PCT route, which makes an initial steep descent north, bridges a sluggish creek, and then quickly arrives at a very good campsite on the south bank of Miners Creek—a 0.4-mile side trip.

However, the newer PCT continues ¼ mile east to a creek and then ¼ mile north to Miners Creek (4490–0.5). You can camp nearby. From the creek's horse bridge, the PCT makes an initial jog downstream and then passes more than half a dozen creeks and creeklets as it climbs east. Switchbacks ultimately take you 400 feet higher to a junction with the old PCT route (5280–1.5). You continue to climb eastward, soon getting southwest views of majestic Glacier Peak and southern views of Fortress Mountain and the deep, glaciated canyon below it. The route turns north and soon reaches a spur trail (5790–0.7) that goes about 150 yards east to a two-tent site. Climbing, you reach a second trail in 0.1 mile, this one a footpath northeast over to the Railroad Creek Trail, which vaults Cloudy Pass. Immediately before Suiattle Pass, you meet a minor trail that climbs to the crest above the PCT. On the crest (5990–0.3), you meet an abandoned trail that starts east across the pass.

Five Mile Camp

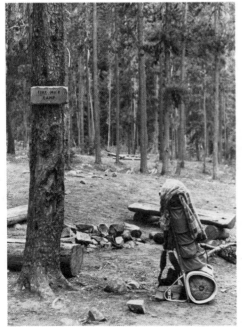

Switchbacks, often accompanied by snow patches, descend to a creeklet (5730–0.3) from which a spur trail climbs north-northwest to a hemlock/meadow campsite. More switchbacks take you down to a junction with the Railroad Creek Trail (5550–0.2), bound for Cloudy Pass and Holden. If you've been having snow problems, you may want to start down this trail rather than stay on the official PCT; we present it as an alternate route, below.

The official PCT route takes you on a fairly scenic, rollercoaster route in and out of two deep side canyons. The route is downhill all the way to the first of these (4980–1.3), with a campsite. Leaving this cirque and its giant, rockfall boulders, which have buried the creek, you switchback—needlessly?—high up on the

See map K11

Agnes Creek canyon wall. After a northward traverse, the trail bends into the second side canyon, and you immediately encounter a spur trail (5450–1.4); this one climbs 110 yards to a poor, heatherbound, one-tent site. In 100 more yards, the PCT meets two more spur trails, one descending 60 yards to a two-tent site and the other climbing 90 yards to another poor, heather-bound, one-tent site. A trickling creeklet flows between these three exposed sites.

You pass up to a dozen more creeklets as you descend to a bridged creek on the floor of the second side canyon. About 300 yards past it, you meet yet another spur trail (4810–1.6), this one climbing 140 yards to a sheltered, two-tent site, with view and spring-fed creeklet. The PCT then drops east, briefly switchbacks west, turns east again, and in 60 yards reaches the last spur trail (4680–0.2) on this stretch; the spur crosses the adjacent creek and ends at some small sites among firs of a nearby ridge.

Now the PCT makes a generally moderate descent to Agnes Creek, the forested route being punctuated with some bushy, wildflowered patches that present views. At last you bridge Agnes Creek and in about 150 yards reach Hemlock Camp (3560–2.0), where the older PCT route, given as an alternate below, rejoins the newer PCT. This camp comes equipped with benches, a table, and a fire ring.

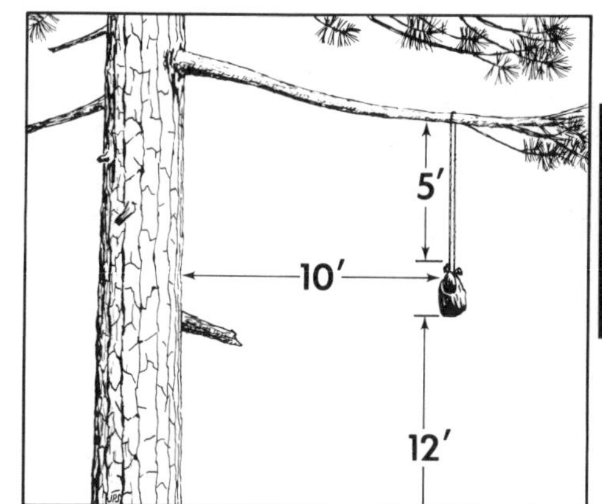

Recommended minimum distances for bearbagging your food

Alternate route. The Railroad Creek Trail forks in about 0.1 mile. The 4.8-mile-long north branch,

See maps K11, K12

View up Lake Chelan, from Stehekin resort

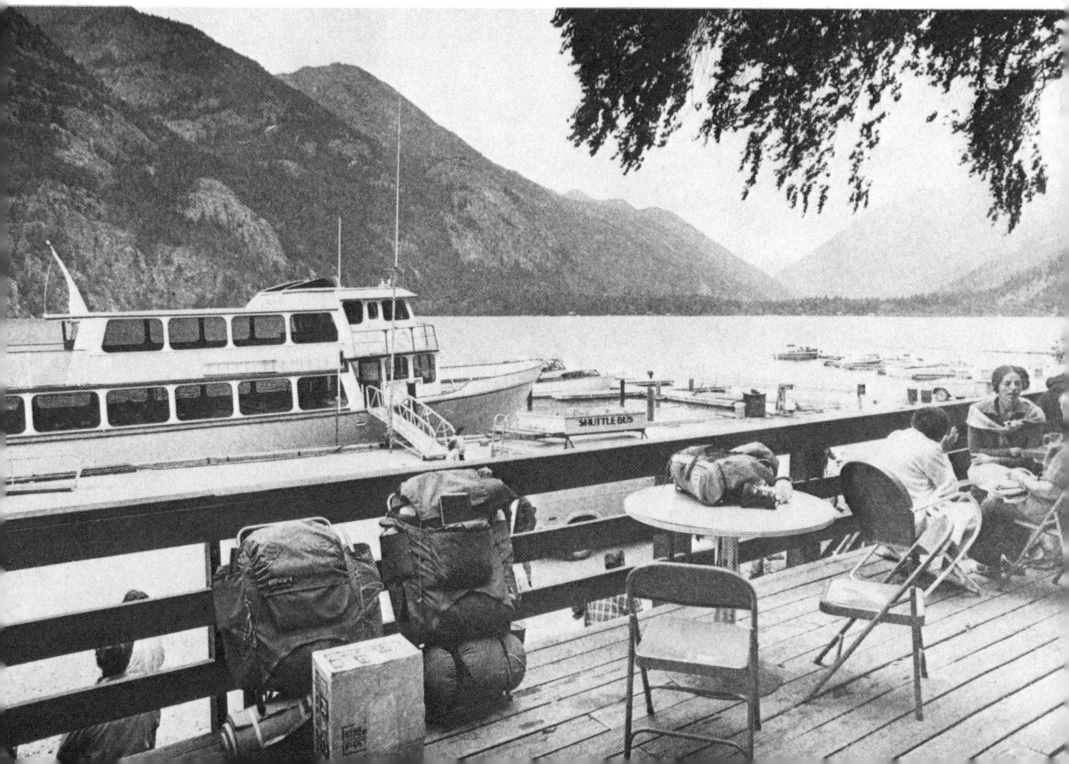

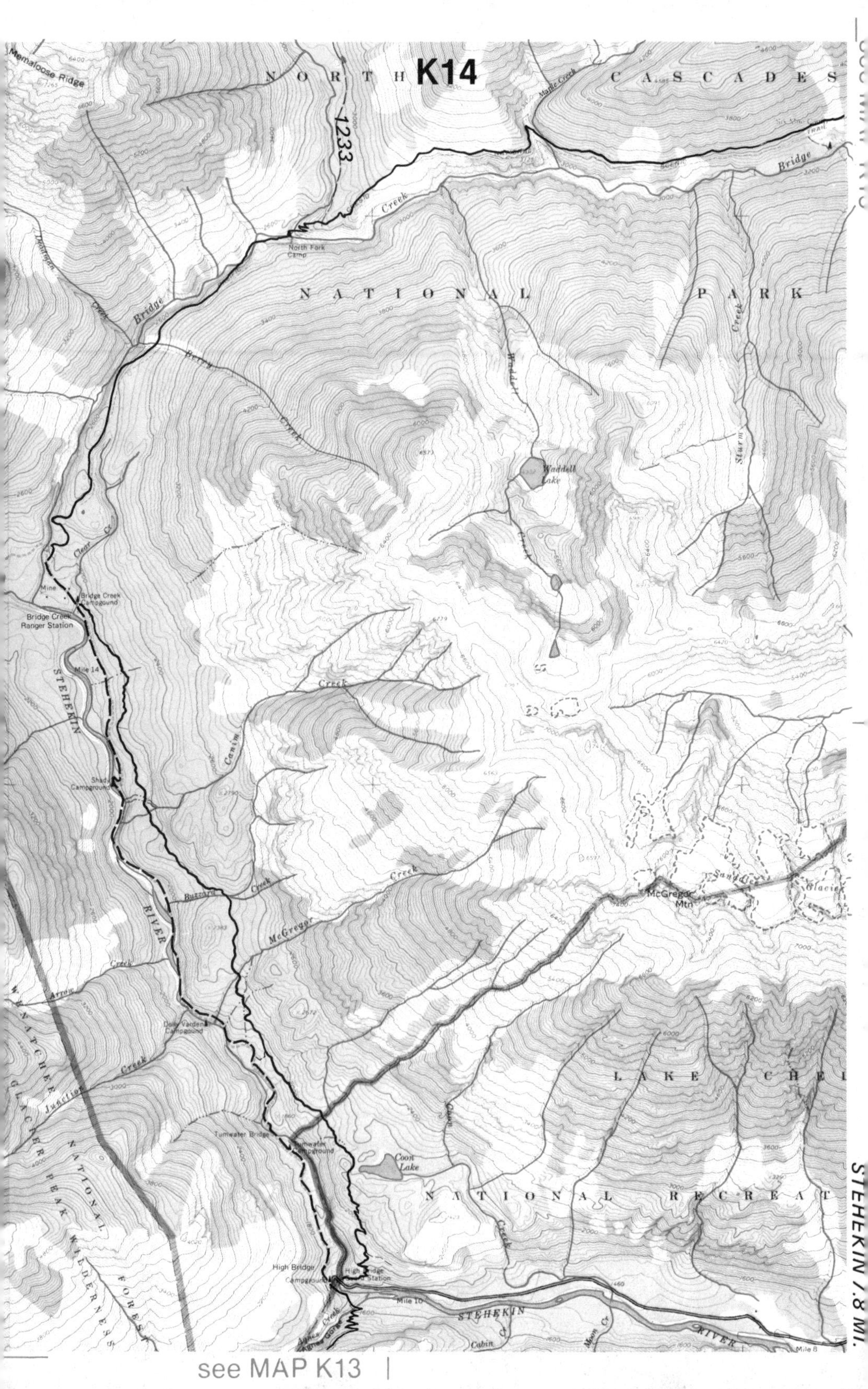
K14
NORTH CASCADES
NATIONAL PARK
1233
Memaloose Ridge
North Fork Camp
Bridge
Creek
Berry Creek
Waddell Lake
Waddell Creek
Maple Creek
Storm Creek
Clear Cr.
Mine
Bridge Creek Campground
Bridge Creek Ranger Station
Mile 14
STEHEKIN
Canim Creek
Shady Campground
Buzzard Creek
McGregor Creek
McGregor Mtn
Sandalee
Glacier
RIVER
Arrow Creek
Dolly Varden Campground
Junction Creek
WENATCHEE
GLACIER PEAK WILDERNESS
FOREST
Tumwater Bridge
Tumwater Campground
Coon Lake
Coon Creek
LAKE CHEL
NATIONAL RECREAT
High Bridge Campground
High Bridge Ranger Station
Mile 10
STEHEKIN
Agnes Creek
Agnes Gorge
Cabin Cr.
Boulder
Moon Cr.
RIVER
Mile 8
STEHEKIN 7.8 MI.
see MAP K13

see MAP K16

see MAP K14

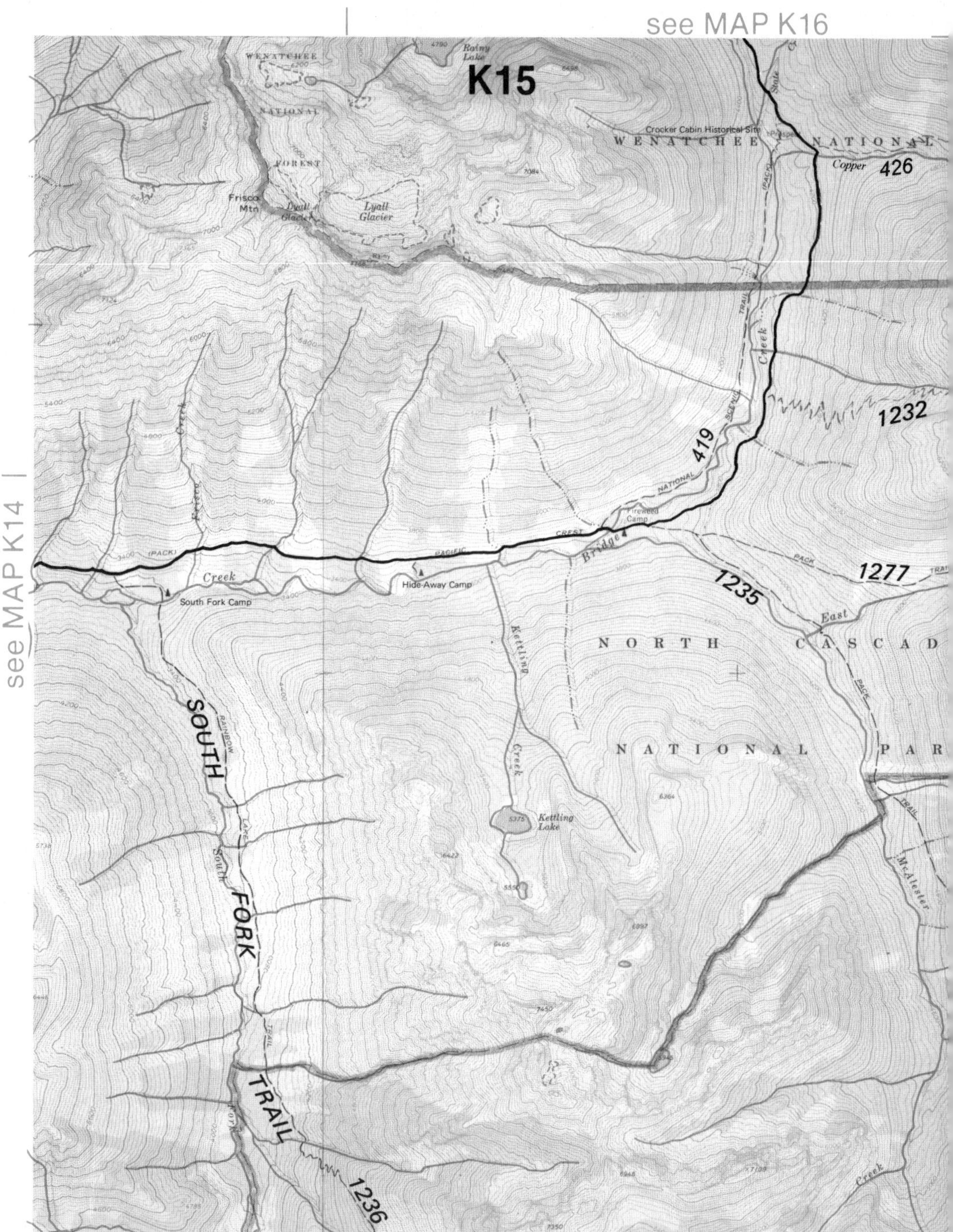

down Agnes Creek, is the older PCT route, and it rejoins the newer 6.5-mile-long PCT segment at Hemlock Camp.

Official PCT route and alternate route rejoined. Continuing north along this near-the-creek route through a forest of western hemlock, Engelmann spruce, western redcedar, Douglas-fir, and western white pine, you descend past Mt. Blankenship (5926) to the west and Needle Peak (7885) to the east before reaching Spruce Creek Camp (2900–2.7). ▮ *At this site, you'll find only log stumps around a fire pit, but it's still quite a nice camp.* ▮

See map K12

The canyon grows ever deeper as you trek northward, catch a glimpse of the blue-green waters of the South Fork, and then contour over to well-equipped Swamp Creek Camp (2780–1.3).

Side route. Here, beside the 7-yard-wide torrent, Swamp Creek Trail 712 begins a 3-mile climb up the creek toward Dark Glacier, which is tucked in a deep amphitheater.

Leaving this very good campsite, you cross the creek on a sturdy horse bridge, progress north to the rim of the inner gorge of South Fork Agnes Creek (2570–1.6) and then gradually curve down to a junction with West Fork Agnes Creek Trail 1272 (2160–1.4), which descends west-northwest to that creek. Several fair campsites are just west of this junction, but much better ones are at Five Mile Camp, about 100 yards east, above the west bank of Pass Creek. These are the last campsites you'll see within Glacier Peak Wilderness.

▮ *You'll soon leave the granitic rocks of the Cloudy Pass batholith behind and walk upon schist and gneiss that date back to Jurassic times or earlier. The overpowering canyon that you are hiking through bears a strong resemblance to deep Kings Canyon in the Sierra Nevada of California, except that this one supports a much denser growth of flowers, shrubs, and trees.* ▮

See map K12

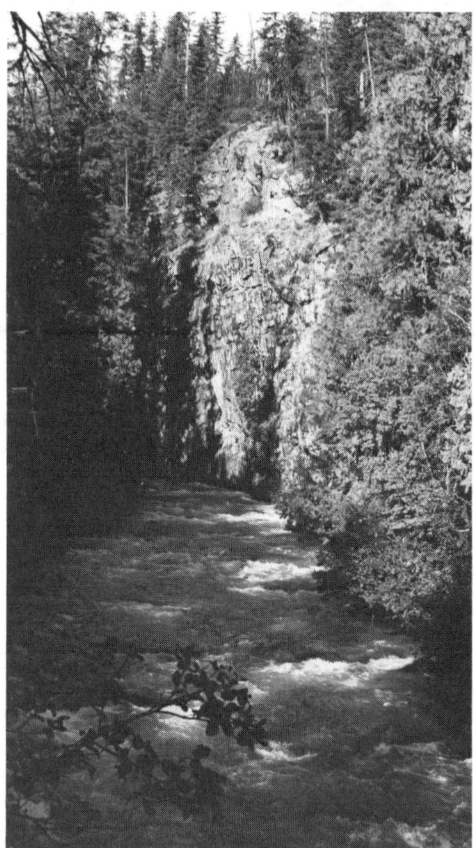

Inner Gorge of Agnes Creek

View up South fork Bridge Creek canyon

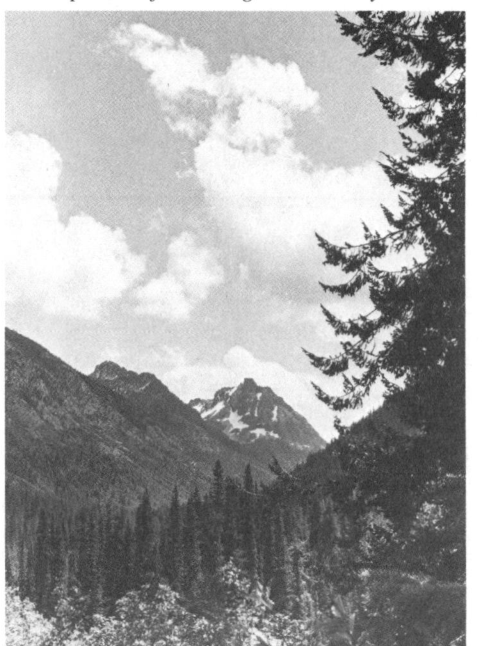

Hiking northeast, you pass by seasonal Trapper Creek (2070–1.2) and then approach Agnes Creek which, like its South Fork, possesses an inner gorge. The undulating trail goes right out to the gorge's brink at several spots and then descends to switchback down to a massive bridge 40 feet above roaring Agnes Creek (1550–3.6) which, at this point, is larger than most rivers you've seen along the PCT. Now within the Lake Chelan National Recreation Area, you cross the 27-yard-long bridge, climb a low ridge, and then contour northwest to the Agnes Creek trailhead at a bend in the Stehekin River Road (1650–0.2).

See maps K12, K13, K14

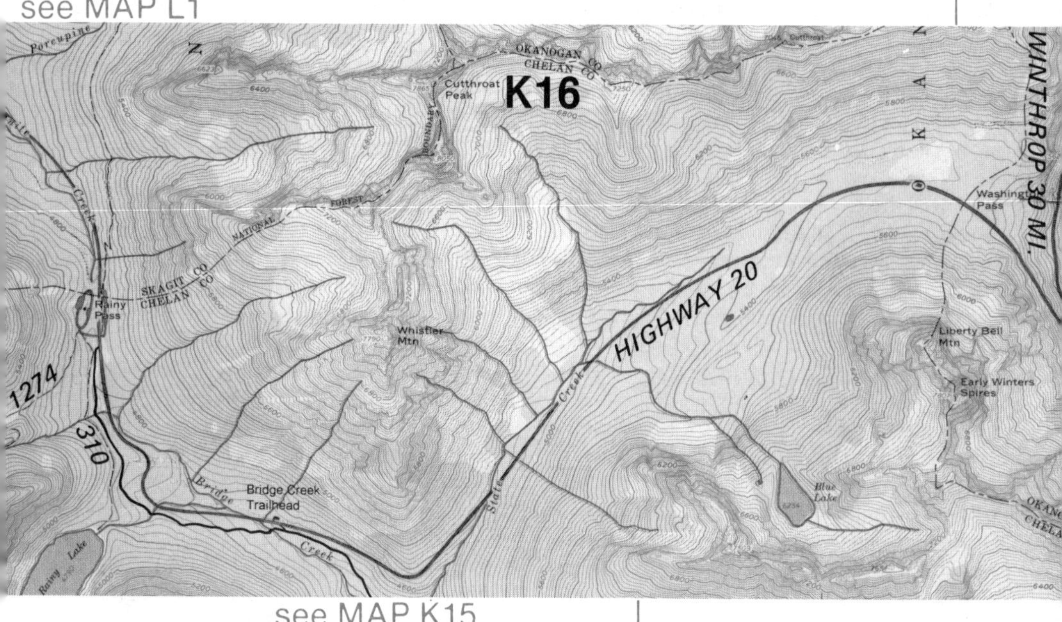

Side route. Just 35 yards up the road is High Bridge Campground, with a shelter and outside tables. Water can be obtained by walking back down the road to the high bridge and then descending steep, short switchbacks northward to the west bank of the Stehekin River.

Side route. You can descend the road 200 yards to the High Bridge Ranger Station, which is immediately northeast of a bend in the Stehekin River. During the summer, shuttle buses from the Stehekin resort area, 10.6 miles downstream, depart about four times daily. The schedule changes from year to year, and even during the season, so check at the High Bridge Ranger Station (or on a posted sign nearby) for the current schedule. The shuttle buses take about an hour to reach the High Bridge stop, and the one-way fee between Stehekin and High Bridge was $5.00 in 1999. Bus service continues north from here to Cottonwood Camp, 11.4 miles up-river, so it's possible to ride a total distance of 22 miles.

If you're like most hikers, you'll be weary by the time the PCT reaches the Agnes Creek trailhead, and you'll welcome the opportunity to relax overnight in Stehekin. The North Cascades Lodge dominates the Stehekin complex, providing good meals and accommodations. The old Golden West Lodge has been transformed into the Park Service's Golden West Visitor Center, where you can get wilderness permits and information. Nearby are a public shower, laundromat, and, in the Stehekin Ranger Station, the Stehekin Post Office (98852). Just southeast of the lodge is McGregor Mountain Outdoor Supply, which should have basic backpacker needs.

You'll find camping ¼ mile north of the complex at Purple Point Campground. ▮ *It is possible, though very unlikely, that you'll encounter western rattlesnakes here, for they are quite common in the Stehekin area, though they become less common up-canyon. More likely, however, you'll meet black bears, which have become an increasing nuisance as they've grown bolder in recent years. You can expect to see them at any of the nine roadside campgrounds. Be sure you know how to "bearbag" your food.* ▮

Many backpackers hiking from Stevens Pass through Glacier Peak Wilderness to High Bridge end their hike there and take the shuttle bus to Stehekin. They can then take one of three boats that ply between Stehekin and Chelan, a popular resort town at the far end of Lake Chelan. The slowest and cheapest boat

See maps K14

takes about 4 hours, the fastest and most expensive, about 1 hour. In 2000, the round-trip rates ranged from $22 to $79. *In its deepest spot, this 50-mile-long lake is 1486 feet deep, or in other words, its deepest point is about 386 feet below sea level. If the lake were drained, its lowest floor would be the lowest land surface in the western United States. This has caused many, including author Schaffer, to believe that the past glaciers, flowing through the enormous canyon to Chelan, must have performed major erosion, but now this does not appear to be so. The eastern part of this range is fault-ridden, and glaciers may have merely flowed through a graben (a valley formed by down-faulting).*

The advantage of ending at Chelan rather than at Rainy Pass is that you are much closer to Stevens Pass, your starting point for this section. The drive from Stevens Pass to Chelan is 90 miles, but it is an *additional* 103 miles to Rainy Pass. For non-through PCT hikers, that additional shuttle is not worth the generally viewless hike along the last stretch of this section.

To complete this stretch on the PCT from the Agnes Creek trailhead, walk down to the nearby bridge over the Stehekin River, immediately beyond which you'll find another trailhead by the High Bridge Ranger Station (1600–0.1). Take this trail, which starts initially east and then switchbacks up to a granitic bench with a trail junction (1860–0.4); this trail descends southeast to the Cascade Corral on the Stehekin River Road. The PCT climbs northward, topping a low, bedrock ridge and reaching a junction at the west arm of swampy Coon Lake (2180–0.7).

Side route. From this junction, a rigorously switchbacking trail climbs about 7 miles to the top of McGregor Mountain.

The PCT heads northwest, passing two seasonal creeklets on a mostly descending grade to yet another junction (1940–0.8).

Side route. From here, the Old Wagon Trail winds 200 yards west down to the Stehekin River Road. Dolly Varden Campground, with two sites, lies 0.4 miles up it.

The PCT coincides with a stretch of the Old Wagon Trail, and you cross two seasonal creeklets before climbing to McGregor Creek (2195–0.6). The ascent abates, and soon the trail fords Buzzard Creek (2260–0.4) and, later, two-branched Canim Creek (2160–0.7). In about ⅓ mile, you leave the Old Wagon Trail and make an undulating traverse that ends about 50 yards before Clear Creek, roughly opposite the Bridge Creek Ranger Station (2105–1.3). Just beyond it, you pass Bridge Creek Campground with its shelter. After a few more minutes of walking, you arrive at the PCT Bridge Creek trailhead (2180–0.3), located 240 yards southeast of Road 3505's crossing of Bridge Creek.

Back on a trail again, you climb up a wandering path that passes a small, lily-pad pond on a bench, winds to the edge of the Bridge Creek gorge, and climbs its slopes to jump-across Berry Creek (2720–1.7). Watching out for western toads, you climb a little higher on the slope before descending to a horse bridge above wild, roaring Bridge Creek (2540–1.0). Climbing a few yards north of the bridge, you reach dusty, rustic North Fork Camp atop a rocky bluff that overlooks the junction of the North Fork with Bridge Creek. *The camp's resident landlords, golden-mantled ground squirrels, may exact "rent" from your backpack while you're not looking.*

From this site, the trail switchbacks east up to a junction with North Fork Bridge Creek Trail 1233 (2810–0.3), which climbs northward. Climb east up a bushy, aromatic slope, reach a point several hundred feet above Bridge Creek, and take in gorgeous views below as you descend slightly to a small, stonewall campsite immediately before a saddle. Beyond it, the trail descends north to wide, alder-lined Maple Creek (3070–1.5), which has a suspension-bridge crossing it 25 yards upstream. Be careful climbing the talus boulders to and from the bridge. Then follow the level, relaxing path east and come to a 250-yard-long spur trail (3130–1.7)

Side route. This spur descends southeast, steeply at first, through a meadow of tall cow parsnips, to Six Mile Camp, a well furnished site designed with equestrians in mind.

See map K14

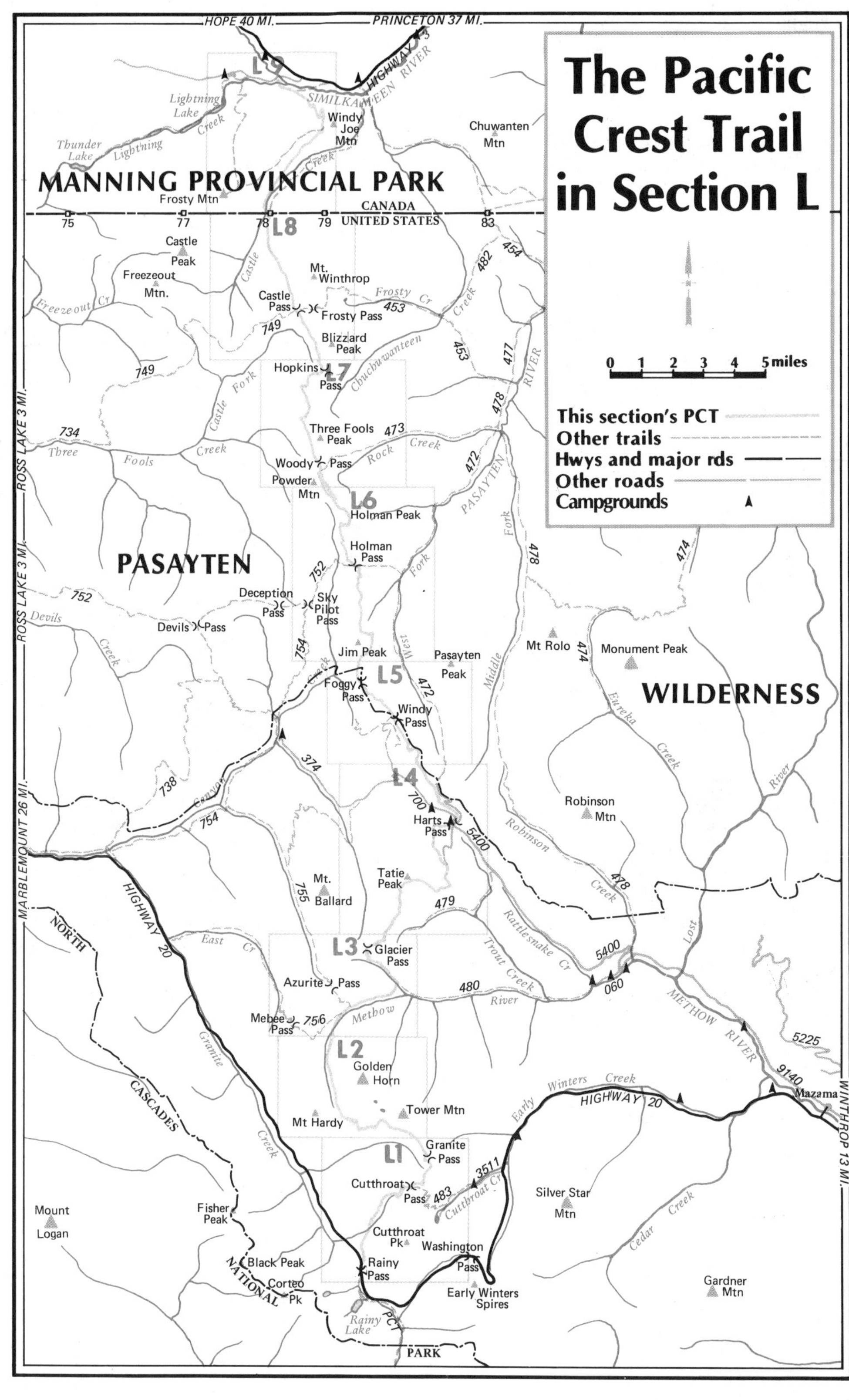
The Pacific Crest Trail in Section L
0 1 2 3 4 5 miles
This section's PCT
Other trails
Hwys and major rds
Other roads
Campgrounds
HOPE 40 MI.
PRINCETON 37 MI.
HIGHWAY 3
SIMILKAMEEN RIVER
MANNING PROVINCIAL PARK
Lightning Lake
Thunder Lake
Lightning Creek
Windy Joe Mtn
Chuwanten Mtn
Frosty Mtn
CANADA
UNITED STATES
Castle Peak
Freezeout Mtn.
Mt. Winthrop
Castle Pass
Frosty Pass
Blizzard Peak
Hopkins Pass
Three Fools Peak
Woody Pass
Powder Mtn
Holman Peak
Holman Pass
PASAYTEN
WILDERNESS
Deception Pass
Sky Pilot Pass
Devils Pass
Jim Peak
Pasayten Peak
Mt Rolo
Monument Peak
Foggy Pass
Windy Pass
Robinson Mtn
Harts Pass
Mt. Ballard
Tatie Peak
Glacier Pass
Azurite Pass
Mebee Pass
Golden Horn
Tower Mtn
Mt Hardy
Granite Pass
Cutthroat Pass
Cutthroat Pk
Washington Pass
Early Winters Spires
Silver Star Mtn
Gardner Mtn
Rainy Pass
Rainy Lake
Black Peak
Corteo Pk
Fisher Peak
Mount Logan
Mazama
HIGHWAY 20
METHOW RIVER
NORTH CASCADES NATIONAL PARK
ROSS LAKE 3 MI.
MARBLEMOUNT 26 MI.
WINTHROP 13 MI.
PCT

Not far beyond this spur trail, the Rainbow Lake Trail (3240–0.7) peels off from the PCT.

Side route. Just 330 yards down this trail is South Fork Camp beside Bridge Creek. The trail descends southeast and then climbs up South Fork Canyon to Pass 6230, immediately west of domineering Bowan Mountain (7895) and Rainbow Lake south of the pass.

From the junction, the PCT continues east through alternating forest and brush cover and then reaches a junction with a 110-yard-long spur trail (3510–1.5).

Side route. This spur trail descends first southwest and then southeast to the loveliest Bridge Creek campsite: Hide-Away Camp. Strictly for backpackers, this shady, creekside campsite has log stumps and a fire ring.

Continuing east within hearing distance of the creek, the PCT leaves this junction and eventually turns northeast just before reaching a junction with Twisp Pass Trail 1277 (3635–0.9). Ahead, the old (pre-1990s) PCT route continues north as Trail 419. The newer PCT route branches right, curving east to quickly bridge, in 70 yards, Bridge Creek. About 40 yards onward, the trail meets a fork to the right, going about 30 yards to large, well-furnished Fireweed Camp. Just beyond, the PCT leaves Trail 1277 and Trail 1234, which branches from it bound for McAlester Pass. The trail parallels Bridge Creek up-canyon at a distance, soon curving north and passing unmaintained, east-climbing Stiletto Peak Trail 1232 about ½ mile before the PCT exits North Cascades National Park (4180–1.9). After an easy ascent for about ⅔ mile, you cross swift-flowing Copper Creek and over the next ⅓ mile first pass Trail 426, heading up that creek, and then reach the north end of the old PCT route, Trail 419 (4300–1.0).

You quickly reach and cross swift-flowing State Creek and then parallel Bridge Creek at a closer distance as you arc from north to west to an important junction (4510–0.9).

Side route. If you're not going on through Section L, you'll want to end your Section-K hike here. Take a spur trail 70 yards northwest up to Highway 20. From there, you walk 90 yards west on the highway to the PCT trailhead parking area for southbound hikers. This trailhead parking area is 70 yards east of where the highway crosses Bridge Creek, and also is 1.2 miles before the highway tops out at Rainy Pass.

Staying on the official PCT route, you take slightly longer, first bridging Bridge Creek immediately past the spur trail and then heading west, gradually up and away from the creek, to Rainy Lake's outlet creek (4705–0.5). From it, your path climbs gently north, levels off, and strikes a course through the soggy headwaters of Bridge Creek immediately before it ends beside Highway 20 at the entrance to spacious Rainy Pass Picnic Area (4855–0.9), Road 700. Here you'll find tables and outhouses but no tap water. Rainy Lake Trail 310 also starts south from here. Just across Highway 20 from the picnic area's entrance road is short, north-curving Road 600, which goes to the PCT trailhead parking area and equestrian area for northbound trekkers (for Section L).

See maps K15, K16

Section L: Highway 20 at Rainy Pass to Highway 3 in Manning Park

Introduction: The final leg of the PCT leads from the North Cascades Highway (Washington 20) at Rainy Pass to Manning Provincial Park, British Columbia. In this relatively short trek, there is vehicle access only at Harts Pass (30 miles north), where gravel Road 5400 crosses the crest to serve a turn-of-the-century—19th to 20th—mining district.

In this entire section, the PCT is well east of much of the Cascade Range. To the west, Mt. Baker, Mt. Shuksan, and the Picket Range receive the brunt of any bad weather. Overall snow accumulation along the PCT route here is much less than it is at Mt. Baker, and PCT hikers may enjoy sunshine when Puget Sound and the western mountains are cloud- and rain-bound. Nonetheless, until midsummer, hikers should be prepared for a snow-covered and icy trail. After the snow melts, the mosquitoes have a heyday, so the most pleasant month to hike this section is, usually, September. Typically, the winter snows do not start in earnest until at least October (but beware the exception!).

Near Rainy Pass, the scenery is spectacular, and many mountains are crowned with craggy spires of Golden Horn granodiorite. Consequently, the PCT only occasionally follows the crest of the Cascades exactly: much of the mileage is in long traverses and river valleys. Even if backpackers were as surefooted and agile as mountain goats, they would not choose a route true to the divide. Then, as the intrusive rocks give way to lower Cretaceous graywackes, the terrain becomes hilly, so the PCT can follow the crest more closely than before.

North of Harts Pass, the PCT offers a variety of scenery and terrain. High meadows, wooded slopes and valleys, as well as rugged, precipitous ridges make up the bulk of this section, which traverses the backbone of the 790-square-mile Pasayten Wilderness. In good weather, the views are frequently spectacular, particularly in the fall when larch, spruce, and scrub maple splash gold, green, and red across the slopes.

Declination: 20°E

Mileages:	**S→N**	**Mi. Btwn. Pts.**	**N→S**
Highway 20 at Rainy Pass	0.0		7.03
Cutthroat Pass	5.1	5.1	65.2
Methow Pass	10.6	5.5	59.7
Glacier Pass	21.2	10.6	49.1
Harts Pass	30.5	9.3	39.8
Windy Pass	35.7	5.2	34.6
Holman Pass	44.3	8.6	26.0
Woody Pass	50.5	6.2	19.8
Hopkins Pass	55.6	5.1	14.7
U.S.-Canadian border at Monument 78	66.2	6.6	8.1
Highway 3 in Manning Park	70.3	8.1	0.0

Supplies: No supply points are found until northbound hikers reach trail's end, in Manning Provincial Park. In it, just west of the trailhead, you'll find Manning Park Lodge, with food and lodging, and the park headquarters, where you can get information. Greyhound Bus service is available to and from Vancouver, B.C.

Problems: Very early and very late season hikers should be ready for treacherous, precipitous snow slopes, avalanche hazards, and dangerously exposed hiking along parts of this PCT section. It is also wise to acquaint yourself with the border-crossing information in Chapter 2 to avoid unpleasant hassles associated with customs and immigration regulations of both the United States and Canada.

Maps:

Washington Pass, WA
Mount Arriva, WA
Azurite Peak, WA (PCT barely enters map)
Slate Peak, WA
Pasayten Peak, WA
Shull Mountain, WA
Castle Peak, WA

THE ROUTE

A large, off-road rest area equipped with "plush" toilet facilities has been built west of the North Cascades Highway. Ample trailhead parking for horse packers and hikers parallels the shoulder of the road. Nearby outhouses are smaller than those in the rest area. The northbound PCT bisects the narrow peninsula of wilderness between the highway and an eastern parking lot. At the north end of the parking lot, you enter Douglas-fir forest to begin a climbing, northward traverse. One creek draining Cutthroat Peak (7865) cascades across the path even in September and October. Numerous other streams are of nuisance value early in the season but typically dry up by late August. The grade levels as the trail nears Porcupine Creek

See map L1

Black Peak (right) stands high above Granite Creek canyon Hartline

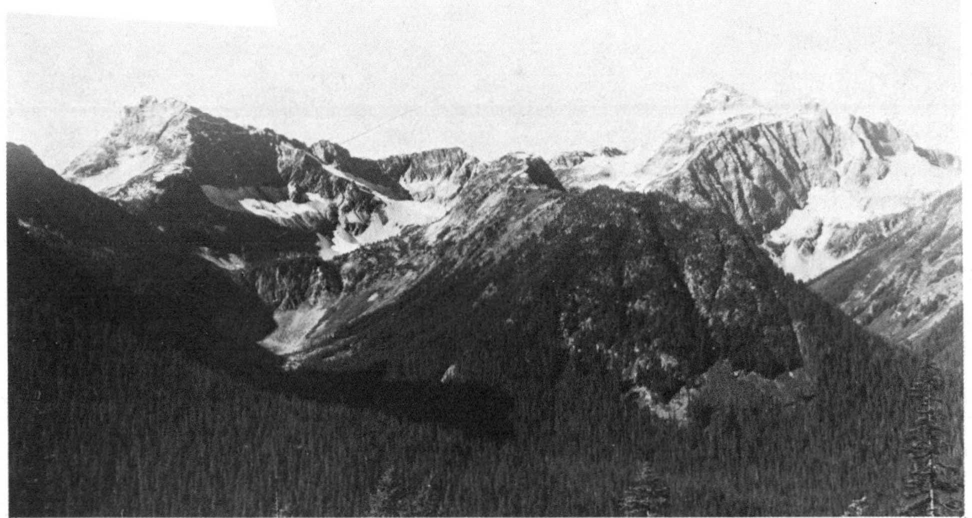

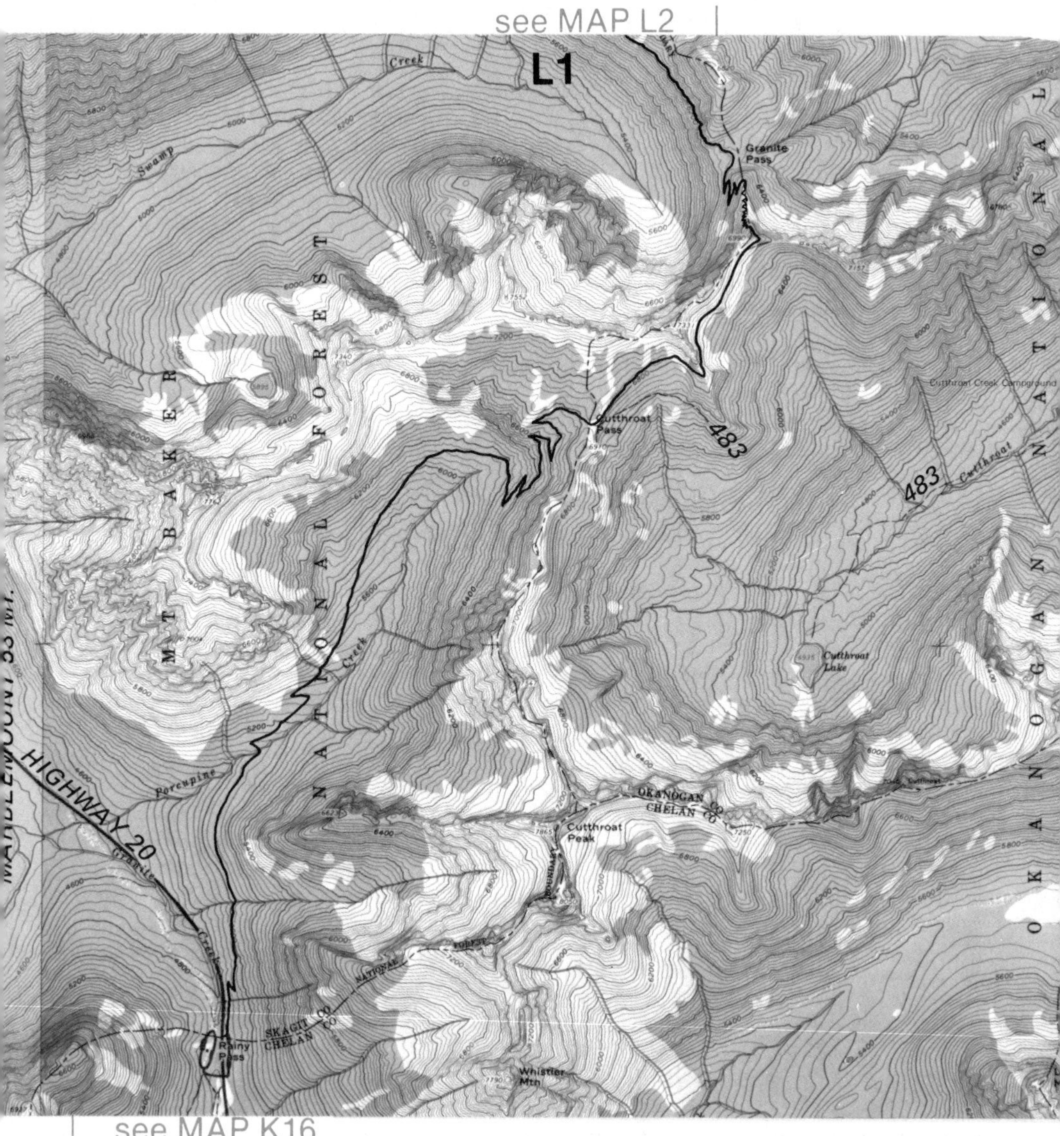

(5080–1.5) and bridges it. Then you turn northeast to parallel it and resume the ascent. A pair of switchbacks lifts the path away from the streambed and guides you onto a steep, open slope where avalanches sweeping down from Peaks 7004 and 7762 may threaten May and June hikers. After traversing higher to contour around the headwaters bowl of Porcupine Creek, you switchback up the steep, glacier-formed basin wall. ▮ *Deciduous larches, the poetic tamaracks, add foreground to the rugged panorama unfolding before you. Black Peak (8970) and Corteo Peak (8100) across the highway front the more distant North Cascades. Scrub huckleberry and heather compose the basic ground cover that "springtime" (July) flowers eloquently embroider.* ▮

You pass campsites that are inviting, though lacking late-season water, as the PCT levels to the west of grassy, granitic Cutthroat Pass (6820–3.6). Here, Cutthroat Lake Trail 483 forks east to begin its traversing descent to Cutthroat Lake (4935), visible in the valley below. Liberty Bell Mountain (7720), a favorite rock climb, peeks above the ridge across the lake. Head northeast to arc around two bowls, contouring across steep scree slopes beneath precipitous cliffs. Before leaving the second cirque, you choose the upper and more traveled of two trails; the lower trail

See map L1

dead-ends on the ridge 100 yards ahead. Climbing slightly, you reach a crest and pause to enjoy a picturesque view of Tower Mountain (8444).

The route continues northward, balancing precariously across a precipice before executing several short, tight switchbacks down the rugged north ridge. Avoiding the rock walls above Granite Pass, you descend south to zigzag above beautiful, glacier-carved Swamp Creek valley. Then, at Granite Pass (6290–2.4), you reach "terra flata" and are welcomed into a sheltered camp. Don't expect convenient late-season water here.

From the camp, the PCT makes a long traverse of the open, lower slopes of Tower Mountain on the way to Methow Pass. Scrub subalpine fir, western white pine, mountain ash, and heather provide little protection for sun-beaten or windswept walkers. ▮ *Outcrops of the Golden Horn granodiorite are clearly exposed by the trail cut.* ▮ Upon reaching the bowl below Snowy Lakes, you lose some precious elevation as the trail drops into an idyllic park where a bubbling stream, grassy flowerlands, larch, and spruce all recommend a large campsite (6300–2.2). ▮ *Shed your pack, don your sweater, and settle in. Firewood in this delicate alpine valley is in limited supply, and it is better left unburned.* ▮ A cross trail from the campsite heads north, up-valley, to Upper and Lower Snowy Lakes in a higher cirque.

From the camp, a pair of switchbacks help you climb out of the bowl to set up the approach to Methow Pass (6600–0.9) (pronounced MET-how). Views of Mt. Arriva (8215) and Fisher Peak (8050) are the last you'll have of the mountains west of Granite Creek. Mt. Hardy (7197) just west of the pass and Golden Horn (8366) to the north will stay with you during the trek down the valley of the Methow River's West Fork. Like most high-elevation "campsites," Methow Pass is waterless when it is not swampy.

Leaving Methow Pass on a northward traverse, you spy below a backpackers' campsite on a level bench with an uncertain water supply. Now zigzagging into the valley, the PCT crosses a few infant streams and then straightens to parallel the West Fork of the Methow. ▮ *From here at sunset, Golden Horn glows spectacularly against the deep blue-black of the eastern sky.* ▮ A long, slight but steady downgrade takes the trail to Golden Creek and Willis Camp (4570–4.2). Nimbly rock-hopping the stream, you have only a short stint before bridging the West Fork Methow River (4390–0.7). A small camp by the bridge on the east bank is the best trailside camp between here and Brush Creek. Within 200 yards, the level path enters the first of several avalanche paths.

At a PCT mileage sign, the trail merges onto the route of the old Cascade Crest Trail (now Trail 756) (4380–0.8).

See maps L1, L2, L3

Playground by Manning Hartline

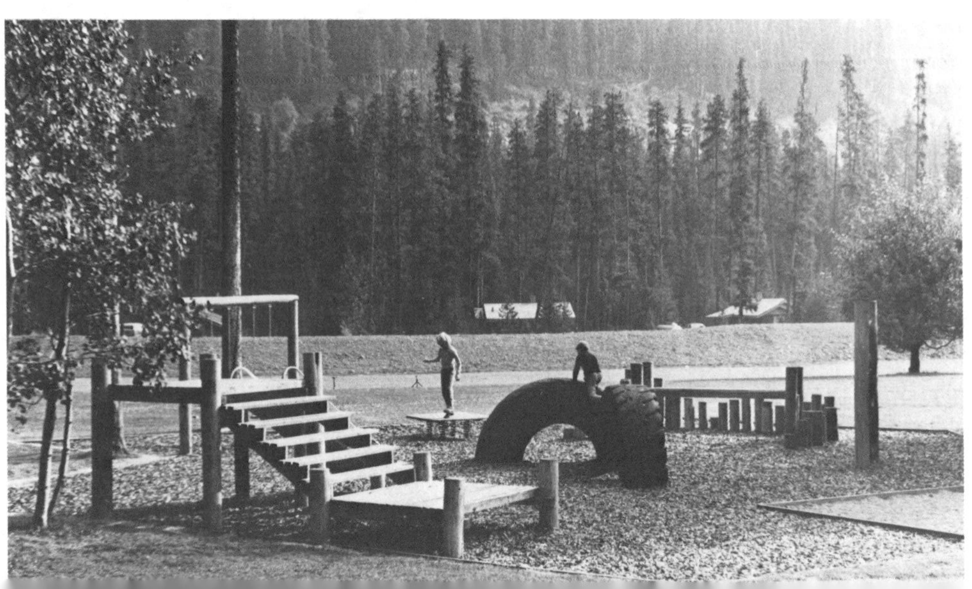

Side route. Westbound, this overgrown trail climbs out of the Methow Valley via Mebee Pass to descend along East Creek, pass the Gold Hill Mine, and meet Granite Creek and Washington Highway 20. This trail also extends diagonally 0.2 mile downhill to riverside Horse Heaven Camp.

The PCT, bending east and crossing what the map calls Jet Creek, reaches a junction with Mill Creek Trail 755 (4380–0.2), which looks like a rocky streambed in the grass of the clearing. Almost immediately, you cross signed Jet Creek, dry in late season.

From here, the trail continues east. The scree fields change in character and composition as the trail heads east out of the granodiorite body and into a zone of lower Cretaceous graywackes ("muddy" sandstones), conglomerates, argillites, and shales. Then the trail turns northeast to enter the mouth of beaver-inhabited Brush Creek's canyon. After passing a small campsite, you cross Brush Creek on a bridge and, in 50 yards, meet West Fork Methow Trail 480 (4280–1.9). Here, the trail zigs once and starts climbing in earnest along steep, brushy Brush Creek. A few small campsites line the trail in this fairly hospitable and picturesque valley, and, high in the west, some small glaciers cling between the rugged upper cliffs of Azurite Peak (8400). A few switchbacks ease the grade of the final climb to Glacier Pass (5520–2.8), where campsites without nearby late-season water are found in the forest-sheltered gap. Two trails, the first heading north and the second trending west, are separated by 100 PCT trail yards.

Ambling on, you gear down for a long, zigzagging climb to a grassy pass. ▮ *Dwindling scrub subalpine fir, spruce, and larch accompany the trail up the slope.* ▮ Pausing for breath, you appreciate the view of three little lakes nestled near the head of South Fork Slate Creek's glacial valley, as well as the broadening panorama of the North Cascades. At last the trail tops off the climb and descends slightly along the ridge into an alpine-garden pass (6750–2.6) above South Fork Trout Creek.

See maps L3, L4

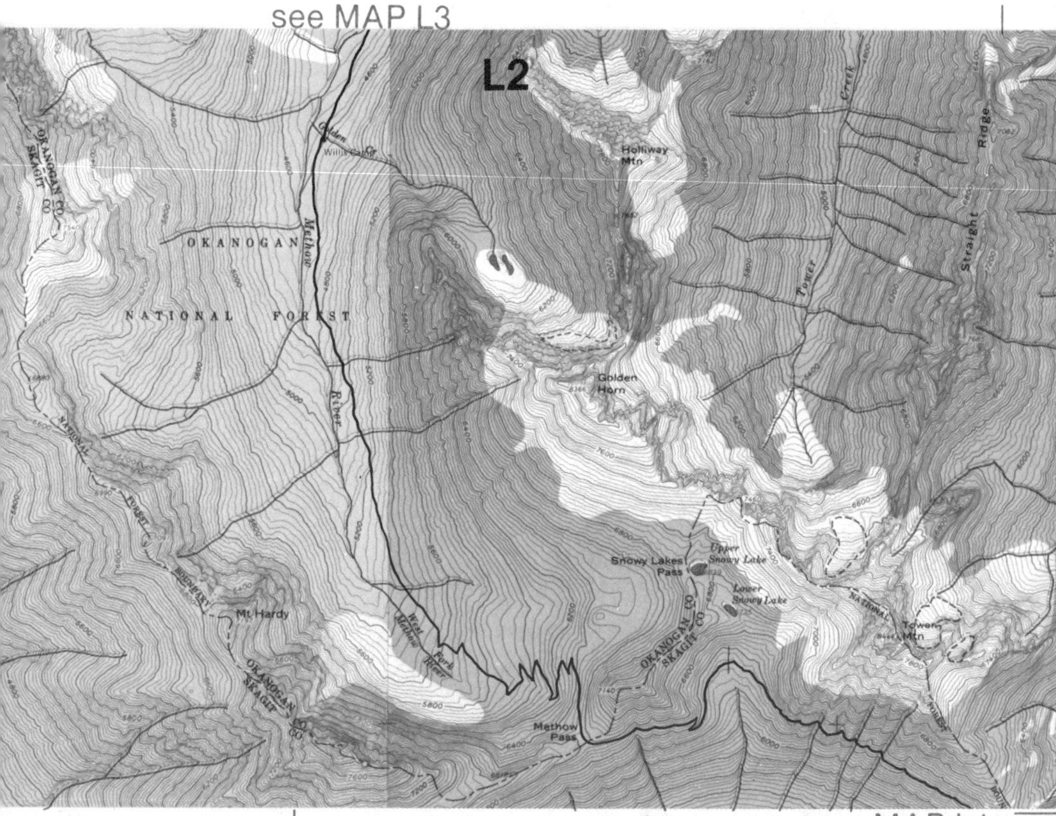

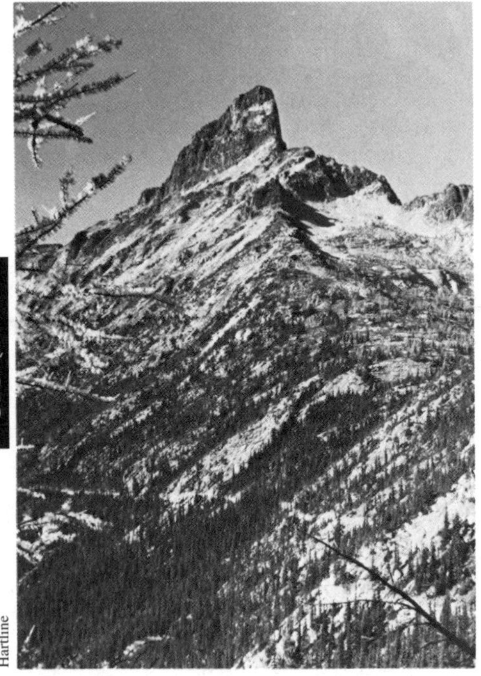
Hartline

Tower Mountain, from above Tower Pass

Here, the trail begins a long traverse northeastward. Beyond the first ridge you round is a pleasant trailside campsite with water (6600–1.0). Continuing, you climb to a windy, viewful pass (6900–0.9) on the southwest shoulder of Tatie Peak (7386). As the trail contours around the peak, it passes stratified outcrops of alternating shale and conglomerate and then approaches a knife-edge saddle above Ninetynine Basin, beyond which the Slate Peak Lookout Tower (7440) is prominent. A descending traverse guides you around Peak 7405 through a gap in a side ridge. ■ *Both the Harts Pass Road and the Brown Bear Mine house remains can be seen from here.* ■

Angling down, the trail passes below the sites of the mine tunnels—not obvious from the trail—and approaches dirt Road 500. Twenty yards short of the road (6440–2.8), PCT emblems guide you onto a newer stretch of trail that avoids that road. In 150 yards, you cross the jeep-trail access to the Brown Bear tunnels, and then you continue to traverse above Road 500. A trail from the road joins the

See map L4

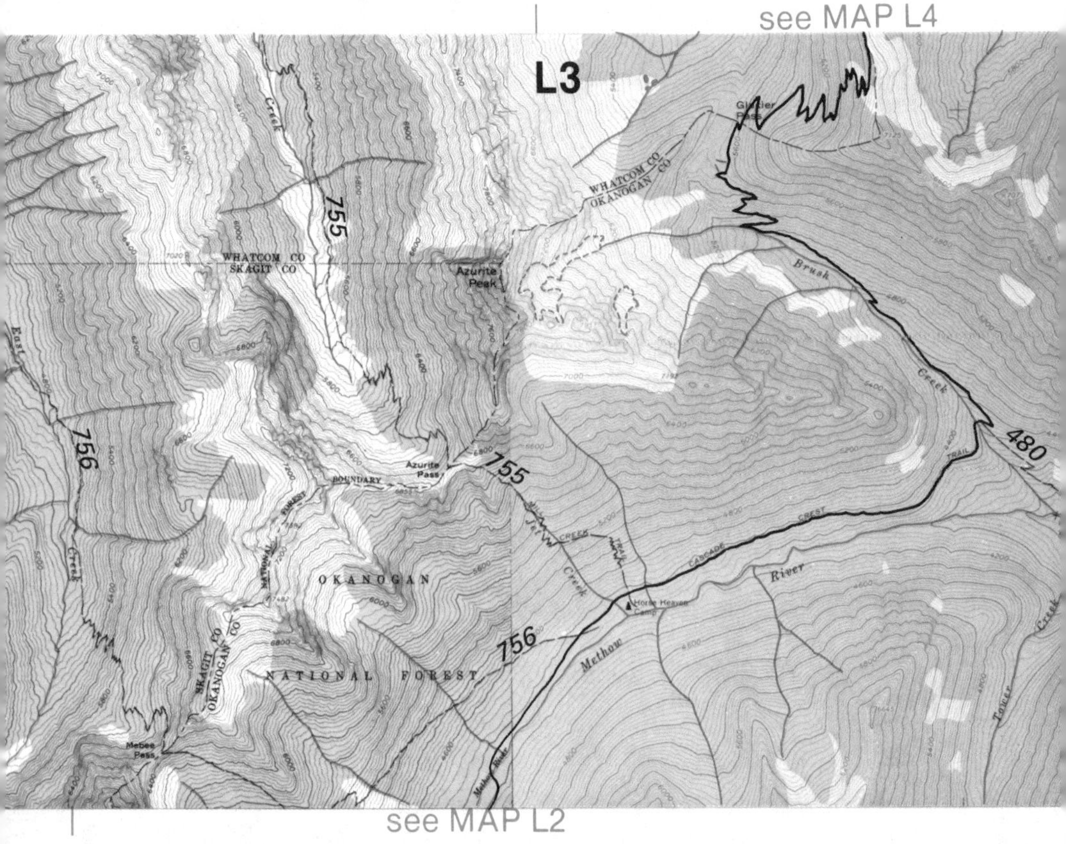

see MAP L4

L3

see MAP L2

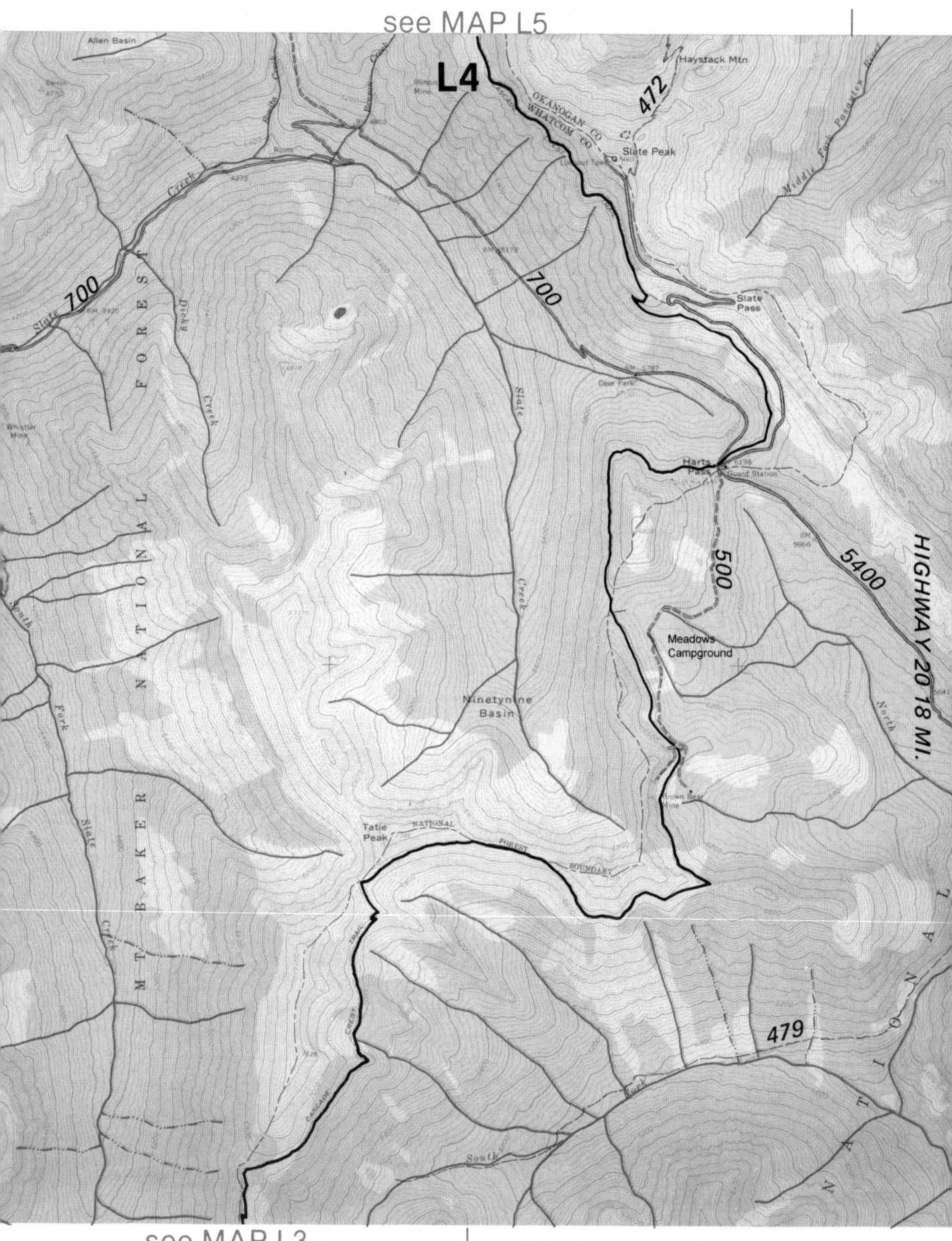

PCT as it approaches and threads a minor gap (6390–0.7).

Water access. This trail descends briefly to the environs of Meadows Campground, near which you can get water. When the North Cascades dry up, which isn't too often, your route ahead can be waterless all the way to Shaw Creek, a full 10 miles beyond Harts Pass.

Beneath exposed outcrops of banded argillite and gray sandstone, the trail traverses north along a steep hillside before turning to

See map L4

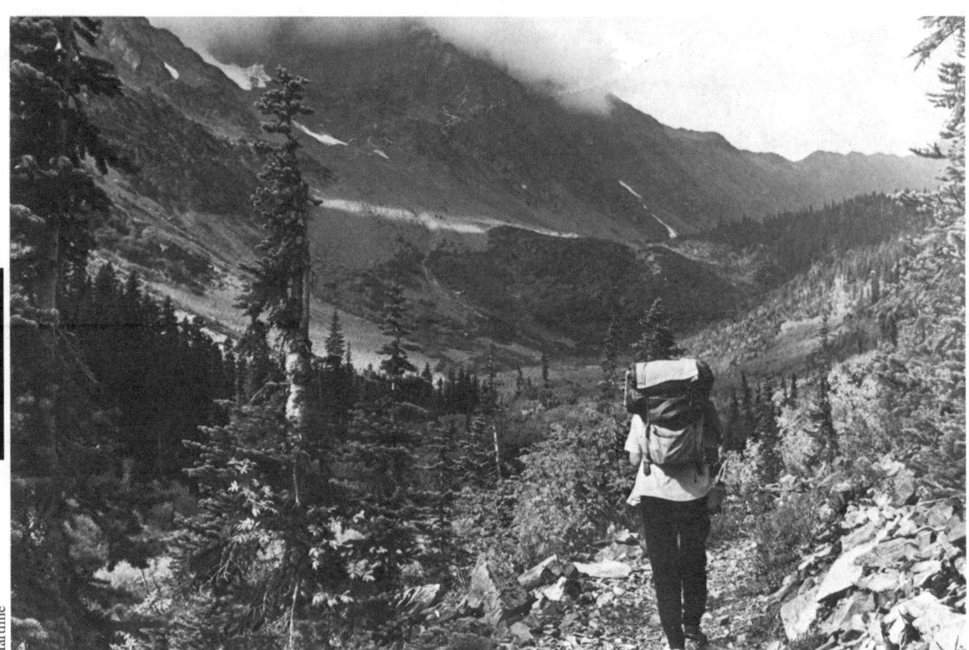

Hartline

Climbing toward Glacier Pass

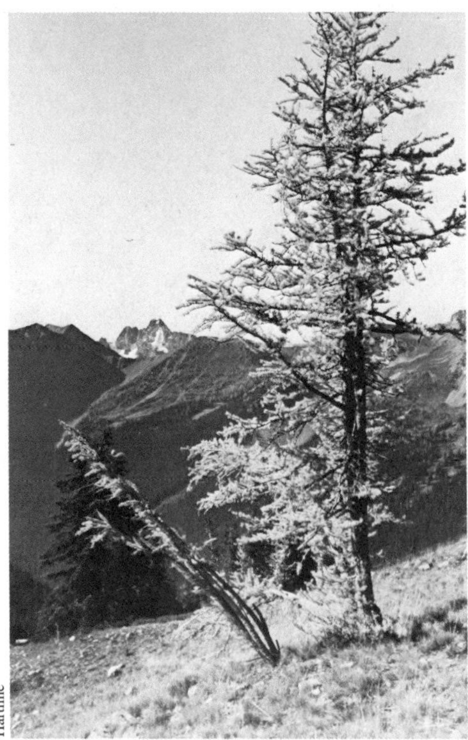

Hartline

Tatie Peak, from Slate Peak area

traverse down to Harts Pass (6198–1.3). *An infrequently manned Forest Service Guard Station, on the east side of Harts Pass Road 5400 across from a trailhead parking lot, sometimes has a backcountry register for hikers to sign.*

Side routes. The small community of Mazama is 18.7 miles east on Road 5400. Also at the pass, a road branches east-northeast from Road 5400 to parallel the PCT for 1.3 miles before switchbacking up to Slate Peak Lookout.

The Slate Creek mining district was a relatively rich mining area in the State of Washington. Boom camps were fairly populated in the early 1890s until word of the Klondike bonanza lured all the miners away. Del Hart, who owned some mines near Slate Creek, commissioned Charles H. Ballard in 1895 to survey a road from Mazama to the mining area. The pass through which the road was routed now bears Hart's name. The road today is a favorite summer-recreation route and one of the best access roads to Pasayten Wilderness, which you'll soon enter. Gold, silver, copper, lead, and zinc are among the metals whose

See map L4

ores were mined in the Slate Creek District. An interesting sidelight to the history of this area is that the first hydroelectric powerplant in the high Cascades was installed here. O.B. Brown designed, paid for, and supervised construction of the 350-kilowatt plant that he located on the South Fork of Slate Creek. ▮

From the PCT crossing of Road 5400, a scant 35 yards north-northwest of the pass proper, you proceed east-northeast through partly open spruce-fir woods, parallelling a Forest Service road and about 100 feet below it. Beyond a meadow, the trail switchbacks up onto a small shoulder with an adequate camp, where you come to a junction (6880–1.4) with a spur trail to the road; it is about 0.1 mile east-southeast down this spur to parking spaces.

Continuing west-northwest on the PCT, you ascend gradually past scattered Lyall larches, common on this small shoulder. Soon the shoulder gives out, leaving the trail hanging on the side of Slate Peak, with spectacular views down the Slate Creek valley, dominated by Mt. Baker (10,778) and other peal[illegible]

Mt. Baker is a living volcano, anu[illegible] 1975, it increased its thermal activity, w[illegible] led many to suspect it would soon erupt. Since the end of the Ice Age, about 10,000 years ago, it has erupted violently at least four times, and on at least four other occasions it has produced enough steam to melt glaciers and trigger large mudflows. Some future PCT hikers may just witness a full-scale eruption. ▮

Passing occasional outcrops of gray and green slate, you descend gradually to the pass (6700–2.2) just above Benson Creek Camp. Still on the west side of the divide, the trail climbs up around an arm and descends past Buffalo Pass (6550–0.7) to Windy Pass (6257–0.9), from which a trail crosses the PCT to descend south-southwest to Indiana Basin. In about 35 yards, you pass a sign heralding your entrance into Pasayten Wilderness.

The PCT continues north-northwest, leading out of true-to-its-name Windy Pass and around to the northeast cirque of Tamarack

See maps L4, L5

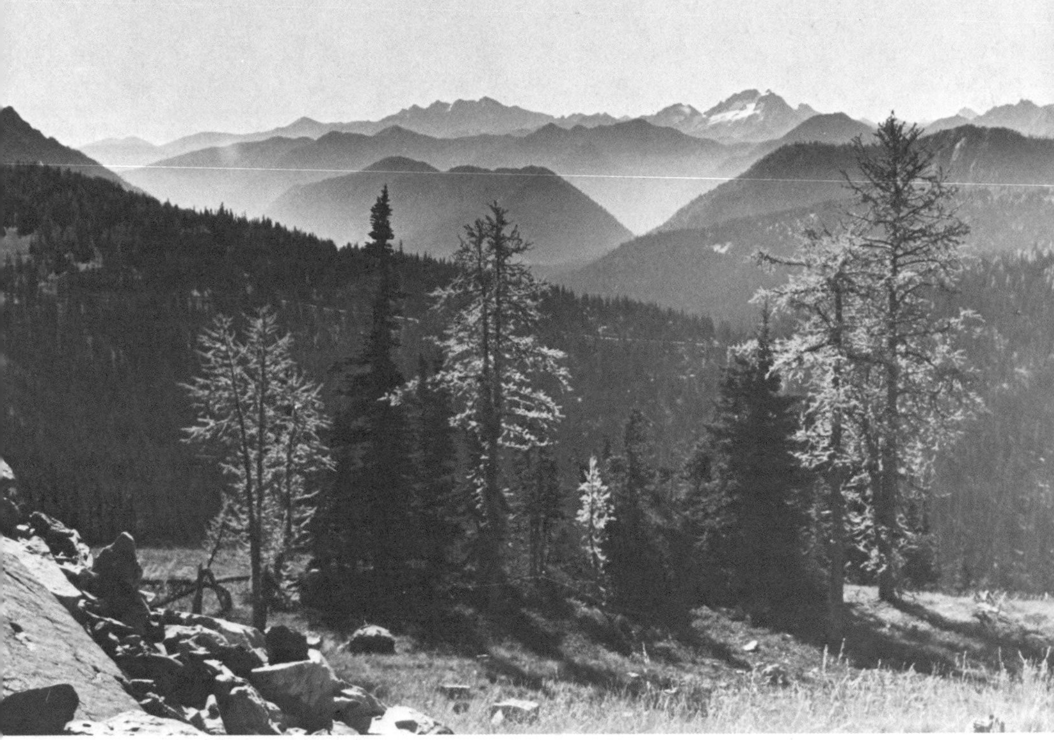

Hartline

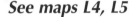

Silver Star Mountain, viewed from Harts Pass area

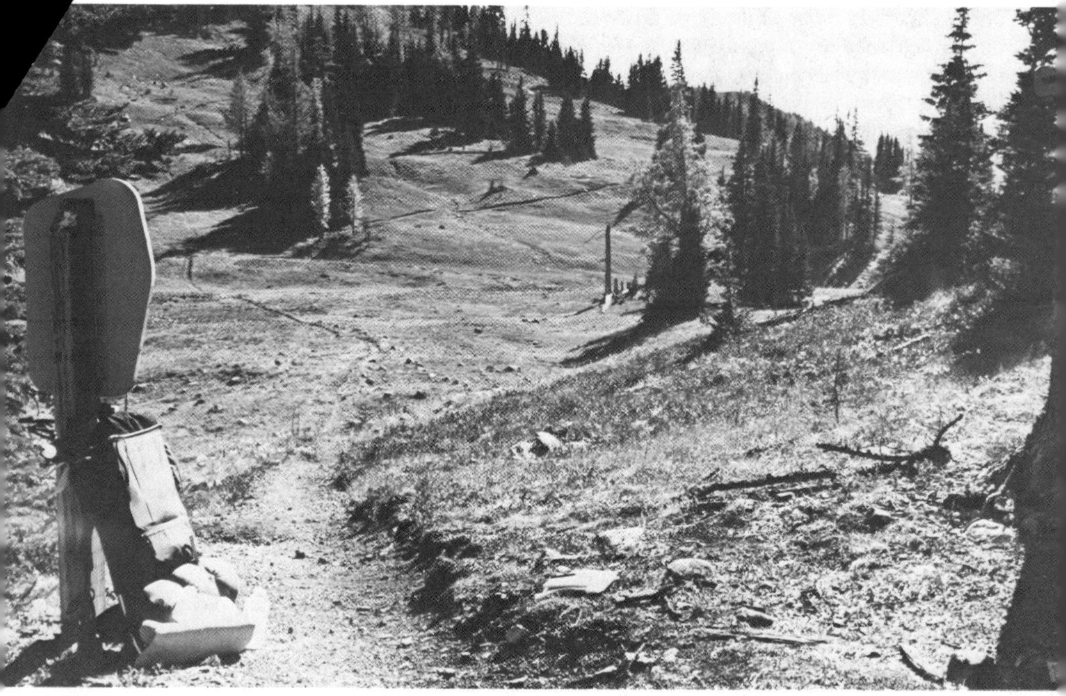

Windy Pass Hartline

see MAP L6

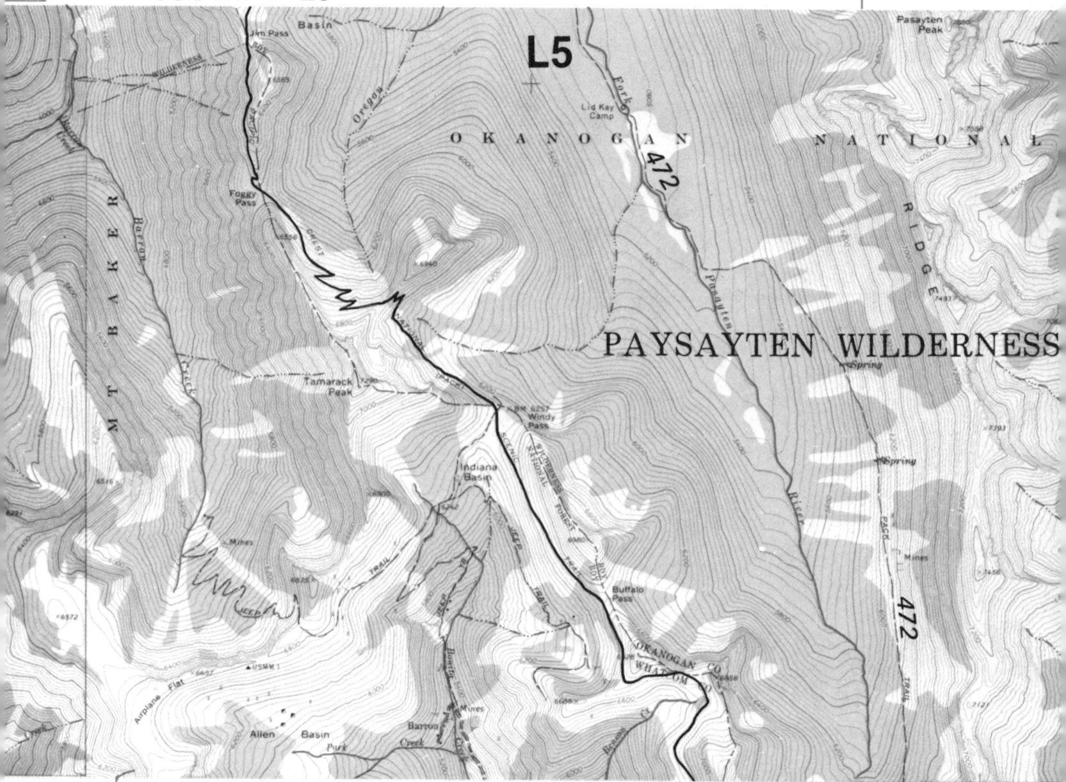

L5

OKANOGAN NATIONAL

PAYSAYTEN WILDERNESS

see MAP L4

Peak (7290), clad in tamarack, or larch. After crossing a small basin with water and an adequate camp, the trail switchbacks up to and over an arm of Tamarack Peak, descends the open north cirque, and finally traverses the northwest arm of the mountain to Foggy Pass (6180–2.2). From this pass, the PCT crosses to the west side of the divide for a brief, wooded

See map L5

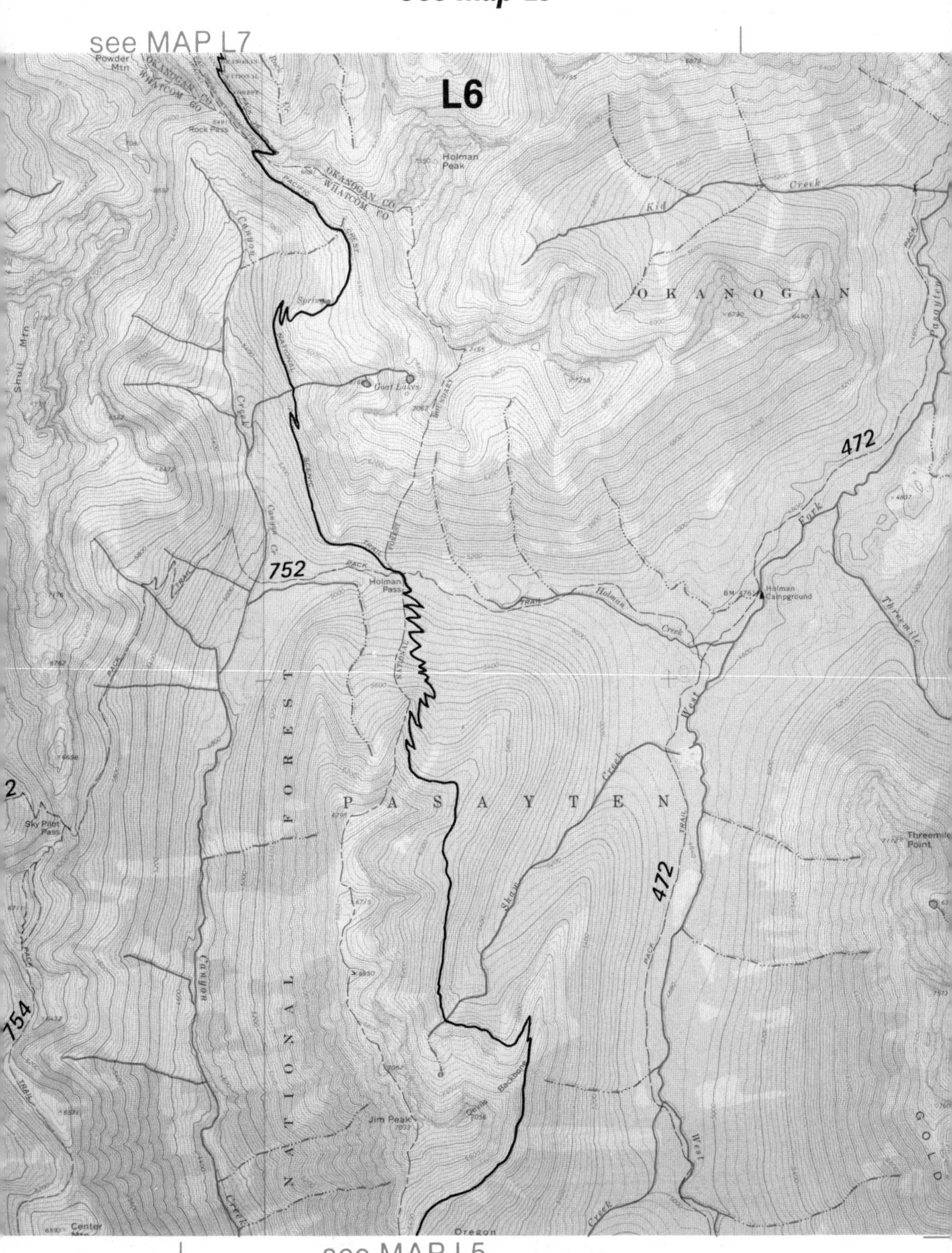

hike to Jim Pass (6270–0.7). Then, back on the east side of the divide, it traverses around Jim Peak (7033) to the rocky shoulder called Devils Backbone (6180–1.3). Descending into the north cirque of Jim Peak, the PCT crosses the head of Shaw Creek and ascends gradually, passing, in ¾ mile, a campsite with a seasonal water supply. About ¼ mile farther, the route begins a plunge down switchbacks to a junction with Trail 752 at Holman Pass (5050–4.4). This pass is heavily wooded and not particularly nice for camping, although wildlife abounds in the vicinity.

Climb northwest out of Holman Pass, crossing the outlet stream from Goat Lakes in about a mile, and switchback up a grassy knoll to a never-failing spring (6200–2.4) and a good but much-used camp. From here, the trail traverses up the steep, grassy slopes bounding Canyon Creek to top a narrow crest (6560-1.0), about 300 yards southeast of a minor gap, Rock Pass. ▌*For a time, the PCT used to continue on a high route northwest toward that pass, but since the 1990s, the "new" route is along the original route.* ▌The trail now makes a switchback east, often through snow, and then takes a descending route northwest. It soon levels off, and then, from a crossing of a tributary of Rock Creek, it climbs briefly to a junction with the high route (6120–1.4). Now you switchback briefly up to

See maps L5, L6, L7

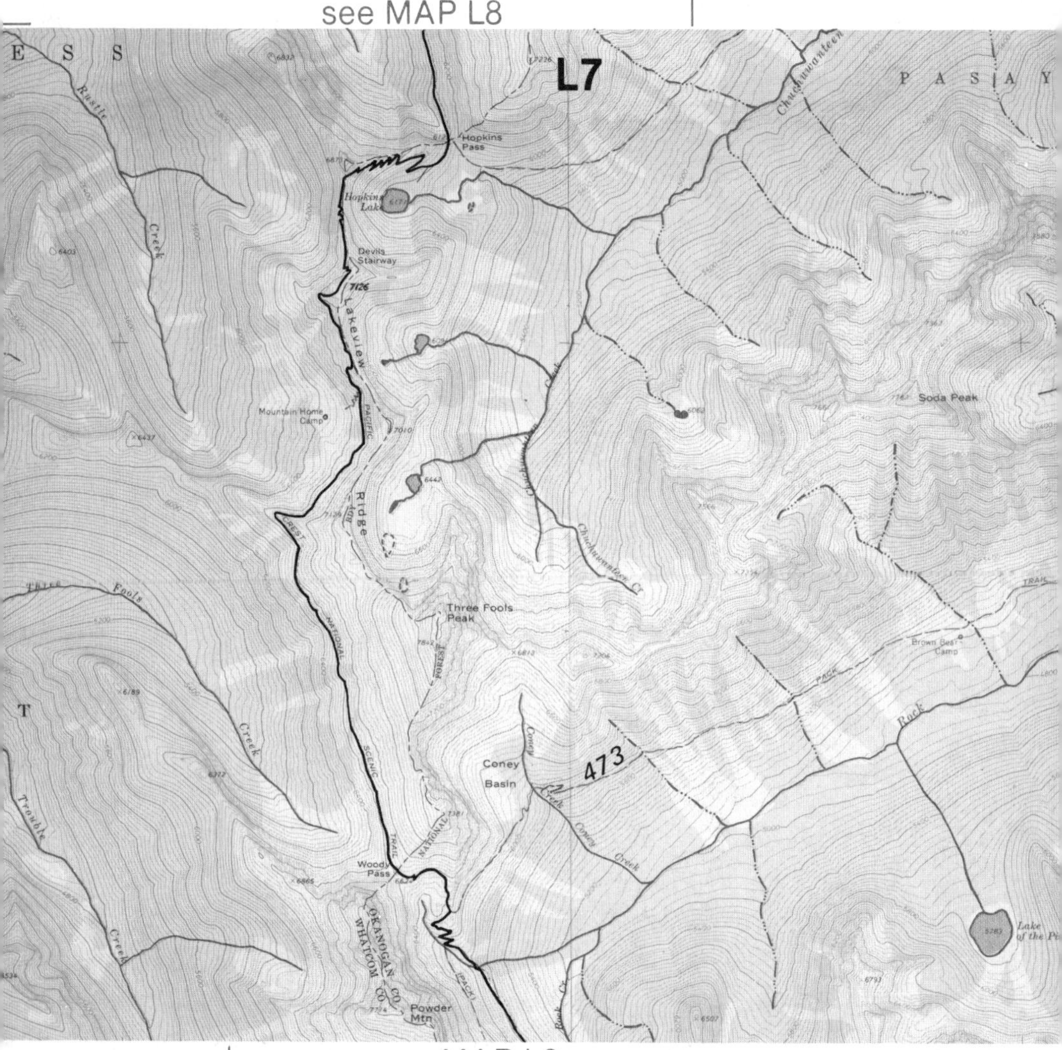

a junction with Trail 473 (6360–0.3), which descends Rock Creek canyon about 7 miles east to the Pasayten River. Keeping high, you curve counterclockwise up to misnamed, rock-strewn Woody Pass (6624–0.5).

From here, you traverse open slopes with a few wooded fingers—the least spectacular side of Three Fools Peak (7930)—until the trail rounds the south arm of the cirque that cradles Mountain Home Camp, a flat, grassy bench with good camping. Beyond, the trail begins to climb steadily as it traverses the grassy headwall of the cirque. Shortly after you arc to the north, climbing through occasional stands of scrub conifers, a faint trail (6800–2.5) takes off down a more or less open gully to the flat bench of Mountain Home Camp, now 400 feet directly below.

Continuing on the PCT, a short switchback brings you to the crest of Lakeview Ridge, on which a short spur trail takes you to an enticing view of a nestled lake 1000 feet below and the valley of Chuchuwanteen Creek beyond. The PCT continues along the crest for a short dis-

See map L7

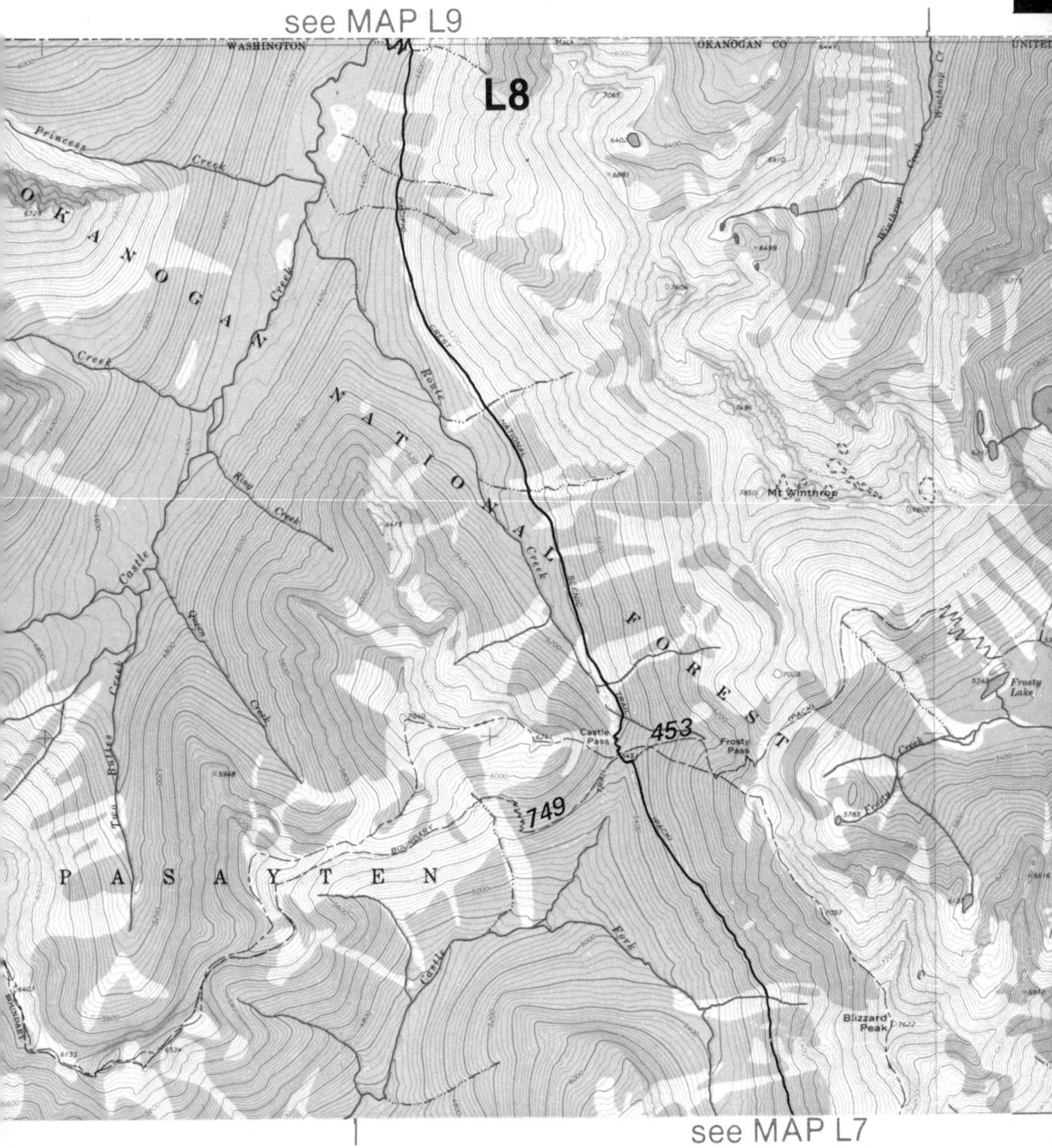

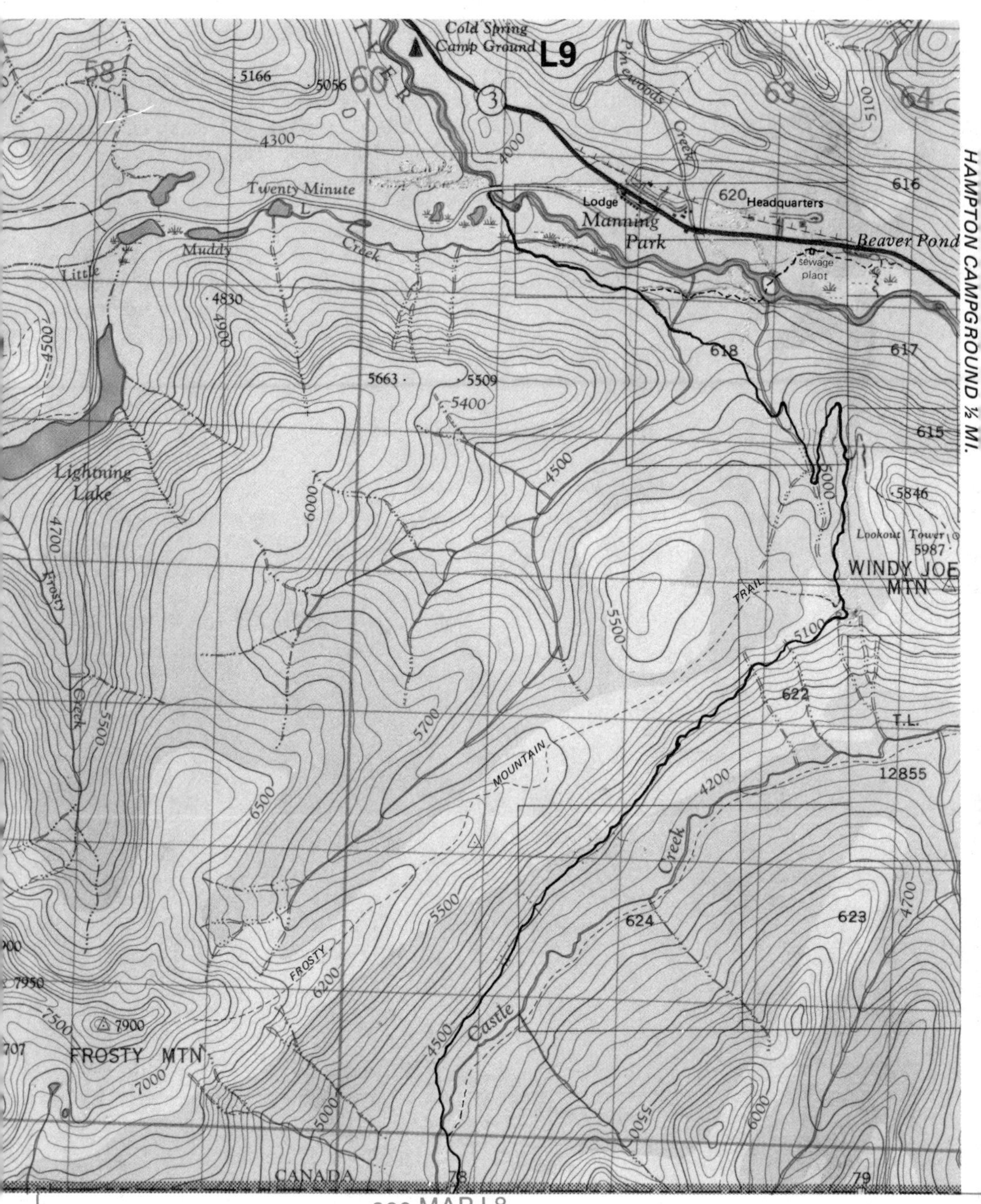

see MAP L8

tance before it is forced to the west just long enough to switchback once more before climbing to an unnamed summit (7126–0.7) on Lakeview Ridge. ▮ *From here, at the highest PCT point in Washington, you have views on all sides, weather permitting: to the south, the very rugged Three Fools Peak; to the north, your first glimpse of Hopkins Lake; and farther north and west, the rugged Cascades of Washington and Canada.* ▮

Now heading down toward Hopkins Pass, the trail sticks to the ridgecrest most of the time until it is forced by Peak 6873 on the ridge to pass east of that peak. Then the route switchbacks around the north side of the amphitheater for which Hopkins Lake is the "stage."

See map L7

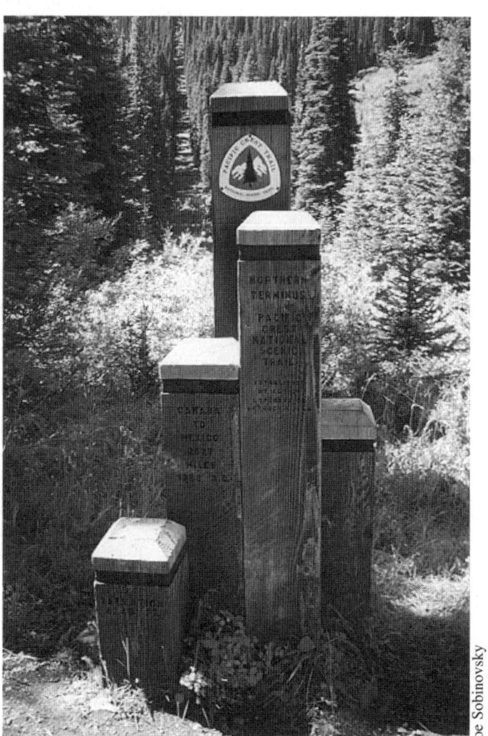
Joe Sobinovsky

Monument 78 on U.S.-Canada border

Several short switchbacks and two longer ones bring you down nearly to the level of the lake, to a point where a trail (6220–1.7) to dependable campsites at Hopkins Lake (6171) takes off to the southwest. The trail then continues almost eastward for a few hundred yards to Hopkins Pass (6122–0.2).

The PCT continues north-northwest from Hopkins Pass, traversing the mostly wooded west slopes of Blizzard Peak (7622). After a mile, you reach a stream and its clearing and then re-enter woods and continue the traverse about 0.4 mile before starting a gradual descent toward Castle Pass. Shortly before the pass, you join Boundary Trail 749, turn sharply left, and follow it around a small hummock to Castle Pass (5451–2.5), where you might lunch in the sunshine of a small, open area. Then, after meandering northward down a quarter mile of lush alpine gardens, the trail becomes firmly established on the east slope of the Route Creek watershed. You cross two seasonal streams and two avalanche paths, one from the east and one from the west.

Side route. A reasonable camp lies 200 yards off the trail on the edge of one avalanche track; don't stay there if there is still much snow on the slopes above. This is quite spacious, has adjacent water, and is about ¾ mile below Castle Pass—a good place to spend your last night in the wilderness before reaching civilization at trail's end. However, if you want to camp in Canada, continue to a campsite about 3¾ miles north of the border.

SECTION L

Continuing the traverse, you come to two reliable streams in about a mile and then leave the woods for more-open slopes with rounded granite outcrops. After passing two more streams and a stock gate across the trail, you finally pound down the last four switchbacks to Monument 78 on the United States-Canada border (4240–4.1). ▮ *The monument is a greatly scaled-down version of the Washington Monument, and beside it are some inscribed wooden posts. One marks this spot as the northern terminus of the United States' Pacific Crest National Scenic Trail. Ahead, in Canada, it is merely the Pacific Crest Trail. Another gives the mileage from Canada to Mexico as exactly 2627. However, this accuracy to the nearest mile assumes that every step of the way has been mapped to within about 99.99% accuracy, which it has not. Furthermore, every decade since the trail's inception has seen reroutes—which changes the total mileage—and more reroutes are planned for the Third Millennium.* ▮

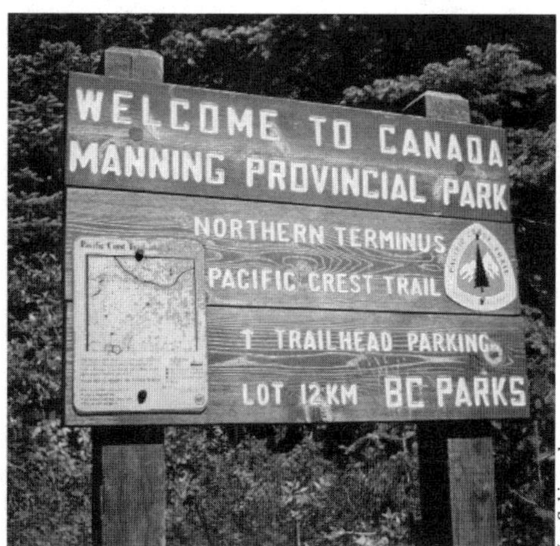
WELCOME TO CANADA
MANNING PROVINCIAL PARK
NORTHERN TERMINUS
PACIFIC CREST TRAIL
↑ TRAILHEAD PARKING
LOT 12KM BC PARKS
Joe Sobinovsky

At U.S.-Canada border

See maps L7, L8, L9

Just north of the monument is a junction with the Castle Creek/Monument 78 Trail, veering right.

Side route. This provides a mostly downhill route out to Highway 3, but you end up about 2½ miles east of Manning Park Lodge (though only ½ mile southwest of Hampton Campground). However, this trail is often boggy and can be in poor shape after too much horse use.

Plunging into the dense, wet, valley-bottom woods, you quickly reach, just ¼ mile into Canada, a bridge across seasonally raging Castle Creek. Still in the woods, the trail winds through a dense spruce-fir forest and soon begins a mostly viewless climb steadily but gently northeast. As the path climbs, you cross from granite to slate and back again, plod up a short switchback leg, cross a few ravines, jump a few creeklets, and arrive at the southwest base (5070–3.7) of Windy Joe Mountain. Here, by a spring, you'll find the PCT's northernmost campsite, about 4 miles from the Canadian trailhead. The PCT soon turns north and climbs briefly to a saddle and a junction with the Mt. Frosty Trail (5120–0.3), which starts to climb southwest.

From here, the PCT makes an undulating traverse north across Windy Joe Mountain's west slopes. Soon you hear the traffic on Canada's main east-west thoroughfare, Route 3, cutting a swath through the dense forest on the unseen, deep canyon floor below you. The trail ends at a hairpin turn on the closed Windy Joe Trail (5220-0.7). You may have encountered mountain bikes on the PCT at various spots along your journey, and you may encounter them here. Whereas in the United States they are banned, here in Canada, along the Windy Joe Trail, they are allowed. On this trail—a closed road—you first descend north and then south, down to a creek crossing. You immediately recross the creek, descend ½ mile, and then cross it for the last time.

The moderately descending route soon winds down gentler, still-viewless slopes ⅔ mile northwest to a crossing of a larger creek, and, just beyond it, you reach a junction (4100-2.1). Through much of the 1990s, the PCT headed northeast to a Highway 3 trailhead at Beaver Pond, but too much flooding of the bottomlands of the Similkameen River made this route often boggy and impassable. A better route now exists, one that crosses only its major tributary, Little Muddy Creek. On a mostly gentle descent westward, you go about a mile to bridge that creek and then head north about ¼ mile to a trailhead parking area (3980-1.3). ***Congratulations on completing your trek!***

This trailhead is situated along the Gibson Pass Road immediately west of the Similkameen River.

Side route. West, this road goes about 2 miles to the Lightning Lake Campground, in the popular Lightning Lake area. East, the road goes about ⅔ mile to Highway 3, where you'll find Manning Park Lodge. You may want to stay at the lodge to shower and get a warm meal. It also has tempting accommodations, but they are beyond the budget of many backpackers. From the lodge, the economy-minded backpacker can trek 1¼ miles west on Highway 3 to Coldspring Campground and then later return to catch a bus from Manning Park Lodge west to Vancouver, B.C. The official bus stop is at the park's East Gate entrance station, but lodge personnel will phone the station if you want to have the bus make a stop at the lodge. You'll need exact change to pay the bus driver for the fare, so get it at the lodge. In years past, summer buses have passed west through the park in late morning and in late afternoon.

We hope you arrived in good spirits and in good health. And we also hope that your hike through Section L was, despite the odds, warm, dry, and insect-free. If you have hiked all or most of the way from Mexico to Canada, won't you please write us and tell us about your experiences and about the usefulness of this guidebook? The letters we received from your predecessors helped make this edition more useful for PCT trekkers, and we'd like to see the tradition continue.

See map L9

Recommended Reading and Source Books

Pacific Crest Trail

Clarke, Clinton C. 1945. *The Pacific Crest Trailway.* Pasadena: The Pacific Crest Trail System Conference.

Croot, Leslie C. 1999. *Pacific Crest Trail Town Guide.* Sacramento, CA: Pacific Crest Trail Association.

Go, Ben. 1997. *Pacific Crest Trail Data Book.* Sacramento, CA: Pacific Crest Trail Association.

Gray, William R. 1975. *The Pacific Crest Trail.* Washington, D.C.: National Geographic Society.

Green, David. 1979. *A Pacific Crest Odyssey.* Berkeley: Wilderness Press.

Holtel, Bob. 1994. *Soul, Sweat and Survival on the Pacific Crest Trail.* Livermore, CA: Bittersweet Publ. Co.

Ryback, Eric. 1971. *The High Adventure of Eric Ryback.* San Francisco: Chronicle Books.

Schaffer, Jeffrey P., and Ben Schifrin, Thomas Winnett, Ruby Jenkins. 1995. *The Pacific Crest Trail, Volume 1: California.* Berkeley: Wilderness Press.

Sutton, Ann, and Myron Sutton. 1975. *The Pacific Crest Trail: Escape to the Wilderness.* Philadelphia: Lippincott.

Backpacking and Mountaineering

Aadland, Dan. 1993. *Treading Lightly with Pack Animals: a Guide to Low-Impact Travel in the Backcountry.* Missoula, MT: Mountain Press.

Back, Joe. 1987. *Horses, Hitches and Rocky Trails: The Packer's Bible.* Boulder, CO: Johnson Books.

Beckey, Fred. 1974. *Cascade Alpine Guide, Climbing & High Routes, Volume 1: Columbia River to Stevens Pass.* Seattle: The Mountaineers.

Beckey, Fred. 1978. *Cascade Alpine Guide, Climbing & High Routes, Volume 2: Stevens Pass to Rainy Pass.* Seattle: The Mountaineers.

Beckey, Fred. 1981. *Cascade Alpine Guide, Climbing & High Routes, Volume 3: Rainy Pass to Fraser River.* Seattle: The Mountaineers.

Darvill, Fred T. 1998. *Mountaineering Medicine.* Berkeley: Wilderness Press.

Drummond, Roger. 1998. *Ticks And What You Can Do About Them.* Berkeley: Wilderness Press.

Fleming, June. 1994. *Staying Found; The Complete Map & Compass Handbook.* Seattle: The Mountaineers.

Graydon, Don, and Kurt Hanson, eds. 1997. *Mountaineering: The Freedom of the Hills.* Seattle: The Mountaineers.

Harmon, David, and Amy S. Rubin. 1992. *Llamas on the Trail: A Packer's Guide.* Missoula, MT: Mountain Press.

Latimer, Carole. 1991. *Wilderness Cuisine.* Berkeley: Wilderness Press.

Miles, John C., ed.. 1996. *Impressions of the North Cascades.* Seattle: Mountaineers Books.

Reifsnyder, William E. 1980. *Weathering the Wilderness: the Sierra Club Guide to Practical Meteorology.* San Francisco: Sierra Club.

Schaffer, Jeffrey P. 1983. *Crater Lake National Park and Vicinity.* Berkeley: Wilderness Press.

Thomas, Jeff. 1983. *Oregon Rock: A Climber's Guide.* Seattle: The Mountaineers.

Winnett, Thomas, with Melanie Findling. 1994. *Backpacking Basics.* Berkeley: Wilderness Press.

Geology

Alt, David D., and Donald W. Hyndman. 1995. *Northwest Exposures, a Geologic Story of the Northwest.* Missoula, MT: Mountain Press.

American Geological Institute. 1984. *Dictionary of Geological Terms.* New York: Doubleday.

Bacon, Charles R. 1983. "Eruptive History of Mount Mazama and Crater Lake Caldera, Cascade Range, U.S.A." *Journal of Volcanology and Geothermal Research,* v. 18, p. 57-115.

Baldwin, Ewart M. 1981. *Geology of Oregon.* Dubuque: Kendall/Hunt.

Crandell, Dwight R. 1969. *Surficial Geology of Mount Rainier National Park, Washington* (U.S. Geological Survey Bulletin 1288). Washington, D.C.: U.S. Government Printing Office.

Crandell, Dwight R. 1969. *The Geologic Story of Mount Rainier* (U.S. Geological Survey Bulletin 1292). Washington, D.C.: U.S. Government Printing Office.

Crandell, Dwight R. 1980. *Recent Eruptive History of Mount Hood, Oregon, and Potential Hazards from Future Eruptions* (U.S. Geological Survey Bulletin 1492). Washington, D.C.: U.S. Government Printing Office.

Harris, Ann G., and Esther Tuttle, Sherwood D. Tuttle. 1997. *Geology of National Parks.* Dubuque: Kendall/Hunt.

Harris, Stephen L. 1988. *Fire Mountains of the West: the Cascade and Mono Lake Volcanoes.* Missoula, MT: Mountain Press.

Luedke, Robert G., and Robert L. Smith. 1982. *Map Showing Distribution, Composition, and Age of Late Cenozoic Volcanic Centers in Oregon and Washington* (U.S. Geological Survey Miscellaneous Investigations Series Map I-1091-D). Washington, D.C.: U.S. Government Printing Office.

Nelson, C. Hans, et al. 1994. "The volcanic, sedimentologic, and paleolimnologic history of the Crater Lake caldera floor, Oregon: Evidence for small caldera evolution." *Geological Society of America Bulletin,* v. 106, p. 684-704.

Tabor, Roland, and Ralph Haugerud, *Geology of the North Cascades.* Seattle: Mountaineers Books, 1999.

Wells, Francis G., and Dallas L. Peck. 1961. *Geologic Map of Oregon West of the 121st meridian* (U.S. Geological Survey Miscellaneous Investigations Series Map I-325). Washington, D.C.: U.S. Government Printing Office.

Biology

Arno, Stephen F., and Ramona P. Hammerly. 1977. *Northwest Trees.* Seattle: The Mountaineers.

Burt, William H., and Richard P. Grossenheider. 1976. *A Field Guide to the Mammals.* Boston: Houghton Mifflin.

Franklin, Jerry F., and C.T. Dyrness. 1973. *Natural Vegetation of Oregon and Washington* (USDA Forest Service General Technical Report PNW-8). Washington, D.C.: U.S. Government Printing Office.

Hitchcock, C. Leo, and Arthur Cronquist. 1973. *Flora of the Pacific Northwest; an Illustrated Manual.* Seattle: University of Washington Press.

Horn, Elizabeth L. 1972. *Wildflowers 1: The Cascades.* Beaverton, OR: Touchstone Press.

Ingles, Lloyd G. 1965. *Mammals of the Pacific States.* Stanford: Stanford University Press.

Keator, Glenn. 1978. *Pacific Coast Berry Finder.* Berkeley: Nature Study Guild.

Larrison, Earl J., and Grace W. Patrick, William H. Baker, James A. Yaich. 1974. *Washington Wildflowers.* Seattle: Seattle Audubon Society.

Murie, Olaus J. 1975. *A Field Guide to Animal Tracks.* Boston: Houghton Mifflin.

Niehaus, Theodore F., and Charles L. Ripper. 1981. *A Field Guide to Pacific States Wildflowers.* Boston: Houghton Mifflin.

Peterson, Roger T. 1990. *A Field Guide to Western Birds.* Boston: Houghton Mifflin.

Stebbins, Robert C. 1985. *A Field Guide to Western Reptiles and Amphibians.* Boston: Houghton Mifflin.

Sudworth, George B. 1967 (1908 reprint with new Foreword and Table of Changes in Nomenclature). *Forest Trees of the Pacific Slope.* New York: Dover.

Watts, Tom. 1973. Pacific *Coast Tree Finder.* Berkeley: Nature Study Guild.

Whitney, Stephen R. 1983. *A Field Guide to the Cascades & Olympics.* Seattle: The Mountaineers.

Index

The italic letter-number combinations (A1, B1, etc.) refer to this book's topographic maps.

Gamma Creek 305, *K10*
Gamma Hot Springs 305, *K10*
Garfield Peak Trail 110, *C10*